D1265890

Adult Acute Lymphocytic Leukemia

CONTEMPORARY HEMATOLOGY

Judith E. Karp, MD, Series Editor

For other titles published in the series, go to
www.springer.com/series/7681

Adult Acute Lymphocytic Leukemia

Biology and Treatment

Edited by

Anjali S. Advani, MD

Cleveland Clinic
Taussig Cancer Center
Cleveland, OH
USA

Hillard M. Lazarus, MD

Case Western Reserve University
University Hospitals Case Medical Center
Case Comprehensive Cancer Center
Cleveland, OH
USA

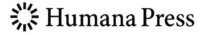 Humana Press

Editors
Anjali S. Advani, MD
Cleveland Clinic
Taussig Cancer Center
Cleveland, OH
USA
advania@ccf.org

Hillard M. Lazarus, MD
Case Western Reserve University
University Hospitals Case Medical Center
Case Comprehensive Cancer Center
Cleveland, OH
USA
hillard.lazarus@case.edu

ISBN 978-1-60761-706-8   e-ISBN 978-1-60761-707-5
DOI 10.1007/978-1-60761-707-5
Springer New York Dordrecht Heidelberg London

Printed on acid-free paper

Humana Press is part of Springer Science+Business Media (www.springer.com)

To my mother and father for their unwavering support,
understanding, and love.
To my mentors Matt Kalaycio, Fred Appelbaum,
Jon Gockerman, and Brice
Weinberg for their knowledge, advice, and support.
To our patients, who give us the inspiration to learn and develop better treatments
for leukemia.
To our nurses, who are there with our patients every step of the way.

– Anjali S. Advani, MD

To my wife Joan and our sons Jeffrey and Adam for their
continued and steadfast
support.
To my mentors Oscar D. Ratnoff, MD and Nathan A. Berger, MD for their patience,
guidance and encouragement.
To our patients and their families for their courage and trust.

– Hillard M. Lazarus, MD

Preface

Childhood acute lymphoblastic leukemia (ALL) is the "poster child" for the story of success in treating cancer patients. Over the past five decades, this essentially uniformly fatal disease has been eradicated in 80% of young patients. Cures were realized only as a result of slow and painstaking work that involved investigators pursuing a series of studies using radiation therapy and drugs such as vincristine, prednisone, cyclophosphamide, anthracyclines, L-asparaginase, methotrexate, and 6-mercapto-purine. ALL in adults is less common and clearly has a different disease biology. For example, only 3% of childhood ALL cases are BCR-ABL positive, in contrast to 20–30% in adults; despite emulating the pediatric approach, the cure rate in this population is only half that of childhood ALL.

In this tome, we rely upon some of the world's ALL experts to enlighten the reader in all facets on the continuing progress in the diagnosis and treatment of this disorder. The reader will receive in-depth updates ranging from the epidemiology and causation, to pathobiology including cytogenetic and specific gene abnormalities, to pharmacology and pharmacogenetics. Our contributors address new paradigms for classifying disease subsets as well as techniques for detecting and monitoring minimal residual disease and the implications thereof. Further, these extremely knowledgeable investigators present and discuss the many clinical and biologic factors that form the basis of risk assessment for the entire constellation of patient-, disease- and treatment-related factors for the various patient subsets. For example, they discuss the need for approaching adolescents and young adults differently than older adults. We review the different treatment strategies from remission induction, consolidation/intensification and maintenance, including the use of novel agents such as monoclonal antibodies, tyrosine kinase inhibitors, and agents that appear to have selectivity in specific T-cell and B-cell lineage. Finally, we address the pros and cons of hematopoietic stem cell transplantation as a therapeutic modality.

What is the future likely to hold for patients and investigators alike? We can look forward to continued progress in this uncommon but very important disorder that has stood as a model for the success of combination chemotherapy. Already monoclonal antibodies alone or in combination are in clinical trials and have shown great promise. The tyrosine kinase inhibitors, particularly the more potent SRC-ABL inhibitors, add significantly to chemotherapy effect. The introduction of a number of T-cell targeting agents (nelarabine) and "anti-ALL drugs" (clofarabine) already have been shown to improve patient outcome. Modified formulations of the older agents L-asparaginase (pegylated formulation), vincristine (liposomal formulation), and cytarabine (liposomal formulation for CNS disease) may provide enhanced efficacy as well. New NOTCH inhibitors are being developed that soon will enter the clinical arena. Finally, reduced-intensity conditioning transplantation procedures, especially with greater use of alternative donors such as umbilical cord blood grafts, may provide positive anti-ALL effect with significantly less toxicity. The future holds great promise and undoubtedly the cure rate in this malignant disorder will continue to increase.

Cleveland, OH   Anjali S. Advani, MD
Cleveland, OH   Hillard M. Lazarus, MD

Acknowledgement

I would like to thank my assistant Shendra Smith for her help in compiling this textbook. This book would not have been possible without her.

Anjali S. Advani, MD

My most sincere thanks to Michelle Rose for her expertise and help in compiling this textbook.

Hillard M. Lazarus, MD

Contents

Contributors

Camille N. Abboud
Division of Oncology, Washington University School of Medicine,
Saint Louis, Missouri, USA

Fredrick R. Appelbaum
Division of Hematology and Medical Oncology, Department of Medicine,
University of Washington and Clinical Research Division,
Fred Hutchinson Cancer Research Center, Seattle, Washington, USA

David Avigan
Division of Hematology/Oncology, Department of Medicine,
Beth Israel Deaconess Medical Center, Harvard Medical School,
Boston, Massachusetts, USA

Paul M. Barr
Department of Medicine, Case Comprehensive Cancer Center,
Center for Science, Health and Society, Case Western Reserve University School
of Medicine and University
Hospitals Case Medical Center, Cleveland, Ohio, USA

Nathan A. Berger
Department of Medicine, Case Comprehensive Cancer Center,
Center for Science, Health and Society, Case Western Reserve University School
of Medicine and University
Hospitals Case Medical Center, Cleveland, Ohio, USA

Nicolas Boissel
Hematology Department, Saint-Louis Hospital, Paris Diderot University, Paris, France

Michael J. Borowitz
Department of Pathology, Johns Hopkins Medical Institute, Baltimore, Maryland, USA

Edward Copelan
Department of Hematologic Oncology and Blood Disorders,
Taussig Cancer Center, The Cleveland Clinic, Cleveland, Ohio, USA

Kevin A. David
Department of Medicine, Division of Hematology/ Oncology,
Northwestern University Feinberg School of Medicine, Robert H. Lurie Comprehensive
Cancer Center, Chicago, Illinois, USA

Daniel J. DeAngelo
Department of Medical Oncology/Hematologic Malignancies,
Harvard Medical School, Dana-Farber Cancer Institute, Boston, Massachusetts, USA

Herve Dombret
Hematology Department, Saint-Louis Hospital, Paris, France

Andrew M. Evens
Department of Medicine, Division of Hematology/Oncology, Northwestern University Feinberg
School of Medicine, Robert H. Lurie Comprehensive Cancer Center, Chicago, Illinois, USA

Stefan Faderl
Department of Leukemia, The University of Texas M. D. Anderson
Cancer Center, Houston, Texas, USA

Adele K. Fielding
Haematology Department, University of College London,
United Kingdom

Christopher A. Fox
School of Cancer Sciences, University of Birmingham, United Kingdom

Olga Frankfurt
Department of Medicine and Pathology, Northwestern University Feinberg School of Medicine,
Robert H. Lurie Comprehensive Cancer Center, Chicago, Illinois, USA

Anthony H. Goldstone
Department of Haematology, University College of London, United Kingdom

Christine J. Harrison
Division of Cancer Sciences, University of Southampton, United Kingdom

Matthew J. Hourigan
Department of Haematology, University College of London, United Kingdom

Francoise Huguet
Hematology Department, Purpan Hospital, Toulouse, France

Hagop Kantarjian
Department of Leukemia, The University of Texas M. D. Anderson
Cancer Center, Houston, Texas, USA

Vaishalee P. Kenkre
Department of Medicine and Cancer Research Center, University of Chicago,
Chicago, Illinois, USA

Maja Krajinovic
Research Center Charles Bruneau, Research Center CHU Sainte-Justine Quebec, Canada Department
of Pediatrics, Department of Pharmacology, University of Montreal, Canada

Richard J. Creger
Department of Medicine, Case Comprehensive Cancer Center,
Center for Science, Health and Society, Case Western Reserve University School of Medicine and
University Hospitals Case Medical Center, Cleveland, Ohio, USA

Richard A. Larson
Department of Medicine and Cancer Research Center, University of Chicago, Chicago, Illinois, USA

Mark R. Litzow
Department of Hematology, Mayo Clinic, Rochester, Minnesota, USA

Selina M. Luger
Department of Hematology and Medical Oncology, University
of Pennsylvania Medical Center, Philadelphia, Pennsylvania, USA

David I. Marks
Department of Oncology, University Hospitals of Bristol,
Bristol Children's Hospital, United Kingdom

Mike G. Martin
Division of Oncology, Washington University School of Medicine,
Saint Louis, Missouri, USA

Anthony R. Mato
Department of Haematology and Medical Oncology, University
of Pennsylvania Medical Center, Philadelphia, Pennsylvania, USA

A.K. McMillan
Department of Haematology, Nottingham University Hospital,
United Kingdom

Anthony V. Moorman
Leukaemia Research Cytogenetics Group, Northern Institute
of Cancer Research, University of Newcastle, United Kingdom

Alicia K. Morgans
Department of Hematology and Medical Oncology, University
of Pennsylvania Medical Center, Philadelphia, Pennsylvania, USA

Susan O'Brien
Department of Leukemia, The University of Texas M. D. Anderson
Cancer Center, Houston, Texas, USA

Elisabeth Paietta
Department of Oncology, Montefiore Medical Center-North Division,
Bronx, New York, USA

LoAnn C. Petersen
Department of Pathology, Northwestern University Feinberg School
of Medicine, Robert H. Lurie Comprehensive Cancer Center,
Chicago, Illinois, USA

Jerald Radich
Department of Medical Oncology, Fred Hutchinson Cancer Research Center,
Seattle, Washington, USA

Mark Roberts
Department of Pathology, Northwestern University Feinberg School
of Medicine, Robert H. Lurie Comprehensive Cancer Center,
Chicago, Illinois, USA

Jacalyn Rosenblatt
Department of Medicine, Beth Israel Deaconess Medical Center,
Harvard Medical School, Boston, Massachusetts, USA

Olga Sala
Department of Medical Oncology, Fred Hutchinson Cancer Research Center, Seattle, Washington

Charles A. Schiffer
Department of Medicine, Division of Oncology, Karmanos Cancer Center, Wayne State University School of Medicine, Detroit, Michigan, USA

Andrei R. Shustov
Division of Hematology and Medical Oncology, Department of Medicine,
University of Washington and Clinical Research Division, Fred Hutchinson Cancer Research Center, Seattle, Washington, USA

Christy J. Stotler
Department of Hematologic Oncology and Blood Disorders,
Taussig Cancer Center, The Cleveland Clinic, Cleveland, Ohio, USA

Martin S. Tallman
Department of Medicine and Pathology, Northwestern University Feinberg School of Medicine, Robert H. Lurie Comprehensive Cancer Center, Chicago, Illinois, USA

Deborah A. Thomas
Department of Leukemia, The University of Texas, M.D. Anderson
Cancer Center, Houston, Texas, USA

John S. Welch
Division of Oncology, Washington University School of Medicine,
Saint Louis, Missouri, USA

Patrick A. Zweidler-McKay
The Children's Cancer Hospital at the University of Texas M.D. Anderson Cancer Center, Houston, Texas, USA

Chapter 1
A Perspective on the Treatment of Acute Lymphoblastic Leukemia in Adults

Charles A. Schiffer

The progressive improvement in the outcome of children treated for acute lymphoblastic leukemia (ALL) represents one of the major achievements of clinical cancer research and is frequently singled out as an example of the progress to be hoped for in other cancers. More than 80% of children with ALL are expected to be long-term disease-free survivors (DFS) and many of the current clinical trials focus on means of decreasing the intensity of therapy so as to achieve the same results with fewer short- and longer-term side effects [1]. Of note is that these improvements occurred:

- Despite the fact that no significant new chemotherapy agents were introduced in the last 20 years;
- Before the recent remarkable expansion of knowledge about the biology of the disease;
- Often as a result of sequential phase II, rather than randomized clinical trials.

Although trials in adults have attempted to build upon these observations, the results have been relatively disappointing with DFS of 30–35% in B lineage ALL and ~50–60% in patients with T-cell lineage, with modest improvements in the past 15–20 years [2–7]. Differences in disease and patient characteristics account for some of the disparities in outcome including:
The distribution of cytogenetic and molecular subtypes

- Philadelphia chromosome [t(9,22)] – found in ~30% of adults with B lineage ALL and increasing with patient age vs. 2–3% in children
- Very low incidence of hyperdiploidy and TEL/AML fusion (both of which confer a favorable outcome) in adults compared with children [8–12]
- Better outcome in children with FAB L3 (Burkitt's type, c-myc mutated) mature B cell ALL

In addition, it has become clear in recent years that clones molecularly identical to the eventual ALL can be detected antenatally, with the supposition that additional mutagenic "hits" result in the development of ALL in some such children [13–16]. Indeed, it appears that the majority of childhood ALL cases share this pathogenesis. It is unlikely that ALL in adults has a similar derivation. Whether this difference in the age and immunologic "experience" of the cell from which the ALL clone derives can affect the response to treatment, is also unknown.
Tolerance of therapy

- Other complicating medical conditions in adults
- Potential effects of subclinical organ dysfunction in adults on drug disposition as well as other drug metabolism differences that may change with age [17]
- More confounding medications in adults

C.A. Schiffer (✉)
Division of Hematology/Oncology, Karmanos Cancer Institute,
Wayne State University School of Medicine, Detroit, MI 48302, USA
e-mail: schiffer@karmanos.org

A.S. Advani and H.M. Lazarus (eds.), *Adult Acute Lymphocytic Leukemia*, Contemporary Hematology,
DOI 10.1007/978-1-60761-707-5_1, © Springer Science+Business Media, LLC 2011

- Better organ tolerance in children with ability to deliver repetitive courses more easily
- Possible differences in compliance

Multiple differing, albeit overlapping, regimens have been used in adult cooperative group trials with apparent similar overall results. Few randomized trials have been done, however, and it is difficult to attribute with confidence any possible differences to specific alterations in regimens. The paucity of large clinical trials is partially explained by the relatively low incidence of the disease in adults but the fact remains that a substantial fraction of patients are cared for by oncologists and hematologists who are more akin to "generalists" (at least in the USA) compared to the treatment of children, most of whom are entered on clinical trials and treated by subspecialists for whom ALL is generally the most common cancer they treat. In addition, the care of patients with ALL differs in many respects from the treatments provided to other adults with cancer. Differences include:

- ALL regimens are very complex, with multiple drugs given intravenously, subcutaneously, intrathecally and orally over a prolonged period of time
- Protocols demand "on time" therapy
- Most of the treatment is outpatient with substantial use of oral agents, raising issues of compliance
- Involves many specialists (radiation oncologists, interventional radiology for lumbar punctures)
- ALL is a small fraction of adult oncologists' patients (even among adult leukemia specialists)
- Less experienced nursing and ancillary staff compared to pediatric subspecialists

How Can Results Be Improved in Adults?

Focus on Subgroups of Patients

ALL is a heterogeneous disease with recent gene expression studies emphasizing differences even amongst seemingly homogeneous immunophenotypic subtypes. Certain relatively well-characterized subtypes benefit from unique treatment approaches, which will be covered in detail in other chapters of this book.

Briefly, patients with *mature B lineage* (so called Burkitt's or L3 ALL) benefit from the application of intensive regimens incorporating fractionated cyclophosphamide, high dose methotrexate, and high dose cytarabine delivered over a period of a few months without maintenance therapy [18, 19]. Recent studies suggest that the addition of rituximab may improve results further with cure rates perhaps approaching what can be seen in children [20].

The treatment of *Philadelphia chromosome positive ALL* now routinely includes the simultaneous administration of imatinib [21] and more recently dasatinib [22], with a preliminary suggestion in both children and adults that some patients may enjoy sustained disease free survival without the need for allogeneic transplantation [23]. Since the incidence of Philadelphia chromosome positivity increase markedly with patient age, refinements of these regimens is of particular importance for these patients for whom transplantation is not an option.

What Can Be Learned from Pediatric Protocols and Can This Be Applied to Adults?

The majority of patients have *pre-B or T lineage ALL* however, and adult trials have not identified discrete treatment approaches for these subtypes. Certainly, the factors listed earlier contribute to the substantial differences in outcome between children and adults, with an even greater disparity in outcome in patients>50–60 years of age, an important group because there is a second "mini-peak" in incidence in older adults.

Some clues may be derived from a series of recent studies from cooperative groups around the world, which compared outcomes in adolescents with similar demographic and biologic characteristics treated on childhood and adult protocols [24–28]. The results were remarkably consistent; although initial complete remission rates were similar, there were marked differences in disease-free and overall survival favoring the patients treated on pediatric protocols. This has resulted in increased collaboration between pediatric and adult groups and pilot studies in which adults up to the age of 30 are being treated by adult cooperative groups using pediatric protocols. One report from Spain has shown that these regimens can be delivered safely to patients up to 30 years of age with apparent improvement compared to older studies [29], while other institutions are attempting to extend this approach to adults up to 50 years of age [30].

If these results are verified and these regimens become standard, then the overall results in younger adults may improve. Because most protocols did not carefully track actual drug delivery, it is currently impossible to distinguish between differences in patient and physician adherence to protocol and the impact of the differences in the protocols themselves. This is obviously critical in designing new approaches.

Assuming that ALL in children and adults have sufficient biologic similarities to permit extrapolation from one experience to the other, it would seem reasonable to try to identify features of pediatric protocols, which might be applied to adults, remembering however, that pediatric trials already formed the backbone of most adult protocols designed in the past. Pediatric protocols are quite complex and there are often separate treatment algorithms for different "risk" groups, generally defined clinically both at the time of diagnosis (age, WBC count, lineage) and at distinct intervals during the course of treatment (rapidity of response, minimal residual disease). Arguably, most adults would a priori be considered "high" risk according to pediatric standards. Pediatric regimens generally use more intensive dosing of non-myelosuppressive drugs such as corticosteroids, L-asparaginase and vincristine as well as earlier and more intensive central nervous system prophylaxis. Because of the higher incidence of comorbidities such as diabetes mellitus and hypertension, it is likely that older adults will be less tolerant of the side effects of these agents with the consequence that the delivery of cytotoxic therapy could be compromised as well. Thus, totally different, perhaps more biologically oriented approaches may be needed for older adults with ALL.

Recent pediatric studies have shown the negative prognostic impact of the quantification of *minimal residual disease* (MRD) by flow cytometry at the end of induction therapy with many protocols evaluating further dose intensification for such patients [31]. Although these evaluations are currently done in centralized research-oriented laboratories, it is likely that such assays could become more widely available if shown to be clinically relevant. The problem, of course, is how to change therapy to overcome this early predictor of treatment failure, coupled with the realization that most adults are likely to have MRD given their observed high rate of relapse *and* the fact that they should already be being treated on studies designed to maximize their long-term outcome.

Enter *allogeneic transplantation*, the default refuge for all high-risk situations. This topic is reviewed elsewhere in this book but a few comments seem relevant.

- In general, the outcome of transplantation in ALL is inferior to the results in acute myeloid leukemia, possibly related to a less vigorous graft vs. leukemia effect.
- As in all diseases in which transplantation is applied, results are poorer in patients in higher-risk groups primarily due to higher rates of leukemia relapse. This generalization would almost certainly apply to patients transplanted for MRD as well.
- Concerns about higher relapse rates might make the use of reduced intensity transplants less attractive in older patients.

- In the few randomized trials which have been done [32], it has been difficult to demonstrate an overall benefit from allogeneic transplant in first remission. Somewhat counterintuitively, in what some (but not all) consider to be a recent "positive" trial [6], any possible benefit was confined to a "standard" risk group defined in a somewhat "nonstandard" fashion. Interpretation of this trial is also complicated by the fact that many patients intended to receive allogeneic transplantation did not actually receive this treatment. However, in another recently published trial comparing autologous and allogeneic transplantation, almost all patients with matched siblings actually did receive the transplant, and there was an overall survival benefit for those with available donors [33].

Thus, although allogeneic transplantation is currently certainly appropriate for many adult patients with ALL in first remission, the results from published trials clearly also define the limitations of this approach and emphasize the need for other treatment improvements, which can be applied more widely.

Future Considerations

The adult ALL glass is at best half full and stagnant, and it is arguable whether we can turn adults into children even with rigorous application of pediatric regimens to a larger fraction of adults. New drugs which have a possible selectivity against T lineage ALL, such as nelarabine [34, 35] and the gamma secretase inhibitors (the latter affecting the notch signaling pathway) [36–38] are under evaluation, as are more preliminary studies with liposomal vincristine [39], which has the potential to increase vincristine dose intensity.

My sense, however, is that cytotoxic chemotherapy has reached its approximate limits and that the next big "jump" is more likely to derive from other approaches, including the intercalation of monoclonal antibodies (either "naked" or "armed") into chemotherapy regimens [40–42]. Further understanding of the poorly characterized phenotypic and molecular nature of the ALL stem cell as well as potential interactions with the supporting stroma are likely to be of importance as well [43].

Efforts at molecular characterization of adult ALL have lagged behind the studies of gene expression profiling of childhood ALL. The latter have identified a number of genes and pathways, which are distinctively affected in different ALL subtypes and correlate with prognosis [44–46]. It is critical that similar studies be done in adults to further address the question of the degree of fundamental biologic overlap between the diseases in different age groups. Discovering candidate genes and pathways is a first step, but still a far cry from identifying drugs or small molecules which safely inhibit these potential "weaknesses," particularly given the redundancy of signaling pathways of most therapy-resistant tumors.

Why Are Patients with Leukemia Cured?

There have been hundreds of investigations of factors predictive of treatment failure in patients with leukemia. These studies have almost invariably focused on mechanisms of drug resistance, with evaluations of biochemical and cytokinetic parameters of the cells and pharmacokinetic and pharmacodynamic assessments of the patients. In contrast, there has been remarkably little attention paid to the question of why certain patients and leukemia subtypes do well following treatment.

Given the large number of distinct subgroups of patients with ALL as well as those yet to be discovered, and the fact that cancer (leukemia) stem cells have redundant pathways capable of bypassing drug induced blockage of one signaling "route," one would think that curing leukemia patients would be impossible. Yet, >80% of children with ALL are cured, as are a real fraction of adults, accomplishments achieved by empiric manipulation of a small number of older drugs, with little understanding of the biology by which cure occurs. Lessons can be learned from these responders as well as from individuals who enjoyed long-term disease-free survival with standard treatment despite the presence of multiple "high risk" characteristics. Molecular or cellular pharmacology experiments focused on those in whom the unexpected has occurred could provide clues pointing the way to new treatment approaches.

Some possible explanations for drug "sensitivity" include:

- Sufficient cytoreduction by chemotherapy
- Unique sensitivity of certain types of clonogenic leukemia stem cell
- Re-expression of genes suppressed by mutations or epigenetic silencing
- Differentiation of leukemia: "clonal remissions" (in AML) [47]
- Recovery of immune surveillance – elimination/suppression of residual disease

First, although it is conceivable that chemotherapy simply kills "all" the leukemia cells, this seems to be an unlikely scenario for most leukemias. There may however, be differences in the sensitivity of the clonogenic stem cells in subsets of leukemia patients, particularly those with a more differentiated phenotype, such as mature B cell ALL. Another possibility is that intensive chemotherapy somehow causes re-expression of genes that were suppressed by mutations or epigenetic silencing that affect transcription and differentiation. Somewhat forgotten is the observation that in some patients in long-term CR of AML, standard chemotherapy in some way overcame the block in differentiation, producing apparently normal, but clonally derived hematopoiesis, resulting in what has been termed a "clonal remission" [47].

A final and very appealing possibility is that crude chemotherapy somehow restored the immune surveillance which had failed when the leukemia started to develop. There is technology that can detect small clones of T-cells from patients in remission which are reactive to the original leukemic clone [48, 49] with the possibility that these cells eliminate or suppress residual disease post-chemotherapy, analogous to the graft vs. leukemia effect following allogeneic transplantation. This hypothesis can be tested experimentally in patients with AML and ALL and such studies would be of great interest, with the hope that interventions could be developed to augment this "autoimmune" reactivity.

Conclusions

The treatment of adult ALL is frustrating but also rewarding, since we should not ignore the fact that a substantial fraction of patients are cured with current treatment paradigms. Further improvements will not come easily, but will hopefully be accelerated by the impressive array of biologic data derived from gene array and proteomic experiments, currently being done largely in the pediatric population. Since ALL is a relatively uncommon disease in adults, further coordination amongst cooperative groups around the world would be desirable in order to more efficiently perform focused studies in different subgroups of patients.

References

1. Pui, C. H., Robison, L. L., & Look, A. T. (2008). Acute lymphoblastic leukaemia. *Lancet, 371*, 1030–1043.
2. Hoelzer, D., Gokbuget, N., Digel, W., et al. (2002). Outcome of adult patients with T-lymphoblastic lymphoma treated according to protocols for acute lymphoblastic leukemia. *Blood, 99*, 4379–4385.
3. Hoelzer, D., Thiel, E., Loffler, H., et al. (1984). Intensified therapy in acute lymphoblastic and acute undifferentiated leukemia in adults. *Blood, 64*, 38–47.

4. Larson, R. A., Dodge, R. K., Burns, C. P., et al. (1995). A five-drug remission induction regimen with intensive consolidation for adults with acute lymphoblastic leukemia: Cancer and leukemia group B study 8811. *Blood, 85,* 2025–2037.

5. Ellison, R. R., Mick, R., Cuttner, J., et al. (1991). The effects of postinduction intensification treatment with cytarabine and daunorubicin in adult acute lymphocytic leukemia: A prospective randomized clinical trial by Cancer and Leukemia Group B. *Journal of Clinical Oncology, 9,* 2002–2015.

6. Goldstone, A. H., Richards, S. M., Lazarus, H. M., et al. (2008). In adults with standard-risk acute lymphoblastic leukemia, the greatest benefit is achieved from a matched sibling allogeneic transplantation in first complete remission, and an autologous transplantation is less effective than conventional consolidation/maintenance chemotherapy in all patients: Final results of the International ALL Trial (MRC UKALL XII/ECOG E2993). *Blood, 111,* 1827–1833.

7. Rowe, J. M., Buck, G., Burnett, A. K., et al. (2005). Induction therapy for adults with acute lymphoblastic leukemia: Results of more than 1500 patients from the International ALL trial: MRC UKALL XII/ECOG E2993. *Blood, 106,* 3760–3767.

8. Pullarkat, V., Slovak, M. L., Kopecky, K. J., Forman, S. J., & Appelbaum, F. R. (2008). Impact of cytogenetics on the outcome of adult acute lymphoblastic leukemia: Results of Southwest Oncology Group 9400 study. *Blood, 111,* 2563–2572.

9. Wetzler, M., Dodge, R. K., Mrozek, K., et al. (1999). Prospective karyotype analysis in adult acute lymphoblastic leukemia: The cancer and leukemia Group B experience. *Blood, 93,* 3983–3993.

10. Pui, C. H. (2005). Impact of molecular profiling and cytogenetics in acute lymphoblastic leukemia. *Hematology, 10*(Suppl 1), 176–177.

11. Raimondi, S. C., Behm, F. G., Roberson, P. K., et al. (1988). Cytogenetics of childhood T-cell leukemia. *Blood, 72,* 1560–1566.

12. Raimondi, S. C., Behm, F. G., Roberson, P. K., et al. (1990). Cytogenetics of pre-B-cell acute lymphoblastic leukemia with emphasis on prognostic implications of the t(1, 19). *Journal of Clinical Oncology, 8,* 1380–1388.

13. Greaves, M. (1993). A natural history for pediatric acute leukemia. *Blood, 82,* 1043–1051.

14. Greaves, M. F., Maia, A. T., Wiemels, J. L., & Ford, A. M. (2003). Leukemia in twins: Lessons in natural history. *Blood, 102,* 2321–2333.

15. Taub, J. W., Konrad, M. A., Ge, Y., et al. (2002). High frequency of leukemic clones in newborn screening blood samples of children with B-precursor acute lymphoblastic leukemia. *Blood, 99,* 2992–2996.

16. Taub, J. W., Mundschau, G., Ge, Y., et al. (2004). Prenatal origin of GATA1 mutations may be an initiating step in the development of megakaryocytic leukemia in Down syndrome. *Blood, 104,* 1588–1589.

17. Cunningham, L., & Aplenc, R. (2007). Pharmacogenetics of acute lymphoblastic leukemia treatment response. *Expert Opinion on Pharmacotherapy, 8,* 2519–2531.

18. Lee, E. J., Petroni, G. R., Schiffer, C. A., et al. (2001). Brief-duration high-intensity chemotherapy for patients with small noncleaved-cell lymphoma or FAB L3 acute lymphocytic leukemia: Results of cancer and leukemia group B study 9251. *Journal of Clinical Oncology, 19,* 4014–4022.

19. Thomas, D. A., Cortes, J., O'Brien, S., et al. (1999). Hyper-CVAD program in Burkitt's-type adult acute lymphoblastic leukemia. *Journal of Clinical Oncology, 17,* 2461–2470.

20. Thomas, D. A., Faderl, S., O'Brien, S., et al. (2006). Chemoimmunotherapy with hyper-CVAD plus rituximab for the treatment of adult Burkitt and Burkitt-type lymphoma or acute lymphoblastic leukemia. *Cancer, 106,* 1569–1580.

21. de Labarthe, A., Rousselot, P., Huguet-Rigal, F., et al. (2007). Imatinib combined with induction or consolidation chemotherapy in patients with de novo Philadelphia chromosome-positive acute lymphoblastic leukemia: Results of the GRAAPH-2003 study. *Blood, 109,* 1408–1413.

22. Ottmann, O., Dombret, H., Martinelli, G., et al. (2007). Dasatinib induces rapid hematologic and cytogenetic responses in adult patients with Philadelphia chromosome positive acute lymphoblastic leukemia with resistance or intolerance to imatinib: Interim results of a phase 2 study. *Blood, 110,* 2309–2315.

23. Wassmann, B., Pfeifer, H., Goekbuget, N., et al. (2006). Alternating versus concurrent schedules of imatinib and chemotherapy as front-line therapy for Philadelphia-positive acute lymphoblastic leukemia (Ph + ALL). *Blood, 108,* 1469–1477.

24. Boissel, N., Auclerc, M. F., Lheritier, V., et al. (2003). Should adolescents with acute lymphoblastic leukemia be treated as old children or young adults? Comparison of the French FRALLE-93 and LALA-94 trials. *Journal of Clinical Oncology, 21,* 774–780.

25. de Bont, J. M., Holt, B., Dekker, A. W., van der Does-van den Berg, A., Sonneveld, P., & Pieters, R. (2004). Significant difference in outcome for adolescents with acute lymphoblastic leukemia treated on pediatric vs adult protocols in the Netherlands. *Leukemia, 18,* 2032–2035.

26. Hallbook, H., Gustafsson, G., Smedmyr, B., Soderhall, S., & Heyman, M. (2006). Treatment outcome in young adults and children >10 years of age with acute lymphoblastic leukemia in Sweden: A comparison between a pediatric protocol and an adult protocol. *Cancer, 107,* 1551–1561.

27. Ramanujachar, R., Richards, S., Hann, I., & Webb, D. (2006). Adolescents with acute lymphoblastic leukaemia: Emerging from the shadow of paediatric and adult treatment protocols. *Pediatric Blood & Cancer, 47*, 748–756.
28. Stock, W., La, M., Sanford, B., et al. (2008). What determines the outcomes for adolescents and young adults with acute lymphoblastic leukemia treated on cooperative group protocols? A comparison of Children's Cancer Group and Cancer and Leukemia Group B studies. *Blood, 112*, 1646–1654.
29. Ribera, J. M., Oriol, A., Sanz, M. A., et al. (2008). Comparison of the results of the treatment of adolescents and young adults with standard-risk acute lymphoblastic leukemia with the Programa Espanol de Tratamiento en Hematologia pediatric-based protocol ALL-96. *Journal of Clinical Oncology, 26*, 1843–1849.
30. Barry, E., DeAngelo, D. J., Neuberg, D., et al. (2007). Favorable outcome for adolescents with acute lymphoblastic leukemia treated on Dana-Farber Cancer Institute Acute Lymphoblastic Leukemia Consortium Protocols. *Journal of Clinical Oncology, 25*, 813–819.
31. Borowitz, M. J., Devidas, M., Hunger, S. P., et al. (2008). Clinical significance of minimal residual disease in childhood acute lymphoblastic leukemia and its relationship to other prognostic factors: A Children's Oncology Group study. *Blood, 111*, 5477–5485.
32. Fiere, D., Lepage, E., Sebban, C., et al. (1993). Adult acute lymphoblastic leukemia: A multicentric randomized trial testing bone marrow transplantation as postremission therapy The French Group on Therapy for Adult Acute Lymphoblastic Leukemia. *Journal of Clinical Oncology, 11*, 1990–2001.
33. Cornelissen, J. J., van der Holt, B., Verhoef, G. E., et al. (2009). Myeloablative allogeneic versus autologous stem cell transplantation in adult patients with acute lymphoblastic leukemia in first remission: A prospective sibling donor versus no-donor comparison. *Blood, 113*, 1375–1382.
34. DeAngelo, D. J., Yu, D., Johnson, J. L., et al. (2007). Nelarabine induces complete remissions in adults with relapsed or refractory T-lineage acute lymphoblastic leukemia or lymphoblastic lymphoma: Cancer and Leukemia Group B study 19801. *Blood, 109*, 5136–5142.
35. Kurtzberg, J. (2007). The long and winding road of the clinical development of Nelarabine. *Leukaemia & Lymphoma, 48*, 1–2.
36. Armstrong, F., de la Grange, P. B., Gerby, B., et al. (2009). NOTCH is a key regulator of human T-cell acute leukemia initiating cell activity. *Blood, 113*, 1730–1740.
37. Grabher, C., von Boehmer, H., & Look, A. T. (2006). Notch 1 activation in the molecular pathogenesis of T-cell acute lymphoblastic leukaemia. *Nature Reviews Cancer, 6*, 347–359.
38. Grosveld, G. C. (2009). Gamma-secretase inhibitors: Notch so bad. *Natural Medicines, 15*, 20–21.
39. Leonetti, C., Scarsella, M., Semple, S. C., et al. (2004). In vivo administration of liposomal vincristine sensitizes drug-resistant human solid tumors. *International Journal of Cancer, 110*, 767–774.
40. Stanciu-Herrera, C., Morgan, C., & Herrera, L. (2008). Anti-CD19 and anti-CD22 monoclonal antibodies increase the effectiveness of chemotherapy in Pre-B acute lymphoblastic leukemia cell lines. *Leukemia Research, 32*, 625–632.
41. Raetz, E. A., Cairo, M. S., Borowitz, M. J., et al. (2008). Chemoimmunotherapy reinduction with epratuzumab in children with acute lymphoblastic leukemia in marrow relapse: A Children's Oncology Group Pilot Study. *Journal of Clinical Oncology, 26*, 3756–3762.
42. Thomas, D. A., O'Brien, S., Jorgensen, J. L., et al. (2009). Prognostic significance of CD20 expression in adults with de novo precursor B-lineage acute lymphoblastic leukemia. *Blood, 113*(25), 6330–6337.
43. Cox, C. V., Martin, H. M., Kearns, P. R., Virgo, P., Evely, R. S., & Blair, A. (2007). Characterization of a progenitor cell population in childhood T-cell acute lymphoblastic leukemia. *Blood, 109*, 674–682.
44. Mullighan, C. G., Su, X., Zhang, J., et al. (2009). Deletion of IKZF1 and prognosis in acute lymphoblastic leukemia. *The New England Journal of Medicine, 360*, 470–480.
45. Kuiper, R. P., Schoenmakers, E. F., van Reijmersdal, S. V., et al. (2007). High-resolution genomic profiling of childhood ALL reveals novel recurrent genetic lesions affecting pathways involved in lymphocyte differentiation and cell cycle progression. *Leukemia, 21*, 1258–1266.
46. Mullighan, C. G., Goorha, S., Radtke, I., et al. (2007). Genome-wide analysis of genetic alterations in acute lymphoblastic leukaemia. *Nature, 446*, 758–764.
47. Fearon, E. R., Burke, P. J., Schiffer, C. A., Zehnbauer, B. A., & Vogelstein, B. (1986). Differentiation of leukemia cells to polymorphonuclear leukocytes in patients with acute nonlymphocytic leukemia. *The New England Journal of Medicine, 315*, 15–24.
48. Molldrem, J. J., Lee, P. P., Wang, C., et al. (2000). Evidence that specific T lymphocytes may participate in the elimination of chronic myelogenous leukemia. *Natural Medicines, 6*, 1018–1023.
49. Molldrem, J. J. (2006). Vaccination for leukemia. *Biology of Blood and Marrow Transplantation, 12*, 13–18.

Uncertainty may remain with either technique as to whether cells found to have a leukemic genotype/phenotype are truly clonogenic (capable of proliferation with potential to cause relapse).

Clinical Significance of MRD

The largest body of evidence to support the clinical importance of MRD is derived from pediatric studies and has incontrovertibly demonstrated that the level (and course) of MRD is the most powerful predictor of outcome in childhood ALL, in addition to emphasizing the heterogeneity of response to initial therapy. The international BFM group recently reported a 10-year EFS of 93% for those children with MRD <0.01% on days 33 and 78, compared with 16% if MRD >0.1% at both time points [12]. Employing an MRD cut-off of 0.1%, the Dana-Farber group has reported similar differences in relapse-free survival at 5 years [16]. In the Children's Oncology Group series [10], the detection of MRD >0.01% in the bone marrow on day 29 was the strongest predictor of survival.

MRD in adults has been studied less extensively but has demonstrated similar results, at least in affirming its prognostic power, albeit from mainly retrospective studies. In contrast to studies in childhood ALL where as many as 44% of patients achieved MRD negativity (<0.01% BM blasts) by D19 [32], only 10% of adults are thought to demonstrate similar kinetics of blast clearance [5] (Figs. 11.1 and 11.2)

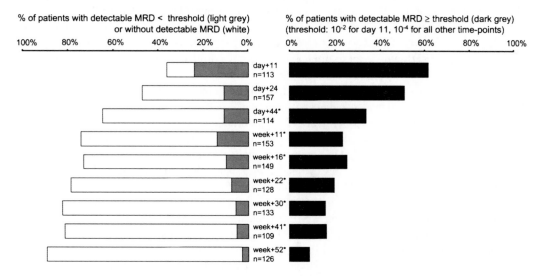

Fig. 11.1 Proportion of patients with detectable MRD represented by time-point of assessment (this research was originally published in Blood [5]. © The American Society of Hematology)

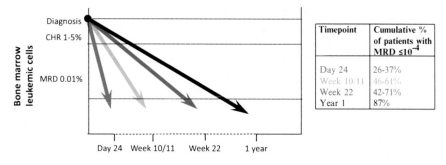

Fig. 11.2 Approximate cumulative percentages of adults achieving MRD≤ 10^{-4} according to published time-points [5, 9, 14]

The early and rapid reduction in MRD observed frequently in children following induction is associated with low relapse but MRD levels fall more slowly in adults and fewer patients become MRD negative [5, 13, 32]. A landmark study in adult ALL, from the GMALL group, quantified target genes IgH, IgK, and TCR rearrangements with high sensitivity ($<10^{-4}$) and defined "low risk" if MRD was negative on D11 and D24 of induction using two molecular markers with an assay sensitivity of at least 10^{-4}. High risk was defined as detectable MRD greater than 10^{-4} at two time points after induction. Three-year DFS probabilities for these two risk groups were markedly divergent, at 100% and 5.8%, respectively, although only 11 patients fulfilled the low-risk criteria. It should also be noted that this study identified a large number of intermediate patients (50%) who could not be assigned to either of these groups due to either a lack of a second molecular marker, insufficient sensitivity or an inconclusive course of MRD. The DFS for this "intermediate" group was 53.2% and their relapse risk was no different from the study population as a whole. It is likely that further methodological improvements will allow clearer stratification of relapse risk for patients within this group.

In terms of assessment *following* induction therapy, the available data suggests that current MRD strategies can reliably identify those at high risk of relapse, but not those with a genuinely low relapse risk. It may be that the longitudinal course of MRD is more important in adults in delineating risk groups [14]. Further data from the GMALL study group [5, 17] has shown that the predictive value of high levels of MRD after induction, in terms of relapse risk, is higher at later time points. The latter observation has been recently reiterated by data published from the NILG-ALL 09/00 study [9]. These authors evaluated an MRD risk model based on the MRD results of week 16 and week 22(by quantitative RT-PCR with ≥ 1 case-specific probe at a sensitivity of $\leq 10^{-4}$ for the majority) and showed that MRD status at these time points strongly correlated with DFS and superseded the prognostic power afforded by traditional risk classification.

The utility of flow cytometry to detect residual leukemia has been well established in pediatric ALL and has provided good evidence that end-induction MRD may be the most important prognostic variable currently available for assessment [10, 11]. Although less well studied than PCR in adult patients, similar results have been observed in studies using an immunophenotypic approach to MRD monitoring. Vidriales et al. [15] studied a relatively large series of adolescent and adult patients with ALL using three color flow cytometry with standardized and reproducible methodology. They found that detection of MRD, using a cut-off 0.05% (i.e., $10^{-3.3}$), had strong discriminating power on day 35 of induction therapy and was associated with a significantly increased relapse risk. This study suggested that a single early MRD evaluation may be sufficient to identify patients requiring intensification of treatment. However, it must be noted that the study group was somewhat heterogeneous, with 13 patients with Philadelphia positive disease and 10 classified with FAB L3 morphology. Given the age range of the patients studied (14–80 years) it is also likely that the treatment protocols were not uniform, particularly with regard to indications for allogeneic SCT.

More recent data derived from the Polish PALG 4-2002 multicenter study also demonstrated the prognostic significance of MRD using a standardized three-color flow cytometric approach. One hundred and fifteen adult patients were studied of whom 72% were classified as standard risk (SR) or high risk (HR), as defined by conventional parameters (age >35 years, WBC at diagnosis $>30 \times 10^9$ /L, adverse immunophenotype, i.e., pro-B, early-T or mature-T, or late achievement of CHR.) At least two aberrant phenotypes were identified in 98.5% of cases, with a sensitivity of 0.01% (10^{-4}). MRD >0.1% (10^{-3}) at the end of induction was significantly associated with shorter leukemia-free survival and was the strongest independent predictor of treatment failure in this study. Its prognostic value was demonstrable in both SR and HR groups. Prospective trials of uniformly stratified and treated patients are required to further delineate the role of this technique for MRD monitoring and clinical decision-making. It may be that MRD assessment using a combined approach of patient-specific qRT-PCR and flow cytometry will provide the optimal sensitivity and specificity, although this would represent a major challenge to be widely incorporated and standardized across protocols.

MRD: Redefining Remission?

The GMALL data, when considered in terms of risk of relapse, suggests a "low risk" group can be defined by an MRD level of less than 10^{-4} (or undetectable) in the bone marrow, before the start of consolidation on day 29. It might be more meaningful in the future to redefine the term complete remission and apply it only to this small group of patients, whose MRD level is low enough to be considered compatible with sustaining long-term remission, but this would currently be premature on the basis of existing evidence.

Cautions of MRD Interpretation

In common with all methods of response assessment, it is imperative that MRD data should be interpreted in the context of:

- Time-point of assessment
- Treatment protocol prescribed (and whether this was adhered to – including drug omissions, dose modifications and treatment delays)
- Sensitivity of method (GMALL data suggests (for PCR) ≥ 2 molecular markers with sensitivity $\geq 10^{-4}$)

Each of these factors may impact upon the definition of MRD risk groups. Precise MRD "cut-offs" for assignation of risk need to be thoughtfully defined before MRD-based risk stratification can be implemented for a given protocol.

How to Respond to MRD Data – Therapeutic Decisions

MRD-Based Early Treatment Response

Can treatment intensity be reduced in a low-risk population of patients as defined by MRD and conversely, can further post-remission intensification improve outcome for an MRD-defined high risk group?

In pediatric ALL, a protocol incorporating reduction in treatment intensity for patients with negative MRD in bone marrow on day 19 as determined by flow cytometry [47] is currently being tested [32]. UKALL 2003 (this UK study includes adolescents and young adults) is currently testing the hypothesis that de-intensification of therapy will not compromise outcome for a MRD-defined low-risk group (negative or $\leq 10^{-4}$ on day 29 and negative at week 11) who will be assigned either one or two delayed intensifications.

Conversely, if a patient is appropriately assigned to "high-risk MRD" the question remains as to what is the most optimal therapy/intensification? Allogeneic SCT, for example, provides a definite graft versus leukemia effect (refer to Chaps. 18 and 19) but its undoubted ability to prevent relapse should be balanced against significant procedure-related morbidity and mortality. Employing MRD in this manner may result in over-treatment of some patients according to the assigned risk threshold and sensitivity/specificity of MRD methodology. An alternative to SCT is to intensify or prolong post-induction intensification (PII) for those perceived to be at risk. In pediatric ALL, the Children's Cancer Group study (CCG-1961) examined the relative contribution of "length" and "strength" of PII for children with higher risk ALL and a rapid marrow response to induction therapy [48]. This large study showed that *stronger* intensification resulted in a highly statistically significant improvement in event-free survival (EFS) compared with the standard intensity therapy whereas *longer* PII provided no EFS benefit. The authors suggest that a window of opportunity may exist to allow eradication of resistant clones by early intensification of therapy. Several study groups are currently addressing this important therapeutic principle in adult ALL by means of post-induction MRD risk stratification.

MRD Monitoring During Follow-Up to Detect Early Relapse

The UKALL XII/ECOG study permitted analysis of a large series of patients with adult ALL experiencing relapse after a uniform approach to initial therapy [2]. The vast majority of patients relapsed within the bone marrow, with isolated extramedullary relapse recorded as 8% of this large cohort. Of the patients destined to relapse, the majority (81%) of cases were witnessed within 2 years of diagnosis, although a significant proportion (19%) relapsed more than 2 years following diagnosis.

In the absence of conventional risk factors for relapse, adults treated on modern protocols can expect a greater than 50% expectation of long-term survival with chemotherapy alone. Intensification and/or prolongation of therapy will therefore expose many patients to unnecessary toxicity and attendant risks. On the other hand, the outcome of patients with relapsed ALL is extremely poor, even if a second remission is achieved [2, 4].

Raff et al. [17] prospectively monitored MRD by real-time quantitative PCR in 105 patients to evaluate its ability to predict disease relapse in the early post-consolidation phase, for patients considered to be in hematological and molecular remission. They reported that 28 of the 105 patients converted to MRD positivity, 17 of whom had experienced frank relapse at the time of analysis. In 15 of these patients, MRD was detected within the *quantitative* range of PCR (prior to morphological relapse) and 13 of these patients (89%) relapsed after a median interval of 4.1 months. The sensitivity of the PCR assay in this study was designed in order not to miss true positives. Of the 77 continuously MRD negative patients, only 5 (6%) have experienced relapse; one case was thought to be missed as consequence of leukemic clonal evolution.

In principle, molecular detection of an impending relapse provides an opportunity to initiate salvage therapy prior to frank hematological relapse, with a lower tumor burden, fewer disease-related complications and a potentially improved outcome. Whereas there are good data in acute promyelocytic leukemia (APL) suggesting that re-initiating therapy early in the course of molecular relapse may improve prognosis [49], similar data are not yet available in adult ALL.

MRD-Based Post-Consolidation Therapy and SCT

The recently published NILG-ALL 09/00 study [9] asked whether prospectively monitoring MRD in the post consolidation phase of adult ALL therapy could spare a proportion of (traditionally defined) "high risk" (HR) patients from the morbidity and mortality of SCT in addition to identifying "standard risk" (SR) patients for whom standard chemotherapy is likely to fail. The experimental phase of this study allocated maintenance therapy for MRD-negative patients, and high-dose therapy with allogeneic or tandem-autologous SCT for MRD-positive patients (very-high risk patients e.g., BCR/ABL or MLL-AF4 positive were excluded). Applying this strategy in unselected SR/HR patients who achieved MRD negativity at weeks 16 and 22, the BM relapse rate was <20% and the 5-year DFS nearly 80%, without remission mortality. For MRD-positive patients, the data indicated that allogeneic SCT can indeed "rescue" a proportion of patients, although one-third of this group did not adhere to the protocol and failed to proceed to SCT. Importantly, however, this study confirmed that the majority of patients on standard protocols will not relapse prior to the informative MRD timepoints and that it is feasible to employ this data to individually optimize therapy.

Chapter 12
T-Cell Acute Lymphoblastic Leukemia

Andrei R. Shustov and Frederick R. Appelbaum

Introduction

T-cell acute lymphoblastic leukemia (T-ALL) is a highly aggressive neoplasm of lymphoblasts committed to the T-cell lineage. In 1994, the WHO Classification of Hematologic Malignancies defined T-ALL as precursor T lymphoblastic leukemia/lymphoblastic lymphoma underscoring the unity between the two entities in biology, natural history and outcomes. When the process is confined to a mass lesion and/or lymph nodes without any or with minimal involvement (<25%) of peripheral blood and/or bone marrow, the diagnosis is lymphoblastic lymphoma (LBL). When peripheral blood and/or bone marrow are extensively involved (>25%), the appropriate term is lymphoblastic leukemia regardless of the mass/lymphadenopathy. This designation is admittedly arbitrary.

T-ALL represents about 15% of childhood ALL, being more common in adolescents than in younger children and more common in males than in females. In adults, T-ALL comprises approximately 25% of ALL diagnoses. In contrast to its leukemic counterpart, T-cell LBL represents 85–90% of lymphoblastic lymphomas. It is most common in adolescent males.

Morphologically, both T-ALL and T-LBL are typically composed of small/medium-sized blast cells with scant cytoplasm, moderately condensed to dispersed chromatin and inconspicuous nucleoli (Fig. 12.1). Because morphologically T-ALL is indistinguishable from B-cell ALL, additional testing including immunohistochemistry and flow cytometry is necessary to establish the correct pathologic diagnosis. Table 12.1 outlines the place of ALL in the current WHO classification.

T-ALL Classification

T-ALL is a heterogeneous group of diseases with regard to immunophenotype, cytogenetics, molecular genetic abnormalities, clinical features, response to therapy, and prognosis, comprising several clinico-biological entities. Among several classifications, the most commonly used European Group for the Immunological Characterization of Leukemias (EGIL) classification is based predominantly on the expression of imunophenotypic markers on T-lymphoblasts, reflecting the stage of thymic maturation/development [1]. Four subgroups are identified: TI – the most immature subgroup or pro-T-ALL with expression of only CD7; TII – less immature, pre-T-ALL that also expresses CD2 and/or CD5 and/or CD8; TIII – cortical T-ALL defined by co-expression of CD1a;

A.R. Shustov (✉)
Seattle Cancer Care Alliance, 825 Eastlake Ave E, G3-200, Seattle, WA 98109-1024, USA
e-mail: ashustov@fhcrc.org

A.S. Advani and H.M. Lazarus (eds.), *Adult Acute Lymphocytic Leukemia*, Contemporary Hematology, 157
DOI 10.1007/978-1-60761-707-5_12, © Springer Science+Business Media, LLC 2011

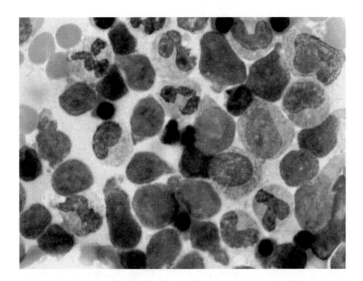

Fig. 12.1 T-cell acute lymphoblastic leukemia. Bone marrow aspirate from a patient with T-cell acute lymphoblastic leukemia. There is prominent infiltration by immature lymphoid blasts (Wright-Giemsa; oil emersion; ×1,000) (Courtesy of Dr. S. Cherian, University of Washington, Seattle, WA)

Table 12.1 World Health Organization classification of acute lymphoblastic leukemia

WHO classification	Frequency in adults (%)	Frequency in children (%)
Precursor B-cell ALL	70–75	85
Mature B-cell ALL	5	2
Precursor T-cell ALL	20–25	13

and TIV – mature T-ALL characterized by the presence of surface CD3 and CD1a-negativity. Based on mutually exclusive expression of $\alpha\beta$ or $\gamma\delta$ TCR chains, group a and group b designations are applied (TIIa, TIIIb, etc.). A multitude of clinical trials have demonstrated relevance of this classification to outcomes in T-ALL and even suggested risk stratification based on T-ALL subtype to identify patients who might benefit from either standard or intensified protocols, including allogeneic hematopoietic cell transplantation (HCT). Other proposed classifications are less commonly used and did not appear to bear on clinical outcomes at this time [2].

Molecular Genetics and Pathogenesis

Heterogeneity of T-ALL derives from its complex genetic and molecular pathophysiology. Standard cytogenetic analysis of lymphoid blasts reveals recurrent translocations responsible for activation of a small number of oncogenes in 25–50% of T-ALL [3]. In addition, fluorescent in situ hybridization (FISH) frequently demonstrates cytogenetically cryptic abnormalities. Among these, microdeletions leading to the loss of tumor suppressor genes are most frequent. In many T-ALL patients, T-cell oncogenes are over-expressed in the absence of specific chromosomal abnormalities in the corresponding genetic loci, suggesting the role for epigenetic alterations. DNA-array analysis has identified several gene expression signatures indicative of leukemic arrest at specific stages of normal thymocyte development [4–6]. Finally, mutational analysis of oncogenes implicated in T-cell development has shown activating mutations of NOTCH1 gene in high proportions of T-ALL [7].

These recent developments preliminarily identified several major signaling pathways that may be responsible for neoplastic transformation.

Genetic aberrations in T-ALL can be divided into five subgroups: (1) translocations involving TCR loci; (2) generation of fusion genes; (3) deletions (cryptic microdeletions) with loss of tumor suppressor genes; (4) activating mutations in signaling pathways; and (5) over-expression of cell cycle associated and signaling genes without associated chromosomal aberrations (suggestive of epigenetic deregulations). Table 12.2 summarizes more frequent genetic changes observed in T-ALL. More complete description can be found elsewhere [8].

Translocations involving TCR loci. The breakpoints in TCR loci occur on 14q11 (TCR*A/D*) and 7q34 (TCR*B*). V(D)J recombination taking place during T-cell development ensures open chromatin configuration in a number of genes making them vulnerable to the action of the recombinase enzymes. This facilitates "illegitimate" recombinations that may juxtapose transcription factor genes with strong promoter and enhancer elements of the TCR genes. Overexpression of transcription factors resulting from such recombinations gives rise to differentiation blocks at different stages of thymocyte development and eventually T-ALL [9]. The most common translocation so far identified in over 20% of childhood T-ALL and over 10% of adult T-ALL is a cryptic t(5;14)(q35;q32) [10]. *HOX11Like2*, an orphan homeobox gene was mapped to the breakpoint on chromosome 5 and *CTIP2*, a highly expressed gene during T-cell development, was localized to the vicinity of the chromosome 14 breakpoint. The *HOX11L2* gene was found to be transcriptionally activated under the influence of the strong *CTIP2* transcriptional regulation elements suggesting an important role for *HOX11* family member activation in T-ALL leukemogenesis [10]. Translocations involving the TCR loci are found in approximately 35% of T-ALL patients [9].

Table 12.2 Common genetic alterations in T-cell acute lymphoblastic leukemia

Chromosomal aberrations	Involved genes	Function of fusion gene	Frequency (%)	
			Children	Adults
Translocations/deletions				
t(7;10)(q34;q24)	TLX1 (*HOX11*)	TF	7	31
t(10;14)(q24;q11)				
t(5;14)(q35;q32)	TLX3 (*HOX11L2*)	TF	20	13
inv(7)(p15;q34)	*HOXA* cluster	TF	5	
t(7;7)				
t(1;14)(p32;q11)	*TAL1*	TF	3	
t(1;7)(p32;q34)				
t(11;14)(p15;q11)	*LMO1*	PPI	2	
t(11;14)(p13;q11)	*LMO2*	PPI	3	
t(7;11)(q35;p13)				
d(1p32)	*SIL-TAL1*	TF	9–30	U/K
t(10;11)(p13;q14)	*CALM-AF10*	TF	10	
t(11;x)(q23;x)	*MLL-*	TR	8	
t(9;9)(q34;q34)	NUP214-ABL1	ST	≤6	
9p21 (homozygous/ hemizygous)	P16	TSG	65/15	
d(6q)	U/K	TSG	20–30	
Mutations				
NOTCH1	*NOTCH1*	Differentiation	56	
FLT3 ITD	*FLT3*	Stem cell Development	5	
N-RAS	*N-RAS*	ST	<10	U/K

TF Transcription factor, *PPI* protein–protein interaction, *TR* transcriptional regulator, *TSG* tumor suppressor gene, *ST* signal transduction, *U/K* unknown

Translocations/deletions resulting in generation of fusion genes. During these rearrangements, parts of two genes located at the chromosomal breakpoints are fused "*in-frame*" and encode a new chimeric protein with oncogenic properties. Cryptic interstitial deletion at 1p32 results in the *SIL-TAL1* fusion gene and is found in 9–30% of childhood T-ALL; its frequency decreases with age in adult T-ALL [11]. *TLX1*, a transcription factor generally associated with favorable outcomes in T-ALL, was found to be over-expressed in at least 13% of childhood [12] and up to 30% adult [13] T-ALL. *TLX1* gene is localized to 10q24. Molecular analysis of 10q24 locus in T-ALL samples with over-expression of *TLX1* identified either a split locus by FISH, suggestive of translocation (in the majority of samples), or a *TCR-TLX1* junction (in the minority of samples). *CALM-AF10* fusion gene is found in 10% of ALL and results from t(10;11)(p13;q14) translocation [14]. Only half of the translocations were identified by conventional karyotyping while the other half required molecular analysis (RT-PCR) for detection. Interestingly, this aberration was restricted to TCRγδ but not TCRαβ T-ALL. Furthermore, it has conferred favorable survival outcome for mature TCRγδ but not immature TCRγδ T-ALL. Translocations, involving *MLL* gene at chromosome band 11q23 with different partners are found in about 8% of T-ALL cases [4, 15]. Translocation (4;11)(q21;q23) resulting in the overexpression of *MLL-AF4* fusion protein is seen in approximately 50% of cases in infants, 2% of cases in children, and 5–6% of cases in adults. Translocation (11;19)(q23;p13.3) encoding *MLL-ENL* is found in young adolescents and portends a better prognosis then usually associated with other *MLL* rearrangements [16, 17]. Remaining translocations are rare. Taken as a group, *MLL* translocations represent a distinct molecular subtype with unique expression profile, characterized by upregulation of a subset of *HOX* genes (*HOXA9, HOXA10, HOXC6*) and of *MEIS1*, differentiation arrest at an early stage of thymocyte development and commitment to γδ lineage [4]. Recently, translocations of *ABL1* were identified in approximately 6% of T-ALL patients, with *ABL1-NUP214* fusion being most common [18, 19]. This leads to extrachromosomal (episomal) amplification of the *ABL1* gene and might represent the basis for targeted therapy with tyrosine kinase inhibitors, such as imatinib mesylate. Several other translocations resulting in fusion genes and chimeric proteins are identified but represent less than 1% of T-ALL cases.

Deletions leading to loss of tumor suppressor genes. The most frequent deletion observed in up to 80% of T-ALL is loss of the p16^{INK4A}/p15^{INK4B} (also termed multi-tumor suppressor (MTS)-1 and MTS-2) locus at 9p21–22 leading to loss of cell cycle control and arrest in G1 [20]. Another common deletion site is 6q where variable sizes of DNA can be deleted without known target gene in 20–30% of T-ALL patients. The commonly deleted region focuses around 6q16, implicating *GRIK2* (*glutamate receptor ionotropic kainite 2*) as candidate tumor suppressor gene [21]. Other deletions are much less common.

Gene expression signatures. Several T-cell oncogenes (*HOX11, TAL1, LYL1, LMO1, and LMO2*) were recently found to be aberrantly expressed in T-ALL patients without demonstrable chromosomal abnormalities [5]. Oligonucleotide microarrays methodology identified several gene expression signatures suggestive of cell cycle arrest at specific stages of a normal thymocyte development: *LYL1*⁺ signature (pro-T ALL, TI), *HOX11*⁺ signature (early cortical thymocyte, TII), and *TAL1*⁺ (late cortical thymocyte, TIII). These findings have clinical significance since *HOX11* activation as discussed above, is associated with favorable prognosis [13], while *TAL1* and *LYL1* expression is linked to inferior responses to therapy and poor outcomes [5].

Deregulation of signaling pathways. NOTCH1 signaling deregulation is the most studied pathway in T-ALL leukemogenesis to date. *NOTCH1* signaling plays an important role in thymocyte transformation in animal (murine) [22, 23], paraclinical in vitro (T-ALL cell lines and patient-derived leukemic T-lymphoblasts) [24, 25] and clinical (therapeutic trials) setting. *NOTCH1* is an important regulator in T-cell commitment decisions of the earliest common lymphocyte progenitor (CLP) [26, 27] and in the assembly and signaling of the pre-TCR in immature thymocytes [28, 29]. Additionally, it could also play a role in controlling the turnover of the E2A cyclin-dependent kinase, a crucial cell cycle regulator [30].

Table 2.3 Genetic anomalies in adult T-ALL

Cytogenetic abnormality	Genetic lesion	Frequency (%)
1p32 [51–53]	TAL1	20–30
t(v;11q23) [54]	MLL	8–10
10q24 [55, 56]	HOX11	30
5q35 [57]	HOX11L2	10–15
t(8;14), t(8;22), t(2;8) [58]	MYC	4
19p13 [59]	LYL1	3
11p15 [60]	RBTN1(LMO1)	<1
11p13	RBTN2(LMO2)	<1
1p34.3–35	LCK	<1
t(10;11) (p13;q14)	PICALM-MLLT10	10
del(9p)	Loss CDKN2A	>30
	NOTCH1 activation	50

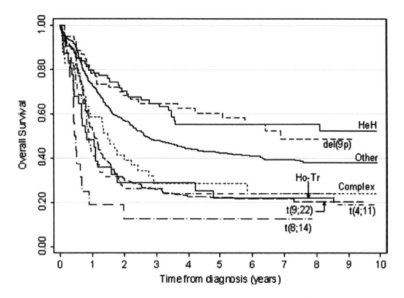

Fig. 2.5 Overall survival by cytogenetic subgroup of patients registered on MRC UKALLXII/ECOG 2993 (Reprinted with permission from [49]) HeH=high hyperdiploidy, Ho-Tr=low hypodiploidy, near triploidy

predictors of inferior outcome irrespective of age, gender, and WBC on presentation. A detailed risk stratification algorithm, based on the cytogenetic and molecular abnormalities, has been recently proposed by the Southwestern Oncology Group (SWOG) based on the outcome analysis of 200 ALL patients treated on the SWOG9400 study [48] (Fig. 2.6).

The majority of B-ALL and 20% of T-ALL cases have clonal DJ rearrangements of the immuno-globulin heavy chain (IgH) gene. The T-cell receptor (TCR) rearrangement has been documented in almost all T-ALL and up to 70% of B-ALL cases [61, 62]. Hence, these antigen receptor gene rearrange-ments are not helpful in lineage assessment. Although gene rearrangement studies may not be essential for the ALL diagnosis, they can be valuable in assessment of minimal residual disease (MRD).

The most recent WHO classification (2008) recognizes several specific entities among patients with B-cell ALL, defined by the presence of particular chromosomal abnormalities associated with unique phenotypic and prognostic features (Table 2.4). They include t(9;22), t(v;11q23), t(12;21), B-ALL with hyperdiploidy, B-ALL with hypodiploidy, t(5;14), and t(1;19). Other chromosomal abnor-malities, such as del(6q), del(9p), and del(12p) do not appear to impact the outcome of ALL patients.

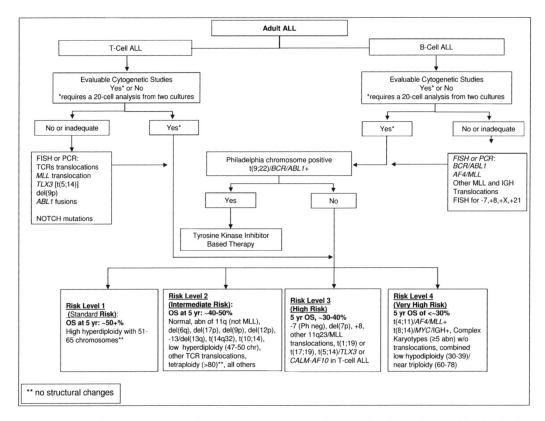

Fig. 2.6 Proposed cytogenetic and molecular genetic prognostic risk grouping for adult ALL (Reprinted with permission from [48])

Table 2.4 WHO classification of ALL

Precursor B lymphoblastic leukemia/lymphoma not otherwise specified (NOS)
Precursor B lymphoblastic leukemia/lymphoma with recurrent genetic abnormalities
    t(9;22) (q34;q11.2); BCR-ABL1
    t(v;11q23); MLL rearranged
    t(12;21) (p13;q22); TEL/AML 1 (ETV6-RUNX1)
    B-ALL with hyperdiploidy
    B-ALL with hypodiploidy
    t(5;14) (q31;q32); IL3-IGH
    t(1;19) (q23;p13.3); E2A-PBX1 (TCF-PBX1)
Precursor T-cell acute lymphoblastic leukemia

Among patients with T-ALL the most common recurrent cytogenetic translocations involve the α and δ TCR loci at 14q11.2, the β locus at 7q35, and the γ locus at 7p14–15 with a variety of partner genes [59, 63]. In most cases, these translocations lead to an inappropriate activation of *structurally intact* transcription factor proto-oncogenes such as HOX11(TLX1) (10q24), HOX11L2 (TLX3) (5q35), MYC (8q24.1), TAL1 (1p32), RBTN1 (LMO1) (11p15), RBTN2 (LMO2) (11p13), LYL1 (19p13) and LCK (cytoplasmic tyrosine kinase) (1p34.3–35). Some translocations result in a creation of *fusion genes*, such as PICALM-MLLT10 t(10;11) (p13;q14) and MLL-ENL t(11;19) (q23;p13) [63]. Activating mutations in the NOTCH1 gene, important for T cell development, are detected in 50% of adult T-ALL patients and are associated with a shorter survival [64, 65].

In some cases translocations not detected by routine karyotyping can be identified by molecular genetic studies. For example the TAL1 locus is altered by translocation in 20–30% of T-ALL. However, the actual t(1;14) (p32;q11) translocation can only be identified in 3% [60, 66]. Deletion del(9p), resulting in loss of the tumor-suppressor gene CDKN2A, is discovered in 30% of T-ALL patients.

Gene Expression Profiling

Completion of the human genome project and the development of high throughput technologies allowed for the simultaneous measurement of the quantitative expression of thousands of genes, using complementary DNA (cDNA) microarrays [67]. This technique is effective in deciphering the biological and clinical diversity of ALL and other malignant disorders [68].

The underlying principle of gene array analysis relies on the fact that only a fraction of the genes encoded in the genome of each cell is actively transcribed into messenger RNA (mRNA) and hence, expressed. Messenger RNA, extracted from a cell, is copied enzymatically to create a fluorescent cDNA probe representing the expressed genes in that cell. The probe is then incubated on the surface of a DNA microarray, which contains spots of DNA derived from thousands of distinct human genes. During the incubation, each cDNA molecule in the probe hybridizes to the microarray spot that represents its respective gene. The *extent* of hybridization of fluorescent cDNA to each microarray spot is quantitated with use of a scanning fluorescent microscope [69]. In pediatric B-cell ALL, certain gene expression signatures correlate with specific chromosomal aberrations with 96–100% accuracy [70, 71]. Several studies demonstrated that gene expression profiling is able to distinguish ALL without known chromosomal abnormalities from other known ALL subtypes [72, 73].

Although still a research technique, gene expression profiling can not only accurately identifies major subtypes of ALL but also implicates single genes and signaling pathways as important determinants of clinical outcome [74, 75]. The technique is able to identify distinct sets of genes that are associated with resistance to various classes of anti-leukemic agents [76–78]. Once these methods have been refined, prospectively validated and made cost effective, they will likely replace some of the current diagnostic techniques.

Minimal Residual Disease

In improved understanding of the molecular characteristics of ALL has lead to the development of novel methods for the detection of morphologically occult leukemia or minimal residual disease (MRD). Both molecular and immunophenotypic methods can reliably detect MRD at the levels of less than 0.01% [79, 80]. In adult ALL, identification of clonally rearranged immunoglobulin and T-cell receptor genes, chromosomal abnormalities and fusion proteins by polymerase chain reaction (PCR) are commonly utilized [81–84]. The role of flow cytometry, identifying aberrant protein expression on the leukemic cells, is less well established in adults compared to that in pediatric ALL [85–87]. Presence of MRD early in the course of therapy is strongly associated with poor treatment response and increased relapse rate (RR) [83, 88–93]. In the pediatric population, it is *the most* powerful predictor of overall outcome [94–97, 101]. Prospective analysis of MRD in 196 adult patients with "standard risk" ALL, conducted by the German study group, identified a subset of patients with a particularly high risk of relapse. These patients (23%) had an MRD level of 0.01% or higher at 16 weeks of therapy and had an RR of 94% [83]. Only a minority (10%) of patients cleared (<0.01%) MRD by day 11 or 22; however, of those who became MRD negative, none relapsed within 3-years of follow-up.

Since early clearance of MRD indicates high chemosensitivity of the leukemic clone, it could be used not only as a predictive factor, but as a guide to intensification or reduction in the intensity of the intended therapy [98]. Measuring MRD may help to establish an optimal timing for hematopoietic stem cell transplant (HSCT), guide modulation of immunosuppression after an allogeneic HSCT, and provide an important end-point for phase II clinical trials.

Differential Diagnosis

The initial presentation of ALL must be distinguished from a variety of the malignant (AML, lymphoma, CML in lymphoid blast crisis) and benign (ITP, aplastic anemia) hematological disorders, infections etiologies (mononucleosis), rheumatoid diseases and reactive processes. The acute onset of ecchymosis, petechiae, and bleeding may suggest ITP. However, the presence of the large platelets, normal hemoglobin, and absence of leukocytes anomalies in the blood and marrow – will help to differentiate these disorders. Pancytopenia and clinical consequences of bone marrow failure can be presenting features of both aplastic anemia and ALL, particularly, rare cases of ALL with a hypocellular or necrotic marrow, later replaced by lymphoblasts. ALL should be considered in the differential diagnosis of hypereosinophilia, which may be a presenting feature of ALL or precede its diagnosis by several months [99, 100].

Various viral infections (mononucleosis, pertussis, and parapertussis) may have similar clinical presentation to that of ALL, particularly if present with leukocytosis, thrombocytopenia and hemolytic anemia. However, lymphocytosis associated with viral infections is expected to be due to the increase in mature lymphocytes counts rather than leukemic blasts.

Arthralgia and bone pain may mimic collagen vascular disease, such as rheumatoid arthritis.

Ideally, in a patient suspected of having ALL, disease-specific therapy should be initiated as soon as possible to minimize complications. However, it might be delayed and supportive care instituted until a definitive diagnosis is established. In most cases, an adequate bone marrow biopsy from which appropriate morphologic, immunophenotypic, and molecular studies are performed, allows the definitive diagnosis to be established.

References

1. Lazarus, H. M., et al. (2006). Central nervous system involvement in adult acute lymphoblastic leukemia at diagnosis: Results from the international ALL trial MRC UKALL XII/ECOG E2993. *Blood, 108*(2), 465–472.
2. Reman, O., et al. (2008). Central nervous system involvement in adult acute lymphoblastic leukemia at diagnosis and/or at first relapse: Results from the GET-LALA group. *Leukemia Research, 32*(11), 1741–1750.
3. Larson, R. A., et al. (1995). A five-drug remission induction regimen with intensive consolidation for adults with acute lymphoblastic leukemia: Cancer and leukemia group B study 8811. *Blood, 85*(8), 2025–2037.
4. Kantarjian, H. M., et al. (2000). Results of treatment with hyper-CVAD, a dose-intensive regimen, in adult acute lymphocytic leukemia. *Journal of Clinical Oncology, 18*(3), 547–561.
5. Cortes, J., et al. (1995). The value of high-dose systemic chemotherapy and intrathecal therapy for central nervous system prophylaxis in different risk groups of adult acute lymphoblastic leukemia. *Blood, 86*(6), 2091–2097.
6. Petersdorf, S. H., et al. (2001). Comparison of the L10M consolidation regimen to an alternative regimen including escalating methotrexate/L-asparaginase for adult acute lymphoblastic leukemia: A Southwest Oncology Group Study. *Leukemia, 15*(2), 208–216.
7. Schattner, A., et al. (2001). Facial diplegia as the presenting manifestation of acute lymphoblastic leukemia. *The Mount Sinai Journal of Medicine, 68*(6), 406–409.

8. Mayo, G. L., Carter, J. E., & McKinnon, S. J. (2002). Bilateral optic disk edema and blindness as initial presentation of acute lymphocytic leukemia. *American Journal of Ophthalmology, 134*(1), 141–142.

9. Pui, C. H. (2006). Central nervous system disease in acute lymphoblastic leukemia: Prophylaxis and treatment. *Hematology American Society of Hematology. Education Program, 2006*, 142–146.

10. Beslac-Bumbasirevic, L., et al. (1996). Neuroleukemia in adults. *Srpski Arhiv za Celokupno Lekarstvo, 124*(3–4), 82–86.

11. Kay, H. E. (1983). Testicular infiltration in acute lymphoblastic leukaemia. *British Journal Haematology, 53*(4), 537–542.

12. Storti, S., et al. (1988). Emergency abdominal surgery in patients with acute leukemia and lymphoma. *The Italian Journal of Surgical Sciences, 18*(4), 361–363.

13. Ferrara, F., et al. (1998). Spontaneous splenic rupture in a patient with acute lymphoblastic leukemia of Burkitt type. *Leukaemia & Lymphoma, 29*(5–6), 613–616.

14. Choo-Kang, L. R., et al. (1999). Cerebral edema and priapism in an adolescent with acute lymphoblastic leukemia. *Pediatric Emergency Care, 15*(2), 110–112.

15. Kim, H. R., et al. (2006). Arthritis preceding acute biphenotypic leukemia. *Clinical Rheumatology, 25*(3), 380–381.

16. Gur, H., et al. (1999). Rheumatic manifestations preceding adult acute leukemia: Characteristics and implication in course and prognosis. *Acta Haematologica, 101*(1), 1–6.

17. Guven, G. S., et al. (2005). Knee arthritis as a rare inaugural manifestation of adult leukemia. *Rheumatology International, 25*(4), 317–318.

18. Sinigaglia, R., et al. (2008). Musculoskeletal manifestations in pediatric acute leukemia. *Journal of Pediatric Orthopedics, 28*(1), 20–28.

19. Ali, R., et al. (2006). Leukaemia cutis in T-cell acute lymphoblastic leukaemia. *Cytopathology, 17*(3), 158–161.

20. Porcu, P., et al. (2000). Hyperleukocytic leukemias and leukostasis: A review of pathophysiology, clinical presentation and management. *Leukaemia & Lymphoma, 39*(1–2), 1–18.

21. Maurer, H. S., et al. (1988). The effect of initial management of hyperleukocytosis on early complications and outcome of children with acute lymphoblastic leukemia. *Journal of Clinical Oncology, 6*(9), 1425–1432.

22. Rosenbluth, M. J., Lam, W. A., & Fletcher, D. A. (2006). Force microscopy of nonadherent cells: A comparison of leukemia cell deformability. *Biophysical Journal, 90*(8), 2994–3003.

23. Strauss, R. A., et al. (1985). Acute cytoreduction techniques in the early treatment of hyperleukocytosis associated with childhood hematologic malignancies. *Medical and Pediatric Oncology, 13*(6), 346–351.

24. Sarris, A. H., et al. (1992). High incidence of disseminated intravascular coagulation during remission induction of adult patients with acute lymphoblastic leukemia. *Blood, 79*(5), 1305–1310.

25. Solano, C., et al. (1992). Acute lymphoblastic leukemia: Hypofibrinogenemia with a low incidence of clinical complications is often found during induction remission therapy. *Blood, 80*(5), 1366–1368.

26. Higuchi, T., et al. (1998). Disseminated intravascular coagulation in acute lymphoblastic leukemia at presentation and in early phase of remission induction therapy. *Annals of Hematology, 76*(6), 263–269.

27. O'Regan, S., et al. (1977). Electrolyte and acid-base disturbances in the management of leukemia. *Blood, 49*(3), 345–353.

28. Jeha, S. (2001). Tumor lysis syndrome. *Seminars in Hematology, 38*(4 Suppl 10), 4–8.

29. Fukasawa, H., et al. (2001). Hypercalcemia in a patient with B-cell acute lymphoblastic leukemia: A role of proinflammatory cytokine. *The American Journal of the Medical Sciences, 322*(2), 109–112.

30. Schneider, T., et al. (2001). Life threatening hypercalcemia in a young man with ALL. *Deutsche Medizinische Wochenschrift, 126*(1–2), 7–11.

31. Lankisch, P., et al. (2004). Hypercalcemia with nephrocalcinosis and impaired renal function due to increased parathyroid hormone secretion at onset of childhood acute lymphoblastic leukemia. *Leukaemia & Lymphoma, 45*(8), 1695–1697.

32. Esbrit, P. (2001). Hypercalcemia of malignancy – new insights into an old syndrome. *Clinica y Laboratorio, 47*(1–2), 67–71.

33. Tan, A. W., et al. (2004). Extensive calcinosis cutis in relapsed acute lymphoblastic leukaemia. *Annals of the Academy of Medicine, Singapore, 33*(1), 107–109.

34. Sillos, E. M., et al. (2001). Lactic acidosis: A metabolic complication of hematologic malignancies: Case report and review of the literature. *Cancer, 92*(9), 2237–2246.

35. Mazurek, S., Boschek, C. B., & Eigenbrodt, E. (1997). The role of phosphometabolites in cell proliferation, energy metabolism, and tumor therapy. *Journal of Bioenergetics and Biomembranes, 29*(4), 315–330.

36. Mathupala, S. P., Rempel, A., & Pedersen, P. L. (1997). Aberrant glycolytic metabolism of cancer cells: A remarkable coordination of genetic, transcriptional, post-translational, and mutational events that lead to a critical role for type II hexokinase. *Journal of Bioenergetics and Biomembranes, 29*(4), 339–343.

37. Elmlinger, M. W., et al. (1996). Insulin-like growth factor binding protein 2 is differentially expressed in leukaemic B- and T-cell lines. *Growth Regulation, 6*(3), 152–157.

38. Cohick, W. S., & Clemmons, D. R. (1993). The insulin-like growth factors. *Annual Review of Physiology, 55*, 131–153.
39. Werner, H., & LeRoith, D. (1996). The role of the insulin-like growth factor system in human cancer. *Advances in Cancer Research, 68*, 183–223.
40. Burger, B., et al. (2003). Diagnostic cerebrospinal fluid examination in children with acute lymphoblastic leukemia: Significance of low leukocyte counts with blasts or traumatic lumbar puncture. *Journal of Clinical Oncology, 21*(2), 184–188.
41. Gilchrist, G. S., et al. (1994). Low numbers of CSF blasts at diagnosis do not predict for the development of CNS leukemia in children with intermediate-risk acute lymphoblastic leukemia: A Childrens Cancer Group report. *Journal of Clinical Oncology, 12*(12), 2594–2600.
42. Pui, C. H., et al. (2004). Improved outcome for children with acute lymphoblastic leukemia: Results of Total Therapy Study XIIIB at St Jude Children's Research Hospital. *Blood, 104*(9), 2690–2696.
43. Gajjar, A., et al. (2000). Traumatic lumbar puncture at diagnosis adversely affects outcome in childhood acute lymphoblastic leukemia. *Blood, 96*(10), 3381–3384.
44. Swerdlow, S., Campo, E., Harris, N. L., & Jaffe, E. S. (2008). *WHO classification of tumors of haematopoietic and lymphoid tissues.* Lyon, France: IARC Press.
45. Al Khabori, M., et al. (2008). Adult precursor T-lymphoblastic leukemia/lymphoma with myeloid-associated antigen expression is associated with a lower complete remission rate following induction chemotherapy. *Acta Haematologica, 120*(1), 5–10.
46. Pui, C. H., Robison, L. L., & Look, A. T. (2008). Acute lymphoblastic leukaemia. *Lancet, 371*(9617), 1030–1043.
47. Faderl, S., et al. (1998). Clinical significance of cytogenetic abnormalities in adult acute lymphoblastic leukemia. *Blood, 91*(11), 3995–4019.
48. Pullarkat, V., et al. (2008). Impact of cytogenetics on the outcome of adult acute lymphoblastic leukemia: Results of Southwest Oncology Group 9400 study. *Blood, 111*(5), 2563–2572.
49. Moorman, A. V., et al. (2007). Karyotype is an independent prognostic factor in adult acute lymphoblastic leukemia (ALL): Analysis of cytogenetic data from patients treated on the Medical Research Council (MRC) UKALLXII/Eastern Cooperative Oncology Group (ECOG) 2993 trial. *Blood, 109*(8), 3189–3197.
50. Mancini, M., et al. (2005). A comprehensive genetic classification of adult acute lymphoblastic leukemia (ALL): Analysis of the GIMEMA 0496 protocol. *Blood, 105*(9), 3434–3441.
51. François, S., Delabesse, E., Baranger, L., Dautel, M., Foussard, C., Boasson, M., et al. (1998). Deregulated expression of the TAL1 gene by t(1;5)(p32;31) in patient with T-cell acute lymphoblastic leukemia. *Genes, Chromosomes & Cancer, 23*(1), 36–43.
52. van der Burg, M., et al. (2002). A single split-signal FISH probe set allows detection of TAL1 translocations as well as SIL-TAL1 fusion genes in a single test. *Leukemia, 16*(4), 755–761.
53. Curry, J. D., & Smith, M. T. (2003). Measurement of SIL-TAL1 fusion gene transcripts associated with human T-cell lymphocytic leukemia by real-time reverse transcriptase-PCR. *Leukemia Research, 27*(7), 575–582.
54. Brassesco, M. S., et al. (2009). Cytogenetic and molecular analysis of MLL rearrangements in acute lymphoblastic leukaemia survivors. *Mutagenesis, 24*(2), 153–160.
55. Bergeron, J., et al. (2007). Prognostic and oncogenic relevance of TLX1/HOX11 expression level in T-ALLs. *Blood, 110*(7), 2324–2330.
56. Ferrando, A. A., et al. (2004). Prognostic importance of TLX1 (HOX11) oncogene expression in adults with T-cell acute lymphoblastic leukaemia. *Lancet, 363*(9408), 535–536.
57. Baak, U., et al. (2008). Thymic adult T-cell acute lymphoblastic leukemia stratified in standard- and high-risk group by aberrant HOX11L2 expression: Experience of the German multicenter ALL study group. *Leukemia, 22*(6), 1154–1160.
58. Palomero, T., & Ferrando, A. (2008). Oncogenic NOTCH1 control of MYC and PI3K: Challenges and opportunities for anti-NOTCH1 therapy in T-cell acute lymphoblastic leukemias and lymphomas. *Clinical Cancer Research, 14*(17), 5314–5317.
59. Han, X., & Bueso-Ramos, C. E. (2007). Precursor T-cell acute lymphoblastic leukemia/lymphoblastic lymphoma and acute biphenotypic leukemias. *American Journal of Clinical Pathology, 127*(4), 528–544.
60. Brown, L., et al. (1990). Site-specific recombination of the tal-1 gene is a common occurrence in human T cell leukemia. *The EMBO Journal, 9*(10), 3343–3351.
61. Szczepanski, T., et al. (1999). Ig heavy chain gene rearrangements in T-cell acute lymphoblastic leukemia exhibit predominant DH6-19 and DH7-27 gene usage, can result in complete V-D-J rearrangements, and are rare in T-cell receptor alpha beta lineage. *Blood, 93*(12), 4079–4085.
62. van der Velden, V. H., et al. (2004). TCRB gene rearrangements in childhood and adult precursor-B-ALL: Frequency, applicability as MRD-PCR target, and stability between diagnosis and relapse. *Leukemia, 18*(12), 1971–1980.
63. Graux, C., et al. (2006). Cytogenetics and molecular genetics of T-cell acute lymphoblastic leukemia: From thymocyte to lymphoblast. *Leukemia, 20*(9), 1496–1510.

64. Weng, A. P., et al. (2006). c-Myc is an important direct target of Notch1 in T-cell acute lymphoblastic leukemia/lymphoma. *Genes & Development, 20*(15), 2096–2109.
65. Zhu, Y. M., et al. (2006). NOTCH1 mutations in T-cell acute lymphoblastic leukemia: Prognostic significance and implication in multifactorial leukemogenesis. *Clinical Cancer Research, 12*(10), 3043–3049.
66. Hebert, J., et al. (1994). Candidate tumor-suppressor genes MTS1 (p16INK4A) and MTS2 (p15INK4B) display frequent homozygous deletions in primary cells from T- but not from B-cell lineage acute lymphoblastic leukemias. *Blood, 84*(12), 4038–4044.
67. Schena, M., et al. (1995). Quantitative monitoring of gene expression patterns with a complementary DNA microarray. *Science, 270*(5235), 467–470.
68. Alizadeh, A. A., et al. (2000). Distinct types of diffuse large B-cell lymphoma identified by gene expression profiling. *Nature, 403*(6769), 503–511.
69. Staudt, L. M. (2003). Molecular diagnosis of the hematologic cancers. *The New England Journal of Medicine, 348*(18), 1777–1785.
70. Armstrong, S. A., et al. (2002). MLL translocations specify a distinct gene expression profile that distinguishes a unique leukemia. *Nature Genetics, 30*(1), 41–47.
71. Yeoh, E. J., et al. (2002). Classification, subtype discovery, and prediction of outcome in pediatric acute lymphoblastic leukemia by gene expression profiling. *Cancer Cell, 1*(2), 133–143.
72. Ross, M. E., et al. (2004). Gene expression profiling of pediatric acute myelogenous leukemia. *Blood, 104*(12), 3679–3687.
73. van Delft, F. W., et al. (2005). Prospective gene expression analysis accurately subtypes acute leukaemia in children and establishes a commonality between hyperdiploidy and t(12;21) in acute lymphoblastic leukaemia. *British Journal Haematology, 130*(1), 26–35.
74. Mi, S., et al. (2007). MicroRNA expression signatures accurately discriminate acute lymphoblastic leukemia from acute myeloid leukemia. *Proceedings of the National Academy of Sciences of the United States of America, 104*(50), 19971–19976.
75. Kawamata, N., et al. (2008). Molecular allelokaryotyping of pediatric acute lymphoblastic leukemias by high-resolution single nucleotide polymorphism oligonucleotide genomic microarray. *Blood, 111*(2), 776–784.
76. Tissing, W. J., et al. (2007). Genomewide identification of prednisolone-responsive genes in acute lymphoblastic leukemia cells. *Blood, 109*(9), 3929–3935.
77. Cheok, M. H., et al. (2003). Treatment-specific changes in gene expression discriminate in vivo drug response in human leukemia cells. *Nature Genetics, 34*(1), 85–90.
78. Holleman, A., et al. (2004). Gene-expression patterns in drug-resistant acute lymphoblastic leukemia cells and response to treatment. *The New England Journal of Medicine, 351*(6), 533–542.
79. de Haas, V., et al. (2000). Accurate quantification of minimal residual disease at day 15, by real-time quantitative polymerase chain reaction identifies also patients with B-precursor acute lymphoblastic leukemia at high risk for relapse. *Blood, 96*(4), 1619–1620.
80. Malec, M., et al. (2001). Flow cytometry and allele-specific oligonucleotide PCR are equally effective in detection of minimal residual disease in ALL. *Leukemia, 15*(5), 716–727.
81. Foroni, L., & Hoffbrand, A. V. (2002). Molecular analysis of minimal residual disease in adult acute lymphoblastic leukaemia. *Best Practice & Research. Clinical Haematology, 15*(1), 71–90.
82. Mortuza, F. Y., et al. (2002). Minimal residual disease tests provide an independent predictor of clinical outcome in adult acute lymphoblastic leukaemia. *Journal of Clinical Oncology, 20*(4), 1094–1104.
83. Bruggemann, M., et al. (2006). Clinical significance of minimal residual disease quantification in adult patients with standard-risk acute lymphoblastic leukemia. *Blood, 107*(3), 1116–1123.
84. Raff, T., et al. (2007). Molecular relapse in adult standard-risk ALL patients detected by prospective MRD monitoring during and after maintenance treatment: Data from the GMALL 06/99 and 07/03 trials. *Blood, 109*(3), 910–915.
85. Coustan-Smith, E., et al. (2002). Prognostic importance of measuring early clearance of leukemic cells by flow cytometry in childhood acute lymphoblastic leukemia. *Blood, 100*(1), 52–58.
86. Krampera, M., et al. (2003). Outcome prediction by immunophenotypic minimal residual disease detection in adult T-cell acute lymphoblastic leukaemia. *British Journal Haematology, 120*(1), 74–79.
87. Vidriales, M. B., Orfao, A., & San-Miguel, J. F. (2003). Immunologic monitoring in adults with acute lymphoblastic leukemia. *Current Oncology Reports, 5*(5), 413–418.
88. Jacquy, C., et al. (1997). A prospective study of minimal residual disease in childhood B-lineage acute lymphoblastic leukaemia: MRD level at the end of induction is a strong predictive factor of relapse. *British Journal Haematology, 98*(1), 140–146.
89. van Dongen, J. J., et al. (1998). Prognostic value of minimal residual disease in acute lymphoblastic leukaemia in childhood. *Lancet, 352*(9142), 1731–1738.
90. Coustan-Smith, E., et al. (1998). Immunological detection of minimal residual disease in children with acute lymphoblastic leukaemia. *Lancet, 351*(9102), 550–554.

91. Ciudad, J., et al. (1998). Prognostic value of immunophenotypic detection of minimal residual disease in acute lymphoblastic leukemia. *Journal of Clinical Oncology, 16*(12), 3774–3781.
92. Biondi, A., et al. (2000). Molecular detection of minimal residual disease is a strong predictive factor of relapse in childhood B-lineage acute lymphoblastic leukemia with medium risk features. A case control study of the International BFM study group. *Leukemia, 14*(11), 1939–1943.
93. Bjorklund, E., et al. (2003). Flow cytometric follow-up of minimal residual disease in bone marrow gives prognostic information in children with acute lymphoblastic leukemia. *Leukemia, 17*(1), 138–148.
94. Dworzak, M. N., et al. (2002). Prognostic significance and modalities of flow cytometric minimal residual disease detection in childhood acute lymphoblastic leukemia. *Blood, 99*(6), 1952–1958.
95. Nyvold, C., et al. (2002). Precise quantification of minimal residual disease at day 29 allows identification of children with acute lymphoblastic leukemia and an excellent outcome. *Blood, 99*(4), 1253–1258.
96. Zhou, J., et al. (2007). Quantitative analysis of minimal residual disease predicts relapse in children with B-lineage acute lymphoblastic leukemia in DFCI ALL Consortium Protocol 95-01. *Blood, 110*(5), 1607–1611.
97. Flohr, T., et al. (2008). Minimal residual disease-directed risk stratification using real-time quantitative PCR analysis of immunoglobulin and T-cell receptor gene rearrangements in the international multicenter trial AIEOP-BFM ALL 2000 for childhood acute lymphoblastic leukemia. *Leukemia, 22*(4), 771–782.
98. Coustan-Smith, E., et al. (2006). A simplified flow cytometric assay identifies children with acute lymphoblastic leukemia who have a superior clinical outcome. *Blood, 108*(1), 97–102.
99. D'Angelo, G., Hotz, A. M., & Tooeschin, P. (2008). Acute lymphoblastic leukemia with hypereosinophilia and 9p21 deletion: Case report and review of the literature. *Laboratory Hematology, 14*(1), 7–9.
100. Wilson, F., & Tefferi, A. (2005). Acute lymphocytic leukemia with eosinophilia: Two case reports and a literature review. *Leukaemia & Lymphoma, 46*(7), 1045–1050.
101. Cave, H., et al. (1998). Clinical significance of minimal residual disease in childhood acute lymphoblastic leukemia. European Organization for Research and Treatment of Cancer – Childhood Leukemia Cooperative Group. *The New England Journal of Medicine, 339*(9), 591–598.

Chapter 3
The Biology of Adult Acute Lymphoblastic Leukemia

Jerald P. Radich and Olga Sala

Introduction

The evolution of treatment in pediatric acute lymphoblastic leukemia (ALL) is a well-documented success story. Indeed, treatments have improved to a point that some pediatric ALL protocols strive to reduce therapy for selected subgroups of patients. It is interesting that much of these improvements in outcome came before the proliferation of modern molecular biological techniques that we now rely upon to study the underlying biology of disease.

Meanwhile, in the adult world we have struggled to make incremental gains. There is an ongoing debate (discussed in later chapters), whether the superior outcome in pediatric ALL compared to adult ALL is from differences in the biology of the disease, the treatment regimens, or the delivery of the care. These elements are certainly not mutually exclusive. In this chapter, we will present an overview of the biology of adult ALL. Given that more work has been done in pediatric ALL, we will naturally refer to the pediatric variation with some regularity.

Epidemiology

The age distribution of ALL shows a dramatic increase during the first decade of life, followed by a precipitous decline, and ending with a slow and steady increase of the last decades of life [1]. ALL is increased in certain genetic syndromes, such as Bloom's syndrome, Fanconi anemia, and Down syndrome [2–8]. Associations with petrochemicals (including pesticides) have been noted [9–13], as well as excess radiation (e.g., Hiroshima, but not Chernobyl) [14–16]. Thus, we are left with the strongest determinants of ALL being age and bad luck. Unfortunately, both are difficult to address with reliable or acceptable public health measures.

Biology of ALL

Much of what is known about the biology of ALL has been gleaned through the study of cases with recurrent chromosomal changes, especially translocations. Approximately 80% of adult ALL cases have evidence of clonal cytogenetic abnormalities at diagnosis [17]. Several of these genetic lesions

J.P. Radich (✉)
Clinical Research Division, Fred Hutchinson Cancer Research Center,
Seattle, WA 98109, USA
e-mail: jradich@fhcrc.org

A.S. Advani and H.M. Lazarus (eds.), *Adult Acute Lymphocytic Leukemia*, Contemporary Hematology,
DOI 10.1007/978-1-60761-707-5_3, © Springer Science+Business Media, LLC 2011

Table 3.1 Common cytogenetic abnormalities detected in acute lymphoblastic leukemia

Chromosomal	Lineage	Frequency in adults (%)	Frequency in children (%)	Genes involved	Functions affected
t(9;22)	B	25	3	BCR-ABL	Cell cycle, apoptosis, differentiation
11q23	B	10	8	MLL, AF4 and others	Transcription activation of certain HOX genes and MEIS1 cofactor
t(1;19)	B	3	5	E2A, PBX1	Transcriptional activator [18]
t(12;21)	B	2	22	TEL, and AML1	Transcriptional repressor [19]
t(8;14), t(2;8), t(8;22)	B	4	2	IGH, IG kappa or IG lambda, and MYC	Transcription (target proteins involved in cell cycle regulation and apoptosis)
Hyperdiploidy	B	7	25	Unknown but chromosomes X, 4, 6, 10, 14, 17, 18, and 21 are commonly involved	
Hypodiploidy	B	2	1		
t(5;14)	T	1	2.5	BCL11B, HOX11L2	Transcription
t(7;19)	T	2.5	1.5	TCRB, LYL1	Transcription
t(1;7), t(1;14), 1p32 cryptic deletion	T	12	7	TCRB or TCR A/D, or SIL and TAL1	Transcription
t(7;10), t(10;14)	T	8	0.7	TCRB or TCR A/D and HOX11	Transcription

TF transcription factors

define specific therapeutic targets and treatment outcomes (Table 3.1). In a current survey of karyotype "low hypodipoidy/near triploidy," or the translocations t(9;22), t(4;11), or t(8;14) did relatively poorly, while those patients with "high" hyperdiploidy or del (9q) did relatively well [20].

The Philadelphia Chromosome, t(9;22)

The Philadelphia chromosome (Ph) results from the reciprocal translocation of the long arms of chromosomes 9 and 22. While chromosome 9 breaks occur in the 5′ region of the Abelson murine leukemia viral oncogene homolog 1 (ABL1), the break point in chromosome 22 may occur in the major (M-BCR) or the minor (m-BCR) breakpoint cluster regions of the BCR gene. Thus, two fusion BCR-ABL variants occur, the larger p210 or the shorter p190 (designated by the molecular weights of their respective protein products [21–24]). The Ph is found in virtually all cases of chronic myeloid leukemia (CML), where the p210 variant dominates. The Ph is found in 25% of adult ALL, representing the most common translocation found in adult ALL. More than half of Ph+ ALL patients express the p190 variant.

ABL1 is a non-receptor tyrosine kinase found predominantly in the nucleus [25]. When fused to BCR, it is tetramerized through the BCR coiled-coil domain, autophosphorylated, and translocated to the cytoplasm [26, 27]. Additionally, in the chimeric protein BCR-ABL1, ABL1 is capable to associate to a broader protein spectrum than wild type ABL1 through BCR protein–protein domains. The result is the loss of ABL1 tightly regulated activity, and the activation of a complex signaling network that results in blocked differentiation, apoptosis inhibition and activation of survival signals, increased proliferation, and altered cell adhesion (Fig. 3.1).

The activation of phosphoinositide-3 kinase (PI3K) is required for the malignant transformation by BCR-ABL [28]. AKT is the main downstream target for PI3K, and its activation results in survival advantage through the inhibition of proapoptotic molecules BIM, TRAIL, and BAD.

BCR-ABL expression also leads to constitutive activation of RAS, through adapter proteins. RAS activation results also in inhibition of apoptotic signaling, and activation of proliferation [29, 30].

BCR-ABL phosphorylates signal transducer and activator of transcription (STAT) proteins independent of cytokines, which also results in the upregulation of several antiapoptotic proteins, such as MCL-1 and BCL-XL [31, 32], and the activation of cyclin D1 that activates cell cycle. Mouse models suggest that STAT5a/b is required for lymphoid transformation by BCR-ABL [33, 34]. Interestingly, STAT6 is preferentially phosphorylated by p190 over p210 BCR-ABL, thus potentially explaining the predilection of p190 BCR-ABL for lymphoid transformation [32].

Finally, BCR-ABL reduces cell adhesion through altering focal adhesion proteins like FAK and paxillin [35].

BCR-ABL+ leukemia is characterized by a high degree of genomic instability, as is demonstrated by the increased frequency of DNA insertions and deletions present in BCR-ABL preleukemic mice [36]. BCR-ABL increases polymerase-ß expression [37], downregulates DNA-repair enzymes (DNA-PKcs) [38], and deregulates RAD51 [39] and BRCA-1 [40], thus leading to increased mutations.

Ph+ ALL typically presents as a pre-B phenotype, reflecting an arrest in B-cell maturation with aberrant co-expression of myeloid cell surface markers and myeloid specific genes. Aberrant splicing of key genes in lymphoid development such as Bruton's tyrosine kinase (*BTK*), and B-cell linker (*BLNK*), as well as deletions of *IKZF1*, the gene that encodes the zinc-finger transcription factor Ikaros, are also typically present [41–45]. The aberrant splicing of *SLP65* and *BTK* in B cell precursors results in shorter transcripts that halt lymphoid maturation [46]. Treatment with ABL kinase inhibitor restores the normal *BLNK* splice variant in some of these cells and allows progression to

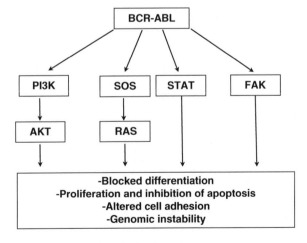

Fig. 3.1 Signaling pathways downstream of BCR-ABL. Schematic representation of the signaling network activated by BCR-ABL

a more differentiated phenotype [41]. Common additional mutations in patients with Ph+ ALL are deletions on chromosome 9p21. This particular locus encodes the *INK4A-ARF* gene. Deletions of this gene have been detected in up to 30% of adult and pediatric patients in some cohorts [47, 48]. Activation of p14^{ARF} induces cell cycle arrest and apoptosis through p53 activation. ARF-null BCR-ABL+ cells induce more severe leukemia when transplanted in irradiated mice recipients, and with reduced latency when compared to ARF-positive BCR-ABL transformed cells. Additionally, ARF-null p210 or p190 positive mice leukemias are resistant to ABL kinase inhibitors in vivo [49].

In the murine model of Ph+ ALL, BCR-ABL transformation is also dependent on the SRC kinases LYN, HCK, and FGR that are not required for the induction of CML [50]. BCR-ABL activates SRC kinases in a kinase-independent manner, and the inhibition of BCR-ABL by imatinib does not decrease SRC activation [51]. At the same time, the specific inhibition of SRC kinases (without inhibition of BCR-ABL), induces apoptosis in leukemia cells and extends survival in mice with Ph+ ALL, suggesting a role for both SRC kinases and BCR-ABL in the transformation of lymphoid cells [51].

CML progression to lymphoid blast crisis may also be dependent on the activation of SRC kinases [51], as lymphoid blast crisis cells are dependent on LYN for survival (in a higher extent than myeloid blasts), [52]. SRC kinases activate ß-catenin in an in vitro model, a molecule with a role in self-renewal of tumor cells. The specific inhibition of SRC kinases in BCR-ABL+ leukemic cells inhibits this activation, suggesting SRC inhibition may impact the leukemia stem cells [53].

The remarkable ability of BCR-ABL to influence pathways regulating proliferation, differentiation, and apoptosis is also the Achilles' heel of Ph+ leukemia, since blocking the tyrosine kinase activity of ABL, via tyrosine kinase inhibitors (TKI) such as imatinib, nilotinib, or dasatinib inhibits the multiple pathways needed for leukemogenesis.

Are p210 and p190 BCR-ABL Different?

As noted above, p190 and p210 Bcr-Abl are both found in Ph+ ALL as compared to CML, whereas p190 Bcr-Abl is found only in ALL. Several lines of data indicate that p190 and p210 diseases may be subtly different. First, p190 and p210 differ in their in vitro kinase activity, with p190 exhibiting higher kinase activity than p210 [54, 55]. Additionally, although both proteins transform murine IL-3 dependent cell lines from myeloid (32D cl3) and lymphoid (Ba/F3) lineage, p190 transformation of Ba/F3 results in a higher proliferation rate [54]. P190 and p210 BCR-ABL also produce different effects in murine models. While p190 transgenic mice develop a rapidly progressive pre-B leukemia [56, 57], p210 transgenic mice develop B, T, and myeloid diseases with more chronic features and longer median survival [58]. In the murine transplant model, mice transplanted with bone marrow transduced with p190 or p210 BCR-ABL and treated with 5-FU (which enriches the marrow for myeloid precursors) developed a myeloproliferative disease arising from a pluripotential cell resembling CML that transformed to acute leukemia similar to blast crisis [54, 59]. However, when the transduced marrow was not enriched for myeloid progenitors, differences among diseases were displayed, with p210 generating a CML-like disease originating in a pluri-potential cell in 50% of the animals, whereas p190 produced a B-cell leukemia arising from a lineage-committed progenitor with shorter latency in most of the animals, and rapid death [54]. Moreover, a study involving cell sorting of primary Ph+ ALL samples showed that cases with p210 Bcr-Abl had evidence of the translocation in CD34+ CD38+, CD34+CD38−CD19+, and CD34+CD38−CD19− cell populations [60]. On the other hand, p190 Bcr-Abl samples had evidence of the translocation only in the committed CD34+CD38−CD19+ cell population.

Studies of human Ph+ ALL are inconsistent in regards to the effect of p190 versus p210 BCR-ABL and outcome. Several studies have shown no difference in prognosis at the time of diagnosis [20, 61, 62], while others have demonstrated a worse prognosis with p190 disease, especially in the context of detection in the setting of minimal residual disease [63–65].

Ikaros

Ikaros is a member of a family of zinc-finger-containing transcription factors, and was initially described in 1992. It possesses N-terminal zinc fingers with DNA binding activity, and C-terminal fingers that mediate dimerization of the protein. Ikaros is transcribed into different isoforms through alternative splicing. The proportion of these splice variants influences Ikaros function. It appears that in these various isoforms, certain exons are essential for normal lymphocyte development [66, 67].

Previously, in vitro experiments suggested that BCR-ABL induction causes a shift in Ikaros splicing, and encourages isoforms lacking DNA-binding domains [43]. However, a more recent paper demonstrates actual deletion of key DNA binding domains. In a genome wide screen of deletions and additions in ALL, Mullighan et al. found an exceptionally high loss of the *IKZF1* gene (coding for Ikaros) in Ph+ ALL cases [45]. Of the 43 Ph+ cases studied, 36 (84%) had deletions in *IKZF1*. In 19 cases, the deletion was restricted to the region coding Ikaros exons 3–6 (designated the *IK6* variant). This isoform lacks the DNA binding domain while retaining the dimerization domains in exon 7, and acts as a dominant negative inhibitor of Ikaros, halting B-cell differentiation and contributing to the aberrant expression of myeloid specific genes [43].

The authors examined 159 ALL cases looking for *IK6* mRNA expression, and found it only in cases that harbored the exon 3–6 deletion, strongly suggesting that *IK6* expression was based on DNA structural changes, rather than a splicing variation. No alterations in the *IKZF1* site were found in chronic phase CML. However, 4 out of 15 blast crisis samples demonstrated an *IKZF1* deletion. Sequence analysis of the *IKZF1* deletion suggested that exons 3–6 were potentially deleted by aberrant function of the lymphoid RAG-mediated recombination machinery, which normally creates V(D)J rearrangements in lymphocyte differentiation. Thus, this study implicates non-DNA binding Ikaros variants with the pathogenesis of Ph+ lymphoid malignancy.

The presence of the IK6 variant may be important in understanding the resistance of Ph+ ALL to tyrosine kinase inhibition [68]. At diagnosis, nearly 50% of Ph+ ALL expresses only the non-DNA binding Ik6 isoform. *In vitro*, the Ik6 variant is associated with an impaired apoptotic response to tyrosine kinase inhibitor exposure, increased DNA synthesis, and more robust colony growth.

Ikaros dominant negative isoforms (*IK4* to *IK8*) have also been identified in Ph negative B-ALL and T-ALL [69], and deletions or mutations of Ikaros have been recently associated with adverse outcome, independent of *BCR-ABL* or other known prognostic factors, in two different cohorts or children with B-ALL [70]. The expression profile of leukemia with genetic alterations of Ikaros resembles that of Ph+ ALL with enrichment of stem-cell progenitor cells and underrepresentation of B-lymphoid genes consistent with differentiation arrest [70].

Induced expression of *IK6* in the cytokine-dependent murine pro-B cell lines enhances survival after cytokine withdrawal, associated with increased BCL-xL (an antiapoptotic molecule), probably through activation of the JAK2-STAT5 pathway [71, 72], and the expression of IK6 in CD34+ hematopoietic progenitors impairs B-lineage differentiation [73].

In sum, these studies suggest an important role of Ikaros in the pathogenesis of Ph+, and a subgroup of Ph–, lymphoid malignancies.

Mixed Lineage Leukemia

Mixed lineage leukemia (MLL) accounts for ~80% of infant acute leukemia and occurs in ~10% of adult ALL [74]. Its name derives from a distinctive phenotype, which marks as an ALL with co-expression of the myeloid CD15 and CD65 markers [75]. Besides its high prevalence in infant leukemia, it often arises in the setting of a secondary leukemia following chemotherapy (specifically following treatment with topoisomerase II inhibitors). Chromosomal rearrangements can fuse the

MLL gene from chromosome 11q23 to any of approximately 50 partner genes. Conceptually, and in murine models, leukemia may evolve from a gain of function, depending on the partner gene involved, or a disruption of normal MLL function. The most common translocation is the t(4;11), which fuses *MLL* to *AF4*. ALL with t(4;11) has a dismal prognosis in both infants and adults [76].

Gene expression studies have demonstrated that MLL is transcriptionally distinct compared to AML and ALL [77]. Since *MLL* gene shares significant homology to the drosophila *Homeobox* (*Hox*) control gene *Trithorax* (*Trx*), it is not surprising that MLL shows dysregulation of several *HOX* genes, particularly *HOXA9* and *HOXA5*. In addition, there is a dramatic upregulation of FMS-like tyrosine kinase 3 (*FLT3*) in MLL [78]. The involvement of FLT3 in *MLL* points to a particular biological pathway that may be targeted with tyrosine kinase inhibitors. Multiple other genes are downregulated in MLL leukemia and may represent potential therapeutic targets [78].

Chromosomal Changes Affecting Multiple Other Genes Involved with the Cell Cycle

Cyclin-dependent kinase inhibitors (CDKI) play a major role in the control of the cell cycle. Dysregulation of their function, leading to inappropriate cell cycle entry, plays an important role in the biology of ALL. The *CDKI*s p16^{INK4a}/p14^{ARF} and p15^{INK4b} are located on chromosome 9p21, and this region is frequently deleted in both B and T-ALLs. Tumor suppressor genes also play a role in cell cycle progression, dictating entry or exit at defined "checkpoints." The tumor suppressor genes *RB1* and *p53* are frequently altered in adult ALL, with *RB1* deletions found in more than 50% of patients with newly diagnosed ALL, and *p53* mutations occurring in 10–20% of cases [79]. In a study of patients with deletions of the above *CDKI* and tumor suppressor genes, 85% of cases had a lesion in one of the genes, and 33% had lesions in at least two of the genes [80]. Patients with multiple genetic abnormalities had a terrible prognosis compared to cases with one or no mutations (median overall survival 8 months v. 25 months). In pediatric T-ALL, abrogation of p15 and p16 is virtually universal (DNA, RNA, or protein level), and promoter hypermethylation is an important mechanism contributing to inactivation of p15 [81].

MYC in Mature B Cell Leukemia

MYC is a nuclear phosphoprotein that acts as a potent transcription factor, influencing cell cycle control and apoptosis. The t(8;14) translocation, occurs in <5% of adult ALL, and is found in patients with Burkitts leukemia/lymphoma. The *MYC* gene, located on chromosome 8q, is placed in juxtaposition to the *IgH* gene on chromosome 14q. A less common variant moves *MYC* to the Ig kappa locus on chromosome 2p, yielding the t(2;8) translocation.

Genome-Wide Expression Analysis

Since the first report on the ability of microarray technology to discriminate primary leukemia specimens according to lineage [82], multiple studies have used gene expression profiling (GEP) in pediatric ALL to improve molecular disease classification, and prediction of outcome or response to drugs. In the pediatric setting, GEP studies have been used to delineate the transcriptome of known subtypes of ALL [77, 83, 84], define new subtypes [83, 85], identify treatment-specific changes in leukemia cells [86], predict response to treatment [87, 88], and predict treatment outcome [89, 90].

From initial studies, it became clear that GEP was able to segregate different known subtypes of ALL based on gene expression signatures providing significant insight into specific mechanisms of transformation [82, 83, 85, 91–93]. Additionally, multiple reports highlighted the capability of GEP to improve current molecular disease classification by identifying a novel group of leukemias that do not bear consistent cytogenetic abnormalities [83–85]. For example, a novel group of pediatric precursor B-ALL cases (representing 15–20% of analyzed cases) was identified that resembles Ph+ ALL by both GEP and poor clinical outcome. Genetic characterization of this group revealed deletions in genes involved in B-cell development in about 80% of cases, similar to that seen in Ph+ ALL [85]. The transcription profile of this poor prognosis group was also similar to that seen in Ph+ ALL [70].

Conversely, GEP studies have yielded somewhat limited results in predicting outcome in other groups of ALL patients. Transcription profiles associated with outcome have not succeeded in adding additional predictive information to clinical and genetic factors already used in risk assessment in pediatric patients [94], or have failed inter-study validation [95–97]. The limitations of the technique in this context may merely reflect the heterogeneity of the disease. Gene expression profile may be driven primarily by karyotype, and uncovering specific gene signature predictors may require stratification by known prognosis factors and treatment protocols to allow more subtle differences to standout. However, genes involved in apoptosis and cell proliferation are clearly underexpressed in leukemia resistant to chemotherapy [89, 94, 97, 98].

There have been relatively few studies examining global gene expression in adult ALL [91, 99, 100], likely due to the rarity of the disease in older patients and the lower enrollment in clinical trials. However, findings in pediatric leukemia are likely relevant to adults, as shown by the validation of pediatric gene expression signatures for different leukemia subtypes in an independent adult cohort [100].

A recent GEP study has uncovered a gene that may be both a prognostic marker and a treatment target [101]. Connective tissue growth factor (CTGF) expression is heterogeneously expressed in B-ALL, and its expression correlates with poor clinical outcome. Patients with the highest tertile of CTGF expression have a significantly worse outcome compared to those adult ALL cases with lower expression levels. The role of CTGF in the pathogenesis of ALL is unknown. Clinical studies with a CTGF antibody in pancreatic cancer and diabetes are ongoing, so a drug suitable for study in ALL may soon be available.

T-ALL

T-ALL comprises 15% and 25% of pediatric and adult ALL, respectively [74]. It is a heterogeneous group of diseases that arises from the transformation of T-lymphocyte precursors at different stages of normal development. Up to 50% of T-ALL cases have an abnormal karyotype with recurrent translocations [102]. FISH studies frequently uncover micro-deletions and other cryptic abnormalities.

Recurrent Translocations in T-ALL

The promoter and enhancer elements of the T cell receptor genes, *TCR A/D* (14q11), and *TCR B* (7p32), are involved in translocations in 35% of T-ALL cases. Fusion of transcription factors (TF) to enhancer elements results in deregulated expression of the associated partner genes.

TAL1, a TF essential for hematopoiesis is a member of the class-II basic helix-loop-helix (bHLH) family of TFs that contains a HLH or dimerization domain, and a DNA-binding domain. *TAL1* is a recurrent target for translocation to *TCR* genes, (i.e., t(1;14)). However, constitutive activation of *TAL1* in T-ALL more often results from the generation of the chimeric gene *SIL-TAL*.

Through an, often cryptic, deletion of 1p32 the regulatory region of TAL1 is replaced with the *SIL* regulatory region in 25% of pediatric T-ALLs. The mechanism of leukemia transformation driven by unscheduled *TAL1* expression remains unclear. TAL1 inhibits the transcriptional activity of class-I bHLH (E2A, HEB) through formation of heterodimers. Mice models that show the induction of T-ALL by suppression of E2A [103, 104], or the dispensability of the DNA-binding domain of TAL1 for transformation [105, 106], support the relevance of this inhibition for the induction of leukemia. However, deregulated *TAL1* expression in mice has inconsistently succeeded in generating leukemia on its own [107–110], suggesting the requirement of a secondary genetic hit. *TAL2*, *LYL1*, and *BHLH1* are other class-II bHLH that partner with *TCR* genes in the infrequent translocations t(7;9)(q34;q32), t(7;19)(q34;p13), and t(14;21)(q11.2;q22).

LIM domain proteins are the second group of proteins overexpressed in chromosomal transloca-tions to *TCR* genes in T-ALL: *LIM domain only-1* (*LMO1*) was in fact discovered because of its involvement in the translocations t(11;14)(p15;q11), and *LIM domain only-2* (*LMO2*) is involved in t(11;14)(p13;q11). Additionally, *LMO2* expression can also be activated by the deletion of a nega-tive regulatory element immediately upstream of *LMO2* [111]. LIM domain proteins are involved in protein–protein interactions, and LMO2 is expressed in early hematopoietic progenitors. Four out of 5 patients who developed T-ALL in 2 gene therapy trials for X-linked SCID had retroviral inte-gration in proximity to *LMO2*, with subsequent *LMO2* activation [112–114]. Other cooperating genetic abnormalities were also present. Transgenic mice with *LMO1* or *LMO2* overexpression develop T-ALL with long latency, suggesting *LMO* overexpression is not sufficient for the develop-ment of leukemia and that a second genetic hit is needed [107, 115]. Also consistent with this is the observation that the time span to develop leukemia is shorter in double transgenic mice with *TAL1* and *LMO2* mutations [116].

Homeobox (*HOX*) genes are highly conserved transcription factors, organized in clusters in 4 different chromosomes, key in embryonic development and hematopoiesis regulation. *HOXA* genes expression is upregulated in a subgroup of ALL that includes leukemias with *TCRB-HOXA* rear-rangements resulting from inv(7) [117] or t(7;7), but also leukemias with *MLL* rearrangements [78] and *CALM-AF10* fusion gene [118, 119]. *CALM-AF10* results from t(10;14) (p13;q14), and *MLL* can rearrange with multiple different partners. Significantly, *CALM-AF10* T-ALLs are also charac-terized by increased expression of *BMI1*, a gene that inhibits the tumor suppressor *CDKN2A* that is frequently inactive T-ALL (but not in *CALM-AF10* T-ALL) [119].

Orphan *HOX* genes, so named because they are not part of a cluster but are dispersed through the genome that are involved in T-ALL are *HOX11* (*TLX1*) and *HOX11L2* (*TLX3*). *HOX11* is juxtaposed to *TCR* locus in t(10;14) and t(7;10), and *HOX11L2* is juxtaposed to *BCL11B* in t(5;14). *HOX11* is not expressed in normal T-lymphocyte precursors and when overexpressed in mice it results in T-cell leukemia after a long latency [120].

Less frequently, translocations in T-ALL result in the generation of chimeric genes with oncogenic properties. In addition to *CALM-AF10* and *MLL* translocated T-ALLs mentioned above, *ABL1* is fused to *NUP214* in 6% of T-ALL cases. *NUP214-ABL1* is usually fused in episomes and thus escapes normal cytogenetic analysis [121]. Patients present this fusion gene amplified, and with coexisting genetic abnormalities, and in some cases only in a percentage of blasts pointing at a late event in leu-kemogenesis [122]. Of clinical interest, *NUP214-ABL* is sensitive to imatinib and other Abl-kinase inhibitors [121, 123] and their potential use for treatment in this disease should be considered.

Deletions, Duplications, and Mutations in T-ALL

Other frequent genetic lesions in T-ALL include deletions and duplications. Deletion of the long arm of chromosome 6 (6q) has been described in 23% of adult T-ALL [124], but is also present in by alternate *c-myc* and *IgH* gene breakpoints, cytogenetically indistinguishable. These breakpoints lie between *c-myc* exons 1 and 2 on chromosome 8 and within the *IgH* switch region on chromosome 14 [14]. The pro-transcription effects of the Eμ enhancer are eliminated in the sporadic variant, indicating that other *IgH* enhancers may be responsible for *c-myc* up-regulation [14, 16, 18–21].

Role of Epstein-Barr Virus (EBV)

EBV is a ubiquitous DNA herpes virus infecting the vast majority of the world's population, usually causing a relatively innocuous infection of B lymphocytes. EBV infection drives polyclonal B cell activation and proliferation, which is normally regulated in part by a cytotoxic T cell response. Unregulated B cell proliferation, for which immunodeficiency may be a possible predisposing factor, could augment B cell susceptibility to oncogenic mutations, such as those involving *c-myc* [22, 23].

The EBV life cycle is characterized by lytic and latent phases. The lytic cycle features replication of releasable infectious viral particles and is regulated by key intermediates such as transcriptional activators, DNA replication factors, and viral capsid antigens. BZLF1 and BRLF1 proteins play a key role in the switch from latency to the lytic cycle [24]. During the latent phase, viral replication does not occur. Rather, the viral machinery assumes control of B cell growth and replication, leading to B cell immortalization. The viral DNA is maintained as an episome within the infected cell, replicates with the assistance of DNA polymerase, and is passed on to daughter cells following cell division. The expression of six EBV nuclear antigens (Epstein-Barr virus nuclear antigens (EBNA) 1, 2, 3A, 3B, 3C, and EBNA leader protein) is associated with the latent phase, which also manifests the expression of three viral membrane proteins – latent membrane protein (LMP) 1, 2A, and 2B, and two small nonpolyadenylated Epstein-Barr virus–encoded small RNAs (EBER1 and EBER2). Three patterns of latent EBV gene expression exist – latency I (latency program), II (default program), and III (growth program). Latency III is characterized by expression of all latency genes and occurs during primary B cell infection. Latency I is characterized by expression of a smaller gene panel – EBER and EBNA1 and is associated with chronic infection [23, 25].

EBV derives its name from two scientists, Anthony Epstein and Yvonne Barr, who, along with Bert Achong, discovered the virus after investigating lymphoma cell samples provided by Denis Burkitt from equatorial Africa [26]. Endemic Burkitt lymphoma and leukemia appear to be associated with EBV infection in over 95% of cases, whereas the sporadic and immunodeficiency-related variants less frequently have this association [25]. Twenty percent to 35% of sporadic Burkitt lymphoma and leukemia cases in the USA and Europe show EBV-positivity [27], while this increases up to 50–80% in parts of the Middle East and South America [28, 29]. The precise mechanisms by which EBV contributes to Burkitt lymphoma and leukemia pathogenesis remain to be completely elucidated. There is evidence that EBNA-1 inhibits cellular apoptosis [30] and enhances B cell immortalization [31]. EBER has been shown in some studies to upregulate bcl-2, thereby contributing to apoptosis inhibition [32]. Additionally, Niller et al. identified a *c-myc* binding site in the promoter region of the *EBER1* gene, suggesting a possible cooperative role for these two genes in inhibiting apoptosis and spurring lymphomagenesis [33].

LMP2A signaling has been shown to be an important component of the development of Burkitt lymphoma. Longnecker and colleagues showed that LMP2A was able to allow a complete bypass of normal B cell developmental checkpoints allowing B cells to colonize the spleen that do not express a functional B cell receptor (BCR) as measured by Ig expression [34]. Typically, B cells without a functional BCR undergo apoptosis; however, with upregulated LMP2A, normal B cell development is altered by the transmission of signals normally attributed to the pre-BCR, allowing LMP2A to drive B cell development even in recombinase activating gene 1 (RAG)-deficient mice, demonstrating that LMP2A provides a BCR-like signal that supplants the requirement for signals from the BCR in normal B cell development. RAG-1 null animals are unable to rearrange immuno-globulin genes and are characterized by a block in B cell development at the CD43+ pro B stage [35, 36]. Further, in vivo data have shown that LMP2A promotes lymphocyte differentiation and survival by inducing constitutive signaling of varied oncogenic pathways. Longnecker and col-leagues showed that LMP2A induces Lyn and Syk activity, which is absolutely essential for LMP2A signaling [37–39]. Further, they and others have shown that LMP2A constitutively activates Bruton's tyrosine kinase (Btk), B-cell linker protein (SLP-65/BLNK), and the RAS/PI3K/AKT pathway [40–44]. LMP2A-mediated activation of Akt is linked to suppression of the pro-apoptotic cytokine, transforming growth factor-β1 (TGF-β1) and the activation of mammalian target of rapamycin (mTOR) in a PI3Kinase/Akt-dependent manner [41, 45].

The Germinal Center

Many investigators believe that Burkitt lymphoma and leukemia cells derive from the germinal center, although controversy surrounds this, with other evidence supporting derivation from mem-ory B cells [25]. Burkitt cells classically display germinal center phenotype markers, such as CD10 and bcl-6, but interestingly, classic anatomic sites of the disease, such as the jaw and ovary, do not normally contain germinal centers. Burkitt lymphoma and leukemia cells have been shown to har-bor evidence of somatic hypermutation with Ig V(D)J recombination, characteristic of the germinal center; in particular, translocations involving *c-myc* are thought to involve V(D)J recombination events [46–48]. Bellan et al. have shown that the cell of origin may differ according to the clinical Burkitt lymphoma and leukemia variant and tumor EBV status. Semi-nested polymerase chain reac-tion (PCR) analysis of immunoglobulin heavy chain V(D)J gene rearrangements identified a dif-ferentiation pattern corresponding to early centroblasts in sporadic, EBV-negative tumors. In contrast, a pattern corresponding to post-germinal-center memory B cells was found in EBV-positive endemic and AIDS-related Burkitt lymphomas [49].

Diagnosis of Burkitt Lymphoma and Burkitt Leukemia

The diagnostic approach to Burkitt lymphoma and Burkitt leukemia involves the combination of clinical and laboratory findings, including an assessment of morphology by routine histology and immunophenotyping by immunohistochemistry and/or flow cytometry. Genetic analysis, including karyotyping with Giemsa banding and fluorescence in situ hybridization (FISH), is important for detecting a *c-myc* translocation, especially in cases where classic tumor morphology is not observed. Recent advances in transcriptional profiling have allowed for an initial characterization of distinc-tive patterns of gene expression in Burkitt lymphoma and leukemia [50, 51]. Future approaches to the diagnosis of challenging cases that have features lying between Burkitt lymphoma and diffuse large B-cell lymphoma (DLBCL) may utilize microarray-based gene expression analysis.

Particular morphologic and immunophenotypic findings are necessary for a diagnosis of Burkitt lymphoma and leukemia. A classically distinct morphology is seen in most endemic and a large percentage of sporadic cases [2, 52]. The malignant lymphocytes are monomorphic with a diffuse growth pattern often appearing as a monotonous sheet of cells. Burkitt lymphoma and leukemia cells are medium-sized (10–25 μM) with round to oval non-cleaved, non-folded nuclei [2, 53]. Nuclei demonstrate immature, finely granular chromatin and multiple paracentric basophilic small to medi-um-sized nucleoli (Fig. 13.1). The cytoplasm is deeply basophilic, owing to an abundance of polyri-

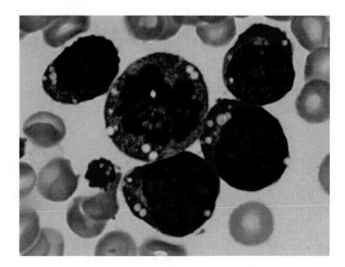

Fig. 13.1 Morphology of Burkitt lymphoma and leukemia cells. Burkitt lymphoma and leukemia cells, bone marrow aspirate, 100× magnification. The malignant cells shown here have a high nuclear to cytoplasmic ratio, coarse granular chromatin, multiple nucleoli, deep basophilic cytoplasm and multiple lipid vacuoles. A mitotic figure is present

bosomes [53]. Cytoplasmic vacuoles are often present and are best seen in touch preparations or aspirate smears. The tumor has a very high proliferation fraction – among the highest of human tumors – which is evidenced by numerous mitotic figures and apoptotic bodies. At low microscopic power, a "starry sky" pattern results from tingible body macrophages containing darkly staining ingested apoptotic tumor cell debris (Figs. 13.2a, b) [2]. The morphologic spectrum of Burkitt lymphoma and leukemia includes a subset of cases with eccentrically located nuclei and a single prominent central nucleolus and is known as Burkitt lymphoma with plasmacytoid differentiation [2]. This variant is seen mostly in states of immunodeficiency and occasionally in children [54].

Immunopheotyping by immunohistochemistry or flow cytometry is also necessary for diagnoses of Burkitt lymphoma and leukemia. B cell-associated antigens CD19, CD20, CD22, and CD79a are present, as well as markers common to cells of germinal center origin, including CD10, Bcl-6, Tcl1, and CD38 [2, 53, 55]. Mum-1 and CD138 are negative [53]. Bcl-2 is usually negative, although weak staining may be observed in 20% of cases [56]. Terminal deoxynucleotidyl transferase (TdT) is uniformly negative [2]. Malignant cells also express moderate to strong monotypic surface IgM, best appreciated by flow cytometric immunophenotyping. Invariably, the nuclear protein antigen Ki-67 (MIB-1) stains positive between 95% and 100% of cells demonstrating the high mitotic rate of the tumor (Fig. 13.3) [3]. In practice, this proliferation fraction marker is usually assessed by immunohistochemical staining.

Genetics studies, including routine karyotype preparation with Giemsa banding and FISH, may be included in the initial workup of suspected Burkitt lymphoma and leukemia. Malignant cells harbor *c-myc* translocations, which are detectable in more than 90% of cases. The most common translocation, t(8;14)(q24;q32), is readily detectable with a dual-color, dual-fusion FISH probe. The less common t(2;8)(p12;q24) and t(8;22)(q24;q11) translocations can be detected with break-apart probes, which are useful in the event that only one partner in a translocation is known. The dual-color dual-fusion FISH probe employs two DNA probes of differing color, usually red and green, which hybridize to breakpoint regions near 8q24 on chromosome 8 and 14q32 on chromosome 14 (Fig. 13.4). Two hundred interphase nuclei are usually counted, although more may be included in the analysis depending on the testing facility. With a reciprocal *c-myc* translocation, red and green hybridization signals will be separated and juxtaposed in the participant chromosomes, resulting in a yellow signal. Correspondingly, a t(8;14)(q24;q32) will generate two yellow, one red, and one

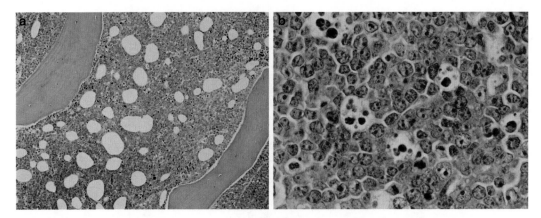

Fig. 13.2 Burkitt lymphoma and leukemia. (**a**) Burkitt lymphoma/leukemia extensively involving the bone marrow, 10× magnification. This bone marrow core biopsy is 80% cellular and largely replaced by a monomorphic population of malignant lymphocytes with a diffuse pattern of infiltration. (**b**) Burkitt lymphoma/leukemia involving the bone marrow, 60× magnification. Malignant cells are medium-sized (10–25 μM) with round nuclei containing coarse granular chromatin and multiple basophilic small to medium-sized paracentric nucleoli. The cytoplasm is deeply basophilic secondary to an abundance of polyribosomes. The tumor has a very high proliferation fraction evidenced by numerous mitotic figures and apoptotic bodies. A "starry sky" pattern results from tingible body macrophages stippled with darkly staining ingested apoptotic tumor cell debris.

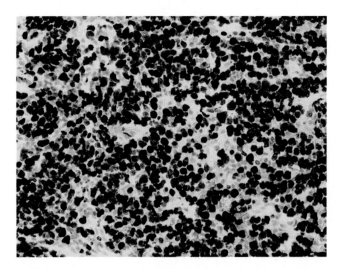

Fig. 13.3 Ki-67 proliferative index in Burkitt lymphoma and leukemia. Burkitt lymphoma involving the rectum, Ki-67 immunohistochemical stain, 20× magnification. Ki-67 is a nuclear protein antigen expressed during mitotic activity. It stains positive in 95–100% of malignant cells and is an important diagnostic tool in the differentiation of Burkitt lymphoma and leukemia from other types of non-Hodgkin lymphoma

green signal in the malignant cell nucleus being examined. For detection of the less common t(2;8) (p12;q24) and t(8;22)(q24;q11) translocations, the "break-apart" probe utilizes flanking red and green probes across the 8q24 region, which are visible as a yellow signal. A reciprocal translocation separates the adjacent red and green probes (removing the yellow signal) leading to one yellow, one red, and one green signal in the abnormal interphase nucleus. Dual-color dual fusion probes have also been synthesized and validated for the t(2;8)(p12;q24) and t(8;22)(q24;q11) translocations [57].

share an ancestor, but independent lines of evolution. Of note is that in many cases the relapsed clone was present at a very low level at the time of diagnosis. Why is this study important? First, it expands on previous work in ALL, AML, and CML suggesting that genetic evolution is a relatively common feature of relapse. Thus, chemotherapy may act as a selective force to foster the outgrowth of rare resistance clones, or from the spawn of a more primitive, ancestral (pre)-leukemia cell. The understanding of the diverse paths to resistance, and the genes recruited in this task, may eventually expose the therapeutic targets to control or abort relapse.

Conclusion

ALL is characterized by a myriad of genetic lesions. Thus far, common biological pathways that unify the pathogenesis of adult ALL have escaped detection. Perhaps the best approach for understanding adult ALL is to build upon the success of pediatric ALL, and to use the knowledge of similarities and differences in the biology of the two diseases to devise new strategies of treatment.

References

1. Groves, F. D., Linet, M. S., & Devesa, S. S. (1996). Epidemiology of leukemia: Overview and patterns of occurrence. In E. S. Henderson, T. A. Lister, & M. F. Greaves (Eds.), *Leukemia* (6th ed., pp. 145–159). Philadelphia, PA: W.B. Saunders.
2. Chessells, J. M., Harrison, G., Richards, S. M., et al. (2001). Down's syndrome and acute lymphoblastic leukaemia: Clinical features and response to treatment. *Archives of Disease in Childhood, 85*(4), 321–5.
3. Fong, C. T., & Brodeur, G. M. (1987). Down's syndrome and leukemia: Epidemiology, genetics, cytogenetics and mechanisms of leukemogenesis. *Cancer Genetics and Cytogenetics, 28*(1), 55–76.
4. Janik-Moszant, A., Bubala, H., Stojewska, M., & Sonta-Jakimczyk, D. (1998). Acute lymphoblastic leukemia in children with Fanconi anemia. *Wiadomosci Lekarskie, 51*(Suppl 4), 285–288.
5. Mertens, A. C., Wen, W., Davies, S. M., et al. (1998). Congenital abnormalities in children with acute leukemia: A report from the Children's Cancer Group. *Jornal de Pediatria, 133*(5), 617–623.
6. Robison, L. L., Nesbit, M. E., Jr., Sather, H. N., et al. (1984). Down syndrome and acute leukemia in children: A 10-year retrospective survey from Childrens Cancer Study Group. *Jornal de Pediatria, 105*(2), 235–242.
7. Taub, J. W. (2001). Relationship of chromosome 21 and acute leukemia in children with Down syndrome. *Journal of Pediatric Hematology/Oncology, 23*(3), 175–178.
8. German, J. (1997). Bloom's syndrome. XX. The first 100 cancers. *Cancer Genetics and Cytogenetics, 93*(1), 100–106.
9. Brownson, R. C., Novotny, T. E., & Perry, M. C. (1993). Cigarette smoking and adult leukemia A meta-analysis. *Archives of Internal Medicine, 153*(4), 469–475.
10. Sandler, D. P. (1995). Recent studies in leukemia epidemiology. *Current Opinion in Oncology, 7*(1), 12–18.
11. Lindquist, R., Nilsson, B., Eklund, G., & Gahrton, G. (1991). Acute leukemia in professional drivers exposed to gasoline and diesel. *European Journal of Haematology, 47*(2), 98–103.
12. Shore, D. L., Sandler, D. P., Davey, F. R., McIntyre, O. R., & Bloomfield, C. D. (1993). Acute leukemia and residential proximity to potential sources of environmental pollutants. *Archives of Environmental Health, 48*(6), 414–420.
13. Rudant, J., Menegaux, F., Leverger, G., et al. (2007). Household exposure to pesticides and risk of childhood hematopoietic malignancies: The ESCALE study (SFCE). *Environmental Health Perspectives, 115*(12), 1787–1793.
14. Ichimaru, M., Ishimaru, T., & Belsky, J. L. (1978). Incidence of leukemia in atomic bomb survivors belonging to a fixed cohort in Hiroshima and Nagasaki, 1950–71. Radiation dose, years after exposure, age at exposure, and type of leukemia. *Journal of Radiation Research, 19*(3), 262–282.
15. Preston, D. L., Kusumi, S., Tomonaga, M., et al. (1994). Cancer incidence in atomic bomb survivors. Part III. Leukemia, lymphoma and multiple myeloma, 1950–1987. *Radiation Research, 137*(2 Suppl), S68–S97.
16. Howe, G. R. (2007). Leukemia following the Chernobyl accident. *Health Physics, 93*(5), 512–515.

17. Hematologique GFdC. (1996). Cytogenetic abnormalities in adult acute lymphoblastic leukemia: Correlations with hematologic findings outcome. A Collaborative Study of the Group Francais de Cytogenetique Hematologique. *Blood, 87*(8), 3135–3142.
18. Aspland, S. E., Bendall, H. H., & Murre, C. (2001). The role of E2A-PBX1 in leukemogenesis. *Oncogene, 20*(40), 5708–5717.
19. Hiebert, S. W., Sun, W., Davis, J. N., et al. (1996). The t(12;21) translocation converts AML-1B from an activator to a repressor of transcription. *Molecular and Cellular Biology, 16*(4), 1349–1355.
20. Moorman, A. V., Harrison, C. J., Buck, G. A., et al. (2007). Karyotype is an independent prognostic factor in adult acute lymphoblastic leukemia (ALL): Analysis of cytogenetic data from patients treated on the Medical Research Council (MRC) UKALLXII/Eastern Cooperative Oncology Group (ECOG) 2993 trial. *Blood, 109*(8), 3189–3197.
21. Hermans, A., Heisterkamp, N., von Linden, M., et al. (1987). Unique fusion of bcr and c-abl genes in Philadelphia chromosome positive acute lymphoblastic leukemia. *Cell, 51*(1), 33–40.
22. Hooberman, A. L., Carrino, J. J., Leibowitz, D., et al. (1989). Unexpected heterogeneity of BCR-ABL fusion mRNA detected by polymerase chain reaction in Philadelphia chromosome-positive acute lymphoblastic leukemia. *Proceedings of the National Academy of Sciences of the United States of America, 86*(11), 4259–4263.
23. Kurzrock, R., Shtalrid, M., Gutterman, J. U., et al. (1987). Molecular analysis of chromosome 22 breakpoints in adult Philadelphia-positive acute lymphoblastic leukaemia. *British Journal Haematology, 67*(1), 55–59.
24. Rubin, C. M., Carrino, J. J., Dickler, M. N., Leibowitz, D., Smith, S. D., & Westbrook, C. A. (1988). Heterogeneity of genomic fusion of BCR and ABL in Philadelphia chromosome-positive acute lymphoblastic leukemia. *Proceedings of the National Academy of Sciences of the United States of America, 85*(8), 2795–2799.
25. Taagepera, S., McDonald, D., Loeb, J. E., et al. (1998). Nuclear-cytoplasmic shuttling of C-ABL tyrosine kinase. *Proceedings of the National Academy of Sciences of the United States of America, 95*(13), 7457–7462.
26. McWhirter, J. R., & Wang, J. Y. (1991). Activation of tyrosinase kinase and microfilament-binding functions of c-abl by bcr sequences in bcr/abl fusion proteins. *Molecular and Cellular Biology, 11*(3), 1553–1565.
27. McWhirter, J. R., & Wang, J. Y. (1993). An actin-binding function contributes to transformation by the Bcr-Abl oncoprotein of Philadelphia chromosome-positive human leukemias. *The EMBO Journal, 12*(4), 1533–1546.
28. Kharas, M. G., Deane, J. A., Wong, S., et al. (2004). Phosphoinositide 3-kinase signaling is essential for ABL oncogene-mediated transformation of B-lineage cells. *Blood, 103*(11), 4268–4275.
29. Cortez, D., Stoica, G., Pierce, J. H., & Pendergast, A. M. (1996). The BCR-ABL tyrosine kinase inhibits apoptosis by activating a Ras-dependent signaling pathway. *Oncogene, 13*(12), 2589–2594.
30. Mandanas, R. A., Leibowitz, D. S., Gharehbaghi, K., et al. (1993). Role of p21 RAS in p210 bcr-abl transformation of murine myeloid cells. *Blood, 82*(6), 1838–1847.
31. Horita, M., Andreu, E. J., Benito, A., et al. (2000). Blockade of the Bcr-Abl kinase activity induces apoptosis of chronic myelogenous leukemia cells by suppressing signal transducer and activator of transcription 5-dependent expression of Bcl-xL. *The Journal of Experimental Medicine, 191*(6), 977–984.
32. Ilaria, R. L., Jr., & Van Etten, R. A. (1996). P210 and P190(BCR/ABL) induce the tyrosine phosphorylation and DNA binding activity of multiple specific STAT family members. *The Journal of Biological Chemistry, 271*(49), 31704–31710.
33. Hoelbl, A., Kovacic, B., Kerenyi, M. A., et al. (2006). Clarifying the role of Stat5 in lymphoid development and Abelson-induced transformation. *Blood, 107*(12), 4898–4906.
34. Sexl, V., Piekorz, R., Moriggl, R., et al. (2000). Stat5a/b contribute to interleukin 7-induced B-cell precursor expansion, but abl- and bcr/abl-induced transformation are independent of stat5. *Blood, 96*(6), 2277–2283.
35. Cheng, K., Kurzrock, R., Qiu, X., et al. (2002). Reduced focal adhesion kinase and paxillin phosphorylation in BCR-ABL-transfected cells. *Cancer, 95*(2), 440–450.
36. Brain, J. M., Goodyer, N., & Laneuville, P. (2003). Measurement of genomic instability in preleukemic P190BCR/ABL transgenic mice using inter-simple sequence repeat polymerase chain reaction. *Cancer Research, 63*(16), 4895–4898.
37. Canitrot, Y., Lautier, D., Laurent, G., et al. (1999). Mutator phenotype of BCR–ABL transfected Ba/F3 cell lines and its association with enhanced expression of DNA polymerase beta. *Oncogene, 18*(17), 2676–2680.
38. Deutsch, E., Dugray, A., AbdulKarim, B., et al. (2001). BCR-ABL down-regulates the DNA repair protein DNA-PKcs. *Blood, 97*(7), 2084–2090.
39. Slupianek, A., Schmutte, C., Tombline, G., et al. (2001). BCR/ABL regulates mammalian RecA homologs, resulting in drug resistance. *Molecular Cell, 8*(4), 795–806.
40. Deutsch, E., Jarrousse, S., Buet, D., et al. (2003). Down-regulation of BRCA1 in BCR-ABL-expressing hematopoietic cells. *Blood, 101*(11), 4583–4588.
41. Klein, F., Feldhahn, N., Harder, L., et al. (2004). The BCR-ABL1 kinase bypasses selection for the expression of a pre-B cell receptor in pre-B acute lymphoblastic leukemia cells. *The Journal of Experimental Medicine, 199*(5), 673–685.

42. Jumaa, H., Bossaller, L., Portugal, K., et al. (2003). Deficiency of the adaptor SLP-65 in pre-B-cell acute lymphoblastic leukaemia. *Nature, 423*(6938), 452–456.
43. Klein, F., Feldhahn, N., Herzog, S., et al. (2006). BCR-ABL1 induces aberrant splicing of IKAROS and lineage infidelity in pre-B lymphoblastic leukemia cells. *Oncogene, 25*(7), 1118–1124.
44. Feldhahn, N., Rio, P., Soh, B. N., et al. (2005). Deficiency of Bruton's tyrosine kinase in B cell precursor leukemia cells. *Proceedings of the National Academy of Sciences of the United States of America, 102*(37), 13266–13271.
45. Mullighan, C. G., Miller, C. B., Radtke, I., et al. (2008). BCR-ABL1 lymphoblastic leukaemia is characterized by the deletion of Ikaros. *Nature, 453*(7191), 110–114.
46. Jumaa, H., Mitterer, M., Reth, M., & Nielsen, P. J. (2001). The absence of SLP65 and Btk blocks B cell development at the preB cell receptor-positive stage. *European Journal of Immunology, 31*(7), 2164–2169.
47. Heerema, N. A., Harbott, J., Galimberti, S., et al. (2004). Secondary cytogenetic aberrations in childhood Philadelphia chromosome positive acute lymphoblastic leukemia are nonrandom and may be associated with outcome. *Leukemia, 18*(4), 693–702.
48. Primo, D., Tabernero, M. D., Perez, J. J., et al. (2005). Genetic heterogeneity of BCR/ABL+ adult B-cell precursor acute lymphoblastic leukemia: Impact on the clinical, biological and immunophenotypical disease characteristics. *Leukemia, 19*(5), 713–720.
49. Williams, R. T., Roussel, M. F., & Sherr, C. J. (2006). Arf gene loss enhances oncogenicity and limits imatinib response in mouse models of Bcr-Abl-induced acute lymphoblastic leukemia. *Proceedings of the National Academy of Sciences of the United States of America, 103*(17), 6688–6693.
50. Hu, Y., Liu, Y., Pelletier, S., et al. (2004). Requirement of Src kinases Lyn, Hck and Fgr for BCR-ABL1-induced B-lymphoblastic leukemia but not chronic myeloid leukemia. *Nature Genetics, 36*(5), 453–461.
51. Hu, Y., Swerdlow, S., Duffy, T. M., Weinmann, R., Lee, F. Y., & Li, S. (2006). Targeting multiple kinase pathways in leukemic progenitors and stem cells is essential for improved treatment of Ph+ leukemia in mice. *Proceedings of the National Academy of Sciences of the United States of America, 103*(45), 16870–16875.
52. Ptasznik, A., Nakata, Y., Kalota, A., Emerson, S. G., & Gewirtz, A. M. (2004). Short interfering RNA (siRNA) targeting the Lyn kinase induces apoptosis in primary, and drug-resistant, BCR-ABL1(+) leukemia cells. *Natural Medicines, 10*(11), 1187–1189.
53. Li, S., & Li, D. (2007). Stem cell and kinase activity-independent pathway in resistance of leukaemia to BCR-ABL kinase inhibitors. *Journal of Cellular and Molecular Medicine, 11*(6), 1251–1262.
54. Li, S., Ilaria, R. L., Jr., Million, R. P., Daley, G. Q., & Van Etten, R. A. (1999). The P190, P210, and P230 forms of the BCR/ABL oncogene induce a similar chronic myeloid leukemia-like syndrome in mice but have different lymphoid leukemogenic activity. *The Journal of Experimental Medicine, 189*(9), 1399–1412.
55. Lugo, T. G., Pendergast, A. M., Muller, A. J., & Witte, O. N. (1990). Tyrosine kinase activity and transformation potency of bcr-abl oncogene products. *Science, 247*(4946), 1079–1082.
56. Voncken, J. W., Morris, C., Pattengale, P., et al. (1992). Clonal development and karyotype evolution during leukemogenesis of BCR/ABL transgenic mice. *Blood, 79*(4), 1029–1036.
57. Heisterkamp, N., Jenster, G., ten Hoeve, J., Zovich, D., Pattengale, P. K., & Groffen, J. (1990). Acute leukaemia in bcr/abl transgenic mice. *Nature, 344*(6263), 251–253.
58. Voncken, J. W., Kaartinen, V., Pattengale, P. K., Germeraad, W. T., Groffen, J., & Heisterkamp, N. (1995). BCR/ABL P210 and P190 cause distinct leukemia in transgenic mice. *Blood, 86*(12), 4603–4611.
59. Pear, W. S., Miller, J. P., Xu, L., et al. (1998). Efficient and rapid induction of a chronic myelogenous leukemia-like myeloproliferative disease in mice receiving P210 bcr/abl-transduced bone marrow. *Blood, 92*(10), 3780–3792.
60. Castor, A., Nilsson, L., Astrand-Grundstrom, I., et al. (2005). Distinct patterns of hematopoietic stem cell involvement in acute lymphoblastic leukemia. *Natural Medicines, 11*(6), 630–637.
61. Gleissner, B., Gokbuget, N., Bartram, C. R., et al. (2002). Leading prognostic relevance of the BCR-ABL translocation in adult acute B-lineage lymphoblastic leukemia: A prospective study of the German Multicenter Trial Group and confirmed polymerase chain reaction analysis. *Blood, 99*(5), 1536–1543.
62. Secker-Walker, L. M., Craig, J. M., Hawkins, J. M., & Hoffbrand, A. V. (1991). Philadelphia positive acute lymphoblastic leukemia in adults: Age distribution, BCR breakpoint and prognostic significance. *Leukemia, 5*(3), 196–199.
63. Radich, J., Gehly, G., Lee, A., et al. (1997). Detection of bcr-abl transcripts in Philadelphia chromosome-positive acute lymphoblastic leukemia after marrow transplantation. *Blood, 89*(7), 2602–2609.
64. Cimino, G., Pane, F., Elia, L., et al. (2006). The role of BCR/ABL isoforms in the presentation and outcome of patients with Philadelphia-positive acute lymphoblastic leukemia: A seven-year update of the GIMEMA 0496 trial. *Haematologica, 91*(3), 377–380.
65. Stirewalt, D. L., Guthrie, K. A., Beppu, L., et al. (2003). Predictors of relapse and overall survival in Philadelphia chromosome-positive acute lymphoblastic leukemia after transplantation. *Biology of Blood and Marrow Transplantation, 9*(3), 206–212.

66. Georgopoulos, K., Moore, D. D., & Derfler, B. (1992). Ikaros, an early lymphoid-specific transcription factor and a putative mediator for T cell commitment. *Science, 258*(5083), 808–812.
67. Molnar, A., Wu, P., Largespada, D. A., et al. (1996). The Ikaros gene encodes a family of lymphocyte-restricted zinc finger DNA binding proteins, highly conserved in human and mouse. *Journal of Immunology, 156*(2), 585–592.
68. Iacobucci, I., Lonetti, A., Messa, F., et al. (2008). Expression of spliced oncogenic Ikaros isoforms in Philadelphia-positive acute lymphoblastic leukemia patients treated with tyrosine kinase inhibitors: Implications for a new mechanism of resistance. *Blood, 112*, 3847–3855.
69. Rebollo, A., & Schmitt, C. (2003). Ikaros, Aiolos and Helios: Transcription regulators and lymphoid malignancies. *Immunology and Cell Biology, 81*(3), 171–175.
70. Mullighan, C. G., Su, X., Zhang, J., et al. (2009). Deletion of IKZF1 and prognosis in acute lymphoblastic leukemia. *The New England Journal of Medicine, 360*(5), 470–480.
71. Ruiz, A., Jiang, J., Kempski, H., & Brady, H. J. (2004). Overexpression of the Ikaros 6 isoform is restricted to t(4;11) acute lymphoblastic leukaemia in children and infants and has a role in B-cell survival. *British Journal Haematology, 125*(1), 31–37.
72. Kano, G., Morimoto, A., Takanashi, M., et al. (2008). Ikaros dominant negative isoform (Ik6) induces IL-3-independent survival of murine pro-B lymphocytes by activating JAK-STAT and up-regulating Bcl-xl levels. *Leukaemia & Lymphoma, 49*(5), 965–973.
73. Tonnelle, C., Bardin, F., Maroc, C., et al. (2001). Forced expression of the Ikaros 6 isoform in human placental blood CD34(+) cells impairs their ability to differentiate toward the B-lymphoid lineage. *Blood, 98*(9), 2673–2680.
74. Pui, C. H., Relling, M. V., & Downing, J. R. (2004). Acute lymphoblastic leukemia. *The New England Journal of Medicine, 350*(15), 1535–1548.
75. Pui, C. H., Rubnitz, J. E., Hancock, M. L., et al. (1998). Reappraisal of the clinical and biologic significance of myeloid-associated antigen expression in childhood acute lymphoblastic leukemia. *Journal of Clinical Oncology, 16*(12), 3768–3773.
76. Chen, C. S., Sorensen, P. H., Domer, P. H., et al. (1993). Molecular rearrangements on chromosome 11q23 predominate in infant acute lymphoblastic leukemia and are associated with specific biologic variables and poor outcome. *Blood, 81*(9), 2386–2393.
77. Armstrong, S. A., Staunton, J. E., Silverman, L. B., et al. (2002). MLL translocations specify a distinct gene expression profile that distinguishes a unique leukemia. *Nature Genetics, 30*(1), 41–47.
78. Ferrando, A. A., Armstrong, S. A., Neuberg, D. S., et al. (2003). Gene expression signatures in MLL-rearranged T-lineage and B-precursor acute leukemias: Dominance of HOX dysregulation. *Blood, 102*(1), 262–268.
79. Tsai, T., Davalath, S., Rankin, C., et al. (1996). Tumor suppressor gene alteration in adult acute lymphoblastic leukemia (ALL). Analysis of retinoblastoma (Rb) and p53 gene expression in lymphoblasts of patients with de novo, relapsed, or refractory ALL treated in Southwest Oncology Group studies. *Leukemia, 10*(12), 1901–1910.
80. Stock, W., Tsai, T., Golden, C., et al. (2000). Cell cycle regulatory gene abnormalities are important determinants of leukemogenesis and disease biology in adult acute lymphoblastic leukemia. *Blood, 95*(7), 2364–2371.
81. Omura-Minamisawa, M., Diccianni, M. B., Batova, A., et al. (2000). Universal inactivation of both p16 and p15 but not downstream components is an essential event in the pathogenesis of T-cell acute lymphoblastic leukemia. *Clinical Cancer Research, 6*(4), 1219–1228.
82. Golub, T. R., Slonim, D. K., Tamayo, P., et al. (1999). Molecular classification of cancer: Class discovery and class prediction by gene expression monitoring. *Science, 286*(5439), 531–537.
83. Yeoh, E. J., Ross, M. E., Shurtleff, S. A., et al. (2002). Classification, subtype discovery, and prediction of outcome in pediatric acute lymphoblastic leukemia by gene expression profiling. *Cancer Cell, 1*(2), 133–143.
84. Ross, M. E., Zhou, X., Song, G., et al. (2003). Classification of pediatric acute lymphoblastic leukemia by gene expression profiling. *Blood, 102*(8), 2951–2959.
85. den Boer, M. L., van Slegtenhorst, M., De Menezes, R. X., et al. (2009). A subtype of childhood acute lymphoblastic leukaemia with poor treatment outcome: A genome-wide classification study. *The Lancet Oncology, 10*(2), 125–134.
86. Cheok, M. H., Yang, W., Pui, C. H., et al. (2003). Treatment-specific changes in gene expression discriminate in vivo drug response in human leukemia cells. *Nature Genetics, 34*(1), 85–90.
87. Lugthart, S., Cheok, M. H., den Boer, M. L., et al. (2005). Identification of genes associated with chemotherapy crossresistance and treatment response in childhood acute lymphoblastic leukemia. *Cancer Cell, 7*(4), 375–386.
88. Holleman, A., Cheok, M. H., den Boer, M. L., et al. (2004). Gene-expression patterns in drug-resistant acute lymphoblastic leukemia cells and response to treatment. *The New England Journal of Medicine, 351*(6), 533–542.
89. Flotho, C. (2006). Genes contributing to minimal residual disease in childhood acute lymphoblastic leukemia: Prognostic significance of CASP8AP2. *Blood, 108*(3), 1050–1057.
90. Bhojwani, D., Kang, H., Moskowitz, N. P., et al. (2006). Biologic pathways associated with relapse in childhood acute lymphoblastic leukemia: A Children's Oncology Group study. *Blood, 108*(2), 711–717.

91. Chiaretti, S. (2005). Gene expression profiles of B-lineage adult acute lymphocytic leukemia reveal genetic patterns that identify lineage derivation and distinct mechanisms of transformation. *Clinical Cancer Research, 11*(20), 7209–7219.

92. Fine, B. M., Stanulla, M., Schrappe, M., et al. (2004). Gene expression patterns associated with recurrent chromosomal translocations in acute lymphoblastic leukemia. *Blood, 103*(3), 1043–1049.

93. Rozovskaia, T., Ravid-Amir, O., Tillib, S., et al. (2003). Expression profiles of acute lymphoblastic and myeloblastic leukemias with ALL-1 rearrangements. *Proceedings of the National Academy of Sciences of the United States of America, 100*(13), 7853–7858.

94. Bhojwani, D., Kang, H., Menezes, R. X., et al. (2008). Gene expression signatures predictive of early response and outcome in high-risk childhood acute lymphoblastic leukemia: A Children's Oncology Group Study [corrected]. *Journal of Clinical Oncology, 26*(27), 4376–4384.

95. Catchpoole, D., Guo, D., Jiang, H., & Biesheuvel, C. (2008). Predicting outcome in childhood acute lymphoblastic leukemia using gene expression profiling: Prognostication or protocol selection? *Blood, 111*(4)), 2486–2487. author reply 7-8.

96. Holleman, A. (2006). Expression of the outcome predictor in acute leukemia 1 (OPAL1) gene is not an independent prognostic factor in patients treated according to COALL or St Jude protocols. *Blood, 108*(6), 1984–1990.

97. Flotho, C., Coustan-Smith, E., Pei, D., et al. (2007). A set of genes that regulate cell proliferation predicts treatment outcome in childhood acute lymphoblastic leukemia. *Blood, 110*(4), 1271–1277.

98. Cario, G., Stanulla, M., Fine, B. M., et al. (2005). Distinct gene expression profiles determine molecular treatment response in childhood acute lymphoblastic leukemia. *Blood, 105*(2), 821–826.

99. Juric, D., Lacayo, N., Ramsey, M., et al. (2007). Differential gene expression patterns and interaction networks in BCR-ABL-positive and -negative adult acute lymphoblastic leukemias. *Journal of Clinical Oncology, 25*(11), 1341–1349.

100. Kohlmann, A., Schoch, C., Schnittger, S., et al. (2004). Pediatric acute lymphoblastic leukemia (ALL) gene expression signatures classify an independent cohort of adult ALL patients. *Leukemia, 18*(1), 63–71.

101. Sala-Torra, O., Gundacker, H. M., Stirewalt, D. L., et al. (2007). Connective tissue growth factor (CTGF) expression and outcome in adult patients with acute lymphoblastic leukemia. *Blood, 109*(7), 3080–3083.

102. Graux, C., Cools, J., Michaux, L., Vandenberghe, P., & Hagemeijer, A. (2006). Cytogenetics and molecular genetics of T-cell acute lymphoblastic leukemia: From thymocyte to lymphoblast. *Leukemia, 20*(9), 1496–1510.

103. Bain, G., Engel, I., Robanus Maandag, E. C., et al. (1997). E2A deficiency leads to abnormalities in alphabeta T-cell development and to rapid development of T-cell lymphomas. *Molecular and Cellular Biology, 17*(8), 4782–4791.

104. Yan, W., Young, A. Z., Soares, V. C., Kelley, R., Benezra, R., & Zhuang, Y. (1997). High incidence of T-cell tumors in E2A-null mice and E2A/Id1 double-knockout mice. *Molecular and Cellular Biology, 17*(12), 7317–7327.

105. O'Neil, J., Billa, M., Oikemus, S., & Kelliher, M. (2001). The DNA binding activity of TAL-1 is not required to induce leukemia/lymphoma in mice. *Oncogene, 20*(29), 3897–3905.

106. O'Neil, J., Shank, J., Cusson, N., Murre, C., & Kelliher, M. (2004). TAL1/SCL induces leukemia by inhibiting the transcriptional activity of E47/HEB. *Cancer Cell, 5*(6), 587–596.

107. Aplan, P. D., Jones, C. A., Chervinsky, D. S., et al. (1997). An scl gene product lacking the transactivation domain induces bony abnormalities and cooperates with LMO1 to generate T-cell malignancies in transgenic mice. *The EMBO Journal, 16*(9), 2408–2419.

108. Elwood, N. J., & Begley, C. G. (1995). Reconstitution of mice with bone marrow cells expressing the SCL gene is insufficient to cause leukemia. *Cell Growth & Differentiation, 6*(1), 19–25.

109. Curtis, D. J., Robb, L., Strasser, A., & Begley, C. G. (1997). The CD2-scl transgene alters the phenotype and frequency of T-lymphomas in N-ras transgenic or p53 deficient mice. *Oncogene, 15*(24), 2975–2983.

110. Condorelli, G. L., Facchiano, F., Valtieri, M., et al. (1996). T-cell-directed TAL-1 expression induces T-cell malignancies in transgenic mice. *Cancer Research, 56*(22), 5113–5119.

111. Van Vlierberghe, P., van Grotel, M., Beverloo, H. B., et al. (2006). The cryptic chromosomal deletion del(11) (p12p13) as a new activation mechanism of LMO2 in pediatric T-cell acute lymphoblastic leukemia. *Blood, 108*(10), 3520–3529.

112. Hacein-Bey-Abina, S., Garrigue, A., Wang, G. P., et al. (2008). Insertional oncogenesis in 4 patients after retrovirus-mediated gene therapy of SCID-X1. *The Journal of Clinical Investigation, 118*(9), 3132–3142.

113. Hacein-Bey-Abina, S., Von Kalle, C., Schmidt, M., et al. (2003). LMO2-associated clonal T cell proliferation in two patients after gene therapy for SCID-X1. *Science, 302*(5644), 415–419.

114. Howe, S. J., Mansour, M. R., Schwarzwaelder, K., et al. (2008). Insertional mutagenesis combined with acquired somatic mutations causes leukemogenesis following gene therapy of SCID-X1 patients. *The Journal of Clinical Investigation, 118*(9), 3143–3150.

115. Larson, R. C., Osada, H., Larson, T. A., Lavenir, I., & Rabbitts, T. H. (1995). The oncogenic LIM protein Rbtn2 causes thymic developmental aberrations that precede malignancy in transgenic mice. *Oncogene, 11*(5), 853–862.

116. Larson, R. C., Lavenir, I., Larson, T. A., et al. (1996). Protein dimerization between Lmo2 (Rbtn2) and Tal1 alters thymocyte development and potentiates T cell tumorigenesis in transgenic mice. *The EMBO Journal, 15*(5), 1021–1027.

117. Speleman, F., Cauwelier, B., Dastugue, N., et al. (2005). A new recurrent inversion, inv(7)(p15q34), leads to transcriptional activation of HOXA10 and HOXA11 in a subset of T-cell acute lymphoblastic leukemias. *Leukemia, 19*(3), 358–366.

118. Soulier, J., Clappier, E., Cayuela, J. M., et al. (2005). HOXA genes are included in genetic and biologic networks defining human acute T-cell leukemia (T-ALL). *Blood, 106*(1), 274–286.

119. Dik, W. A., Brahim, W., Braun, C., et al. (2005). CALM-AF10+ T-ALL expression profiles are characterized by overexpression of HOXA and BMI1 oncogenes. *Leukemia, 19*(11), 1948–1957.

120. Hawley, R. G., Fong, A. Z., Reis, M. D., Zhang, N., Lu, M., & Hawley, T. S. (1997). Transforming function of the HOX11/TCL3 homeobox gene. *Cancer Research, 57*(2), 337–345.

121. Graux, C., Cools, J., Melotte, C., et al. (2004). Fusion of NUP214 to ABL1 on amplified episomes in T-cell acute lymphoblastic leukemia. *Nature Genetics, 36*(10), 1084–1089.

122. Graux, C., Stevens-Kroef, M., Lafage, M., et al. (2009). Heterogeneous patterns of amplification of the NUP214-ABL1 fusion gene in T-cell acute lymphoblastic leukemia. *Leukemia, 23*(1), 125–133.

123. Quintas-Cardama, A., Tong, W., Manshouri, T., et al. (2008). Activity of tyrosine kinase inhibitors against human NUP214-ABL1-positive T cell malignancies. *Leukemia, 22*(6), 1117–1124.

124. Kamada, N., Sakurai, M., Miyamoto, K., et al. (1992). Chromosome abnormalities in adult T-cell leukemia/lymphoma: A karyotype review committee report. *Cancer Research, 52*(6), 1481–1493.

125. Hayashi, Y., Raimondi, S. C., Look, A. T., et al. (1990). Abnormalities of the long arm of chromosome 6 in childhood acute lymphoblastic leukemia. *Blood, 76*(8), 1626–1630.

126. Raimondi, S. C. (1993). Current status of cytogenetic research in childhood acute lymphoblastic leukemia. *Blood, 81*(9), 2237–2251.

127. Lahortiga, I., De Keersmaecker, K., Van Vlierberghe, P., et al. (2007). Duplication of the MYB oncogene in T cell acute lymphoblastic leukemia. *Nature Genetics, 39*(5), 593–595.

128. Clappier, E., Cuccuini, W., Kalota, A., et al. (2007). The C-MYB locus is involved in chromosomal translocation and genomic duplications in human T-cell acute leukemia (T-ALL), the translocation defining a new T-ALL subtype in very young children. *Blood, 110*(4), 1251–1261.

129. Pear, W. S., Aster, J. C., Scott, M. L., et al. (1996). Exclusive development of T cell neoplasms in mice transplanted with bone marrow expressing activated Notch alleles. *The Journal of Experimental Medicine, 183*(5), 2283–2291.

130. Weng, A. P., Ferrando, A. A., Lee, W., et al. (2004). Activating mutations of NOTCH1 in human T cell acute lymphoblastic leukemia. *Science, 306*(5694), 269–271.

131. Mansour, M. R., Linch, D. C., Foroni, L., Goldstone, A. H., & Gale, R. E. (2006). High incidence of Notch-1 mutations in adult patients with T-cell acute lymphoblastic leukemia. *Leukemia, 20*(3), 537–539.

132. Lee, S. Y., Kumano, K., Masuda, S., et al. (2005). Mutations of the Notch1 gene in T-cell acute lymphoblastic leukemia: Analysis in adults and children. *Leukemia, 19*(10), 1841–1843.

133. Asnafi, V., Buzyn, A., Le Noir, S., et al. (2008). NOTCH1/FBXW7 mutation identifies a large subgroup with favourable outcome in adult T-cell acute lymphoblastic leukemia (T-ALL): A GRAALL study. *Blood, 113*, 3918–3924.

134. Flex, E., Petrangeli, V., Stella, L., et al. (2008). Somatically acquired JAK1 mutations in adult acute lymphoblastic leukemia. *The Journal of Experimental Medicine, 205*(4), 751–758.

135. Ferrando, A. A., Neuberg, D. S., Staunton, J., et al. (2002). Gene expression signatures define novel oncogenic pathways in T cell acute lymphoblastic leukemia. *Cancer Cell, 1*(1), 75–87.

136. Kees, U. R., Heerema, N. A., Kumar, R., et al. (2003). Expression of HOX11 in childhood T-lineage acute lymphoblastic leukaemia can occur in the absence of cytogenetic aberration at 10q24: A study from the Children's Cancer Group (CCG). *Leukemia, 17*(5), 887–893.

137. Ferrando, A. A., Herblot, S., Palomero, T., et al. (2004). Biallelic transcriptional activation of oncogenic transcription factors in T-cell acute lymphoblastic leukemia. *Blood, 103*(5), 1909–1911.

138. Watt, P. M., Kumar, R., & Kees, U. R. (2000). Promoter demethylation accompanies reactivation of the HOX11 proto-oncogene in leukemia. *Genes, Chromosomes & Cancer, 29*(4), 371–377.

139. Bash, R. O., Hall, S., Timmons, C. F., et al. (1995). Does activation of the TAL1 gene occur in a majority of patients with T-cell acute lymphoblastic leukemia? A pediatric oncology group study. *Blood, 86*(2), 666–676.

140. Baldus, C., Martus, P., Burmeister, T., et al. (2007). Low ERG and BAALC expression identifies a new subgroup of sdult acute T-lymphoblastic leukemia with a highly favorable outcome. *Journal of Clinical Oncology, 25*(24), 3739–3745.

141. Rooney, S., Chaudhuri, J., & Alt, F. W. (2004). The role of the non-homologous end-joining pathway in lymphocyte development. *Immunological Reviews, 200*, 115–131.

142. Raghavan, S. C., Kirsch, I. R., & Lieber, M. R. (2001). Analysis of the V(D)J recombination efficiency at lymphoid chromosomal translocation breakpoints. *The Journal of Biological Chemistry, 276*(31), 29126–29133.
143. Marculescu, R., Le, T., Simon, P., Jaeger, U., & Nadel, B. (2002). V(D)J-mediated translocations in lymphoid neoplasms: A functional assessment of genomic instability by cryptic sites. *The Journal of Experimental Medicine, 195*(1), 85–98.
144. Marculescu, R., Vanura, K., Montpellier, B., et al. (2006). Recombinase, chromosomal translocations and lymphoid neoplasia: Targeting mistakes and repair failures. *DNA Repair (Amst), 5*(9–10), 1246–1258.
145. Hochtl, J., & Zachau, H. G. (1983). A novel type of aberrant recombination in immunoglobulin genes and its implications for V-J joining mechanism. *Nature, 302*(5905), 260–263.
146. Cheng, J. T., Yang, C. Y., Hernandez, J., Embrey, J., & Baer, R. (1990). The chromosome translocation (11;14) (p13;q11) associated with T cell acute leukemia asymmetric diversification of the translocational junctions. *The Journal of Experimental Medicine, 171*(2), 489–501.
147. Yoffe, G., Schneider, N., Van Dyk, L., et al. (1989). The chromosome translocation (11;14)(p13;q11) associated with T-cell acute lymphocytic leukemia: An 11p13 breakpoint cluster region. *Blood, 74*(1), 374–379.
148. Marculescu, R., Vanura, K., Le, T., Simon, P., Jager, U., & Nadel, B. (2003). Distinct t(7;9)(q34;q32) breakpoints in healthy individuals and individuals with T-ALL. *Nature Genetics, 33*(3), 342–344.
149. Aplan, P. D., Lombardi, D. P., Ginsberg, A. M., Cossman, J., Bertness, V. L., & Kirsch, I. R. (1990). Disruption of the human SCL locus by "illegitimate" V-(D)-J recombinase activity. *Science, 250*(4986), 1426–1429.
150. Lewis, S. M. (1994). The mechanism of V(D)J joining: Lessons from molecular, immunological, and comparative analyses. *Advances in Immunology, 56*, 27–150.
151. Boehm, T., Baer, R., Lavenir, I., et al. (1988). The mechanism of chromosomal translocation t(11;14) involving the T-cell receptor C delta locus on human chromosome 14q11 and a transcribed region of chromosome 11p15. *The EMBO Journal, 7*(2), 385–394.
152. Garcia, I. S., Kaneko, Y., Gonzalez-Sarmiento, R., et al. (1991). A study of chromosome 11p13 translocations involving TCR beta and TCR delta in human T cell leukaemia. *Oncogene, 6*(4), 577–582.
153. Kagan, J., Finger, L. R., Letofsky, J., Finan, J., Nowell, P. C., & Croce, C. M. (1989). Clustering of breakpoints on chromosome 10 in acute T-cell leukemias with the t(10;14) chromosome translocation. *Proceedings of the National Academy of Sciences of the United States of America, 86*(11), 4161–4165.
154. Lu, M., Dube, I., Raimondi, S., et al. (1990). Molecular characterization of the t(10;14) translocation breakpoints in T-cell acute lymphoblastic leukemia: Further evidence for illegitimate physiological recombination. *Genes, Chromosomes & Cancer, 2*(3), 217–222.
155. Lu, M., Zhang, N., Raimondi, S., & Ho, A. D. (1992). S1 nuclease hypersensitive sites in an oligopurine/oligopyrimidine DNA from the t(10;14) breakpoint cluster region. *Nucleic Acids Research, 20*(2), 263–266.
156. Shima-Rich, E. A., Harden, A. M., McKeithan, T. W., Rowley, J. D., & Diaz, M. O. (1997). Molecular analysis of the t(8;14)(q24;q11) chromosomal breakpoint junctions in the T-cell leukemia line MOLT-16. *Genes, Chromosomes & Cancer, 20*(4), 363–371.
157. Mullighan, C. G., Goorha, S., Radtke, I., et al. (2007). Genome-wide analysis of genetic alterations in acute lymphoblastic leukaemia. *Nature, 446*(7137), 758–764.
158. Szczepański, T., Beishuizen, A., Pongers-Willemse, M. J., et al. (1999). Cross-lineage T cell receptor gene rearrangements occur in more than ninety percent of childhood precursor-B acute lymphoblastic leukemias: Alternative PCR targets for detection of minimal residual disease. *Leukemia, 13*(2), 196–205.
159. Pongers-Willemse, M. J., Seriu, T., Stolz, F., et al. (1999). Primers and protocols for standardized detection of minimal residual disease in acute lymphoblastic leukemia using immunoglobulin and T cell receptor gene rearrangements and TAL1 deletions as PCR targets: Report of the BIOMED-1 CONCERTED ACTION: Investigation of minimal residual disease in acute leukemia. *Leukemia, 13*(1), 110–118.
160. Langerak, A. W., Szczepanski, T., van der Burg, M., Wolvers-Tettero, I. L., & van Dongen, J. J. (1997). Heteroduplex PCR analysis of rearranged T cell receptor genes for clonality assessment in suspect T cell proliferations. *Leukemia, 11*(12), 2192–2199.
161. de Haas, V., Verhagen, O. J., von dem Borne, A. E., Kroes, W., van den Berg, H., & van der Schoot, C. E. (2001). Quantification of minimal residual disease in children with oligoclonal B-precursor acute lymphoblastic leukemia indicates that the clones that grow out during relapse already have the slowest rate of reduction during induction therapy. *Leukemia, 15*(1), 134–140.
162. Moreira, I., Papaioannou, M., Mortuza, F. Y., et al. (2001). Heterogeneity of VH-JH gene rearrangement patterns: An insight into the biology of B cell precursor ALL. *Leukemia, 15*(10), 1527–1536.
163. Szczepański, T., Willemse, M. J., Brinkhof, B., van Wering, E. R., van der Burg, M., & van Dongen, J. J. (2002). Comparative analysis of Ig and TCR gene rearrangements at diagnosis and at relapse of childhood precursor-B-ALL provides improved strategies for selection of stable PCR targets for monitoring of minimal residual disease. *Blood, 99*(7), 2315–2323.
164. van Dongen, J. J., Seriu, T., Panzer-Grumayer, E. R., et al. (1998). Prognostic value of minimal residual disease in acute lymphoblastic leukaemia in childhood. *Lancet, 352*(9142), 1731–1738.

165. Cave, H., Bosch, J., Suciu, S., et al. (1998). Clinical significance of minimal residual disease in childhood acute lymphoblastic leukemia. European Organization for Research and Treatment of Cancer – Childhood Leukemia Cooperative Group. *The New England Journal of Medicine, 339*(9), 591–598.
166. Rosenquist, R., Thunberg, U., Li, A. H., et al. (1999). Clonal evolution as judged by immunoglobulin heavy chain gene rearrangements in relapsing precursor-B acute lymphoblastic leukemia. *European Journal of Haematology, 63*(3), 171–179.
167. Steward, C. G., Goulden, N. J., Katz, F., et al. (1994). A polymerase chain reaction study of the stability of Ig heavy-chain and T-cell receptor delta gene rearrangements between presentation and relapse of childhood B-lineage acute lymphoblastic leukemia. *Blood, 83*(5), 1355–1362.
168. Germano, G., del Giudice, L., Palatron, S., et al. (2003). Clonality profile in relapsed precursor-B-ALL children by GeneScan and sequencing analyses Consequences on minimal residual disease monitoring. *Leukemia, 17*(8), 1573–1582.
169. Mullighan, C., Phillips, L., Su, X., et al. (2008). Genomic analysis of the clonal origins of relapsed acute lymphoblastic leukemia. *Science, 322*(5906), 1377–1380.

Chapter 4
Minimal Residual Disease in Acute Lymphoblastic Leukemia

Patrick A. Zweidler-McKay and Michael J. Borowitz

Introduction

Response to initial therapy in ALL is a well-known prognostic marker. However, as improvements in therapeutic regimens have led to increasing remission rates, it has become clear that traditional measures of response lack adequate sensitivity, particularly in frontline studies. With >90% of newly diagnosed ALL patients entering morphologic remission by the end of induction and nearly all patients remaining in morphologic remission until frank relapse, the era of using bone marrow blast percentage as the sole measure of therapeutic efficacy is coming to an end [1–5]. Technologic advances that allow us to detect minimal residual disease (MRD), that is, the presence of leukemic cells below the level of morphologic detection, have made it possible to refine our analysis of response to therapy, and raise the possibility of early adjustments in therapy both to intensify treatment for those patients with poor initial response, as well as to de-intensify therapy and reduce toxicity for patients whose early response predicts very good outcome. In this chapter, we will discuss technological methods of MRD detection, describe studies that demonstrate its prognostic value, and indicate how MRD is being and will be used to adjust therapy in clinical trials. We will also address some of the challenges that exist in interpreting results from clinical trials, and in adopting this measure in routine clinical practice.

Techniques for Detecting Minimal Residual Disease

Although traditional measures of leukemia burden following therapy, including bone marrow morphology, cytogenetics, fluorescence in situ hybridization (FISH) and immunohistochemistry have prognostic significance, they lack the sensitivity and/or specificity to detect a significant portion of patients likely to relapse on current therapies. Over the past 10 years, two technologies have presented themselves as sensitive and specific enough to detect low levels of MRD accurately. First, polymerase chain reaction (PCR) amplification of leukemia-specific translocations or rearrangements of antigen receptor genes has become feasible. Second, flow cytometry–based identification of aberrant leukemia populations has become more sophisticated. Each of these technologies can now be applied in a growing number of MRD studies.

M.J. Borowitz (✉)
Department of Pathology, Johns Hopkins Medical Institutions, Johns Hopkins Hospital,
Pathology-Weinberg 2337, 401 N. Broadway, Baltimore, MD 21231, USA
e-mail: mborowit@jhmi.edu

A.S. Advani and H.M. Lazarus (eds.), *Adult Acute Lymphocytic Leukemia*, Contemporary Hematology,
DOI 10.1007/978-1-60761-707-5_4, © Springer Science+Business Media, LLC 2011

PCR Methods

PCR for Recurrent Translocations

With the knowledge that a significant subset of leukemia cells carry defined translocations, PCR primer sets have been developed to detect many of the most common translocations, including E2A-PBX1, MLL-AF4, BCR-ABL1, TEL-AML1, and SIL-TAL1 [6–8]. The principle is that individual tumor-specific RNA transcripts in cells may be detected if they can be amplified sufficiently. The PCR has been used to accomplish this. Briefly, RNA is extracted from cells and converted into cDNA to allow repetitive copying. Then, short oligonucleotides, called primers, are synthesized, which specifically bind to complementary cDNA sequences. These primers allow DNA polymerases to begin copying the cDNA sequences. "Reverse" primers allow copying of the complementary cDNA strand, and this process is repeated 40–60 times. Because the partners in a translocation, such as E2A and PBX1, are physically extremely distant in the genome, only in a cell with a classic t(1;19) translocation will the E2A and PBX1 genes be juxtaposed to allow such a primer combination to produce an amplified product. Since the fusion transcripts are unique to leukemic cells, detection of a fusion RNA provides very high specificity and a low false-positive rate. Since these primers rely on predicting translocation breakpoints, sensitivity depends upon the uniformity of translocation breakpoints for each translocation, e.g., BCR-ABL1 is highly uniform with most breakpoints found in limited regions, whereas TEL-AML1 is not, requiring many primer pairs to detect all possible translocations. Nonetheless, PCR amplification of specific translocation breakpoints is a highly sensitive and specific method to detect MRD with the ability to detect 1 leukemic cell in 100,000 normal cells [5]. However, recurrent translocations occur in less than half of all ALL patients, making their utility somewhat limited in the general ALL patient population.

PCR for Antigen Receptor Rearrangements

To overcome this limitation, additional targets for PCR primers are needed. Several groups pioneered the detection of discrete immunoglobulin (Ig) and T cell receptor (TCR) rearrangements, which can be found in most ALLs [9–16]. Both normal and malignant B and T lymphocytes undergo Ig and/or TCR gene rearrangement and excision in the variable (V), diversity (D), and junction (J) regions. Deletions and insertions in specific regions of these genes lead to unique genomic DNA sequences, which can be identified through the use of multiple PCR primer sets. Similar to the translocation-specific PCR amplification described above, primers are used that bind to specific DNA sequences juxtaposed only in cells in which these regions have been rearranged. When an individual leukemic cell has a rearrangement/deletion that juxtaposes two regions of DNA in which primers can bind, an amplified product is detected. Because ALL is a clonal disease, leukemic cells share the same unique Ig/TCR rearrangements. These specific sequences are abundant in a diagnostic leukemia sample and can therefore be characterized easily. However, selection of primer sets is important, as sensitivity and specificity rely on the frequency and stability of specific rearrangements/deletions. Differences in methodologies between studies make comparisons difficult [17]. To overcome this, standardized primer sets have been developed in multicenter cooperative groups [18, 19]. For example, the BIOMED-2 defines a set of 107 unique primers in 18 multiplex PCR reactions, which are performed to identify informative primer pairs [20]. These generic PCR primer sets can identify unique rearrangement products on >90% of diagnostic samples.

However, these primer sets may bind to sequences in the Ig or TCR gene that are also present in normal cells, so that in addition to amplifying leukemic cell DNA they will also amplify DNA from normal B or T cells that have similar rearranged antigen receptor genes. While residual clonal DNA from leukemic cells will give a larger signal than any individual normal lymphocyte, in practice the sensitivity of detection of leukemic DNA is limited to 1 in 1000 cells (10^{-3}) against this normal lymphocyte background. In order to achieve the greater sensitivities needed to detect lower levels of MRD, the unique diagnostic rearrangements must be sequenced, and patient-specific primers (or probes) must be synthesized. The use of patient-specific reagents in conjunction with generic primer sets yields much higher sensitivities (up to 10^{-5}) than can be achieved with generic reagents alone.

The TCR complex is composed of multiple distinct proteins, of which the alpha, beta, gamma, and delta genes are rearranged in normal and malignant T cells. In patients with T cell ALL, TCR beta and gamma rearrangements can be detected by PCR in >90% of patients [21], and can reach a 10^{-4} level of MRD detection in >90% of patients [22]. Interestingly, the frequency of specific TCR gamma rearrangements may depend on ethnic background and therefore may influence primer set selection for different patient populations [23]. Due to the uniform presence of detectable TCR rearrangements in T-ALL, this is the primary method of PCR-based MRD detection in T-ALL patients.

Similarly, the Ig genes are rearranged in normal and malignant B cells. Both immunoglobulin heavy (IgH) and light (IgL) chain (kappa and lambda) genes may be rearranged, though the former is more common. The V(D)J regions of these genes are rearranged independently to form multiple unique rearrangements or deletions per cell. In B precursor ALL, the IgH genes are rearranged in >80% of patients [24]. These are the most commonly detected Ig rearrangements and specific patterns of rearrangement vary depending on the leukemia subtype and the patient's age [25]. In addition, PCR-based assays can also detect light chain rearrangements in half of pre-B ALL patients [26], and the use of light chain PCR can increase the sensitivity of PCR-based MRD, especially in specific subsets of pre-B ALL patients [27]. Surprisingly, cross-lineage TCR rearrangements are found in >90% of pre-B ALL cases [15]. These aberrant TCR beta rearrangements are particularly seen in specific patient subgroups, e.g., those with TEL-AML1 rearrangements [28]. Using a combination of Ig and TCR rearrangement primer sets, informative PCR amplifications can be found for >90% of B- and T-ALLs.

One of the challenges to MRD testing using PCR technology has been quantitation. Early studies used relatively imprecise dilutional methods, which were not highly reproducible, but even with these relatively simple methods, clinically significant measures of MRD could be made [29]. More recently, with the advent of quantitative PCR methods, quantitation is much more reproducible, although distinctions of less than a factor of 10 are still not very accurate. PCR-based MRD measurements have other limitations as well. Specific rearrangements are often "lost" from diagnosis to relapse, and from first to second relapse [30]. This occurs in the IgH or TCR rearrangements in up to one-half of pre-B ALL cases and may either represent the emergence of a sub-clone lacking that specific rearrangement or further rearrangement of the gene preventing a specific primer pair from yielding the same result seen at diagnosis. In order to avoid such false-negative results, the use of at least two informative primer sets in each patient is required. In contrast to the frequently lost IgH rearrangements, rearrangements of the Ig light chain Kappa-deleting element (IgK-Kde), though found in only half of patients, have been found to be much more stable between diagnosis and relapse and therefore can serve to reduce false-negative results [26, 30–32]. With the use of multiple primer sets, informative markers can theoretically still be found in 90% of cases, though in one large series only about 70% of patients had at least two "sensitive" targets [24]. This allows for the possibility that a significant percentage of patients could be found to be falsely negative. False positives are also a concern, either due to contamination from other PCR reactions because of the very high sensitivity of PCR, or because of the presence of benign lymphocytes with similar rearrangements to the leukemia clone leading to apparent positive MRD. These problems are addressable, but they require more primer sets, more rigorous methodology, and more experienced interpretation.

Flow Cytometry Methods

Another method to detect MRD is multiparameter flow cytometry, which identifies aberrant expression of leukocyte differentiation antigens. Over 300 clusters of differentiation (CD) antigens have been characterized on the surface of leukocytes; these represent a wide array of molecules, including receptors, glycans, adhesion molecules, membrane-bound enzymes, etc. Expression of these antigens can define cell lineages, developmental stages, and functional subsets. It was noted over 25 years ago that leukemic cells commonly have dysregulated expression of one or more surface antigens, allowing for the identification of leukemic cells via antibody staining and detection with flow cytometry. Leukemic cells differ from normal bone marrow B and T lineage populations because of cross-lineage, asynchronous, ectopic, or absence of expression of one or more antigens [33–37]. Whole cells can be stained for multiple antigens simultaneously with highly specific antibodies carrying distinct fluorescent dyes. The flow cytometer excites these dyes with one or more lasers and detects the specific fluorescence emitted by each antibody. The intensity of this signal is proportional to the amount of each antigen on the cells. In most studies, three to four specific antibodies are combined to identify abnormal populations of cells consistent with leukemic blasts, but up to 10 or more simultaneous antigens can be measured. Many thousands or even more than a million cells can be analyzed from the same sample; multiple plots are then used to display antigen expression on various cell populations, with each dot on one of these plots representing a single cell. Software programs permit efficient analysis of the data, often by assigning color to a population of cells satisfying a particular set of requirements with respect to light scatter properties and/or antigen expression. The sensitivity of this technology comes from the large number of cells examined, and the ability to identify discrete abnormal populations that occupy regions of the displays in which normal cells are not found (Fig. 4.1).

Many different combinations of antibodies have been used to distinguish leukemic and normal cells; some combinations are particularly useful. For example, the simple combination of TdT/CD10/CD19 can detect leukemic blasts in over three quarters of pre-B ALL cases [38], and TdT/CD7/cyCD3 can detect over 90% of T-ALL cases [39]. A two-tube system of CD19/CD45/CD10/CD20 and CD19/CD45/CD9/CD34 was used by the Children's Oncology Group (COG) to detect MRD and was found to be informative in nearly 95% of cases of precursor B-ALL [40]. Additional combinations include CD10/CD20/CD19, CD34/CD38/CD19, CD34/CD22/CD19, and CD19/CD34/CD45, together yielding 98% detection of the leukemic blasts [38]. Additional markers may be useful in further combinations. For example, the intensity of CD58 [41] and CD49f [42] is higher in leukemic B cells than normal precursors, while that of CD38 is often lower. Although cross-lineage expression of the myeloid markers CD13 and CD33 is seen in ~40% of pre-B ALL cases [38], the usefulness of this as an aberrant phenotype is limited in many cases because expression is weak. In T cell ALL, several additional markers may add sensitivity, such as loss of CD5 and/or CD3, co-expression of CD4 and CD8, co-expression of CD34 and CD7 [39], or overexpression of CD99 [43]. Using one or more of these combinations typically identifies the aberrant leukemia population in >95% of diagnostic ALL samples.

However, flow cytometry–based MRD measurements also have limitations. Studies require large numbers of viable cells, in contrast to PCR studies in which DNA is used. Thus, while DNA can be shipped to many laboratories and inter-laboratory standardization studies carried out, there are only limited data on inter-laboratory variability in flow cytometry [38, 44] because viable cells are more difficult to ship to multiple laboratories. Our experience in the COG has shown that even though extensive sample exchange isn't practical, the frequency of finding MRD positivity is almost identical between two different laboratories (Fig. 4.2), supporting the general reproducibility of the measurement. In addition, as with PCR-based techniques, changes found in leukemic cells during therapy may make detection of MRD difficult, especially if the analysis is designed only to evaluate for the specific abnormalities found at diagnosis [43]. Chemotherapy may induce such phenotypic "drift", which often mimics maturation, with reduction in CD10 and CD34 expression, and increase in

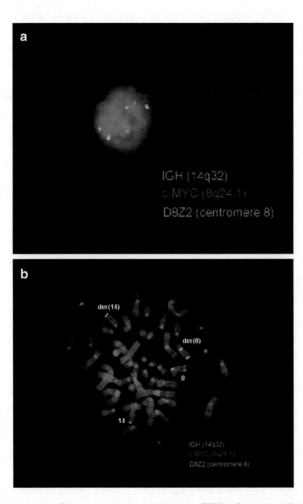

Fig. 13.4 c-MYC translocation by fluorescent in situ hybridation (FISH). Detection of t(8;14)(q24;q32) by FISH involves a dual-color dual-fusion IGH (green) and c-MYC (red) probe set with a centromere 8 control (aqua). (**a**) The typical abnormal metaphase FISH pattern is shown with one normal copy of each of chromosomes 8 and 14 and fusion of c-MYC and IGH on the der(8) and der(14) chromosomes from the t(8;14). (**b**) Interphase FISH demonstrates the corresponding 1R1G2F pattern in nuclei. (Courtesy of Jennelle C. Hodge PhD and Shellie J. Gilbertson, Mayo Foundation for Medical Education and Research, used with permission)

There is evidence that classic Burkitt lymphoma tumors without a detectable *c-myc* translocation (10%) have altered micro RNA (miRNA) expression patterns [58]. Downregulation of the miRNA hsa-mir-34b, a member of the mir-34 family, has been demonstrated in human tumors and cancer cell lines with functional p53 deficiency [58, 59]. Leoncini et al. showed that down-regulation of hsa-mir-34b was correlated with increased *c-myc* expression in five cases of Burkitt lymphoma with classic morphology but without a FISH-detectable *c-myc* translocation. In this study, the 30 Burkitt lymphoma cases with a FISH-detectable *c-myc* translocation did not demonstrate hsa-mir-34b downregulation [58]. This study supports an alternative mechanism for *c-myc* overexpression in *c-myc*-translocation-negative Burkitt lymphoma and leukemia cases, which may be expanded by future miRNA hypermethylation studies.

The differential diagnosis of Burkitt lymphoma and leukemia includes, but is not limited to, diffuse large B-cell lymphoma (DLBCL) and B-cell and T-cell acute lymphoblastic lymphoma/leukemia (B-ALL, T-ALL) (Table 13.1) [2]. In contrast to Burkitt lymphoma and leukemia, DLBCL is typically

Table 13.1 Morphologic, immunophenotypic, and genetic comparisons of Burkitt Lymphoma/Leukemia with other neoplasms

	Morphology	Immunophenotype	Genetics
Burkitt lymphoma/ leukemia	Monomorphic Medium-sized lymphocytes Round to oval non-cleaved, non-folded nuclei Basophilic cytoplasm Starry-sky pattern on low-power (tingible body macrophages)	Ki-67-positive in 95–100% of cells B cell phenotype: CD19+, CD20+, CD22+, CD79a+ Germinal center phenotype: CD10+, Bcl–6+ Mum1–, CD138– Bcl2 usually negative TdT– Moderate to strong surface immunoglobulin expression	c-myc translocations: t(8;14)(q24;q32) t(8;22)(q24;q11) t(2;8)(p12;q24) 10% of cases may exist without a detectable c-myc translocation
Diffuse large B cell lymphoma	Pleomorphic Large-sized cells Irregularly-shaped, often folded nuclei	Lower Ki-67-positivity than Burkitt lymphoma CD10+ (30–60%) – less often than Burkitt lymphoma Bcl-2+ (30–50%) – more often than Burkitt lymphoma	10% may demonstrate a c-myc rearrangement
B-lymphoblastic leukemia/lymphoma	Morphology may be similar to Burkitt lymphoma	Express blastic markers – CD34+ and TdT+ Bcl-6 Surface immunoglobulin usually absent	c-myc translocation not seen Other translocations allow differentiation from Burkitt lymphoma/leukemia: t(9;22)(q34;q11.2) t(v;11q23) t(12;21)(p13;q22) t(1;19)(q23;p13.3)
T-lymphoblastic leukemia/ lymphoma		B-cell markers absent TdT+ Variable expression of CD34, CD1a and T-cell antigens CD2, CD3, CD5, CD7	

characterized by a pleomorphic population of large cells with irregularly shaped, often folded, nuclei and a lower Ki-67-positive proliferation fraction (Fig. 13.5) [2–4]. DLBCLs with a monomorphic population of cells that have round nuclei, prominent nucleoli, scattered histiocytes, and a high proliferative fraction may strongly resemble Burkitt lymphoma and leukemia. However, the Ki-67 proliferation fraction is usually below 80–90% [2, 60]. Furthermore, DLBCL stains for CD10 less often (30–60% of cases), and for bcl-2 more often (30–50% of cases) than Burkitt lymphoma and leukemia [2, 61, 62]. It is important to note that evidence of a *c-myc* translocation by FISH cannot be used to exclude DLBCL [63]. Approximately, 10% of DLBCL cases demonstrate a *c-myc* rearrangement, which is often associated with a complex pattern of genetic alterations [63, 64]. In 60% of *c-myc*-translocation-positive DLBCL cases, the partner is an immunoglobulin gene (*Ig-myc*),

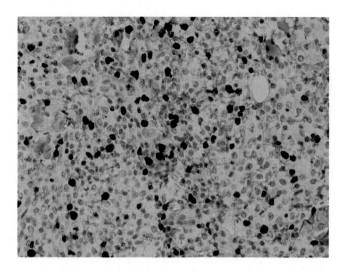

Fig. 13.5 Diffuse large B-cell lymphoma. Diffuse large B-cell lymphoma involving an inguinal lymph node, Ki-67 immunohistochemical stain, 20× magnification. The proliferation fraction in this non-Burkitt lymphoma is approximately 20–30%. The proliferation fraction in this tumor is approximately 20–30%, which is markedly lower than in cases of Burkitt lymphoma.

while in 40% of cases, the translocation partner is a non-immunoglobulin gene [2, 64]. A *c-myc* breakpoint in DLBCL is associated with a substantially lower survival rate, independent of age and Ann Arbor stage [51].

The precursor B-cell neoplasm, B-lymphoblastic leukemia/lymphoma (BLL/L, formerly precursor B acute lymphoblastic leukemia), has morphologic similarities to Burkitt lymphoma and leukemia and may display round regular nuclei, a high nuclear to cytoplasmic ratio, basophilic cytoplasm, multiple prominent nucleoli, and intracellular vacuoles [2]. However, precursor BLL/L is readily distinguished from Burkitt lymphoma and leukemia by the expression of the blastic markers CD34 and TdT and a lack of bcl-6 [2]. In contrast to Burkitt lymphoma and leukemia, kappa and lambda surface immunoglobulins are most often negative [2]. In the event of a complicated case of BLL/L where TdT is underexpressed, genetic studies may be useful; the *c-myc* abnormalities characteristic of Burkitt lymphoma and leukemia are not seen in precursor B cell lesions. Moreover, the finding of a BLL/L associated genetic abnormality such as t(9;22) (q34;q11.2), MLL rearranged t(v;11q23), t(12;21)(p13;q22) and t(1;19)(q23;p13.3) allow for differentiation from Burkitt lymphoma and leukemia [2]. T-lymphoblastic leukemia/lymphoma (TLL/L, formerly precursor T acute lymphoblastic leukemia) is distinguished by a lack of B-cell markers, positive staining with TdT, CD34, and variable expression of CD99, CD1a and pan T-cell antigens including CD2, CD3, CD5, CD7 [2].

A plasmacytoid variant of Burkitt lymphoma with eccentric nuclei and prominent central nucleoli has been described. This morphologic variant is seen more commonly in immunocompromised patients and shares an epidemiologic overlap with immunodeficiency-related Burkitt lymphoma [3, 54]. Plasmablastic lymphoma (PL) is a rare disease with a high incidence in HIV-positive males, but may also occur in other immunodeficiency states [2, 64]. PLs may demonstrate frequent mitotic figures, apoptotic cells, and tingible body macrophages, although the number of macrophages is usually less than DLBCL [65]. PLs can be differentiated from Burkitt lymphoma and leukemia by their plasma cell phenotype. They are positive for CD138 and IRF4/MUM1 and negative for CD20 [2]. The opposite staining profile is characteristic in Burkitt lymphoma and leukemia [2, 53].

B-Cell Lymphoma, Unclassifiable, with Features Intermediate Between Diffuse Large B-Cell Lymphoma and Burkitt Lymphoma

A diagnostic dilemma arises when a B cell lymphoma has features of both DLBCL and Burkitt lymphoma/leukemia. Several challenging case scenarios have emerged and include cases that resemble Burkitt lymphoma and leukemia morphologically, yet demonstrate strong bcl-2 positivity and cases that have a phenotype suggestive of Burkitt lymphoma and leukemia (CD10+, BCL6+, BCL2−, IRF4/MUM1−, Ki-67+ in 95–100% of cells) but have more variation in the size and shape of malignant cells [2, 56]. Diagnostic overlap has led to several names for these entities, including undifferentiated non-Burkitt lymphoma, atypical Burkitt lymphoma, and Burkitt-like lymphoma [2, 3, 56]. The 2008 WHO has categorized these tumors as "B-cell lymphoma, unclassifiable, with features intermediate between diffuse large B-cell lymphoma and Burkitt lymphoma" until their clinical, phenotypic, and molecular features are further characterized [2]. These neoplasms are aggressive, present predominantly in adults, and are generally treatment-resistant [51, 66]. Patients often present with widespread extranodal disease without preferential ileocecal or jaw involvement and frequent CNS and peripheral blood involvement [2, 66]. Tumors in the unclassifiable category have Ig-*myc* translocations and non-Ig-*myc* tranlocations. Approximately 15% of these cases have a concurrent bcl-2 translocation and have been characterized as "double hit lymphomas" [66, 67]. Many were likely characterized previously as Burkitt-like lymphoma. Bcl-6 translocations may also be present with *c-myc* and/or bcl-2; these are the "triple hit lymphomas" [2, 65, 66]. Overall, the presence of additional cytogenetic abnormalities such as bcl-2 and bcl-6 gene rearrangements argues in favor of an aggressive DLBCL with an unfavorable prognosis. Aggressive large cell lymphomas with a sole *c-myc* rearrangement and a lower Ki-67 proliferative fraction (40–80%) should be diagnosed as DLBCL and not considered an unclassifiable tumor [2]. Moreover, an otherwise morphologically classic Burkitt lymphoma with a Ki-67 proliferative fraction of 95–100% but without a FISH-detectable *c-myc* translocation should be considered a Burkitt lymphoma and not an unclassifiable tumor [2].

Gene expression analysis has been used to characterize aggressive large cell lymphomas including Burkitt lymphoma and leukemia, DLBCL and intermediate tumors. Hummel et al. generated a standard Burkitt molecular gene expression signature using Affymetrix U133AA GeneChips on eight core Burkitt lymphoma cases [51]. Gene expression and FISH profiles of 208 aggressive mature B cell lymphomas indicated that patients with tumors having a molecular Burkitt signature (mBL) and "myc-simple" (presence of Ig-*myc* by FISH and low chromosomal complexity by array CGH) genetic profile had a higher overall survival (OS) compared to a non-Burkitt molecular signature (non-mBL). Multivariate analysis in this study, however, failed to show a clear survival benefit in the mBL group independent of patient age. Interestingly, of the 44 mBL cases analyzed, 25% had the morphology of DLBCL and 21% were positive for bcl-2, lending a molecular basis for the broad Burkitt lymphoma morphologic spectrum. In another genomic profiling study, Dave et al. found that among 28 adults and children with a typical Burkitt lymphoma gene expression profile, survival was markedly higher in the group that received intensive chemotherapy regimens compared to the group receiving CHOP (cyclophosphamide, doxorubicin, vinristine, prednisone)-like regimens [50]. It is important to note that the control cases (usually pediatric, and few in number) selected to serve as a "gold standard" for the generation of molecular Burkitt signatures are chosen based on consensus diagnoses rendered by a group of pathologists who used preselected (usually WHO) criteria [50, 53]. It is difficult to ascertain which analysis – morphologic, immunophenotypic, and genetic versus molecular – is truly correct. Regardless, the utility of gene expression analysis in the diagnosis of Burkitt lymphoma and leukemia will continue to increase with subsequent morphologic, immunophenotypic, and genetic validation. Future gene expression studies focusing on the relationship between molecular signature and treatment-based outcomes in patients with intermediate lymphomas will likely allow for more optimal classification and more effective therapies for patients with these diagnostically challenging tumors.

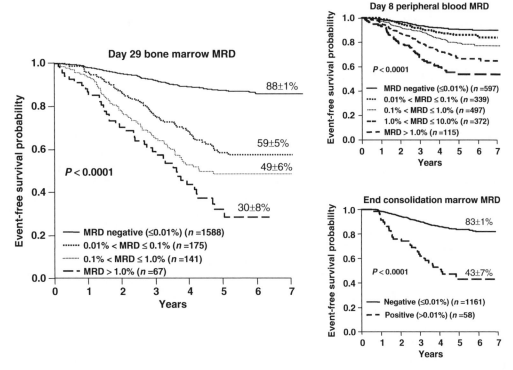

Fig. 4.4 EFS in childhood ALL dependent on MRD level. Nearly 2000 children with ALL had MRD quantitatively measured at three time points by flow cytometry. Day 8 peripheral blood for early response, day 29 at the end of induction, and at the end of consolidation to look for persistent MRD. Five year EFS were calculated based on MRD levels. This research was originally published in [68] (© The American Society of Hematology)

tion) also had strong prognostic ability with 83% and 47% year EFS for patients with MRD less than or greater than 10^{-4}, respectively (Fig. 4.4) [68]. Importantly, the duration of persistent MRD positivity correlates with progressively worse outcome, as a St. Jude's study found that positive MRD at day 43 (week 6), week 14 and week 32 predicted declining RFS of 57%, 34%, and 14% respectively [64]. The AIEOP-BFM study showed that MRD positivity at day 78 (week 11) into therapy predicted particularly poor outcome in their cohort, with a 16% EFS [24].

Although all these studies followed the time course of MRD disappearance, to date only one study has critically evaluated reappearance of MRD after a period of negativity, and showed that it was possible to predict overt relapse far better than routine marrow morphology. In this study, 61% of patients who had MRD positivity at any level after initial molecular remission ultimately relapsed, compared to only 6% of patients who were persistently negative [73]. Interestingly, the median time between MRD positivity and overt relapse was 9.5 months. If this finding is confirmed, it suggests that there might be a window for intervening in patients after MRD recurs to try to prevent relapse.

It is important to note that most of the previously mentioned studies were performed in children. Data in adults are more limited but confirm the prognostic value of MRD. One sentinel study demonstrated not only the prognostic utility of MRD, but also showed that by looking both very early and very late in therapy, it was possible to identify patients with the very best and worst of outcomes. Adults with a day 11 MRD $<10^{-4}$ had a 100% RFS, whereas adults with persistent disease (week 16 $>10^{-4}$) had a dismal prognosis with only 6% RFS [66]. Thus, many different groups, using different PCR or flow-based methodologies, looking at children or adults, have found that at almost all time points, high MRD and particularly persistent MRD is predictive of very poor prognosis, and absence of MRD, particularly at very early time points, predicts excellent outcome. Moreover, when other prognostic factors are taken into consideration, MRD remains highly prognostic [68, 70].

In summary, MRD measurements have proven to be a significant step forward in the identification of ALL patients at low and high risk of relapse. It is now up to individual studies to determine which technology, time points, cutoffs, and interventions will be used.

Efforts to Incorporate MRD into Frontline ALL Trials

Based on the data above, it is generally felt that patients with who are free of MRD within the first 2 weeks of therapy are candidates for relatively low-intensity therapy, for whom questions relating to further treatment intensification are not warranted [29, 34, 71, 72, 74–76]. While de-intensification of therapy might be considered for these patients, this is more controversial because their good outcome at least in part depends upon the intensity of therapy they received. By contrast, there is more consensus that patients with high MRD at end of induction/consolidation require intensified therapies [29, 34, 71, 74, 75]. Although there is precedent that ALL patients with suboptimal response to induction therapy can be salvaged with augmented therapy [77], to date there are no studies which demonstrate that intensifying therapy in response to a high MRD can alter outcomes. Despite this, MRD now plays a pivotal role in the risk assignment in many ALL trials, with some trials using MRD as the primary mode of risk assignment to different treatment arms with only a few other high-risk prognostic factors adding to risk grouping [24]. In other studies, MRD is integrated with traditional prognostic factors such as age, white count, and cytogenetics to establish the best risk grouping. MRD has also been used in some specific high-risk groups, such as Ph+ ALL [78], intra-chromosomal amplification of chromosome 21 [79] and mature B ALL with t(8;14) [80] with the hope that it will add critical information to subgroups currently lacking discriminating prognostic factors.

One question which remains to be answered is whether MRD thresholds found to be prognostic with one treatment regimen, will have the same prognostic ability if the therapy is changed [81]. For example, if MRD values are validated on a 3-drug induction regimen which relies heavily on steroids, would the same MRD values be applicable on a 4-drug induction which also relies on anthracyclines? Importantly, it appears that MRD levels can change based on relatively minor changes in therapy. A mid-study change in the 3-drug induction therapy on POG 9900 was made because of a higher-than-expected induction mortality rate. The initial intrathecal methotrexate was changed to intrathecal cytarabine, and six doses of E. coli asparaginase were changed to a single dose of PEG-asparaginase. These subtle changes affected both day 8 peripheral blood MRD, by increasing the MRD+ subgroup by 17%, and day 29 bone marrow MRD, decreasing the MRD+ subgroup by 19% [82], which would significantly impact MRD-based risk stratification. This example reveals the potential complexity of comparisons across studies that use different therapies.

Applications of MRD Testing in Relapsed ALL

As in frontline studies, there is accumulating evidence to support MRD as an important prognostic factor in relapsed ALL. Indeed, several studies have shown that MRD positivity at the end of re-induction implies lack of chemosensitivity and predicts very poor outcome [83–87]. Similar to the frontline MRD reports, these studies use different patient populations, treatment regimens, technology, and thresholds to predict outcome, making direct comparison difficult. However, the correlation of MRD and outcome in these studies is very consistent.

There are also emerging data on the importance of MRD measurements in the transplant setting. When evaluating the quality of remission prior to stem cell transplant, it is clear that even low levels of detectable MRD are predictive of a higher rate of recurrence following transplant [88–92]. Given these results, pre-transplant measurement of MRD is now generally incorporated into transplant trials [93]. It is still controversial, however, whether patients with MRD prior to transplant should be treated with further conventional therapy in order to induce an MRD-negative remission, or whether MRD after re-induction merely identifies those patients destined to fail.

An intriguing question is whether MRD can be used as a surrogate for therapeutic efficacy. An advantage to MRD measurements is that they are available quickly, without having to wait for long-term outcome. Thus, in theory at least, the effectiveness of a novel therapeutic agent could potentially be assessed by looking at its effect on MRD. To validate such an approach, it is not merely sufficient to show that MRD correlates with outcome; it must also be shown that changes in therapy that affect MRD levels are in turn reflected in changes in outcome. As proof of principle, the COG is testing this in its studies of relapsed ALL. Patients with ALL are treated with three intensive blocks of re-induction therapy, and MRD is assessed after each block. Not surprisingly, MRD correlates with outcome [86]. In the next step, the novel agent epratuzumab is being added to the backbone therapy and its effect on both MRD and outcome will be assessed [94].

Factors Limiting the Use of MRD for Therapeutic Decisions

Given the accumulating evidence for the prognostic utility of MRD measurements in ALL, there is tremendous pressure to incorporate this new variable into therapeutic decision making. However, as discussed above, it is not clear exactly what results should be acted upon, or what actions would be most appropriate to improve patient outcome.

Further complicating the use of results are problems with standardization. In the case of PCR, standardization of techniques allows for replication of results and relatively high sensitivity regardless of where the assay is performed [18, 19], particularly as controls for sample variability and standardization of quantification methods are also employed. However, very few clinical molecular diagnostic labs can afford to synthesize the patient-specific reagents needed to perform these MRD assays. On the other hand, flow cytometry assays, while more widely available, are less well standardized. Although attempts have been made to standardize antibody panels and procedures among multiple institutions [38], data on inter-laboratory reproducibility are limited, and suggest that detection of MRD levels below 10^{-3} (0.1%) may not be reliable [44]. Because most key studies have been from single centralized laboratories [34, 68, 75], further inter-laboratory validation of flow-based MRD assessment is needed. For all these reasons, it is difficult to recommend an intervention based on MRD that should be considered standard of care outside of a clinical trial.

Conclusions

MRD is a powerful tool to identify ALL patients who are at high or low risk of relapse. In spite of the differences in technology used to measure MRD, and the treatment protocols used in different studies, MRD is consistently found to be among the strongest prognostic factors. Many clinical trials in ALL, especially in children, now use measurements of MRD to stratify patients into different risk groups requiring different therapy. However, the impact of MRD-based risk stratification is still unknown, because it is not yet known whether poor risk patients can be rescued with more intensive therapy, or if better risk patients can safely be given less intensive therapy. No single best method to measure or employ MRD has yet emerged from clinical trials, and much more work is needed before standardized MRD measurements are widely available in the routine laboratory. Nevertheless, as therapy evolves to be tailored more to the needs of individual patients, it is clear that MRD will be an important tool used to help direct patient-specific therapy.

References

1. Pieters, R., & Carroll, W. L. (2008). Biology and treatment of acute lymphoblastic leukemia. *Pediatric Clinics of North America, 55*, 1–20. ix.
2. Lamanna, N., & Weiss, M. (2004). Treatment options for newly diagnosed patients with adult acute lymphoblastic leukemia. *Current Hematology Reports, 3*, 40–46.
3. Thomas, X., & Le, Q. H. (2003). Prognostic factors in adult acute lymphoblastic leukemia. *Hematology, 8*, 233–242.
4. Litzow, M. R. (2000). Acute lymphoblastic leukemia in adults. *Current Treatment Options in Oncology, 1*, 19–29.
5. Kantarjian, H. M., O'Brien, S., Smith, T. L., et al. (2000). Results of treatment with hyper-CVAD, a dose-intensive regimen, in adult acute lymphocytic leukemia. *Journal of Clinical Oncology, 18*, 547–561.
6. van Dongen, J. J., Macintyre, E. A., Gabert, J. A., et al. (1999). Standardized RT-PCR analysis of fusion gene transcripts from chromosome aberrations in acute leukemia for detection of minimal residual disease. Report of the BIOMED-1 Concerted Action: Investigation of minimal residual disease in acute leukemia. *Leukemia, 13*, 1901–1928.
7. Gabert, J., Beillard, E., van der Velden, V. H., et al. (2003). Standardization and quality control studies of 'real-time' quantitative reverse transcriptase polymerase chain reaction of fusion gene transcripts for residual disease detection in leukemia – A Europe against cancer program. *Leukemia, 17*, 2318–2357.
8. Beillard, E., Pallisgaard, N., van der Velden, V. H., et al. (2003). Evaluation of candidate control genes for diagnosis and residual disease detection in leukemic patients using 'real-time' quantitative reverse-transcriptase polymerase chain reaction (RQ-PCR) – A Europe against cancer program. *Leukemia, 17*, 2474–2486.
9. Breit, T. M., Wolvers-Tettero, I. L., Hahlen, K., van Wering, E. R., & van Dongen, J. J. (1991). Extensive junctional diversity of gamma delta T-cell receptors expressed by T-cell acute lymphoblastic leukemias: Implications for the detection of minimal residual disease. *Leukemia, 5*, 1076–1086.
10. van Dongen, J. J., Breit, T. M., Adriaansen, H. J., Beishuizen, A., & Hooijkaas, H. (1992). Detection of minimal residual disease in acute leukemia by immunological marker analysis and polymerase chain reaction. *Leukemia, 6*(Suppl 1), 47–59.
11. Beishuizen, A., Verhoeven, M. A., van Wering, E. R., Hahlen, K., Hooijkaas, H., & van Dongen, J. J. (1994). Analysis of Ig and T-cell receptor genes in 40 childhood acute lymphoblastic leukemias at diagnosis and subsequent relapse: Implications for the detection of minimal residual disease by polymerase chain reaction analysis. *Blood, 83*, 2238–2247.
12. van Dongen, J. J., Szczepanski, T., de Bruijn, M. A., et al. (1996). Detection of minimal residual disease in acute leukemia patients. *Cytokines and Molecular Therapy, 2*, 121–133.
13. Szczepanski, T., Langerak, A. W., Wolvers-Tettero, I. L., et al. (1998). Immunoglobulin and T cell receptor gene rearrangement patterns in acute lymphoblastic leukemia are less mature in adults than in children: Implications for selection of PCR targets for detection of minimal residual disease. *Leukemia, 12*, 1081–1088.
14. Pongers-Willemse, M. J., Verhagen, O. J., Tibbe, G. J., et al. (1998). Real-time quantitative PCR for the detection of minimal residual disease in acute lymphoblastic leukemia using junctional region specific TaqMan probes. *Leukemia, 12*, 2006–2014.
15. Szczepanski, T., Beishuizen, A., Pongers-Willemse, M. J., et al. (1999). Cross-lineage T cell receptor gene rearrangements occur in more than ninety percent of childhood precursor-B acute lymphoblastic leukemias: Alternative PCR targets for detection of minimal residual disease. *Leukemia, 13*, 196–205.
16. Pongers-Willemse, M. J., Seriu, T., Stolz, F., et al. (1999). Primers and protocols for standardized detection of minimal residual disease in acute lymphoblastic leukemia using immunoglobulin and T cell receptor gene rearrangements and TAL1 deletions as PCR targets: Report of the BIOMED-1 CONCERTED ACTION: Investigation of minimal residual disease in acute leukemia. *Leukemia, 13*, 110–118.
17. van der Velden, V. H., Hochhaus, A., Cazzaniga, G., Szczepanski, T., Gabert, J., & van Dongen, J. J. (2003). Detection of minimal residual disease in hematologic malignancies by real-time quantitative PCR: Principles, approaches, and laboratory aspects. *Leukemia, 17*, 1013–1034.
18. van der Velden, V. H., Cazzaniga, G., Schrauder, A., et al. (2007). Analysis of minimal residual disease by Ig/TCR gene rearrangements: Guidelines for interpretation of real-time quantitative PCR data. *Leukemia, 21*, 604–611.
19. van der Velden, V. H., Panzer-Grumayer, E. R., Cazzaniga, G., et al. (2007). Optimization of PCR-based minimal residual disease diagnostics for childhood acute lymphoblastic leukemia in a multi-center setting. *Leukemia, 21*, 706–713.
20. van Dongen, J. J., Langerak, A. W., Bruggemann, M., et al. (2003). Design and standardization of PCR primers and protocols for detection of clonal immunoglobulin and T-cell receptor gene recombinations in suspect lymphoproliferations: Report of the BIOMED-2 Concerted Action BMH4-CT98-3936. *Leukemia, 17*, 2257–2317.
21. Szczepanski, T., Langerak, A. W., Willemse, M. J., Wolvers-Tettero, I. L., van Wering, E. R., & van Dongen, J. J. (2000). T cell receptor gamma (TCRG) gene rearrangements in T cell acute lymphoblastic leukemia reflect 'end-stage' recombinations: Implications for minimal residual disease monitoring. *Leukemia, 14*, 1208–1214.

22. Bruggemann, M., van der Velden, V. H., Raff, T., et al. (2004). Rearranged T-cell receptor beta genes represent powerful targets for quantification of minimal residual disease in childhood and adult T-cell acute lymphoblastic leukemia. *Leukemia, 18,* 709–719.
23. Scrideli, C. A., Queiroz, R. G., Kashima, S., Sankarankutty, B. O., & Tone, L. G. (2004). T cell receptor gamma (TCRG) gene rearrangements in Brazilian children with acute lymphoblastic leukemia: Analysis and implications for the study of minimal residual disease. *Leukemia Research, 28,* 267–273.
24. Flohr, T., Schrauder, A., Cazzaniga, G., et al. (2008). Minimal residual disease-directed risk stratification using real-time quantitative PCR analysis of immunoglobulin and T-cell receptor gene rearrangements in the international multicenter trial AIEOP-BFM ALL 2000 for childhood acute lymphoblastic leukemia. *Leukemia, 22,* 771–782.
25. Li, A., Goldwasser, M. A., Zhou, J., et al. (2005). Distinctive IGH gene segment usage and minimal residual disease detection in infant acute lymphoblastic leukaemias. *British Journal Haematology, 131,* 185–192.
26. van der Velden, V. H., Willemse, M. J., van der Schoot, C. E., Hahlen, K., van Wering, E. R., & van Dongen, J. J. (2002). Immunoglobulin kappa deleting element rearrangements in precursor-B acute lymphoblastic leukemia are stable targets for detection of minimal residual disease by real-time quantitative PCR. *Leukemia, 16,* 928–936.
27. van der Velden, V. H., de Bie, M., van Wering, E. R., & van Dongen, J. J. (2006). Immunoglobulin light chain gene rearrangements in precursor-B-acute lymphoblastic leukemia: Characteristics and applicability for the detection of minimal residual disease. *Haematologica, 91,* 679–682.
28. van der Velden, V. H., Bruggemann, M., Hoogeveen, P. G., et al. (2004). TCRB gene rearrangements in childhood and adult precursor-B-ALL: Frequency, applicability as MRD-PCR target, and stability between diagnosis and relapse. *Leukemia, 18,* 1971–1980.
29. van Dongen, J. J., Seriu, T., Panzer-Grumayer, E. R., et al. (1998). Prognostic value of minimal residual disease in acute lymphoblastic leukaemia in childhood. *Lancet, 352,* 1731–1738.
30. Guggemos, A., Eckert, C., Szczepanski, T., et al. (2003). Assessment of clonal stability of minimal residual disease targets between 1st and 2nd relapse of childhood precursor B-cell acute lymphoblastic leukemia. *Haematologica, 88,* 737–746.
31. Beishuizen, A., de Bruijn, M. A., Pongers-Willemse, M. J., et al. (1997). Heterogeneity in junctional regions of immunoglobulin kappa deleting element rearrangements in B cell leukemias: A new molecular target for detection of minimal residual disease. *Leukemia, 11,* 2200–2207.
32. Langerak, A. W., & van Dongen, J. J. (2006). Recombination in the human IGK locus. *Critical Reviews in Immunology, 26,* 23–42.
33. Dworzak, M. N., Fritsch, G., Panzer-Grumayer, E. R., Mann, G., & Gadner, H. (2000). Detection of residual disease in pediatric B-cell precursor acute lymphoblastic leukemia by comparative phenotype mapping: Method and significance. *Leukaemia & Lymphoma, 38,* 295–308.
34. Coustan-Smith, E., Behm, F. G., Sanchez, J., et al. (1998). Immunological detection of minimal residual disease in children with acute lymphoblastic leukaemia. *Lancet, 351,* 550–554.
35. Vidriales, M. B., Orfao, A., & San-Miguel, J. F. (2003). Immunologic monitoring in adults with acute lymphoblastic leukemia. *Current Oncology Reports, 5,* 413–418.
36. Lucio, P., Parreira, A., van den Beemd, M. W., et al. (1999). Flow cytometric analysis of normal B cell differentiation: A frame of reference for the detection of minimal residual disease in precursor-B-ALL. *Leukemia, 13,* 419–427.
37. Szczepanski, T., van der Velden, V. H., & van Dongen, J. J. (2006). Flow-cytometric immunophenotyping of normal and malignant lymphocytes. *Clinical Chemistry and Laboratory Medicine, 44,* 775–796.
38. Lucio, P., Gaipa, G., van Lochem, E. G., et al. (2001). BIOMED-I concerted action report: Flow cytometric immunophenotyping of precursor B-ALL with standardized triple-stainings. BIOMED-1 Concerted Action Investigation of Minimal Residual Disease in Acute Leukemia: International Standardization and Clinical Evaluation. *Leukemia, 15,* 1185–1192.
39. Porwit-MacDonald, A., Bjorklund, E., Lucio, P., et al. (2000). BIOMED-1 concerted action report: Flow cytometric characterization of CD7+ cell subsets in normal bone marrow as a basis for the diagnosis and follow-up of T cell acute lymphoblastic leukemia (T-ALL). *Leukemia, 14,* 816–825.
40. Borowitz, M. J., Pullen, D. J., Winick, N., Martin, P. L., Bowman, W. P., & Camitta, B. (2005). Comparison of diagnostic and relapse flow cytometry phenotypes in childhood acute lymphoblastic leukemia: Implications for residual disease detection: A report from the Children's Oncology Group. *Cytometry Part B: Clinical Cytometry, 68,* 18–24.
41. Veltroni, M., De Zen, L., Sanzari, M. C., et al. (2003). Expression of CD58 in normal, regenerating and leukemic bone marrow B cells: Implications for the detection of minimal residual disease in acute lymphocytic leukemia. *Haematologica, 88,* 1245–1252.
42. Digiuseppe, J. A., Fuller, S. G., & Borowitz, M. J. (2009). Overexpression of CD49f in precursor B-cell acute lymphoblastic leukemia: Potential usefulness in minimal residual disease detection. *Cytometry Part B: Clinical Cytometry, 76(2),* 150–155.
43. Dworzak, M. N., Froschl, G., Printz, D., et al. (2004). CD99 expression in T-lineage ALL: Implications for flow cytometric detection of minimal residual disease. *Leukemia, 18,* 703–708.

44. Dworzak, M. N., Gaipa, G., Ratei, R., et al. (2008). Standardization of flow cytometric minimal residual disease evaluation in acute lymphoblastic leukemia: Multicentric assessment is feasible. *Cytometry Part B: Clinical Cytometry, 74*, 331–340.
45. Gaipa, G., Basso, G., Maglia, O., et al. (2005). Drug-induced immunophenotypic modulation in childhood ALL: Implications for minimal residual disease detection. *Leukemia, 19*, 49–56.
46. van der Sluijs-Gelling, A. J., van der Velden, V. H., Roeffen, E. T., Veerman, A. J., & van Wering, E. R. (2005). Immunophenotypic modulation in childhood precursor-B-ALL can be mimicked in vitro and is related to the induction of cell death. *Leukemia, 19*, 1845–1847.
47. Gaipa, G., Basso, G., Aliprandi, S., et al. (2008). Prednisone induces immunophenotypic modulation of CD10 and CD34 in nonapoptotic B-cell precursor acute lymphoblastic leukemia cells. *Cytometry Part B: Clinical Cytometry, 74*, 150–155.
48. Roshal, M., Fromm, J., Winter, S., Dunsmore, K., & Wood, B. (2008). Precursor T cell acute lymphoblastic leukemia (T-ALL) blasts lose expression of markers of immaturity during chemotherapy: Implications for the detection of minimal residual disease. *Blood, 112*, 541.
49. Malec, M., van der Velden, V. H., Bjorklund, E., et al. (2004). Analysis of minimal residual disease in childhood acute lymphoblastic leukemia: Comparison between RQ-PCR analysis of Ig/TcR gene rearrangements and multicolor flow cytometric immunophenotyping. *Leukemia, 18*, 1630–1636.
50. Kerst, G., Kreyenberg, H., Roth, C., et al. (2005). Concurrent detection of minimal residual disease (MRD) in childhood acute lymphoblastic leukaemia by flow cytometry and real-time PCR. *British Journal Haematology, 128*, 774–782.
51. Neale, G. A., Coustan-Smith, E., Stow, P., et al. (2004). Comparative analysis of flow cytometry and polymerase chain reaction for the detection of minimal residual disease in childhood acute lymphoblastic leukemia. *Leukemia, 18*, 934–938.
52. Robillard, N., Cave, H., Mechinaud, F., et al. (2005). Four-color flow cytometry bypasses limitations of IG/TCR polymerase chain reaction for minimal residual disease detection in certain subsets of children with acute lymphoblastic leukemia. *Haematologica, 90*, 1516–1523.
53. Campana, D., & Coustan-Smith, E. (2002). Advances in the immunological monitoring of childhood acute lymphoblastic leukaemia. *Best Practice & Research. Clinical Haematology, 15*, 1–19.
54. Ryan, J., Quinn, F., Meunier, A., et al. (2009). Minimal residual disease detection in childhood acute lymphoblastic leukaemia patients at multiple time-points reveals high levels of concordance between molecular and immunophenotypic approaches. *British Journal of Haematology, 144*, 107–115.
55. Neale, G. A., Campana, D., & Pui, C. H. (2003). Minimal residual disease detection in acute lymphoblastic leukemia: Real improvement with the real-time quantitative PCR method? *Journal of Pediatric Hematology/Oncology, 25*, 100–102.
56. Pui, C. H., & Campana, D. (2000). New definition of remission in childhood acute lymphoblastic leukemia. *Leukemia, 14*, 783–785.
57. Szczepanski, T., Orfao, A., van der Velden, V. H., San Miguel, J. F., & van Dongen, J. J. (2001). Minimal residual disease in leukaemia patients. *The Lancet Oncology, 2*, 409–417.
58. Donadieu, J., & Hill, C. (2001). Early response to chemotherapy as a prognostic factor in childhood acute lymphoblastic leukaemia: A methodological review. *British Journal Haematology, 115*, 34–45.
59. Gokbuget, N., Kneba, M., Raff, T., et al. (2002). Risk-adapted treatment according to minimal residual disease in adult ALL. *Best Practice & Research. Clinical Haematology, 15*, 639–652.
60. Cazzaniga, G., Gaipa, G., Rossi, V., & Biondi, A. (2003). Minimal residual disease as a surrogate marker for risk assignment to ALL patients. *Reviews in Clinical and Experimental Hematology, 7*, 292–323.
61. van der Velden, V. H., Boeckx, N., van Wering, E. R., & van Dongen, J. J. (2004). Detection of minimal residual disease in acute leukemia. *Journal of Biological Regulators and Homeostatic Agents, 18*, 146–154.
62. Cazzaniga, G., Gaipa, G., Rossi, V., & Biondi, A. (2006). Monitoring of minimal residual disease in leukemia, advantages and pitfalls. *Annali Medici, 38*, 512–521.
63. Szczepanski, T. (2007). Why and how to quantify minimal residual disease in acute lymphoblastic leukemia? *Leukemia, 21*, 622–626.
64. Coustan-Smith, E., Sancho, J., Hancock, M. L., et al. (2000). Clinical importance of minimal residual disease in childhood acute lymphoblastic leukemia. *Blood, 96*, 2691–2696.
65. Coustan-Smith, E., Sancho, J., Hancock, M. L., et al. (2002). Use of peripheral blood instead of bone marrow to monitor residual disease in children with acute lymphoblastic leukemia. *Blood, 100*, 2399–2402.
66. Bruggemann, M., Raff, T., Flohr, T., et al. (2006). Clinical significance of minimal residual disease quantification in adult patients with standard-risk acute lymphoblastic leukemia. *Blood, 107*, 1116–1123.
67. Zhou, J., Goldwasser, M. A., Li, A., et al. (2007). Quantitative analysis of minimal residual disease predicts relapse in children with B-lineage acute lymphoblastic leukemia in DFCI ALL Consortium Protocol 95-01. *Blood, 110*, 1607–1611.

68. Borowitz, M. J., Devidas, M., Hunger, S. P., et al. (2008). Clinical significance of minimal residual disease in childhood acute lymphoblastic leukemia and its relationship to other prognostic factors: A Children's Oncology Group study. *Blood, 111*, 5477–5485.
69. Holowiecki, J., Krawczyk-Kulis, M., Giebel, S., et al. (2008). Status of minimal residual disease after induction predicts outcome in both standard and high-risk Ph-negative adult acute lymphoblastic leukaemia. The Polish Adult Leukemia Group ALL 4-2002 MRD Study. *British Journal of Haematology, 142*(2), 227–237.
70. Motwani, J., Jesson, J., Sturch, E., et al. (2009). Predictive value of flow cytometric minimal residual disease analysis in childhood acute lymphoblastic leukaemia at the end of remission induction therapy – results from a single UK centre. *British Journal of Haematology, 144*(1), 133–135.
71. Cave, H., van der Werff ten Bosch, J., Suciu, S., et al. (1998). Clinical significance of minimal residual disease in childhood acute lymphoblastic leukemia. European Organization for Research and Treatment of Cancer – Childhood Leukemia Cooperative Group. *The New England Journal of Medicine, 339*, 591–598.
72. Coustan-Smith, E., Sancho, J., Behm, F. G., et al. (2002). Prognostic importance of measuring early clearance of leukemic cells by flow cytometry in childhood acute lymphoblastic leukemia. *Blood, 100*, 52–58.
73. Raff, T., Gokbuget, N., Luschen, S., et al. (2007). Molecular relapse in adult standard-risk ALL patients detected by prospective MRD monitoring during and after maintenance treatment: Data from the GMALL 06/99 and 07/03 trials. *Blood, 109*, 910–915.
74. Nyvold, C., Madsen, H. O., Ryder, L. P., et al. (2002). Precise quantification of minimal residual disease at day 29 allows identification of children with acute lymphoblastic leukemia and an excellent outcome. *Blood, 99*, 1253–1258.
75. Dworzak, M. N., Froschl, G., Printz, D., et al. (2002). Prognostic significance and modalities of flow cytometric minimal residual disease detection in childhood acute lymphoblastic leukemia. *Blood, 99*, 1952–1958.
76. Panzer-Grumayer, E. R., Schneider, M., Panzer, S., Fasching, K., & Gadner, H. (2000). Rapid molecular response during early induction chemotherapy predicts a good outcome in childhood acute lymphoblastic leukemia. *Blood, 95*, 790–794.
77. Nachman, J. B., Sather, H. N., Sensel, M. G., et al. (1998). Augmented post-induction therapy for children with high-risk acute lymphoblastic leukemia and a slow response to initial therapy. *The New England Journal of Medicine, 338*, 1663–1671.
78. Cazzaniga, G., Lanciotti, M., Rossi, V., et al. (2002). Prospective molecular monitoring of BCR/ABL transcript in children with Ph+ acute lymphoblastic leukaemia unravels differences in treatment response. *British Journal Haematology, 119*, 445–453.
79. Attarbaschi, A., Mann, G., Panzer-Grumayer, R., et al. (2008). Minimal residual disease values discriminate between low and high relapse risk in children with B-cell precursor acute lymphoblastic leukemia and an intrachromosomal amplification of chromosome 21: The Austrian and German acute lymphoblastic leukemia Berlin-Frankfurt-Munster (ALL-BFM) trials. *Journal of Clinical Oncology, 26*, 3046–3050.
80. Mussolin, L., Pillon, M., Conter, V., et al. (2007). Prognostic role of minimal residual disease in mature B-cell acute lymphoblastic leukemia of childhood. *Journal of Clinical Oncology, 25*, 5254–5261.
81. Dworzak, M. N. (2001). Immunological detection of minimal residual disease in acute lymphoblastic leukemia. *Onkologie, 24*, 442–448.
82. Winick, N., Borowitz, M. J., Devidas, M., et al. (2006). Changes in delivery of standard chemotherapeutic agents during induction affect early Measures of Minimal Residual Disease (MRD): POG 9900 for patients with B-Precursor Low and Standard Risk ALL. *Blood, 108*, 643a.
83. Paganin, M., Zecca, M., Fabbri, G., et al. (2008). Minimal residual disease is an important predictive factor of outcome in children with relapsed 'high-risk' acute lymphoblastic leukemia. *Leukemia, 22*(12), 2193–2200.
84. Szczepanski, T., Flohr, T., van der Velden, V. H., Bartram, C. R., & van Dongen, J. J. (2002). Molecular monitoring of residual disease using antigen receptor genes in childhood acute lymphoblastic leukaemia. *Best Practice & Research. Clinical Haematology, 15*, 37–57.
85. Coustan-Smith, E., Gajjar, A., Hijiya, N., et al. (2004). Clinical significance of minimal residual disease in childhood acute lymphoblastic leukemia after first relapse. *Leukemia, 18*, 499–504.
86. Raetz, E. A., Borowitz, M. J., Devidas, M., et al. (2008). Reinduction platform for children with first marrow relapse of acute lymphoblastic Leukemia: A Children's Oncology Group study [corrected]. *Journal of Clinical Oncology, 26*, 3971–3978.
87. Eckert, C., Biondi, A., Seeger, K., et al. (2001). Prognostic value of minimal residual disease in relapsed childhood acute lymphoblastic leukaemia. *Lancet, 358*, 1239–1241.
88. Mehta, P. A., & Davies, S. M. (2007). Pre-transplant minimal residual disease in children with acute lymphoblastic leukemia. *Pediatric Blood & Cancer, 48*, 1–2.
89. Sramkova, L., Muzikova, K., Fronkova, E., et al. (2007). Detectable minimal residual disease before allogeneic hematopoietic stem cell transplantation predicts extremely poor prognosis in children with acute lymphoblastic leukemia. *Pediatric Blood & Cancer, 48*, 93–100.

90. Bader, P., Hancock, J., Kreyenberg, H., et al. (2002). Minimal residual disease (MRD) status prior to allogeneic stem cell transplantation is a powerful predictor for post-transplant outcome in children with ALL. *Leukemia, 16*, 1668–1672.
91. Spinelli, O., Peruta, B., Tosi, M., et al. (2007). Clearance of minimal residual disease after allogeneic stem cell transplantation and the prediction of the clinical outcome of adult patients with high-risk acute lymphoblastic leukemia. *Haematologica, 92*, 612–618.
92. Krejci, O., van der Velden, V. H., Bader, P., et al. (2003). Level of minimal residual disease prior to haematopoietic stem cell transplantation predicts prognosis in paediatric patients with acute lymphoblastic leukaemia: A report of the Pre-BMT MRD Study Group. *Bone Marrow Transplantation, 32*, 849–851.
93. Goulden, N., Bader, P., Van Der Velden, V., et al. (2003). Minimal residual disease prior to stem cell transplant for childhood acute lymphoblastic leukaemia. *British Journal Haematology, 122*, 24–29.
94. Raetz, E. A., Cairo, M. S., Borowitz, M. J., et al. (2008). Chemoimmunotherapy reinduction with epratuzumab in children with acute lymphoblastic leukemia in marrow relapse: A Children's Oncology Group Pilot study. *Journal of Clinical Oncology, 26*, 3756–3762.

Clinical Presentation of Burkitt Lymphoma and Leukemia

Burkitt Lymphoma

Disease-related symptoms may be due to both the lymphomatous and leukemic aspects of the disease. Unique clinical characteristics have been described in each of the three disease variants – endemic, sporadic, and immunodeficiency-related, although overlap between clinical presentations may certainly exist. The endemic form most commonly occurs in children in equatorial Africa in children, where jaw and facial bone involvement are present in about 50% of patients [1]. Organs less commonly involved include the ileum and cecum, long bones, gonads, kidneys, salivary glands, and breasts [68]. Sporadic presentations, in which jaw tumors are rare, are classically characterized by bulky abdominal lymphadenopathy and gastrointestinal tract involvement (Fig. 13.6) [69]. Breast involvement may also occur, classically during pregnancy or puberty, and tumor cells have been shown to express prolactin receptors [70]. Lymph node involvement is seen more commonly in adults compared with children [2].

Immunodeficiency-related disease is most typically seen in patients with HIV infection. In contrast to opportunistic infections and other malignancies, however, the risk of Burkitt lymphoma development does not correlate with declining CD4 count [11], and the disease has been noted more

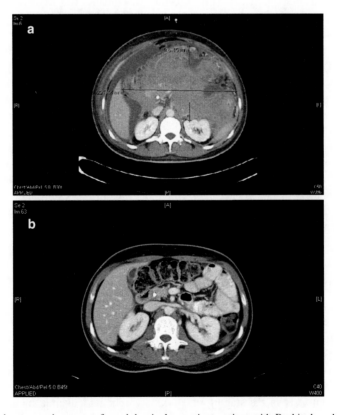

Fig. 13.6 Computed tomography scans of an abdominal mass in a patient with Burkitt lymphoma. (**a**) Computed tomography scan of a 43-year-old man presenting with 3 weeks of abdominal pain and severe fatigue and diagnosed with Burkitt lymphoma. (**b**) Computed tomography scan of the same patient following 2 cycles (of 4 planned) on a clinical trial at Northwestern University adding high-dose rituximab to the Magrath regimen.

commonly in those patients with CD4 counts greater than 200 cells/μL [71]. Like the sporadic variant, immunodeficiency-related Burkitt lymphoma is associated with bulky abdominal masses, precipitating symptoms such as abdominal pain, nausea, vomiting, and gastrointestinal bleeding. Due to the tumor's high proliferative rate, highly elevated lactate dehydrogenase (LDH) levels and uric acid levels are frequently seen.

The CNS is a known sanctuary site in all Burkitt lymphoma subtypes. A recent study by Salzburg et al. that included 1,092 children and adolescents (median age 9.37 years) demonstrated that 8.8% had CNS involvement at diagnosis, a prevalence more than twice that of CNS disease in other NHLs in the group studied (mean 3.6%, $p \leq 0.001$) [72]. Up to 40% of adults, the highest rates being in immunodeficiency-associated Burkitt lymphoma, have leptomeningeal involvement at diagnosis [18, 53, 73].

Burkitt Leukemia

Bone marrow involvement has been reported in 16–70% of Burkitt lymphoma cases and is less commonly seen in endemic Burkitt lymphoma [18, 74, 75]. Immunodeficiency-related Burkitt lymphoma has a high incidence of bone marrow and lymph node involvement, which is related to high tumor burden and the frequent occurrence of widely disseminated disease at presentation [71, 73]. Rarely, patients (mostly male) present with an acute leukemic picture, often with concomitant fever, anemia, bleeding, and adenopathy [2]. This leukemic presentation was referred to as acute lymphocytic leukemia (ALL-L3) in the morphology-based FAB Cooperative Group classification [5, 76]. The leukemic phase of Burkitt lymphoma is now classified as Burkitt lymphoma/leukemia or Burkitt leukemia variant in the 2008 WHO Classification of Tumors of Haematopoietic and Lymphoid Tissues [2]. The somatic mutations present in immunoglobulin heavy genes of ALL-L3 provided the molecular evidence supporting an assignment of this entity to Burkitt lymphoma/leukemia rather than to precursor B-lineage ALL [77]. Currently, no significant morphologic, immunophenotypic, or genetic features distinguish malignant cells in tissue-based Burkitt lymphoma and Burkitt leukemia variants.

Compared to the number of patients with a clinical picture most consistent with Burkitt lymphoma, fewer patients present strictly with Burkitt leukemia. An analysis of patients enrolled in a clinical trial of the hyper-CVAD regimen, described below, for Burkitt leukemia showed that approximately 40% had CNS leukemic involvement, 54% exhibited extramedullary disease outside of the CNS, 31% had gastrointestinal involvement, 77% had thrombocytopenia (platelets < 100 × 10^9/L), and 65% had peripheral blasts.

Staging Systems

The Ann Arbor system is most commonly used for disease staging (Table 13.2) [78]. Alternatively, the St. Jude or Murphy staging system has also been used and, notably, differs from the Ann Arbor system in its more nuanced delineation of extranodal disease (Table 13.3) [79], its classification of Burkitt leukemia as a separate disease entity, and the role of surgical resectability in some of the stage classifications. It is important to note that surgery is a rarely used treatment approach in Burkitt lymphoma. Important tests in the staging of Burkitt lymphoma/leukemia include body computed tomography scans, bone marrow biopsy, PPD with anergy panel, lumbar puncture with CSF analysis, and assessment of ejection fraction, the latter in anticipation of anthracycline-based chemotherapy [80]. There should also be consideration for evaluation of hepatitis B virus (HBV) and hepatitis C

Table 13.2 Cottswolds modification of Ann Arbor staging system [78]

Stage	Area of involvement
I	One lymph node area
II	Multiple lymph node groups on the same side of the diaphragm
III	Multiple lymph node groups on both sides of the diaphragm
IV	Multiple extranodal sites or lymph nodes and extranodal disease
X	Bulk > 10 cm
E	Extranodal extension or single extranodal site
A/B	B symptoms: weight loss > 10%, drenching night sweats, fever

Table 13.3 St. Jude (Murphy) staging system [79]

Stage	Areas of involvement
I	A single tumor (extranodal) or single anatomic area (nodal) with the exclusion of mediastinum or abdomen
II	A single tumor (extranodal) with regional node involvement
	Two or more nodal areas on the same side of the diaphragm
	Two single (extranodal) tumors with or without regional node on the same side of the diaphragm
	A primary gastrointestinal tract tumor with or without mesenteric nodes, grossly and completely excised
III	Two single tumors (extranodal) on opposite sides of the diaphragm
	Two or more nodal areas above and below the diaphragm
	All of the primary intrathoracic tumors (mediastinal, pleural, thymic)
	All extensive primary intraabdominal disease
	All paraspinal or epidural tumors, regardless of the other tumor site(s)
IV	Any of the above with initial central nervous system and/or bone marrow involvement (<25% malignant cells)

virus (HCV) status, especially in patients with risk factors. Patients who are chronic carriers of HBV (i.e., HBV surface antigen (HBsAg) positive) and possibly also patients with prior hepatitis B infection (i.e., HBV core antibody (anti-HBc) positive), should receive empiric HBV prophylactic therapy (e.g., lamivudine 100 mg PO daily) throughout chemotherapy in order to prevent HBV reactivation, which can be fatal [81, 82]. Dental evaluation for identification of possible occult infectious site should also be considered prior to start of chemotherapy. Positron emission tomography (PET) scan may also be considered; PET may be especially helpful in identification of extranodal disease sites as well as for the accurate assessment of disease response for bulky disease.

Treatment: Newly-Diagnosed Disease

Significant advances have been made in the treatment of Burkitt lymphoma and leukemia with contemporary chemotherapeutic regimens yielding long-term disease-free survival (DFS) and OS rates over 60–70% for patients less than 50–60 years of age. The outcomes for older patients are less robust. Many of the early pivotal Burkitt lymphoma studies were from pediatric populations. While many non-Hodgkin lymphoma treatment protocols utilize moderately-dosed chemotherapeutics given over a prolonged period, much of the improvement in Burkitt lymphoma and leukemia outcomes has stemmed from the use of shorter duration, dose-intensive therapeutic schedules. This approach hypothetically weakens the tumor cells' ability to reenter the cell cycle, replicate rapidly, and develop resistance mechanisms during breaks in treatment. In addition, given the propensity of Burkitt lymphoma and leukemia to involve the CNS, aggressive CNS prophylaxis/treatment has been important in improving outcomes. Patients with proven CNS involvement at diagnosis receive aggressive CNS treatment, typically with intrathecal chemotherapy, while even patients with no evidence of CNS disease at diagnosis still receive scheduled/repeated prophylactic intrathecal chemotherapy.

Pediatric Studies

Initial treatments in the 1970s in children included single-agent cyclophosphamide with response rates of approximately 80% [83]. Most children eventually relapsed, however, with systemic or CNS disease. Subsequent regimens employed combinations such as cyclophosphamide, vincristine, methotrexate, and prednisone [84], with higher response rates and longer remission intervals. Among patients with advanced Burkitt lymphoma, clinical trials in the 1970s demonstrated long-term survival rates of only 30–40%, similar to those found in prior African studies [85].

The use of short duration, dose-intense regimens alternating non-cross-resistant agents in pediatric studies yielded a dramatic improvement in outcomes. Murphy et al. devised a novel regimen incorporating four courses of fractionated cyclophosphamide, doxorubicin, vincristine, intrathecal methotrexate, and cytarabine (regimen A) alternating with systemic continuous infusion methotrexate and cytarabine with intrathecal methotrexate and cytarabine (regimen B) [86]. Twenty-nine consecutive patients at St. Jude Children's Research Hospital with stage III ($n = 17$) or IV ($n = 4$) Burkitt lymphoma or B cell ALL ($n = 8$) were enrolled onto this protocol between 1981 and 1985. Ninety-three percent of patients achieved a complete response (CR), one of which required a course of involved-field radiotherapy to a residual abdominal mass. After 2 years, 81% of patients with stage III disease were estimated to be in continuous CR. Outcomes for patients with stage IV Burkitt lymphoma or B cell ALL were poor, with only one of three stage IV patients and one of seven ALL patients who had achieved a remission remaining alive as of January 1986. This regimen formed the backbone of what is known today as hyper-CVAD/MA, which has been explored in subsequent studies as described below. Subsequently, Bowman et al. modified this regimen in a phase II trial in an attempt to improve outcomes, changing the continuous infusion cytarabine of course B to four bolus doses administered 12 h apart and intensifying the intrathecal chemotherapy [87]. The study evaluated 133 patients with L3 B-ALL or stage IV small non-cleaved-cell lymphoma (SNCCL). CR was achieved in 93% of patients. The 4-year event-free survival (EFS) was 65% among patients with L3 B-ALL and approximately 80% for those with stage IV SNCCL and approximately 65% among those with initial CNS involvement. Significant cytopenias were a major treatment toxicity with febrile neutropenia complicating 40% of all treatment phases. Five deaths were due to infection. Due to these toxicities, the protocol was amended in the middle of enrollment to omit the fourth cycle of treatment.

Schwenn et al. conducted a pilot trial of 20 children treated with the HiC-COM regimen, a 2-month course of cyclophosphamide, high-dose methotrexate, high-dose cytarabine, and vincristine with intrathecal chemotherapy [88]. The CR rate was 95% with a 2-year EFS rate of 75%. Similar results were reported by the Berlin-Frankfurt-Munster (BFM) group in a pooled analysis of three separate studies (BFM 81, 83, and 86) evaluating 87 children with L3 ALL or Burkitt lymphoma [89]. Therapy in each of the three separate trials consisted of a cytoreductive prephase consisting of predisone and cyclophosphamide followed by varying combinations of systemic methotrexate, teniposide, cytarabine, doxorubicin, ifosfamide, and intrathecal therapy with methotrexate and/or cytarabine. CNS irradiation was included in BFM 81 and 83. The complete response rate was 82% among all 87 patients in the three studies. Twenty-four patients relapsed. Among patients in the BFM 86 study, 5-year EFS was 78%, a significant improvement over the results seen in the BFM 81 and 83 studies.

Table 5.3 Summary of the main symbols used in the International System for Human Cytogenetic Nomenclature (ISCN) 2005

Symbol	Definition
comma (,)	Separates different elements of the karyotype
cp	Composite karyotype
del	Deletion
der	Derived
dic	Dicentric
dmin	Double minute
dup	Duplication
i	Isochromosome
idem	Denotes stemline karyotype in a sub-clone
idic	Isodicentric chromosome
ins	Insertion
inv	Inversion
ish	In situ hybridization
mar	Marker chromosome
minus sign (−)	Loss of a chromosome
p	Short arm of chromosome
plus sign (+)	Gain of a chromosome
q	Long arm of chromosome
r	Ring chromosome
semicolon (;)	Separates translocated chromosomes or their breakpoints
slash (/)	Separate different clones or sub-clones
square brackets ([])	Number of analyzed cells
t	Translocation
ter	Terminal end of a chromosome

of chromosome 6 resulting in loss of material distal to the breakpoint q21, (2) gain of a normal chromosome 8, and (3) a balanced reciprocal translocation between the long arms of chromosomes 9 and 22, resulting in exchange of material distal to the breakpoints q34 and q11, respectively. In situations where the analysis reveals multiple cell lines, the simplest abnormal cell line is written first, and each cell line is separated by a forward slant. For example, 46,XY,del(6)(q21),t(9;22)(q34;q11) [10]/46,XY[10]. Table 5.3 lists some of the common abbreviations used in cancer cytogenetics.

Fluorescence In Situ Hybridization

Fluorescence in situ hybridization (FISH) is the examination of chromosomes, chromosome sections, or genes by the application of fluorescently labeled DNA probes visualized by fluorescence microscopy. The main types of FISH are listed in Table 5.1 in comparison with cytogenetics and other molecular techniques. There are two main types of probes: whole chromosome paints and locus-specific probes.

Whole chromosome paints are libraries of probes specific for an individual chromosome or chromosomal region. They may be hybridized separately or in pairs for the detection of structural chromosomal abnormalities. Chromosome painting relies on the presence of metaphases and is usually used in association with conventional cytogenetic analysis. Multiplex FISH (M-FISH) uses a mixture of 24 whole chromosome paints probes, each labeled with different combinations of up to three of the fluorochromes: spectrum gold, spectrum red, spectrum far red, spectrum aqua, and spectrum green. Each of the 22 autosomes and the two sex chromosomes can be simultaneously identified in 24 discrete colors generated by sophisticated computer software. It allows for the detection of subtle and complex chromosomal rearrangements, and the identification of marker chromosomes in fixed metaphase spreads. M-FISH has a resolution similar to conventional cytogenetics.

Locus-specific probes target discrete sections of chromosomes, for example, centromeres, subtelomeric regions, or those with complementary DNA sequences, usually genes. The major advantage of locus-specific probes is that they detect abnormalities in interphase as well as metaphase cells and allow for rapid screening of cases. Centromeric probes target the alpha satellite sequences located within the centromeric regions of most chromosomes. They are used to enumerate chromosomes and determine aneuploidy. The human genome mapping project has led to an increased availability of sequence-specific FISH probes for diagnostic or research purposes. They are used to detect deletions, amplifications, and gene fusions. The design of the probe is crucial and depends on the type of abnormality. Deletions and amplifications are usually detected using differentially labeled probes (usually red and green), one to detect the change in copy number and the other to act as a control for the number of chromosomes. A relative change in the number of red and green signals observed indicates the presence of the abnormality. There are two types of probe for detecting gene fusions arising from translocations: fusion probes and break-apart probes. Fusion probes comprise differentially labeled probes that target the two genes involved at the chromosomal breakpoints and colocalize in the presence of the fusion, creating a fusion (yellow) signal. Break-apart probes comprise differentially labeled probes that flank a single gene. They separate into distinct red and green signals when the gene is involved in a rearrangement. Currently, there are numerous commercially available probes designed to detect the significant abnormalities found in acute leukemia. The accurate interpretation of FISH tests depends on an understanding of the probe design in conjunction with the conventional cytogenetics.

Chromosomal Abnormalities in Adult B-Cell Precursor ALL (BCP-ALL)

Table 5.4 lists the six principal cytogenetic subtypes seen in adult BCP-ALL along with the affected genes, incidence and prognosis.

t(9;22)(q34;q11.2)/BCR-ABL1/Philadelphia Chromosome

The translocation, t(9;22)(q34;q11.2), results in the fusion of the 5' part of the *BCR* gene (22q11) with virtually the whole of the *ABL1* gene (9q34). The resultant *BCR-ABL1* fusion gene, which is located on the derived chromosome 22 [der(22)t(9;22)], is a constitutively activated tyrosine kinase. The breakpoints in the *ABL1* gene are scattered across a large area but always upstream of exon 2, such that the resulting fusion transcript always includes exon 2–11 of the gene. The majority of *BCR* breakpoints cluster within the minor (m, exons 1–2) or major (M, exons 12–16) breakpoint regions

Table 5.4 Principal cytogenetic subtypes of adult B-cell precursor acute lymphoblastic leukemia

Chromosomal abnormality	Genes	Incidence (approximate)	Prognosis
t(1;19)(q23;p13)	*TCF3-PBX1*	5%	Standard/poor
t(4;11)(q21;q23)	*MLL-AF4*	5%	Poor
t(9;22)(q34;q11.2)	*BCR-ABL1*	20–25%	Poor
Low hypodiploidy/near triploidy (30–39/60–78 chromosomes)	Unknown	5%	Poor
High hyperdiploidy (51–65 chromosomes)	Unknown	10%	Standard/good
Complex karyotype	Unknown	5%	Poor

and result in differently sized protein products – p190 and p210, respectively. In adult ALL, around two-thirds of *BCR-ABL1* positive patients harbor the minor breakpoint, while the remaining third have the major breakpoint [6].

Although the t(9;22) represents the usual translocation for generating *BCR-ABL1*, rare insertions and three-way translocations have been reported, which are identical at the molecular level [7]. Additional cytogenetic abnormalities are detected in about two-thirds of patients with a t(9;22) [6, 8]. Secondary aberrations, including gain of an additional copy of the Philadelphia chromosome [+der(22)t(9;22)], high hyperdiploidy (51–65 chromosomes), monosomy 7, trisomy 8, gain of chromosome X and abnormalities of 9p, have each been reported in up to 30% of cases. However, a more detailed analysis using genome-wide SNP arrays revealed that deletions of *IKZF1*, which encodes Ikaros and is located on chromosome 7, occur in over 90% of adult ALL patients with t(9;22) [9]. These deletions are frequently monoallelic and exon-specific, resulting in reduced Ikaros expression and/or altered isoform expression. The same study revealed that just over 50% of these patients have deletions of *PAX5* and/or *CDKN2A*, both of which are located on the short arm of chromosome 9.

The t(9;22) is the most prevalent chromosomal abnormality in adult ALL present in 11–30% of patients [6, 10–13]. The incidence is strongly correlated with age, rising from 10% in adolescents (less than 20 years old) to 40% among older patients (more than 40 years old) [6, 10, 14]. Therefore, the variation in overall incidence is probably due to differences in the age distribution of patient cohorts. However, geographic heterogeneity in the incidence of this abnormality has been suggested and remains a possibility [15]. Patients with t(9;22) have a higher white cell count compared to those without the translocation and most leukemic blasts are CD10+. Patients with t(9;22) rarely have T-cell disease, although isolated cases have been reported. Regardless of treatment, the outcome of patients with t(9;22) is significantly worse than patients without this abnormality, even after adjustment for the effects of older age and high white cell count [6, 10–13]. However, the advent of targeted therapy for these patients through the discovery of potent tyrosine kinase inhibitors (e.g. imatinib and dasatinib) shows promise for an improved outlook for these patients (see Chap. 12).

Although the t(9;22) translocation is visible by conventional cytogenetics, given its clinical importance, many laboratories will routinely screen for *BCR-ABL1* using specific FISH probes or by RT-PCR. Such a strategy overcomes the issue of failed cytogenetics and will detect the small proportion of cases where *BCR-ABL1* fusion arises by cryptic insertions.

t(4;11)(q21;q23)/MLL-AF4 and Other 11q23/MLL Translocations

The *MLL* gene, located at 11q23, is known as a promiscuous gene because it forms chimeric fusions with numerous partner genes in all forms of acute leukemia [16]. Within the context of adult ALL, the most prevalent and important translocations are t(4;11)(q21;q23) and t(11;19)(q23;p13.3), which result in fusion of 5' *MLL* with 3' *AF4* or 3' *ENL*, respectively. The breakpoints within the *MLL* gene invariably cluster between exons 5 and 11 within an 8.3 kb region. The essential and pathogenic chimeric oncoprotein comprises the N terminal portion of *MLL* fused to the C terminal portion of the partner gene.

The majority (>75%) of *MLL* translocations in adult ALL are the t(4;11). It is usually observed as the sole genetic abnormality but around 10% harbor an additional X chromosome irrespective of sex [17]. This is an intriguing translocation as it occurs in over 40% of infants with ALL and in around 5% of adult ALL but rarely in childhood ALL [7]. Moreover, it is known to have in utero origins especially when associated with infant leukemia [18]. In adult ALL, patients with a t(4;11) are significantly older, have a higher white cell count, and almost all have a pro-B immunophenotype [6, 19]. Patients with t(4;11) have an inferior outcome with event-free survival rates of less than 25% being reported by recent studies [6, 19].

The second most important *MLL* translocation in adult ALL is t(11;19) which again usually occurs as the sole cytogenetic abnormality [20]. Patients harboring this translocation may present at any age and have pro-B, common or T-ALL [20]. However, they do tend to have higher white cell counts, like all patients harboring an *MLL* translocation [6, 20]. The prognosis of these patients is open to debate as their rarity has generally precluded separate analyses. A recent study, proposing a four tier risk stratification, classified patients with t(4;11) as very high risk and those with other *MLL* translocations as high risk [12].

Although most *MLL* translocations are readily detectable by conventional cytogenetics, some can evade detection especially if the chromosome morphology is poor. FISH using a commercially available dual-color break-apart MLL probe provides a simple and sensitive method for detecting all *MLL* translocations irrespective of the partner genes. If metaphases are present, then the partner chromosome can also be determined.

t(1;19)(q23;p13)/TCF3-PBX1

The translocation, t(1;19)(q23;p13), results in the fusion of the 5′ part of the *TCF3* (formerly known as *E2A*) (19p13) and the 3′ portion of the *PBX1* (1q23). This translocation occurs in two forms: as a balanced translocation – t(1;19) – and as an unbalanced translocation – der(19)t(1;19) – where only one of the derivative chromosomes is present. The crucial gene fusion – 5′*TCF3*–3′*PBX1* – resides on the der(19)t(1;19), hence there is no difference at the molecular level between the two forms. The der(19) t(1;19) is more common and accounts for 75% of cases [7]. While both forms of this abnormality are readily detectable by conventional cytogenetics, only about 90% will result in the *TCF3-PBX1* fusion [21]. Therefore, additional confirmation by FISH or RT-PCR is advisable. The *TCF3-PBX1* fusion is most likely to occur with the balanced form of the translocation [21]. Although other translocations involving *TCF3* have been reported, they are very rare and, to date, have only been observed in children [21].

The t(1;19) occurs in approximately 5% of adults with ALL and is the only major chromosomal abnormality to have an equivalent incidence among children and adults. Patients with this abnormality do not differ in terms of age, sex, or white cell count compared to other patients with ALL. However, virtually all t(1;19) patients have a pre-B immunophenotype and thus express cytoplasmic immunoglobulin. The outcome of adults with t(1;19) is open to some debate. Several small studies reported that they had a poor outcome compared to other patients [13, 19, 22], which led others to classify them as poor risk [12, 23, 24]. However, the largest and most recent study found that their outcome was equivalent to other Philadelphia-negative patients [6].

High Hyperdiploidy (51–65 Chromosomes)

A high hyperdiploid (HeH) clone is defined as one with a modal number of between 51 and 65 chromosomes resulting from the simultaneous gain of between 6 and 19 chromosomes. The process is not random, and chromosomes X, 4, 6, 10, 14, 17, 18, and 21 account for more than 75% of all gains [25]. Intriguingly a proportion of HeH cases will also harbor a t(9;22) translocation (see above). Although the profile of chromosome gains appears to be the same, most patients with t(9;22) and a HeH clone have trisomy of chromosome 2 (unpublished observations). Structural chromosomal abnormalities occur in around half of all HeH cases, with gain of the long arm of chromosome 1 (1q) being the most frequent aberration [25]. In addition to cytogenetically visible abnormalities, several mutations and submicroscopic deletions have been reported to occur in conjunction with high hyperdiploidy: *PAX5* deletions and mutations [26], *RAS* mutations [27], and *CDKN2A* deletion [28]. However, their precise frequency and clinical relevance in adult ALL has yet to be fully determined.

Although HeH is most commonly associated with childhood ALL, where it accounts for around a third of cases, HeH does occur in approximately 10% of adult ALL. However, even within adult ALL, it is associated with a younger age. A recent study showed that these adults with HeH had a median age of 27 years compared to 31 years for the rest of that Philadelphia negative cohort [6]. In accordance with the profile seen in childhood ALL, adults with HeH have a lower white cell count and are less likely to be T-ALL. Several studies have now reported that HeH is associated with a good outcome in adult ALL [6, 10, 12, 13, 19]. However, as HeH correlates with a younger age and lower white cell count, which are both linked to an improved outcome, it is difficult to assess whether or not its prognostic impact is truly independent of traditional risk factors.

Low Hypodiploidy (30–39 Chromosomes)/Near-Triploidy (60–78 Chromosomes)

A low hypodiploid (Ho) clone is defined as one with a modal number of between 30 and 39 chromosomes resulting from the simultaneous loss of between 7 and 16 chromosomes [29]. A particular feature of this type of leukemic clone is its propensity to "double-up" or evolve a subclone with double the number of chromosomes, i.e., a near-triploid clone with 60–78 chromosomes [29, 30]. Conventional cytogenetic analysis can reveal the presence of both the low hypodiploid clone and the near-triploid (Tr) clone or only one of them. However, DNA indexing of these cases always reveals the presence of both clones [30]. The same picture can be detected using a series of FISH probes specific for the centromeres of lost/gained chromosomes (unpublished observations). Therefore, it is now established that Ho and Tr represent a single cytogenetic entity that should be referred to as low hypodiploidy/near-triploidy (Ho-Tr). Moreover, these patients should be grouped together irrespective of which clone is visible by conventional cytogenetics [30]. The loss of chromosomes to generate a low hypodiploid clone is not a random process, and monosomies of chromosomes 2, 3, 4, 7, 13, 15, 16, and 17 are common. As a result, the profile of gained chromosomes in the near-triploidy phase is also nonrandom with tetrasomies of 1, 6, 11, 18, and 21 being most prevalent. Structural abnormalities are not common in this subgroup and no significance secondary aberration has yet emerged [29, 30].

Patients with Ho-Tr do not show any age or sex correlation although they have lower white cell counts and are less likely to be T-ALL [6, 30]. The incidence of Ho-Tr in adult ALL is around 5%. Patients with this abnormality have a significantly increased risk of relapse with 5-year EFS rates of less than 20% and should be regarded as high-risk patients [6, 30].

Based on chromosome number alone, karyotypes with 60–65 chromosomes may be classified as either HeH or Ho-Tr. Given the stark difference in prognosis between HeH and Ho-Tr, discriminating between the two is vital. Fortunately, the pattern of chromosome gains is usually sufficient to differentiate with confidence. In particular, Ho-Tr clones contain a number of tetrasomies, frequently chromosomes 1 and 11, which are rarely gained within the context of HeH. FISH with probes to the centromeres of selected chromosomes provides a useful method to discriminate between HeH and Ho-Tr or detect Ho-Tr among cases with failed or normal cytogenetics.

Complex Karyotype

The concept of a complex karyotype within acute myeloid leukemia (AML) is well established and has been defined variously as karyotypes with more than three or five chromosomal abnormalities. More recently, the definition has been restricted to karyotypes without an established chromosomal abnormality. Few studies have classified ALL karyotypes according to their complexity. The definition used within adult ALL is the presence of five or more chromosomal abnormalities in the absence of an established translocation or ploidy group, which applies to approximately 5% of adults [6]. Although this subgroup does not appear to be associated with age, sex, white cell count, or immunophenotype, it has been reported to indicate a significantly increased risk of relapse and death [6, 31].

Other Chromosomal Abnormalities

The cytogenetically cryptic translocation t(12;21)(p13;q22), which results in *ETV6-RUNX1* fusion (also known as *TEL-AML1*), is predominantly found among young children with ALL and requires FISH or RT-PCR for accurate detection. However, it has been described in a small number of younger adults and more rarely among those over the age of 40 [32, 33]. The *ETV6-RUNX1* fusion is known to arise in utero and give rise to a preleukemic clone, which requires additional abnormalities to transform into full-blown ALL [34]. Too few patients have been reported to accurately assess prognosis in adults.

Recently, a series of translocations involving the *IGH@* gene (14q32) have been reported to up regulate different genes in patients with BCP-ALL. While the juxtaposition of *IGH@* to oncogenes is a well-established mechanism of deregulated expression in mature B-ALL (see below) and lymphoma, it had been rarely described in BCP-ALL, probably due to the cryptic nature of many of the translocations. Five members of the *CEBP* transcription factor family have been shown to be overexpressed as a result of four different translocations involving the *IGH@* locus [35]. A cryptic translocation involving the pseudoautosomal region on the sex chromosomes, t(X;14)(p22;q32) and t(Y;14)(p11;q32), which causes overexpression of the type I cytokine receptor, *CRLF2*, has been reported [36]. Interestingly, *CRLF2* can also be over expressed via juxtaposition to the promoter of the *PR2Y8* gene which lies centromeric of *CRLF2* and occurs as the result of an interstitial deletion [36]. Two further translocations, t(6;14)(p22;q32) and t(14;19)(q32;p13), juxtapose the *ID4* and *EPOR* genes to the *IGH@* promoter causing their overexpression [37, 38]. While accurate incidences and clinical correlations for these translocations have yet to emerge, it is noteworthy that 75% of the reported patients are adolescents or young adults [35, 37, 38].

Many recurrent chromosomal abnormalities in adult ALL are secondary events, including deletions of 6q, 9p, 11q, and 17p. Their incidence varies according to the phenotype and the type of primary abnormality. The assessment of clinical correlations and prognostic relevance of such aberrations is difficult because it requires large datasets and multivariate analysis. Hence, there is little reliable literature available.

Chromosomal Abnormalities in Adult Mature-B ALL

Approximately 5% of adults with ALL have a mature-B immunophenotype and L3 morphology. The majority of these patients harbor a translocation involving the 8q24 locus where the *MYC* gene is located. The translocation results in the juxtaposition of the *MYC* gene to promoter sequences and enhancer elements of one of the immunoglobulin loci, resulting in its overexpression. The three translocations t(8;14)(q24;q32), t(8;22)(q24;q11), and t(2;8)(p11;q24), involving the *IGH@*, *IGL@*, and *IGK@* immunoglobulin loci, account for 85%, 10%, and 5% patients, respectively. Duplication of the long arm of chromosome 1 is found as a secondary abnormality in around one-third patients with an 8q24 translocation and has been reported to confer a poor outcome [39]. Patients with an 8q24 translocation fare very poorly on ALL treatment protocols (like all patients with mature-B) but have a significantly better outcome when treated on lymphoma protocols (see Chap. 13).

Genetic Abnormalities in Adult T-Cell All (T-ALL)

T-ALL is characterized by the activation of a number of transcription factors (e.g., *TLX1*, *TLX3*, *TAL1*, *LYL1*, and *LMO2*) whose over expression blocks T-cell differentiation [40, 41]. Frequently, activation of these oncogenic transcription factors occurs via a chromosomal translocation or abnormality that juxtaposes the oncogene to the promoter and enhancer elements of a gene involved in T-cell development, such as the T-cell receptor. Although some combinations of oncogene/promoter-gene are more prevalent than others, the multiplicity of legitimate permutations has led to the discovery of a plethora of chromosomal translocations in T-ALL [42]. Despite the spectrum of chromosomal translocations, over expression of these oncogenes occurs in the absence of any detectable genetic aberrations [43]. For this reason, there are discrepancies in the literature with respect to the frequency that any one of these oncogenes is involved in T-ALL. In this chapter, we focus on detectable genetic abnormalities in T-ALL.

Activation of TAL1, TLX1, TLX3, and LMO2

Approximately 50% of adult T-ALL patients harbor a genetic abnormality that results in the activation of *TAL1*, *TLX1*, *TLX3*, or *LMO2* (see Table 5.5). Three chromosomal translocations and one chromosomal deletion account for the majority of genetic abnormalities in adult ALL.

In 10–15% of adult T-ALL, a sub-microscopic interstitial deletion of chromosome band 1p32 brings the *TAL1* gene under the regulatory control of the promoter of the *SIL* gene, which lies centromeric of *TAL1*. Although this abnormality cannot be detected by conventional cytogenetics, it is readily identified using a commercially available FISH probe [44].

The translocation, t(10;14)(q24;q11.2), is the most prevalent chromosomal translocation in adult ALL accounting for nearly 15% of T-ALL and 2% of adult ALL overall. The juxtaposition of the *TLX1* (*HOX11*) gene located at 10q24 to the T-cell receptor alpha/delta locus (*TRA@/TRD@*) at 14q11.2 results in its over expression. In comparison to other T-ALL patients, those with this translocation do not appear to have higher white cell counts [6, 45]. Several studies have suggested that the presence of the t(10;14) or over expression of *TLX1* is associated with an improved outcome [12, 13, 43, 45]. Both this translocation and its rare variant, t(7;10)(q36;q24)/*TRB@-TLX1*, are readily detectable by conventional cytogenetic analysis.

The cryptic translocation, t(5;14)(q35;q32), juxtaposes the *TLX3* (*HOX11L2*) gene (5q35) to the promoter of the *BCL11B* gene (14q32) causing its overexpression [46]. This translocation occurs in

Table 5.5 Principal genetic abnormalities in adult T-cell acute lymphoblastic leukemia

Subgroup	Main chromosomal abnormality	Promoters	Incidence
Oncogene over expression			
TAL1	del(1)(p32)/t(1;14)(p32;q11)	*SIL/TRA@/TRD@*	10–15%
TLX1 (*HOX11*)	t(10;14)(q24;q11)/t(7;10)(q35;q24)	*TRA@/TRD@/TRB@*	15%
TLX3 (*HOX11L2*)	t(5;14)(q35;q32)/t(5;14)(q35;q11)	*BCL11B/TRA@/TRD@*	10%
LMO2	t(11;14)(p13;q11)/t(7;11)(q34;p13)/del(11)(p13)	*TRA@/TRD@/TRB@*	5%
Gene fusions			
CALM-AF10	t(10;11)(p13;q14)		5–10%
MLL-ENL	t(11;19)(q23;p13.3)		2%
NUP214-ABL	Episomal 9q34 amplification		5%
Others			
CDKN2A	sub-microscopic deletion of 9p		up to 50%
NOTCH1	Gain of function mutation		up to 70%

10% of adult T-ALL and has been reported by one study to be associated with a very poor outcome [45]. FISH is required for the detection of the t(5;14) translocation and most of its rare variants [46].

The oncogene *LMO2* located at 11p13 is activated by the *TRA@/TRD@* locus via the t(11;14) (p13;q11.2), the *TRB@* locus via the t(7;11)(q34;p13), or a cryptic interstitial deletion that removes the negative regulatory elements upstream of *LMO2* [7]. Collectively, these genetic abnormalities account for 5% of adult T-ALL. The related oncogene, *LMO1*, which lies telomeric of *LMO2* at 11p15 is also known to be activated by the *TRA@/TRD@* locus, but is much rarer in adult T-ALL.

Gene Fusions

The *CALM-AF10* fusion gene, the molecular consequence of the t(10;11)(p13;q14), also impairs T-cell differentiation and occurs in up to 10% of adult T-ALL. Translocations involving the *MLL* gene located at 11q23 occur in T-ALL as well as BCP-ALL (see above). However, within the context of T-ALL, the most prevalent partner gene is *ENL* at 19p13, which also occurs in BCP-ALL. Patients with T-ALL and the t(11;19)(q23;p13.3) tend to be younger adults (<20 years old) and have been reported to have a favorable outcome [20]. The episomal amplification of the *NUP214-ABL1* gene fusion is a secondary event which occurs in 5% of adult T-ALL [47]. Expression of *NUP214-ABL1* promotes cell proliferation and survival [41], and its presence is strongly correlated with the over expression of *TLX1* or *TLX3* and *CDKN2A* deletion [48].

Deletions and Mutations

CDKN2A deletions and *NOTCH1* mutations are the two most common genetic defects in adult T-ALL occurring in 50% and up to 70% of patients respectively (see Table 5.5) (unpublished observations) [49]. Although *CDKN2A* deletions occur in BCP-ALL, they are more prevalent in T-ALL where they are more likely to be homozygous deletions (unpublished observations) [28]. *CDKN2A* deletions disrupt cell cycle control and are a secondary event that associates with particular primary abnormalities [28, 41]. Activating *NOTCH1* mutations are also secondary events [50], which affect the self-renewal capacity of cells [41]. The prognostic relevance of both *CDKN2A* deletions and *NOTCH1* mutations in adult T-ALL is unclear but is likely to be linked to that of the primary event [28].

Summary and Future Directions

The genetic characterization of adult ALL using cytogenetics, FISH and associated molecular techniques is essential for accurate diagnosis and patient management. The presence of the *BCR-ABL1* fusion product now dictates a major change in treatment (see Chap. 12). In addition, several other chromosomal abnormalities are now routinely used to risk stratify patients. The use of state-of-the-art high-resolution technologies (e.g., array-based comparative genomic hybridization (aCGH) and single nucleotide polymorphism (SNP) arrays) has led to the discovery of a plethora of submicroscopic DNA copy number changes. The mean number and targets of these amplifications and deletions correlate with chromosomal translocations and ploidy subgroups, underlying the importance of evaluating new and old data side-by-side [26, 51]. Analysis of some of these new abnormalities is revealing networks of cooperating lesions, which are helping to elucidate the pathogenesis of ALL.

For example, recent studies have revealed frequent focal deletions and mutations of genes involved in B-cell development (e.g., *PAX5*) with many correlating with specific chromosomal translocations [26]. Indeed in *BCR-ABL1* positive adult ALL, Mullighan et al. have demonstrated that virtually all patients harbor a deletion of the Ikaros gene (*IKZF1*), whereas such deletions are very rare among patients in other genetic subtypes [9]. In addition, traditional, hypothesis-based approaches are making significant advances in furthering our knowledge of ALL. The recent identification of a network of translocations involving the *IGH@* gene, which occur predominantly in adolescents and young adults with BCP-ALL, provides not only new diagnostic and prognostic markers but also new therapeutic targets [36]. Continued genetic investigations into adult ALL are vital to ensure that future patients benefit from effective targeted therapy.

References

1. Mitelman, F., Johansson, B., & Mertens, F. (2007). The impact of translocations and gene fusions on cancer causation. *Nature Reviews Cancer, 7*, 233–245.
2. Robinson, H. M., Taylor, K. E., Jalali, G. R., et al. (2004). t(14;19)(q32;q13): A recurrent translocation in B-cell precursor acute lymphoblastic leukemia. *Genes Chromosomes and Cancer, 39*, 88–92.
3. Hawkins, J. M., & Secker-Walker, L. M. (1991). Evaluation of cytogenetic samples and pertinent technical variables in adult acute lymphocytic leukemia. *Cancer Genetics and Cytogenetics, 52*, 79–84.
4. Pedersen, R. K., Kerndrup, G. B., Sorensen, A. G., et al. (2001). Cytogenetic aberrations in adult acute lymphocytic leukemia: Optimal technique may influence the results. *Cancer Genetics and Cytogenetics, 128*, 7–10.
5. Shaffer, L. G., Slovak, M. L., Campbell, L. J. ISCN (2009): *An International System for Human Cytogenetic Nomenclature*. Basel: S. Karger.
6. Moorman, A. V., Harrison, C. J., Buck, G. A., et al. (2007). Karyotype is an independent prognostic factor in adult acute lymphoblastic leukemia (ALL): Analysis of cytogenetic data from patients treated on the Medical Research Council (MRC) UKALLXII/Eastern Cooperative Oncology Group (ECOG) 2993 trial. *Blood, 109*, 3189–3197.
7. Harrison, C. J., & Johansson, B. (2008). Acute lymphoblastic leukemia. In S. M. F. Heim (Ed.), *Cancer cytogenetics* (3rd ed.). New York: Wiley-Liss.
8. Wetzler, M., Dodge, R. K., Mrozek, K., et al. (2004). Additional cytogenetic abnormalities in adults with Philadelphia chromosome-positive acute lymphoblastic leukaemia: A study of the Cancer and Leukaemia Group B. *British Journal Haematology, 124*, 275–288.
9. Mullighan, C. G., Miller, C. B., Radtke, I., et al. (2008). BCR-ABL1 lymphoblastic leukaemia is characterized by the deletion of Ikaros. *Nature, 453*, 110–114.
10. Secker-Walker, L. M., Prentice, H. G., Durrant, J., Richards, S., Hall, E., & Harrison, G. (1997). Cytogenetics adds independent prognostic information in adults with acute lymphoblastic leukaemia on MRC trial UKALL XA. MRC Adult Leukaemia Working Party. *British Journal Haematology, 96*, 601–610.
11. Wetzler, M., Dodge, R. K., Mrozek, K., et al. (1999). Prospective karyotype analysis in adult acute lymphoblastic leukemia: The cancer and leukemia Group B experience. *Blood, 93*, 3983–3993.
12. Pullarkat, V., Slovak, M. L., Kopecky, K. J., Forman, S. J., & Appelbaum, F. R. (2008). Impact of cytogenetics on the outcome of adult acute lymphoblastic leukemia: Results of Southwest Oncology Group 9400 study. *Blood, 111*, 2563–2572.
13. GFCH. (1996). Cytogenetic abnormalities in adult acute lymphoblastic leukemia: Correlations with hematologic findings and outcome. A collaborative study of the Groupe Francais de Cytogenetique Hematologique. *Blood, 87*, 3135–3142.
14. Burmeister, T., Schwartz, S., Bartram, C. R., Gokbuget, N., Hoelzer, D., & Thiel, E. (2008). Patients' age and BCR-ABL frequency in adult B-precursor ALL: A retrospective analysis from the GMALL study group. *Blood, 112*, 918–919.
15. Johansson, B., Mertens, F., & Mitelman, F. (1991). Geographic heterogeneity of neoplasia-associated chromosome aberrations. *Genes, Chromosomes & Cancer, 3*, 1–7.
16. Meyer, C., Schneider, B., Jakob, S., et al. (2006). The MLL recombinome of acute leukemias. *Leukemia, 20*, 777–784.
17. Johansson, B., Moorman, A. V., Haas, O. A., et al. (1998). Hematologic malignancies with t(4;11)(q21;q23) – A cytogenetic, morphologic, immunophenotypic, and clinical study of 183 cases. *Leukemia, 12*, 779–787.
18. Gale, K. B., Ford, A. M., Repp, R., et al. (1997). Backtracking leukemia to birth: Identification of clonotypic gene fusion sequences in neonatal blood spots. *Proceedings of the National Academy of Sciences of the United States of America, 94*, 13950–13954.

19. Mancini, M., Scappaticci, D., Cimino, G., et al. (2005). A comprehensive genetic classification of adult acute lymphoblastic leukemia (ALL): Analysis of the GIMEMA 0496 protocol. *Blood, 105*, 3434–3441.

20. Moorman, A. V., Hagemeijer, A., Charrin, C., Rieder, H., & Secker-Walker, L. M. (1998). The translocations, t(11;19)(q23;p13.1) and t(11;19)(q23;p13.3): A cytogenetic and clinical profile of 53 patients. *Leukemia, 12*, 805–810.

21. Barber, K. E., Harrison, C. J., Broadfield, Z. J., et al. (2007). Molecular cytogenetic characterisation of TCF3 (E2A)/19p13.3 rearrangements in B-cell precursor acute lymphoblastic leukaemia. *Genes Chromosomes and Cancer 46*(5), 478–486.

22. Foa, R., Vitale, A., Mancini, M., et al. (2003). E2A-PBX1 fusion in adult acute lymphoblastic leukaemia: Biological and clinical features. *British Journal Haematology, 120*, 484–487.

23. Faderl, S., Kantarjian, H. M., Talpaz, M., & Estrov, Z. (1998). Clinical significance of cytogenetic abnormalities in adult acute lymphoblastic leukemia. *Blood, 91*, 3995–4019.

24. Gleissner, B., & Thiel, E. (2003). Molecular genetic events in adult acute lymphoblastic leukemia. *Expert Review of Molecular Diagnostics, 3*, 339–355.

25. Moorman, A. V., Richards, S. M., Martineau, M., et al. (2003). Outcome heterogeneity in childhood high-hyperdiploid acute lymphoblastic leukemia. *Blood, 102*, 2756–2762.

26. Mullighan, C. G., Goorha, S., Radtke, I., et al. (2007). Genome-wide analysis of genetic alterations in acute lymphoblastic leukaemia. *Nature, 446*, 758–764.

27. Case, M., Matheson, E., Minto, L., et al. (2008). Mutation of genes affecting the RAS pathway is common in childhood acute lymphoblastic leukemia. *Cancer Research, 68*, 6803–6809.

28. Sulong, S., Moorman, A.V., Irving, J.A., et al. (2008). A comprehensive analysis of the CDKN2A gene in childhood acute lymphoblastic leukaemia reveals genomic deletion, copy number neutral loss of heterozygosity and association with specific cytogenetic subgroups. Blood (in press).

29. Harrison, C. J., Moorman, A. V., Broadfield, Z. J., et al. (2004). Three distinct subgroups of hypodiploidy in acute lymphoblastic leukaemia. *British Journal Haematology, 125*, 552–559.

30. Charrin, C., Thomas, X., Ffrench, M., et al. (2004). A report from the LALA-94 and LALA-SA groups on hypodiploidy with 30 to 39 chromosomes and near-triploidy: 2 possible expressions of a sole entity conferring poor prognosis in adult acute lymphoblastic leukemia (ALL). *Blood, 104*, 2444–2451.

31. Granada, I., Sancho, J.-M., Oriol, A., et al. (2007). The prognostic significance of complex karyotype in Philadelphia chromosome-negative (Ph) acute lymphoblastic leukemia (ALL) in adults is related with risk group. *ASH Annual Meeting Abstracts, 110*, 3501.

32. Aguiar, R. C. T., Sohal, J., Van Rhee, F., et al. (1996). TEL-AML1 fusion in acute lymphoblastic leukaemia of adults. *British Journal Haematology, 95*, 673–677.

33. Jabbar Al Obaidi, M. S., Martineau, M., Bennett, C. F., et al. (2002). ETV6/AML1 fusion by FISH in adult acute lymphoblastic leukaemia. *Leukemia, 16*, 669–674.

34. Greaves, M. F., & Wiemels, J. (2003). Origins of chromosome translocations in childhood leukaemia. *Nature Reviews. Cancer, 3*, 639–649.

35. Akasaka, T., Balasas, T., Russell, L. J., et al. (2007). Five members of the CEBP transcription factor family are targeted by recurrent IGH translocations in B-cell precursor acute lymphoblastic leukemia (BCP-ALL). *Blood, 109*, 3451–3461.

36. Russell, L. J., Capasso, M., Vater, I., et al. (2009). Deregulated expression of cytokine receptor gene, CRLF2, is involved in lymphoid transformation in B-cell precursor acute lymphoblastic leukemia. *Blood, 114*(13), 2688–2698.

37. Russell, L. J., Akasaka, T., Majid, A., et al. (2008). t(6;14)(p22;q32): A new recurrent IGH@ translocation involving ID4 in B-cell precursor acute lymphoblastic leukemia (BCP-ALL). *Blood, 111*, 387–391.

38. Russell, L.J., De Castro, D.G., Griffiths, M., et al. (2009). A novel translocation, t(14;19) (q32;p13), involving IGH@ and the cytokine receptor for erythropoietin. *Leukemia, 23*(3), 614–617

39. Garcia, J. L., Hernandez, J. M., Gutierrez, N. C., et al. (2003). Abnormalities on 1q and 7q are associated with poor outcome in sporadic Burkitt's lymphoma. A cytogenetic and comparative genomic hybridization study. *Leukemia, 17*, 2016–2024.

40. Ferrando, A. A., Neuberg, D. S., Staunton, J., et al. (2002). Gene expression signatures define novel oncogenic pathways in T cell acute lymphoblastic leukemia. *Cancer Cell, 1*, 75–87.

41. De Keersmaecker, K., Marynen, P., & Cools, J. (2005). Genetic insights in the pathogenesis of T-cell lymphoblastic leukemia. *Haematologica, 90*, 1116–1127.

42. Johansson, B., Mertens, F., & Mitelman, F. (2004). Clinical and biological importance of cytogenetic abnormalities in childhood and adult acute lymphoblastic leukemia. *Annali Medici, 36*, 492–503.

43. Ferrando, A. A., Neuberg, D. S., Dodge, R. K., et al. (2004). Prognostic importance of TLX1 (HOX11) oncogene expression in adults with T-cell acute lymphoblastic leukaemia. *Lancet, 363*, 535–536.

44. Van der Burg, M., Poulsen, T. S., Hunger, S. P., et al. (2004). Split-signal FISH for detection of chromosome aberrations in acute lymphoblastic leukemia. *Leukemia, 18*, 895–908.

45. Asnafi, V., Buzyn, A., Thomas, X., et al. (2005). Impact of TCR status and genotype on outcome in adult T-cell acute lymphoblastic leukemia: A LALA-94 study. *Blood, 105*, 3072–3078.
46. Berger, R., Dastugue, N., Busson, M., et al. (2003). t(5;14)/HOX11L2-positive T-cell acute lymphoblastic leukemia. A collaborative study of the Groupe Francais de Cytogenetique Hematologique (GFCH). *Leukemia, 17*, 1851–1857.
47. Graux, C., Cools, J., Melotte, C., et al. (2004). Fusion of NUP214 to ABL1 on amplified episomes in T-cell acute lymphoblastic leukemia. *Nature Genetics, 36*, 1084–1089.
48. Graux, C., Stevens-Kroef, M., Lafage, M., et al. (2009). Heterogeneous patterns of amplification of the NUP214-ABL1 fusion gene in T-cell acute lymphoblastic leukemia. *Leukemia, 23*(1), 125–133.
49. Mansour, M. R., Linch, D. C., Foroni, L., Goldstone, A. H., & Gale, R. E. (2006). High incidence of Notch-1 mutations in adult patients with T-cell acute lymphoblastic leukemia. *Leukemia, 20*, 537–539.
50. Mansour, M. R., Duke, V., Foroni, L., et al. (2007). Notch-1 mutations are secondary events in some patients with T-cell acute lymphoblastic leukemia. *Clinical Cancer Research, 13*, 6964–6969.
51. Paulsson, K., Cazier, J. B., Macdougall, F., et al. (2008). Microdeletions are a general feature of adult and adolescent acute lymphoblastic leukemia: Unexpected similarities with pediatric disease. *Proceedings of the National Academy of Sciences of the United States of America, 105*, 6708–6713.

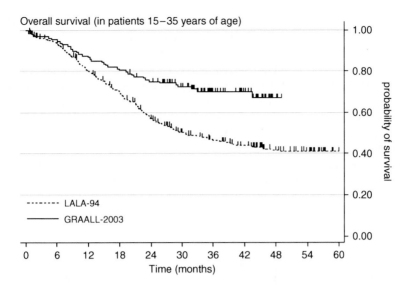

Fig. 14.4 Comparison of the outcome of AYA (15–35 years) treated in the hybrid GRAALL-2003 trial and the historical LALA-94 trial

Dieu Hospital (Paris, France) reported a monocentric historical comparison of 20 adults, mainly AYA with a median age of 23 years (range: 16–54 years), treated according to the pediatric protocol FRALLE 2,000 and 20 adult patients treated in the adult EORTC ALL HR-4 [101]. The 4-year overall survival was 87% in patients treated according to the FRALLE trial vs. 35% in patients treated in EORTC trial. No treatment or infection-related mortality was observed but few data on compliance to scheduled treatment is available.

Several groups have evaluated pediatric treatment approaches in AYA patients or even in older adults. In 2002, the DFCI initiated a phase II study in patients aged 18–50 years old [102]. The backbone of this trial was based on the high-risk arm of the pediatric DFCI Childhood ALL Consortium 00-01. Preliminary results were recently reported in 75 patients (median age: 28 years). The CR rate after 4 weeks was 84% and 2-year overall and event-free survival were 77.1 and 72.5%. Toxicities included 23 neutropenic infections, 1 pancreatitis, and 14 episodes of thrombosis/embolisms. A study by the University of Southern California Hospitals reported the administration of an augmented BFM pediatric regimen in 34 patients aged 19–57 years [103]. The CR rate was 97% and the 3-year event-free survival 61%. Hepatic and pancreatic toxicity secondary to PEG-asparaginase therapy was noted. However, this toxicity was less than that reported by the same group in an adult protocol setting [104].

The CALGB, SWOG, ECOG, and the CCG recently initiated a phase II trial (C-10403) that will evaluate a pediatric CCG approach in patients up to the age of 30 years. The M.D. Anderson Center also reported preliminary results of an augmented BFM protocol feasibility in AYA [105]. The JALSG is currently enrolling patients aged 14–25 years in a pediatric protocol, which was used by the Japan Association of Childhood Leukemia Study.

Long-Term Toxicity

Given the higher intensity regimens and longer overall survival with better therapeutic regimens, adults physicians will have to deal with the long-term toxicities encountered in the AYA population.

Avascular necrosis (AVN) of the bone is a serious complication well identified in pediatric protocols [106–108]. This complication has been attributed to the use of corticosteroids, particularly dexamethasone, and is more frequent in children older than 10 years. Recently, the MRC reported an incidence of AVN in a cohort of adult patients treated on the UKALL XII trial. The incidence of AVN at 10 years was 29% in adolescents (<20 years) compared to 8% in older patients. The risk of developing AVN was significantly higher in patients treated by chemotherapy alone without stem cell transplantation. Other long-term sequelae and complications may be anticipated in ALL survivors, even if precise incidences are unknown after intensified chemotherapy. More limited transplantation indications would probably decrease the incidence of gonadal dysfunction and secondary neoplasms. Two treatment-related AMLs were reported in the GRAALL-2003 trial [50]. Prolonged follow-up of ALL survivors is warranted to detect and manage these adverse events.

Conclusion

A continuum in the frequency of each subtype of ALL is observed, that crosses the line separating adolescence from adulthood. Although there is strong evidence that patients younger than 18–20 years of age should be treated with pediatric therapeutic regimens, some questions concerning the optimal treatment of young adults persist. Pediatric or pediatric-inspired regimens have led to few patients having primary refractory disease, and to overall survival approximating 60% in patients 20–35 years old. At the same time, ASCT has yielded comparable survival rates in the same population of patients, but also comes with long-term toxicities including sterility. If ongoing trials improve the outcome of young adults by employing pediatric therapeutic regimens, indications for ASCT may be reduced. Future challenges in the field of ALL in AYA involve (1) a better care coordination between pediatric and adult medicine, taking into account the unique medical and psychosocial profile of this population, (2) the reduction of early and long-term toxicity, especially through the optimization of supportive care, and (3) better definitions of prognostic factors, including MRD, to optimize risk-adapted strategies.

References

1. Pui, C. H., & Evans, W. E. (1998). Acute lymphoblastic leukemia. *The New England Journal of Medicine, 339*(9), 605–615.
2. Hoelzer, D. (1993). Acute lymphoblastic leukemia–progress in children, less in adults. *The New England Journal of Medicine, 329*(18), 1343–1344.
3. Pui, C. H., & Evans, W. E. (2006). Treatment of acute lymphoblastic leukemia. *The New England Journal of Medicine, 354*(2), 166–178.
4. Gokbuget, N., & Hoelzer, D. (2009). Treatment of adult acute lymphoblastic leukemia. *Seminars in Hematology, 46*(1), 64–75.
5. Perentesis, J. P. (1997). Why is age such an important independent prognostic factor in acute lymphoblastic leukemia? *Leukemia, 11*(Suppl 4), S4–S7.
6. Chessells, J. M., Hall, E., Prentice, H. G., Durrant, J., Bailey, C. C., & Richards, S. M. (1998). The impact of age on outcome in lymphoblastic leukaemia; MRC UKALL X and XA compared: A report from the MRC Paediatric and Adult Working Parties. *Leukemia, 12*(4), 463–473.
7. Plasschaert, S. L., Kamps, W. A., Vellenga, E., de Vries, E. G., & de Bont, E. S. (2004). Prognosis in childhood and adult acute lymphoblastic leukaemia: A question of maturation? *Cancer Treatment Reviews, 30*(1), 37–51.
8. Borkhardt, A., Cazzaniga, G., Viehmann, S., et al. (1997). Incidence and clinical relevance of TEL/AML1 fusion genes in children with acute lymphoblastic leukemia enrolled in the German and Italian multicenter therapy trials. Associazione Italiana Ematologia Oncologia Pediatrica and the Berlin-Frankfurt-Munster Study Group. *Blood, 90*(2), 571–577.

9. Cayuela, J. M., Baruchel, A., Orange, C., et al. (1996). TEL-AML1 fusion RNA as a new target to detect minimal residual disease in pediatric B-cell precursor acute lymphoblastic leukemia. *Blood, 88*(1), 302–308.
10. Copelan, E. A., & McGuire, E. A. (1995). The biology and treatment of acute lymphoblastic leukemia in adults. *Blood, 85*(5), 1151–1168.
11. Goker, E., Lin, J. T., Trippett, T., et al. (1993). Decreased polyglutamylation of methotrexate in acute lymphoblastic leukemia blasts in adults compared to children with this disease. *Leukemia, 7*(7), 1000–1004.
12. Maung, Z. T., Reid, M. M., Matheson, E., Taylor, P. R., Proctor, S. J., & Hall, A. G. (1995). Corticosteroid resistance is increased in lymphoblasts from adults compared with children: Preliminary results of in vitro drug sensitivity study in adults with acute lymphoblastic leukaemia. *British Journal of Haematology, 91*(1), 93–100.
13. Styczynski, J., Pieters, R., Huismans, D. R., Schuurhuis, G. J., Wysocki, M., & Veerman, A. J. (2000). In vitro drug resistance profiles of adult versus childhood acute lymphoblastic leukaemia. *British Journal of Haematology, 110*(4), 813–818.
14. Mattano, L., Jr., Nachman, J., Ross, J., & Stock, W. (2006). Leukemias. In W. Bleyer, M. O'Leary, R. Barr, & L. Ries (Eds.), *Cancer epidemiology in older adolescents and young adults 15 to 29 years of age, including SEER incidence and survival: 1975–2000* (pp. 39–51). Bethesda, MD: National Cancer Institute (NIH Pub. No. 06-5767).
15. Albritton, K. H., Wiggins, C. H., Nelson, H. E., & Weeks, J. C. (2007). Site of oncologic specialty care for older adolescents in Utah. *Journal of Clinical Oncology, 25*(29), 4616–4621.
16. Howell, D. L., Ward, K. C., Austin, H. D., Young, J. L., & Woods, W. G. (2007). Access to pediatric cancer care by age, race, and diagnosis, and outcomes of cancer treatment in pediatric and adolescent patients in the state of Georgia. *Journal of Clinical Oncology, 25*(29), 4610–4615.
17. Nachman, J., Sather, H. N., Buckley, J. D., et al. (1993). Young adults 16-21 years of age at diagnosis entered on Childrens Cancer Group acute lymphoblastic leukemia and acute myeloblastic leukemia protocols. Results of treatment. *Cancer, 71*(10 Suppl), 3377–3385.
18. Stiller, C. A., Benjamin, S., Cartwright, R. A., et al. (1999). Patterns of care and survival for adolescents and young adults with acute leukaemia – a population-based study. *British Journal of Cancer, 79*(3–4), 658–665.
19. Fiere, D., Schaison, G., Bancillon, A., & Sebban, C. (1990). What is the best treatment for patients between 15 years and 20 years with acute lymphoblastic leukemia? Comparative results of two protocols, on for adults, one for children. *Blood, 76*, 270a.
20. Boissel, N., Auclerc, M. F., Lheritier, V., et al. (2003). Should adolescents with acute lymphoblastic leukemia be treated as old children or young adults? Comparison of the French FRALLE-93 and LALA-94 trials. *Journal of Clinical Oncology, 21*(5), 774–780.
21. de Bont, J. M., Holt, B., Dekker, A. W., van der Does-van den Berg, A., Sonneveld, P., & Pieters, R. (2004). Significant difference in outcome for adolescents with acute lymphoblastic leukemia treated on pediatric vs adult protocols in the Netherlands. *Leukemia, 18*(12), 2032–2035.
22. Testi, A. M., Valsecchi, M. G., Conter, V., et al. (2004). Difference in outcome of adolescents with acute lymphoblastic leukemia (ALL) enrolled in pediatric (AIEOP) and adult (GIMEMA) protocols. *Blood (ASH Annual Meeting Abstracts), 104*(11), 1954.
23. Ramanujachar, R., Richards, S., Hann, I., et al. (2007). Adolescents with acute lymphoblastic leukaemia: Outcome on UK national paediatric (ALL97) and adult (UKALLXII/E2993) trials. *Pediatric Blood & Cancer, 48*(3), 254–261.
24. Hallbook, H., Gustafsson, G., Smedmyr, B., Soderhall, S., & Heyman, M. (2006). Treatment outcome in young adults and children >10 years of age with acute lymphoblastic leukemia in Sweden: A comparison between a pediatric protocol and an adult protocol. *Cancer, 107*(7), 1551–1561.
25. Stock, W., La, M., Sanford, B., et al. (2008). What determines the outcomes for adolescents and young adults with acute lymphoblastic leukemia treated on cooperative group protocols? A comparison of children's cancer group and cancer and leukemia group B studies. *Blood, 112*(5), 1646–1654.
26. Usvasalo, A., Raty, R., Knuutila, S., et al. (2008). Acute lymphoblastic leukemia in adolescents and young adults in Finland. *Haematologica, 93*(8), 1161–1168.
27. Pui, C. H., Frankel, L. S., Carroll, A. J., et al. (1991). Clinical characteristics and treatment outcome of childhood acute lymphoblastic leukemia with the t(4;11)(q21;q23): A collaborative study of 40 cases. *Blood, 77*(3), 440–447.
28. Silverman, L. B., Gelber, R. D., Dalton, V. K., et al. (2001). Improved outcome for children with acute lymphoblastic leukemia: Results of Dana-Farber consortium protocol 91-01. *Blood, 97*(5), 1211–1218.
29. Amylon, M. D., Shuster, J., Pullen, J., et al. (1999). Intensive high-dose asparaginase consolidation improves survival for pediatric patients with T cell acute lymphoblastic leukemia and advanced stage lymphoblastic lymphoma: A pediatric oncology group study. *Leukemia, 13*(3), 335–342.
30. Douer, D. (2008). Is asparaginase a critical component in the treatment of acute lymphoblastic leukemia? *Best Practice & Research. Clinical Haematology, 21*(4), 647–658.

31. Wetzler, M., Sanford, B. L., Kurtzberg, J., et al. (2007). Effective asparagine depletion with pegylated asparaginase results in improved outcomes in adult acute lymphoblastic leukemia: Cancer and leukemia group B study 9511. *Blood, 109*(10), 4164–4167.

32. Riehm, H., Gadner, H., Henze, G., et al. (1990). Results and significance of six randomized trials in four consecutive ALL-BFM studies. *Haematology and Blood Transfusion, 33*, 439–450.

33. Tubergen, D. G., Gilchrist, G. S., O'Brien, R. T., et al. (1993). Improved outcome with delayed intensification for children with acute lymphoblastic leukemia and intermediate presenting features: A Childrens Cancer Group phase III trial. *Journal of Clinical Oncology, 11*(3), 527–537.

34. Nachman, J. B., Sather, H. N., Sensel, M. G., et al. (1998). Augmented post-induction therapy for children with high-risk acute lymphoblastic leukemia and a slow response to initial therapy. *The New England Journal of Medicine, 338*(23), 1663–1671.

35. Arico, M., Valsecchi, M. G., Camitta, B., et al. (2000). Outcome of treatment in children with Philadelphia chromosome-positive acute lymphoblastic leukemia. *The New England Journal of Medicine, 342*(14), 998–1006.

36. Balduzzi, A., Valsecchi, M. G., Uderzo, C., et al. (2005). Chemotherapy versus allogeneic transplantation for very-high-risk childhood acute lymphoblastic leukaemia in first complete remission: Comparison by genetic randomisation in an international prospective study. *Lancet, 366*(9486), 635–642.

37. Abrams, A. N., Hazen, E. P., & Penson, R. T. (2007). Psychosocial issues in adolescents with cancer. *Cancer Treatment Reviews, 33*(7), 622–630.

38. Ferrari, A., & Bleyer, A. (2007). Participation of adolescents with cancer in clinical trials. *Cancer Treatment Reviews, 33*(7), 603–608.

39. Spinetta, J. J., Masera, G., Eden, T., et al. (2002). Refusal, non-compliance, and abandonment of treatment in children and adolescents with cancer: A report of the SIOP Working Committee on Phychosocial Issues in Pediatric Oncology. *Medical and Pediatric Oncology, 38*(2), 114–117.

40. Schiffer, C. A. (2003). Differences in outcome in adolescents with acute lymphoblastic leukemia: A consequence of better regimens? Better doctors? Both? *Journal of Clinical Oncology, 21*(5), 760–761.

41. Herold, R., von Stackelberg, A., Hartmann, R., Eisenreich, B., & Henze, G. (2004). Acute lymphoblastic leukemia-relapse study of the Berlin-Frankfurt-Munster Group (ALL-REZ BFM) experience: Early treatment intensity makes the difference. *Journal of Clinical Oncology, 22*(3), 569–570. author reply 70-1.

42. Advani, A. S., Jin, T., Ramsingh, G., et al. (2008). Time to post-remission therapy is an independent prognostic factor in adults with acute lymphoblastic leukemia. *Leukaemia & Lymphoma, 49*(8), 1560–1566.

43. Petersdorf, S. H., Kopecky, K. J., Head, D. R., et al. (2001). Comparison of the L10M consolidation regimen to an alternative regimen including escalating methotrexate/L-asparaginase for adult acute lymphoblastic leukemia: A Southwest Oncology Group Study. *Leukemia, 15*(2), 208–216.

44. Durrant, I. J., Prentice, H. G., & Richards, S. M. (1997). Intensification of treatment for adults with acute lymphoblastic leukaemia: Results of U.K. Medical Research Council randomized trial UKALL XA. Medical Research Council Working Party on Leukaemia in Adults. *British Journal of Haematology, 99*(1), 84–92.

45. Annino, L., Vegna, M. L., Camera, A., et al. (2002). Treatment of adult acute lymphoblastic leukemia (ALL): Long-term follow-up of the GIMEMA ALL 0288 randomized study. *Blood, 99*(3), 863–871.

46. Takeuchi, J., Kyo, T., Naito, K., et al. (2002). Induction therapy by frequent administration of doxorubicin with four other drugs, followed by intensive consolidation and maintenance therapy for adult acute lymphoblastic leukemia: The JALSG-ALL93 study. *Leukemia, 16*(7), 1259–1266.

47. Larson, R. A., Dodge, R. K., Linker, C. A., et al. (1998). A randomized controlled trial of filgrastim during remission induction and consolidation chemotherapy for adults with acute lymphoblastic leukemia: CALGB study 9111. *Blood, 92*(5), 1556–1564.

48. Hunault, M., Harousseau, J. L., Delain, M., et al. (2004). Better outcome of adult acute lymphoblastic leukemia after early genoidentical allogeneic bone marrow transplantation (BMT) than after late high-dose therapy and autologous BMT: A GOELAMS trial. *Blood, 104*(10), 3028–3037.

49. Kantarjian, H., Thomas, D., O'Brien, S., et al. (2004). Long-term follow-up results of hyperfractionated cyclophosphamide, vincristine, doxorubicin, and dexamethasone (Hyper-CVAD), a dose-intensive regimen, in adult acute lymphocytic leukemia. *Cancer, 101*(12), 2788–2801.

50. Huguet, F., Leguay, T., Raffoux, E., et al. (2009). Pediatric-inspired therapy in adults with Philadelphia chromosome-negative acute lymphoblastic leukemia: The GRAALL-2003 study. *Journal of Clinical Oncology, 27*(6), 911–918.

51. Mastrangelo, R., Poplack, D., Bleyer, A., Riccardi, R., Sather, H., & D'Angio, G. (1986). Report and recommendations of the Rome workshop concerning poor-prognosis acute lymphoblastic leukemia in children: Biologic bases for staging, stratification, and treatment. *Medical and Pediatric Oncology, 14*(3), 191–194.

52. Smith, M., Arthur, D., Camitta, B., et al. (1996). Uniform approach to risk classification and treatment assignment for children with acute lymphoblastic leukemia. *Journal of Clinical Oncology, 14*(1), 18–24.

53. Larson, R. A., Dodge, R. K., Burns, C. P., et al. (1995). A five-drug remission induction regimen with intensive consolidation for adults with acute lymphoblastic leukemia: Cancer and leukemia group B study 8811. *Blood, 85*(8), 2025–2037.

observed excess leukemia mortality in newly founded British towns from 1946 to 1950, which brought together new residents from several isolated rural settings. Excess childhood leukemia cases were noted up until 1965 but not for the period from 1966 to 1985. In a study in Italy and Greece, Kinlen and colleagues [46] examined the high mortality in these countries between 1958 and 1987, which was considered to be secondary to high levels of population mixing with large-scale rural to urban migration in years after World War II. In a Canadian study by Koushik and colleagues [47], leukemia incidence was found to be higher in rural areas where the population had grown, while it was lower than expected in growing urban areas.

Smith's hypothesis [42, 43] proposes that high rates of childhood ALL are due to in utero exposure to infections that principally result in cases of precursor B cell ALL. In investigating this hypothesis, study results remain inconclusive. Four recent case-control studies examining maternal infection and risk of childhood leukemia show mixed results. Lehtinen and colleagues [48] reported a significantly increased risk for childhood leukemia associated with lower genital tract infection, while Naumberg and colleagues [49] showed a similar significant increased risk associated with maternal Epstein–Barr virus infection. Conversely, Infante-Rivard and colleagues [50] failed to find any statistically significant association with recurrent maternal infections. Also, McKinney et al.'s [51] Scottish study looked at all infections during pregnancy (respiratory tract, viral, genitourinary, and fungal) and found that this did not significantly affect the risk of ALL in children aged 0–14 years.

The delayed-infection hypothesis of Greaves [44, 45] is based on a minimal two-hits model and suggests that some susceptible individuals with a prenatally acquired preleukemic clone had low or no exposure to common infections early in life because they lived in an affluent hygienic environment. Such infectious insulation predisposes the immune system of these individuals to abnormal or pathological responses after subsequent or delayed exposure to common infections at an age commensurate with increased lymphoid-cell proliferation. This theory is supported by the fact that most cases of ALL diagnosed between 2 and 6 years of age have the TEL-AML1 mutation, and this is considered to be the first of the two hits or mutations in this theory. Some proposed mechanisms for this abnormal immunological response might include direct infection and transformation of precursor B cells or physical characteristics of the virus that stimulate critical receptors for cell growth [45].

Physical Factors

Ionizing Radiation

Since studies by radiologists in the early twentieth century, ionizing radiation has been associated with increased incidence of leukemia including ALL [52, 53]. Survivors of the atomic bomb explosions in Nagasaki and Hiroshima were noted to have a ninefold increase in risk of ALL peaking at 5–10 years after exposure [54]. A similar risk and postexposure peak have also been observed in ankylosing spondylitis patients treated with irradiation [55].

A slightly increased risk for adult leukemia has been found in occupational exposure to low-dose radiation in nuclear workers in Europe and the USA, but findings differ across varied populations [56].

In the 1980s, possible induction of leukemia by emissions from a nuclear processing plant in Seascale, England, was raised. Risk was initially suggested to be associated with the father's employment at the plant and proximity to the plant [57, 58] but later studies did not confirm either [59,60]. Similarly, observations that children living in the vicinity of nuclear power stations have been reported but a direct relationship could not be concluded [61].

Prenatal in utero exposure to diagnostic radiography of the abdomen has been shown to impart a slightly increased risk of ALL in the child, correlating well with the number of exposures [62].

Stewart and colleagues [63] demonstrated a cohort showing an increased risk of all leukemias of 50%. This type of radiation exposure is of negligible relevance today as diagnostic abdominal radiography is avoided in this population.

Nonionizing Radiation

Exposure to high levels of low-frequency electromagnetic fields has been purported to confer an increased risk of ALL, particularly in children [64], but the findings are not clear. Meta-analyses also show conflicting results. There was no significant increase in risk of leukemia in a study by Kheifets and colleagues [65]. However, Wartenberg [66] reported an increased risk of leukemia with high exposure levels. Even if this was true, in the UK fewer than 1 in 25 children would be exposed to such high levels, hence less than 1% of leukemias are likely to be caused by it [67].

Chemical Factors

Hydrocarbons

Benzenes are the most widely recognized hydrocarbon that are used in a variety of industries including leather, rubber, plastics, paint, glue, and printing. Exposure to benzenes has been associated with an increased leukemia risk among workers in these industries. The increased risk of ALL in these occupations where exposure existed is not as excessive as AML [68, 69]. A recent occupational study [70] revealed that even benzene exposure intensities at lower levels (<60 pp-years) than previously reported (up to 220 ppm-years) had an excess risk of leukemia [71].

An association between parental exposures to solvents and childhood ALL has been suggested in a few studies, but these studies have shown generally inconclusive results [72, 73]. Colt and colleagues showed that direct exposure to solvents and motor-vehicle-related occupations are associated with increased risk of leukemia but not childhood ALL [74]. The relationship between parental hobbies and home projects and the incidence of childhood leukemia was investigated in a case-control study of 640 subjects [75]. ALL was shown to have a statistically significant association with prenatal exposure (>4 rooms) (OR = 1.7; 95% CI, 1.1–2.7) and to artwork with solvents (OR = 4.1; 95% CI, 1.1–15.1). It is generally thought that these studies examining parental exposure risks are affected by recall bias of self-reporting exposure assessment.

Pesticides

Several studies have shown a limited association between pesticides (including insecticides, herbicides, and fungicides) and ALL as compared to other hematopoietic malignancies. Most of these studies are also limited by recall bias, small numbers of children, and nonspecific pesticide information. However, some recent studies have suggested a stronger link than first thought. Firstly, Rudant and colleagues, in the French ESCALE study, compared cases of children with hematopoietic malignancies with matched controls [76]. They revealed the maternal household use of any pesticide during pregnancy was significantly more frequent in acute leukemias, both acute myeloid leukemia and ALL (OR = 2.3; 95% CI = 1.9–2.8). Similarly, findings were observed by Infante-Rivard and colleagues, who found an association between indoor and garden pesticides and childhood ALL [77].

Smoking

Cigarette smoke is known to contain several carcinogens including benzene and nitrosamines [78, 79]. Despite being assessed in several studies, there remains no definite link between maternal and paternal cigarette smoking (before or after pregnancy) and developing childhood leukemia. Shu and colleagues showed mixed results [80]. There was an insignificant negative association (OR 0.78, 95% CI =0.51–1.18) between maternal cigarette smoking and ALL. The study also showed that a slightly elevated risk of ALL was associated with paternal smoking in the 1 month prior to pregnancy (OR = 1.56; 95% CI =1.03–2.36). A recent large UK Childhood Cancer Study could not find any significant association between childhood leukemia and parental tobacco smoking [81]. These studies are unfortunately limited by imprecise exposure estimates and limited adjustment for potentially confounding variables.

Maternal Pharmaceutical Use

There remains limited data that address the potential association between maternal medication use and childhood ALL. Wen and colleagues analyzed information from parents of 1842 children with ALL against matched controls [82]. They found that there was an increased risk associated with parental used of antihistamines or diet pills and mind altering drugs (OR 2.8, 99% CI 0.5–15.6). They also found that maternal use of vitamins and iron supplements during the index pregnancy was associated with a decreased risk of ALL. More recently, Kwan and colleagues demonstrated that maternal iron supplementation was associated with reduced ALL risk (OR =0.67, 95% CI: 0.47–0.94) [83].

Maternal Alcohol Use

Excessive maternal alcohol consumption has been shown to be associated with a slightly increased risk of ALL (OR = 1.43, 95% confidence interval [CI] = 1.00–2.04) [80]. The risk of AML among very young children was nearly double (OR 2.64, 95% CI = 1.36–5.06). Paternal alcohol consumption prior to conception did not confer an increased risk of infant leukemia [80].

Outdoor Air Pollution

Several studies have suggested outdoor air pollution as a risk factor for ALL and other leukemias. Benzene, again, is hypothesized to be the agent attributable as it is a component of motor-vehicle exhaust. In most studies that have been conducted, traffic density is used as a surrogate measure for air pollution and this is compared to leukemia incidence or mortality. As with other environmental exposure studies, the results are mixed. Overall, recently reported studies show a positive relationship between outdoor air pollution and childhood leukemia. Most notably, Reynolds and colleagues suggested that children living in areas with high levels of 25 potentially carcinogenic hazardous air pollutants (HAPs), including benzene, perchloroethylene, and trichloroethylene, are at an increased risk of developing leukemia (RR = 1.3; 95% CI, 1.13–1.6) [84]. This study was limited by utilizing group exposure levels to represent individuals and exclusion of indoor HAP sources (e.g., tobacco smoke) as potential confounders of exposure estimates. As suggested by the authors, an assessment of individual-level data is required to better understand the relationships.

Diet

There have been a handful of studies examining the possible link between diet and risk of ALL in adults. Most studies have looked at childhood and maternal diets in childhood ALL.

Kwiatkowski studied 119 adults with acute leukemia (91 acute myeloid leukemia and 28 ALL) and examined selected dietary risk factors and other environmental factors by a case-control study method [85]. It was shown that the diet of patients with acute leukemias had rare consumption of raw vegetables, frequent drinking of milk, frequent consumption of poultry, and drinking of soft water. Shu and colleagues revealed in a Chinese case-control study that childhood consumption of vitamin A and D laden cod-liver oil could reduce the risk of childhood leukemia [86]. As part of the Northern California Childhood Leukemia Study, Kwan and colleagues showed a protective effect of the consumption of oranges, orange juice, and bananas against ALL [87].

Petridou and colleagues used data from a nationwide case-control study in Greece to look at the effect of maternal diet on the risk of ALL in children aged 1–5 years [88]. They found that the risk of ALL was lower with increased maternal intake of fruits, vegetables, fish, and seafood, while the risk increased with the intake of sugars, syrups, meat, and meat products. The Northern California Childhood Leukemia Study showed that maternal consumption of vegetables, protein sources, fruits, as well as provitamin A carotenoids and antioxidant glutathione [89].

Spector and colleagues (2005) also showed that maternal consumption of fruits and vegetables decreases the risk of ALL [90]. They also looked at maternal consumption of foods containing inhibitors of DNA topoisomerase II (an enzyme required for gene transcription, DNA recombination, and replication), such as flavonoids, quinolone, and podophyllin resins, and found that this may increase the risk of AML (MLL positive) cases but had no effect on ALL risk.

References

1. Reis, L. A. G., Melbert, D., Krapcho, M., et al. (Eds.). (2008). *SEER cancer statistics review, 1975–2005.* Bethesda: National Cancer Institute. http://seer.cancer.gov/csr/1975_2005/, based on 2007 SEER data submission, posted to SEER web site 2009.
2. Groves, F. D., Linet, M. S., & Devesa, S. S. (1995). Patterns of occurrence of the leukemias. *European Journal of Cancer, 31A*, 941–949.
3. Gurney, J. G., Davis, S., Severson, R. K., et al. (1996). Trends in Cancer incidence among children in the US. *Cancer, 78*, 532–541.
4. Pui, C.-H. (1996). Acute leukemia in children. *Current Opinion in Hematology, 3*, 249–258.
5. Taylor, P. R., Reid, M. M., Bown, N., et al. (1992). Acute lymphoblastic leukemia in patients aged 60 years and over: A population-based study of incidence and outcome. *Blood, 80*, 1813–1817.
6. Gokbuget, N., Hoelzer, D., Arnold, R., et al. (2000). Treatment of adult ALL according to protocols of the German Multicenter Study Group for Adult ALL (GMALL). *Hematology/Oncology Clinics of North America, 14*, 1307–1325.
7. Linker, C., Damon, L., Ries, C., & Navarro, W. (2002). Intensified and shortened cyclical chemotherapy for adult acute lymphoblastic leukemia. *Journal of Clinical Oncology, 20*, 2464–2471.
8. Annino, L., Vegna, M. L., Camera, A., et al. (2002). Treatment of adult acute lymphoblastic leukemia (ALL): Long-term follow-up of the GIMEMAALL 0288 randomized study. *Blood, 99*, 863–871.
9. Takeuchi, J., Kyo, T., Naito, K., et al. (2002). Induction therapy by frequent administration of doxorubicin with four other drugs, followed by intensive consolidation and maintenance therapy for adult acute lymphoblastic leukemia: the JALSG-ALL93 study. *Leukemia, 16*, 1259–1266.
10. Kantarjian, H., Thomas, D., O'Brien, S., et al. (2004). Longterm follow-up results of hyperfractionated cyclophosphamide, vincristine, doxorubicin, and dexamethasone (Hyper-CVAD), a dose-intensive regimen, in adult acute lymphocytic leukemia. *Cancer, 101*, 2788–2801.
11. Larson, R. A. (2004). The U.S. trials in adult acute lymphoblastic leukemia. *Annals of Hematology, 83*(Suppl 1), S127–S128.
12. Gokbuget, N., & Hoelzer, D. (2006). Treatment of adult acute lymphoblastic leukemia. *Hematology (American Society of Hematology Education Program), 1*, 133–141.

13. Pui, C. H., & Evans, W. E. (2006). Treatment of acute lymphoblastic leukemia. *The New England Journal of Medicine, 354*, 166–178.
14. Ottmann, O. G., Wassmann, B., Pfeifer, H., et al. (2007). Imatinibcompared with chemotherapy as front-line treatment of elderly patients with Philadelphia chromosome-positive acute lymphoblastic leukemia (Ph_ALL). *Cancer, 109*, 2068–2076.
15. Mizuta, S., Kohno, A., Morishita, Y., et al. (2007). Long-term follow-up of 14 patients with Philadelphia chromosome-positive acute lymphoblastic leukemia following autologous bone marrow transplantation in first complete remission. *International Journal of Hematology, 85*, 140–145.
16. Vignetti, M., Fazi, P., Cimino, G., et al. (2007). Imatinib plussteroids induces complete remissions and prolonged survival in elderly Philadelphia chromosome-positive patients with acute lymphoblastic leukemia without additional chemotherapy: Results of the Gruppo Italiano Malattie Ematologiche dell'Adulto (GIMEMA) LAL0201-B protocol. *Blood, 109*, 3676–3678.
17. Carpenter, P. A., Snyder, D. S., Flowers, M. E., et al. (2007). Prophylactic administration of imatinib after hematopoietic cell transplantation for high-risk Philadelphia chromosome-positive leukemia. *Blood, 109*, 2791–2793.
18. Fielding, A. K., Richards, S. M., Chopra, R., et al. (2007). Outcome of 609 adults after relapse of acute lymphoblastic leukemia (ALL); an MRC UKALL12/ ECOG2993 study. *Blood, 109*, 944–950.
19. Zuelzer, W. W. (1964). Implications of long-term survivals in acute stem cell leukemia of childhood treated with composite cyclic therapy. *Blood, 24*, 477–494.
20. Linet, M. S., Wacholder, S., & Zahm, S. H. (2003). Interpreting epidemiologic research: lessons from studies of childhood cancer. *Pediatrics, 112*, 218–232.
21. Swensen, A. R., Ross, J. A., Severson, R. K., Pollock, B. H., & Robison, L. L. (1997). The age peak in childhood acute lymphoblastic leukemia. *Cancer, 79*, 2045–2051.
22. Sandler, D. P., & Ross, J. A. (1997). Epidemiology of acute leukemia in children and adults. *Seminars in Oncology, 24*, 3–16.
23. Ross, J. A., Spector, L. G., & Davies, S. M. (2005). Biological basis of cancer and blood disorder. Etiology of childhood cancer: Recent reports. *Pediatric Blood & Cancer, 45*, 239–241.
24. Ross, J. A., Davies, S. M., Potter, J. D., & Robison, L. L. (1994). Epidemiology of childhood leukemia, with a focus on infants. *Epidemiologic Reviews, 16*, 243–272.
25. Greaves, M. F. (1997). Aetiology of acute leukemia. *Lancet, 349*, 344–349.
26. Greenberg, R. S., & Shuster, J. L., Jr. (1985). Epidemiology of cancer in children. *Epidemiologic Reviews, 7*, 22–48.
27. Poole, C., Greenland, S., Luetters, C., Kelsey, J. L., & Mezei, G. (2006). Socioeconomic status and childhood leukemia: A review. *International Journal of Epidemiology, 35*, 370–384.
28. Vanasse, G. J., Concannon, P., & Willerford, D. M. (1999). Regulated genomic instability and neoplasia in the lymphoid lineage. *Blood, 94*, 3997–4010.
29. Pui, C.-H., Raimondi, S. C., Borowitz, M. J., et al. (1993). Immunophenotypes and karyotypes of leukemic cells in children with Down syndrome and acute lymphoblastic leukemia. *Journal of Clinical Oncology, 11*, 1361–1367.
30. Liberzon, E., Avigad, S., Stark, B., et al. (2004). Germ-line ATM gene alterations are associated with susceptibility to sporadic T-cell acute lymphoblastic leukemia in children. *Genes, Chromosomes & Cancer, 39*, 161.
31. Secker-Walker, L. M., Prentice, H. G., Durrant, J., et al. (1997). Cytogenetics adds independent prognostic information in adults with acute lymphoblastic leukemia on MRC trial UKALL XA. *British Journal Haematology, 96*, 601–610.
32. Charrin, C. (1996). Cytogenetic abnormalities in adult acute lymphoblastic leukemia: Correlations with hematologic findings and outcome. A collaborative study of Groupe Français de Cytogénétique Hématologique. *Blood, 87*, 3135–3142.
33. Borkhardt, A., Cazzaniga, G., Viehmann, S., et al. (1977). Incidence and clinical relevance of TEL/AML1 fusion genes in children with acute lymphoblastic leukemia enrolled in the German and Italian multicenter therapy trials. *Blood, 90*, 571–577.
34. Golub, T. R., Barker, G. F., Bohlander, S. K., et al. (1995). Fusion of the TEL gene on 12p13 to the AML1 gene on 21q22 in acute lymphoblastic leukemia. *Proceedings of the National Academy of Science, 92*, 4917–4921.
35. Mikhail, F. M., Serry, K. A., Hatem, N., et al. (2002). A new translocation that rearranges the AML1 gene in a patient with T-cell acute lymphoblastic leukemia. *Cancer Genetics and Cytogenetics, 135*, 96–100.
36. Mori, H., Colman, S. M., Xiao, Z., et al. (2002). Chromosome translocations and covert leukemic clones are generated during normal fetal development. *Proceedings of the National Academy of Science, 99*, 8242–8247.
37. Rubnitz, J. E., Downing, J. R., Pui, C. H., et al. (1997). TEL gene rearrangement in acute lymphoblastic leukemia: A new genetic marker with prognostic significance. *Clinical Oncology, 15*, 1150–1157.
38. Pui, C. H., Crist, W. M., & Look, A. T. (1990). Biological and clinical significance of cytogenetic abnormalities in childhood acute lymphoblastic leukemia. *Blood, 76*, 1149–1163.
39. Sandler, D. P., & Ross, J. A. (1997). Epidemiology of acute leukemia in children and adults. *Seminars in Oncology, 24*, 3–16.

40. Kinlen, L. J. (1988). Evidence for an infective cause of childhood leukemia: Comparison of a Scottish new town with nuclear reprocessing sites in Britain. *Lancet, ii*, 1323–1327.
41. Kinlen, L. J. (1995). Epidemiological evidence for an infective basis in childhood leukemia [editorial]. *British Journal of Cancer, 71*, 1–5.
42. Smith, M. (1997). Considerations on a possible viral etiology for B precursor acute lymphoblastic leukemia of childhood. *Journal of Immunotherapy, 20*, 89–100.
43. Smith, M. A., Simon, R., Strickler, H. D., et al. (1998). Evidence that childhood acute lymphoblastic leukemia is associated with an infectious agent linked to hygiene conditions. *Cancer Causes & Control, 9*, 285–298.
44. Greaves, M. F. (1988). Speculations on the cause of childhood acute lymphoblastic leukaemia. *Leukemia, 2*, 120–125.
45. Greaves, M. F., & Alexander, F. E. (1993). An infectious etiology for common acute lymphoblastic leukemia in childhood? *Leukemia, 7*, 349–360.
46. Kinlen, L. J., & Petridou, E. (1995). Childhood leukemia and rural population movements: Greece, Italy, and other countries. *Cancer Causes & Control, 6*, 445–450.
47. Koushik, A., King, W. D., & McLaughlin, J. R. (2001). An ecologic study of childhood leukemia and population mixing in Ontario, Canada. *Cancer Causes & Control, 12*, 483–490.
48. Lehtinen, M., Koskela, P., Ogmundsdottir, H. M., et al. (2003). Maternal herpes virus infections and risk of acute lymphoblastic leukaemia in the offspring. *American Journal of Epidemiology, 158*, 207–213.
49. Naumberg, E., Bellocco, R., Cnattingius, S., et al. (2002). Perinatal exposure to infection and risk of childhood leukaemia. *Medical and Pediatric Oncology, 38*, 391–397.
50. Infante-Rivard, C., Fortier, I., & Olson, E. (2000). Markers of infection, breast-feeding and childhood acute lymphoblastic leukaemia. *British Journal of Cancer, 83*, 1559–1564.
51. McKinney, P. A., Juszczak, E., Findlay, E., Smith, K., & Thomson, C. S. (1999). Pre- and perinatal risk factors for childhood leukaemia and other malignancies: A Scottish case control study. *British Journal of Cancer, 80*, 1844–1851.
52. Berrington, A., Darby, S. C., Weiss, H. A., & Doll, R. (2001). 100 years of observation on British radiologists: Mortality from cancer and other causes 1897–1997. *The British Journal of Radiology, 74*, 507–519.
53. Heath, C. W. (1982). Leukemogenesis and low-dose radiation exposure to radiation and chemical agents. In D. S. Yohn & J. R. Blakeslee (Eds.), *Advances in comparative leukemia research* (p. 23). Amsterdam: North Holland/Elsevier.
54. Preston, D. L., Kusumi, S., Tomonaga, M., et al. (1994). Cancer incidence in atomic bomb survivors. Part III: Leukemia, lymphoma and multiple myeloma, 1950–1987. *Radiation Research, 137*, S68–S97.
55. Darby, S. C., Doll, R., Gill, S. K., & Smith, P. G. (1987). Long term mortality after a single treatment course with X-rays in patients treated for ankylosing spondylitis. *British Journal of Cancer, 55*, 179–190.
56. Schuberger-Berigan, M. K., & Wenzl, T. B. (2001). Leukemia mortality among radiation-exposed workers. *Occupational Medicine, 16*, 271–287.
57. Gardner, M. J., Hall, A. J., Downes, S., & Terrell, J. D. (1987). Follow up study of children born elsewhere but attending schools in Seascale, West Cumbria (schools cohort). *British Medical Journal, 295*, 819–827.
58. Gardner, M. J., Snee, M. P., Hall, A. J., Powell, C. A., Downes, S., & Terrell, J. D. (1990). Results of case-control study of leukaemia and lymphoma among young people near Sellafield nuclear plant in West Cumbria. *British Medical Journal, 300*, 423–429.
59. Boice, J. D., Jr., Bigbee, W. L., Mumma, M. T., & Blot, W. J. (2003). Cancer mortality in counties near two former nuclear materials processing facilities in Pennsylvania, 1950–1995. *Health Physics, 85*, 691–700.
60. Laurier, D., Grosche, B., & Hall, P. (2002). Risk of childhood leukaemia in the vicinity of nuclear installations—findings and recent controversies [Review]. [118 refs]. *Acta Oncológica, 41*, 14–24.
61. Haesman, M. A., Kemp, J. W., MacLaren, A. M., et al. (1984). Incidence of leukaemia in young persons in the west of Scotland. *Lancet, 1*, 1188.
62. Doll, R., & Wakeford, R. (1997). Risk of childhood cancer from fetal irradiation. *The British Journal of Radiology, 70*, 130.
63. Stewart, A., Webb, J., & Hewitt, D. (1958). A survey of childhood malignancies. *British Medical Journal, 28*, 1497–1507.
64. Ahlbom, A., Day, N., Feychting, M., et al. (2000). A pooled analysis of magnetic fields and childhood leukemia. *British Journal of Cancer, 83*, 692.
65. Kheifets, L., Afifi, A. A., Buffler, P. A., Zhang, Z., & Matkin, C. (1997). Occupational electric and magnetic field exposure and leukemia. *Journal of Occupational and Environmental Medicine, 39*, 1074–1091.
66. Wartenberg, D. (2001). Residential EMF exposure and childhood leukemia: Meta-analysis and population attributable risk. *Bioelectromagnetics, 5*(Suppl), S86–S104.
67. National Research Council. *Possible health effects of exposure to residential electric and magnetic fields.* Committee on the Possible Effects of Electromagnetic Fields on Biologic Systems (Eds.). Washington, DC: National Academy Press, 1997

68. Kipen, H. M., & Wartenberg, D. (2005). Lymphohematopoietic malignancies. In L. Rosenstock, M. R. Cullen, C. A. Brodkin, & C. A. Redlich (Eds.), *Textbook of clinical occupational and environmental medicine* (pp. 744–756). New York: Elsevier/Saunders.
69. Cronkite, E. P. (1987). Chemical leukemogenesis: Benzene as a model. *Seminars in Hematology, 24*, 2–11.
70. Glass, D. C., Gray, C. N., Jolley, D. J., et al. (2003). Leukemia risk associated with low-level benzene exposure. *Epidemiology, 14*, 569–577.
71. Rushton, L., & Romaniuk, H. (1997). A case-control study to investigate the risk of leukemia associated with exposure to benzene in petroleum marketing and distribution workers in the United Kingdom. *Occupational and Environmental Medicine, 54*, 152–166.
72. Schuz, J., Kaletsch, U., Meinert, R., Kaatsch, P., & Michaelis, J. (2000). Risk of childhood leukemia and parental self-reported occupational exposure to chemicals, dusts, and fumes: Results from pooled analyses of German population-based case-control studies. *Cancer Epidemiology, Biomarkers & Prevention, 9*, 835–838.
73. Shu, X. O., Stewart, P., Wen, W.-Q., Han, D., Potter, J., Buckley, J. D., et al. (1999). Parental occupational exposure to hydrocarbons and risk of acute lymphocytic leukemia in offspring. *Cancer Epidemiology, Biomarkers & Prevention, 8*, 783–791.
74. Colt, J. S., & Blair, S. (1998). Parental occupational exposures and risk of childhood cancers. *Environmental Health Perspectives, 106*(Suppl), 909–925.
75. Freedman, M. D., Stewart, P., Kleinerman, R. A., Wacholder, S., Hatch, E. E., Tarone, R. E., et al. (2001). Household solvent exposures and childhood acute lymphoblastic leukemia. *American Journal of Public Health, 91*, 564–567.
76. Rudant, J., Menegaux, F., Leverger, G., et al. (2007). Household Exposure to Pesticides and Risk of Childhood Hematopoietic malignancies: The ESCALE Study (SFCE). *Environmental Health Perspectives, 115*, 1787–1793.
77. Infante-Rivard, C., Labuda, D., Krajinovic, M., & Sinnett, D. (1999). Risk of childhood leukemia associated with exposure to pesticides and with gene polymorphisms. *Epidemiology, 10*, 481–487.
78. Hecht, S. S., & Hoffmann, D. (1988). Tobacco-specific nitrosamines, an important group of carcinogens in tobacco and tobacco smoke. *Carcinogenesis, 9*, 875–884.
79. Wallace, L. A., & Pellizan, E. D. (1986). Personal air exposures and breath concentration of benzene and other volatile hydrocarbons for smokers and non-smokers. *Toxicology Letters, 35*, 113–116.
80. Shu, X. O., Ross, J. A., Pendergrass, T. W., Reaman, G. H., Lampkin, B., & Robison, L. L. (1996). Parental alcohol consumption, cigarette smoking, and risk of infant leukemia: A Children's CancerGroup study. *Journal of the National Cancer Institute, 88*(1), 24–31.
81. Pang, D., McNally, R. J. Q., & Birch, J. M. (2003). United Kingdom childhood cancer study. Parental smoking and childhood cancer: Results from the United Kingdom childhood cancer study. *British Journal of Cancer, 88*, 373–381.
82. Wen, W., Shu, X. O., Potter, J. D., Severson, R. K., Buckley, J. D., Reaman, G. H., et al. (2002). Parental medication use and risk of childhood acute lymphoblastic leukaemia. *Cancer, 95*(8), 1786–1794.
83. Kwan, M. L., Metayer, C., Crouse, V., & Buffler, P. A. (2007). Maternal illness and drug/medication use during the period surrounding pregnancy and risk of childhood leukemia among offspring. *American Journal of Epidemiology, 165*, 27–35.
84. Reynolds, P., Behren, J. V., Gunier, R. B., Goldberg, D. E., Hertz, A., & Smith, D. F. (2003). Childhood cancer incidence rates and hazardous air pollutants in California: An exploratory analysis. *Environmental Health Perspectives, 111*, 663–668.
85. Kwiatkowski, A. (1993). Dietary and other environmental risk factors in acute leukemias: A case-control study of 119 patients. *European Journal of Cancer Prevention, 2*, 139–146.
86. Shu, X. O., Gao, Y.-T., Brinton, L. A., et al. (1988). A population-based case-control study of childhood leukemia in Shanghai. *Cancer, 62*, 934–937.
87. Kwan, M. L., Block, G., Selvin, S., Month, S., & Buffler, P. A. (2004). Food consumption by children and the risk of childhood acute leukemia. *American Journal of Epidemiology, 160*, 1098–1107.
88. Petridou, E., Ntouvelis, E., Dessypris, N., Terzidis, A., Trichopoulos, D., & the Childhood Hematology-Oncology Group. (2005). Maternal diet and acute lymphoblastic leukemia in young children. *Cancer Epidemiology, Biomarkers & Prevention, 14*(8), 1935–1939.
89. Jensen, C. D., Block, G., Buffler, P., Ma, X., Selvin, S., & Month, S. (2004). Maternal dietary risk factors in childhood acute lymphoblastic leukemia (United States). *Cancer Causes & Control, 15*(6), 559–570.
90. Spector, L. G., Xie, Y., Robison, L. L., Heerema, N. A., Hilden, J. M., Lange, B., et al. (2005). Maternal diet and infant leukemia: The DNA topoisomerase II inhibitor hypothesis: A report from the children's oncology group. *Cancer Epidemiology, Biomarkers & Prevention, 14*(3), 651–655.

Chapter 7
Prognostic Factors in Adult Acute Lymphoblastic Leukemia (ALL)

Adele K. Fielding

Introduction

The treatment of adults with ALL, although not offering the same satisfactory long-term disease-free survivals (DFS) as is afforded to the majority of children, has improved steadily over the past decades. Outcomes have improved for all adult age groups except for the over sixties [1]. Treating physicians are very much aware that age has, arguably, the most significant impact on outcome. To what extent that relates to the changing biology of the disease with age, per se, or whether it results from a different approach to – or tolerance of – therapy is unclear.

Prognostic factors for the outcome of ALL across the age groups have been known for over 20 years. However, it is easier to identify prognostic factors than it is to decide what to do in response to them. Hence, although the major prognostic factors now frequently form the basis for some degree of therapeutic stratification in ALL, there is little convincing evidence that our currently available therapeutic strategies are able to overcome the poorer outcomes predicted by the occurrence of adverse prognostic factors. However, there is some therapeutic comfort in matching a potentially effective – but very toxic – therapy such as allogeneic bone marrow transplant more closely with a patient who is destined to have a high risk of death as a result of his or her disease, and therapeutic stratifications of this type are used both in clinical practice and in clinical trials. As yet, prognostic information cannot be used to define a group of adults at very low risk of relapse, so in contrast to pediatric ALL practice, there is currently no attempt to limit therapy for adults on the basis of an expectation of good outcome.

In this chapter, current prognostic factors for adults with ALL will be reviewed. Where possible, their interrelationships will be explored. An emphasis will be placed on discussion of prognostic factors, where possible therapeutic interventions are available or envisaged.

"Classic" Clinical Diagnostic Prognostic Factors

Presenting White Blood Count (WBC)

The WBC at presentation impacts upon outcome for all subtypes of ALL and at all ages. Although presenting WBC is a continuum, for the purposes of stratification, cutoff levels for poor prognosis have been drawn at levels of 30×10^9/L for those with B precursor ALL and 100×10^9/L for T cell

A.K. Fielding (✉)
University College London Medical School, London, UK
e-mail: a.fielding@medsch.ucl.ac.uk

A.S. Advani and H.M. Lazarus (eds.), *Adult Acute Lymphocytic Leukemia*, Contemporary Hematology, DOI 10.1007/978-1-60761-707-5_7, © Springer Science+Business Media, LLC 2011

ALL [2, 3]. Presenting WBC often predicts for any or all of the outcome measures tested, both for initial response, that is, achievement of complete remission (CR) after initial therapy, and for long-term outcome measures, such as event-free survival (EFS), disease-free survival (DFS), and overall survival (OS).

Age

The outcome of ALL becomes steadily worse with advancing age [4]. This effect is apparent throughout the pediatric, adolescent, adult, and elderly age spectrum. Determining to what extent the reason for this is based on the biology of the disease, the biology of age, or variations in treatment approach with age is the key aim of current research in ALL.

There are evident changes in the biology of the disease with age. Most notably, the incidence of "very high risk" cytogenetic categories, such as Philadelphia chromosome positive (Ph pos) ALL, increases with advancing age. Ph pos ALL accounts for approximately 25% of adults [5], while it is uncommon (approximately 3%) in children [6]. The distribution of presenting white cell counts differs with age; the median presenting white cell counts of patients recruited into pediatric studies is generally much lower than those recruited into adult studies, as demonstrated in the review by Pui and Evans [7].

In addition, the clearly documented biological differences tolerance of treatment is also generally poorer with advancing age. As an example, there is a much higher rate of induction death among adult patients compared to that in children [6].

Impact of Therapy Received on Age-Related Prognosis

There is a body of retrospective evidence, which suggests that a "pediatric" approach to therapy may confer superior survival to an adult approach in those of "adolescent" age group [8–12]. The better of the comparative retrospective datasets are derived from large national studies in which there was overlap between the entry ages to the pediatric and adult studies at the time, enabling some comparison of the different therapeutic approaches in the same age group. It can be reasonably concluded from these studies that a pediatric approach to therapy is superior in those of adolescent age. However, such retrospective studies are subject to considerable selection bias and the data need to be examined carefully and interpreted with caution before extrapolating to older adults. As an example, the study from the UK [13] pediatric and adult groups compared the outcome of patients aged 15–17, who were treated according to either pediatric or adult or national study protocols. On univariate analysis, there was an apparent large and statistically significant survival advantage to having been treated on the pediatric study. However, despite the narrow age range studied, there was also a highly significant age difference between the "adult therapy" and "pediatric therapy" groups, with very few 15 year olds in the "adult therapy" group and very few 17 year olds in the "pediatric therapy" group; age was shown to be a significant prognostic variable among patients in this analysis. On multivariate analysis, only age and Ph status – but not therapy received – remained prognostic for outcome. Despite the difficulties in interpretation, the weight of evidence suggests that for those of "adolescent" age, outcome can be improved by a pediatric therapeutic approach. Based on these data – and in advance of a full understanding of the age-related difference in ALL outcomes – there are several nonrandomized studies in older adults investigating treatment approaches more aligned with those applied in pediatric patients. The outcome of this shift in emphasis remains to be determined. It is becoming clearer that "pediatric style" intensive therapy can be delivered to older patients with standard-risk ALL, at least up to the age of 30, with a reasonably good outcome of approximately

60% OS at 5 years [14]. This outcome is superimposable on the outcome seen for patients of the same age and risk status with a sibling donor in the UKALLXII/ECOG2993 donor vs. no donor analysis [15]. To date, there are currently no data to suggest that the poor prognostic relevance of advanced age can yet be overcome by a "pediatric" therapeutic approach, but this is an active area of study.

Immunophenotype

T Cell Versus B Cell ALL

The stage of differentiation of the precursor cell in both T and B lineage disease can be inferred from the expression of various cell surface markers. These and other immunophenotypic markers, sometimes aberrantly expressed for the cell of origin or stage of differentiation, have been extensively investigated as potential prognostic factors, mostly in childhood ALL. The most useful way in which to evaluate the relevance of these studies is to consider whether the identification of an immunophenotypic marker of potential prognostic value could lead to a different approach to therapy. The most important immunophenotypic and prognostic delineation is between T cell and B cell precursor ALL.

T cell ALL more often occurs in males than females, and in younger as opposed to older individuals. It is more often associated with a higher presenting WBC, and with the presence of a mediastinal mass and central nervous system (CNS) involvement than B cell precursor ALL [16]. Despite this, T cell ALL carries a significantly better prognosis for OS and EFS than B cell ALL, as demonstrated by data from three different large national and international studies [2, 3, 16].

The therapeutic relevance of the differences in associations and outcomes between T ALL and B ALL is increasingly relevant with the advent of more targeted therapeutic strategies. Nelarabine [4] is a prodrug that is rapidly demethylated in the blood by adenosine deaminase to arabinosylguanine (ara-G), a deoxyguanosine analogue. T lymphoblasts are more sensitive than B lymphoblasts to the cytotoxic effects of deoxyguanosine, due to an initial higher accumulation of ara-G. Nelarabine has potential when used specifically in the therapy of T ALL; in adults, there was a 31% CR rate to single agent nelarabine when used in the setting of relapsed or resistant disease [17].

The aberrant expression of myeloid markers CD13 and CD33 on either T or B cell blasts does not appear to confer a poor prognosis in adult ALL. A study from the GIEMEMA ALL 0496 trial found aberrant expression of myeloid antigens in approximately 30% of patients' blasts, but more often in B cell (38%) than T cell (24%) disease. The study did not identify a correlation between myeloid antigen expression and any of the outcome measures studied [18].

Other Immunophenotypic Markers

The prognostic significance of specific immunophenotypic markers of B-precursor ALL is also of increasing therapeutic relevance with the advent of monoclonal antibodies against targets present on B-ALL blasts. Recent evidence suggests that the expression of CD20 on ALL blasts may be associated with a particularly poor prognosis – duration of CR and OS were both poor for the group whose ALL cells expressed high levels of CD20, regardless of chemotherapy received [19]. Intriguingly, recent data from childhood ALL suggested that CD20 – although expressed at low levels in the majority of cases – increased considerably in expression, both in antigen density and in the number of cells expressing the antigen, following initial induction therapy. In vitro work indicated that glucocorticoids were the likely agent responsible for this effect and showed that the increased CD20 expression correlated with an increased in vitro responsiveness to anti-CD20 antibody treatment [20].

The value of identifying certain immunophenotypic markers as prognostic factors is that it generates specific hypotheses about the therapy of ALL, which are immediately testable with clinically available agents. Several groups are already investigating the role of anti-CD20 antibodies in the treatment of ALL in adults.

Specific Clinical Features

CNS Disease at Diagnosis

Approximately 5% of adults have ALL involving the CNS at the time of diagnosis. Survival is generally worse in this situation. Among 1,508 patients enrolled in UKALLXII/ECOG2993, OS at 5 years was 29% for those with vs. 38% for those without CNS involvement [21].

Cytogenetics

The poor prognostic impact of the finding of t(9;22), the Philadelphia chromosome (Ph pos ALL) – in approximately 25% of adults with ALL – has long been recognized. Patients with Ph pos ALL are less likely to enter CR with CR rates of approximately 70–80% and OS of around 15–20%. ALL treatment protocols have typically assigned patients with Ph pos ALL to "very high risk" protocols and myeloablative transplant has typically been offered, even when sibling donors were not available. t(4;11) has also been recognized as carrying a poor prognosis [22]. Recently, 2 large studies have further refined cytogenetic risk factors for adult ALL. In an analysis of data from 1,522 adult patients participating in the UKALLXII/ECOG2993 study [5], patients with t(9;22), t(4;11), complex karyotype (defined as 5 or more chromosomal abnormalities), or low hypodiploidy/near triploidy all had markedly inferior rates of EFS and OS when compared with other patients. Among patients with Ph negative ALL, the prognostic relevance of complex karyotype and low hypodiploidy/near triploidy was independent of the known prognostic factors listed above such as age and presenting WBC. This was the first demonstration that cytogenetic subgroups other than the Ph chromosome can be used for risk-stratification of adults with ALL. A report from SWOG-9400 [23] on the outcome of 200 patients (140 evaluable for cytogenetics) in relation to cytogenetic abnormalities recapitulated the findings of the UKALLXII/ECOG2993 study and a previous GIMEMA study [24]. Importantly, it raised the possibility that when the effect of cytogenetics on OS was accounted for, age was not a significant prognostic factor. This suggests that the worsening prognosis with advancing age in adult ALL could at least in part be a manifestation of the age-related increase in unfavorable cytogenetics.

Response to Therapy

Time to CR

Achievement of CR at an early time-point after the start of treatment – in adults, typically conceived as being 4 weeks, that is, following one course of induction therapy – has long been seen as an important prognostic factor for adult patients with ALL [3]. However, achievement of CR after one course of induction therapy was not confirmed as an independent prognostic factor in the UKALLXII-ECOG2993 international study, which is the largest study of adult ALL to date. However, many patients in this study received myeloablative transplant as a post-induction therapy, which perhaps mitigated against the possible fate accompanying a poor early response to treatment. It was certainly the case that people who had no response to two courses of induction therapy fared very poorly. Recent reports in childhood ALL have suggested that a response within 7–14 days is associated with the best prognosis [25]. However, this has never been prospectively confirmed in adult ALL.

Minimal Residual Disease (MRD)

Morphological detection of remission has very limited sensitivity and a patient in CR may still bear a considerable disease burden. It is now possible to quantitate treatment response very accurately and reproducibly, to the level of one leukemic cell in ten thousand using well-standardized molecular methods [26] to identify patient-specific immunoglobulin and T cell receptor gene rearrangements, which can then be quantified by real-time PCR after therapy. Flow cytometry can also be used to determine a disease-associated immunophenotype at diagnosis, which can then be quantified post-therapy. A diagnostic sample is required in both cases. Where there is a known molecular abnormality such as *BCR-ABL*, this can also be quantified, using a housekeeping gene as a reference standard, to determine the level of residual ALL with similar sensitivity. Studies in both childhood and adult ALL have shown a significant correlation between MRD levels and subsequent relapse risk [27, 28]. In adults, molecular methods have predominated, although there is one report from the Polish Adult Leukemia Group of a correlation between outcome and MRD as quantified by flow cytometry [29]. Reports have generally focused on the prognostic importance of MRD in the standard therapy setting, consisting of protracted consolidation/maintenance chemotherapy after remission attainment [27]. It is not known whether high-risk interventions such as bone marrow transplant can overcome the poor prognostic significance of residual MRD. It is also possible to use MRD analysis to monitor the progress of patients in remission in order to detect impending relapse – the time-window between molecular and hematological relapse is in the order of a few months, possibly yielding an opportunity for early intervention [30]. However, the clinical potential of treatment prior to hematological relapse is not yet clear.

Pharmacogenetics

Normal genetic variations – polymorphisms – can interact to influence treatment outcome in ALL and can be potentially important determinants of response. Polymorphisms in enzymes of the folic acid cycle, immune surveillance, drug metabolism, and drug transport have all been investigated to account for the variations seen in treatment response, recently reviewed by Cunningham and Aplenc [31]. While many of these investigations are at an early stage and there is no immediate clinical impact, it is already possible to take action on the basis of some of these, resulting in the possibility of optimizing therapy on an individual basis. It is also important to bear in mind that pharmacogenetic factors have been studied widely in childhood ALL but rarely, to date, in adult ALL. The best known and used is a genetic polymorphism in the thiopurine S-methyltransferase (TPMT) gene conferring differing levels of enzyme activity. The effect of low enzyme activity is to confer a particular sensitivity to the effects of 6-mercaptopurine (6-MP) as a result of the accumulation of higher cellular concentrations of thioguanine nucleotides. This can be an important determinant of 6-MP

Table 7.1 Summary of prognostic factors in adult ALL

Type of factor	Factor	Impact on outcome
Clinical		
	Presenting WBC	Higher WBC at diagnosis; worse outcome
	Age	Older age; worse outcome
Laboratory		
	Immunophenotype	T cell disease better than B
	Cytogenetic	Several cytogenetic abnormalities correlate with better or worse prognosis
Treatment related		
	Time to CR1	Relationship with outcome less clear than in children
	Minimal residual disease presence at protocol-defined time point	Clear but protocol-specific relationship with outcome
Genetic/genomic		
	Pharmacogenetic	Polymorphisms in many enzymes may affect outcome
	Genomic	Abnormalities in key pathways in lymphocyte biology are increasingly being related to outcome

toxicity, even among patients who are heterozygous for the trait [32]. If the doses of 6-MP are not modified to limit toxicity, delivery of concomitant therapy can also be compromised by the 6-MP toxicity [33].

In a subsequent study, the St Jude's group determined the relationship between 16 genetic polymorphisms affecting the pharmacodynamics of antileukemic agents and outcome. [34] Both a non-null genotype of glutathione S-transferase (GSTM1) and a 3/3 genotype of thymidylate synthetase (TYMS) were predictive of relapse among a high-risk group of children and this was linked to drug resistance conferred by the polymorphisms.

Genomics

Microarray-based analyses of DNA copy number abnormalities (CNAs) has identified a high frequency of common genetic alterations in both B-progenitor and T-lineage ALL. Abnormalities in key pathways, including lymphoid differentiation, cell cycle regulation, and tumor suppression, have all been identified as relating to outcome [35–37]. For example, genetic alteration of IKZF1, a gene that encodes the lymphoid transcription factor IKAROS, is associated with a very poor outcome in B-cell-progenitor ALL in patients who are otherwise characterized as standard-risk patients [38]. Furthermore, the nature and frequency of CNAs differ markedly among ALL genetic subtype [37]. To date, the majority of work has been carried out in pediatric ALL. There is no reason to suppose similar approaches will not yield exciting information in adult ALL, but data are presently lacking (Table 7.1).

Prognosis of Relapsed ALL

Once ALL has relapsed in adults, survival is generally very poor. Although salvage is often attempted, it is very worthwhile to know which patients are most likely to benefit from conventional salvage therapy and which are likely to fare so poorly that they should be directed, if possible, toward studies of novel therapies. Two large studies of patients who relapsed following initial therapy on UKALLXII/ECOG2993 [39] and LALA94 [40] have recently been carried out. It is evident that once relapse has occurred, it is generally features at relapse, rather than at original diagnosis, which determines outcome [40]. Factors predicting poor outcome from relapse included older age, a short duration of first remission, and relapse in the CNS. Treatment received in CR1, that is, chemotherapy or bone marrow transplant, did not predict for outcome after relapse [39].

Conclusions

The most important thing in the therapy of adult ALL is to prevent relapse, since salvage is rarely possible. Increased insight into the innate and acquired factors predicting outcome from both diagnosis and initial therapeutic response will ultimately permit therapy, which is more in keeping with individual risk factors for poor outcome, and will allow us to use appropriate therapies at the optimal times, minimizing risk wherever possible.

References

1. Pulte, D., Gondos, A., & Brenner, H. (2009). Improvement in survival in younger patients with acute lymphoblastic leukemia from the 1980s to the early 21st century. *Blood, 113*(7), 1408–1411.
2. Rowe, J. M., Buck, G., Burnett, A. K., et al. (2005). Induction therapy for adults with acute lymphoblastic leukemia: Results of more than 1500 patients from the international ALL trial: MRC UKALL XII/ECOG E2993. *Blood, 106*, 3760–3767.
3. Hoelzer, D., Thiel, E., Loffler, H., et al. (1988). Prognostic factors in a multicenter study for treatment of acute lymphoblastic leukemia in adults. *Blood, 71*, 123–131.
4. Chessells, J. M., Hall, E., Prentice, H. G., Durrant, J., Bailey, C. C., & Richards, S. M. (1998). The impact of age on outcome in lymphoblastic leukaemia; MRC UKALL X and XA compared: A report from the MRC Paediatric and Adult Working Parties. *Leukemia, 12*, 463–473.
5. Moorman, A. V., Harrison, C. J., Buck, G. A., et al. (2007). Karyotype is an independent prognostic factor in adult acute lymphoblastic leukemia (ALL): Analysis of cytogenetic data from patients treated on the Medical Research Council (MRC) UKALLXII/Eastern Cooperative Oncology Group (ECOG) 2993 trial. *Blood, 109*, 3189–3197.
6. Jones, L. K., & Saha, V. (2005). Philadelphia positive acute lymphoblastic leukaemia of childhood. *British Journal Haematology, 130*, 489–500.
7. Pui, C. H., & Evans, W. E. (2006). Treatment of acute lymphoblastic leukemia. *The New England Journal of Medicine, 354*, 166–178.
8. Boissel, N., Auclerc, M. F., Lheritier, V., et al. (2003). Should adolescents with acute lymphoblastic leukemia be treated as old children or young adults? Comparison of the French FRALLE-93 and LALA-94 trials. *Journal of Clinical Oncology, 21*, 774–780.
9. Ramanujachar, R., Richards, S., Hann, I., & Webb, D. (2006). Adolescents with acute lymphoblastic leukaemia: Emerging from the shadow of paediatric and adult treatment protocols. *Pediatric Blood & Cancer, 47*, 748–756.
10. de Bont, J. M., Holt, B., Dekker, A. W., van der Does-van den Berg, A., Sonneveld, P., & Pieters, R. (2004). Significant difference in outcome for adolescents with acute lymphoblastic leukemia treated on pediatric vs adult protocols in the Netherlands. *Leukemia, 18*, 2032–2035.
11. Hallbook, H., Gustafsson, G., Smedmyr, B., Soderhall, S., & Heyman, M. (2006). Treatment outcome in young adults and children >10 years of age with acute lymphoblastic leukemia in Sweden: A comparison between a pediatric protocol and an adult protocol. *Cancer, 107*, 1551–1561.
12. Stock, W., La, M., Sanford, B., et al. (2008). What determines the outcomes for adolescents and young adults with acute lymphoblastic leukemia treated on cooperative group protocols? A comparison of Children's Cancer Group and Cancer and Leukemia Group B studies. *Blood, 112*, 1646–1654.
13. Ramanujachar, R., Richards, S., Hann, I., et al. (2007). Adolescents with acute lymphoblastic leukaemia: Outcome on UK national paediatric (ALL97) and adult (UKALLXII/E2993) trials. *Pediatric Blood & Cancer, 48*, 254–261.
14. Ribera, J. M., Oriol, A., Sanz, M. A., et al. (2008). Comparison of the results of the treatment of adolescents and young adults with standard-risk acute lymphoblastic leukemia with the Programa Espanol de Tratamiento en Hematologia pediatric-based protocol ALL-96. *Journal of Clinical Oncology, 26*, 1843–1849.
15. Goldstone, A. H., Richards, S. M., Lazarus, H. M., et al. (2008). In adults with standard-risk acute lymphoblastic leukemia, the greatest benefit is achieved from a matched sibling allogeneic transplantation in first complete remission,

and an autologous transplantation is less effective than conventional consolidation/maintenance chemotherapy in all patients: Final results of the International ALL Trial (MRC UKALL XII/ECOG E2993). *Blood, 111*, 1827–1833.

16. Boucheix, C., David, B., Sebban, C., et al. (1994). Immunophenotype of adult acute lymphoblastic leukemia, clinical parameters, and outcome: An analysis of a prospective trial including 562 tested patients (LALA87). French Group on Therapy for Adult Acute Lymphoblastic Leukemia. *Blood, 84*, 1603–1612.

17. DeAngelo, D. J., Yu, D., Johnson, J. L., et al. (2007). Nelarabine induces complete remissions in adults with relapsed or refractory T-lineage acute lymphoblastic leukemia or lymphoblastic lymphoma: Cancer and Leukemia Group B study 19801. *Blood, 109*, 5136–5142.

18. Vitale, A., Guarini, A., Ariola, C., et al. (2007). Absence of prognostic impact of CD13 and/or CD33 antigen expression in adult acute lymphoblastic leukemia. Results of the GIMEMA ALL 0496 trial. *Haematologica, 92*, 342–348.

19. Thomas, D. A., O'Brien, S., Jorgensen, J. L., et al. (2009). Prognostic significance of CD20 expression in adults with de novo precursor B-lineage acute lymphoblastic leukemia. *Blood, 113*, 6330–6337.

20. Dworzak, M. N., Schumich, A., Printz, D., et al. (2008). CD20 up-regulation in pediatric B-cell precursor acute lymphoblastic leukemia during induction treatment: Setting the stage for anti-CD20 directed immunotherapy. *Blood, 112*, 3982–3988.

21. Lazarus, H. M., Richards, S. M., Chopra, R., et al. (2006). Central nervous system involvement in adult acute lymphoblastic leukemia at diagnosis: Results from the international ALL trial MRC UKALL XII/ECOG E2993. *Blood, 108*, 465–472.

22. Wetzler, M., Dodge, R. K., Mrozek, K., et al. (1999). Prospective karyotype analysis in adult acute lymphoblastic leukemia: The cancer and leukemia Group B experience. *Blood, 93*, 3983–3993.

23. Pullarkat, V., Slovak, M. L., Kopecky, K. J., Forman, S. J., & Appelbaum, F. R. (2008). Impact of cytogenetics on the outcome of adult acute lymphoblastic leukemia: Results of Southwest Oncology Group 9400 study. *Blood, 111*, 2563–2572.

24. Mancini, M., Scappaticci, D., Cimino, G., et al. (2005). A comprehensive genetic classification of adult acute lymphoblastic leukemia (ALL): Analysis of the GIMEMA 0496 protocol. *Blood, 105*, 3434–3441.

25. Laughton, S. J., Ashton, L. J., Kwan, E., Norris, M. D., Haber, M., & Marshall, G. M. (2005). Early responses to chemotherapy of normal and malignant hematologic cells are prognostic in children with acute lymphoblastic leukemia. *Journal of Clinical Oncology, 23*, 2264–2271.

26. van der Velden, V. H., Cazzaniga, G., Schrauder, A., et al. (2007). Analysis of minimal residual disease by Ig/TCR gene rearrangements: Guidelines for interpretation of real-time quantitative PCR data. *Leukemia, 21*, 604–611.

27. Bruggemann, M., Raff, T., Flohr, T., et al. (2006). Clinical significance of minimal residual disease quantification in adult patients with standard-risk acute lymphoblastic leukemia. *Blood, 107*, 1116–1123.

28. Mortuza, F. Y., Papaioannou, M., Moreira, I. M., et al. (2002). Minimal residual disease tests provide an independent predictor of clinical outcome in adult acute lymphoblastic leukemia. *Journal of Clinical Oncology, 20*, 1094–1104.

29. Holowiecki, J., Krawczyk-Kulis, M., Giebel, S., et al. (2008). Status of minimal residual disease after induction predicts outcome in both standard and high-risk Ph-negative adult acute lymphoblastic leukaemia. The Polish Adult Leukemia Group ALL 4-2002 MRD Study. *British Journal of Haematology, 142*, 227–237.

30. Raff, T., Gokbuget, N., Luschen, S., et al. (2007). Molecular relapse in adult standard-risk ALL patients detected by prospective MRD monitoring during and after maintenance treatment: Data from the GMALL 06/99 and 07/03 trials. *Blood, 109*, 910–915.

31. Cunningham, L., & Aplenc, R. (2007). Pharmacogenetics of acute lymphoblastic leukemia treatment response. *Expert Opinion on Pharmacotherapy, 8*, 2519–2531.

32. Relling, M. V., Hancock, M. L., Rivera, G. K., et al. (1999). Mercaptopurine therapy intolerance and heterozygosity at the thiopurine S-methyltransferase gene locus. *Journal of the National Cancer Institute, 91*, 2001–2008.

33. Relling, M. V., Hancock, M. L., Boyett, J. M., Pui, C. H., & Evans, W. E. (1999). Prognostic importance of 6-mercaptopurine dose intensity in acute lymphoblastic leukemia. *Blood, 93*, 2817–2823.

34. Rocha, J. C., Cheng, C., Liu, W., et al. (2005). Pharmacogenetics of outcome in children with acute lymphoblastic leukemia. *Blood, 105*, 4752–4758.

35. Mullighan, C. G., Goorha, S., Radtke, I., et al. (2007). Genome-wide analysis of genetic alterations in acute lymphoblastic leukaemia. *Nature, 446*, 758–764.

36. Mullighan, C. G., Flotho, C., & Downing, J. R. (2005). Genomic assessment of pediatric acute leukemia. *Cancer Journal, 11*, 268–282.

37. Mullighan, C. G., & Downing, J. R. (2009). Global genomic characterization of acute lymphoblastic leukemia. *Seminars in Hematology, 46*, 3–15.

38. Mullighan, C. G., Su, X., Zhang, J., et al. (2009). Deletion of IKZF1 and prognosis in acute lymphoblastic leukemia. *The New England Journal of Medicine, 360*, 470–480.

39. Fielding, A. K., Richards, S. M., Chopra, R., et al. (2007). Outcome of 609 adults after relapse of acute lymphoblastic leukemia (ALL); an MRC UKALL12/ECOG 2993 study. *Blood, 109*, 944–950.

40. Tavernier, E., Boiron, J. M., Huguet, F., et al. (2007). Outcome of treatment after first relapse in adults with acute lymphoblastic leukemia initially treated by the LALA-94 trial. *Leukemia, 21*, 1907–1914.

Chapter 8
The Generalized Care of the Patient with Acute Lymphoblastic Leukemia

Anthony R. Mato, Alicia K. Morgans, and Selina M. Luger

Introduction

Caring for the patient with *acute lymphoblastic leukemia* (*ALL*) can be challenging. From the time the diagnosis of ALL is suspected, there is no organ system that is immune from the consequences of this disease or its therapies. Patients may develop complications such as arrhythmias, infection, hyperleukocytosis, bleeding, or thrombosis before treatment can even be initiated. Moreover, the disease, by virtue of its acuity and risks as well as the prolonged duration of treatment, is psychologically very difficult for patients and their families. This is further complicated by some of the treatment modalities used in this disease. In this chapter, we will focus on the most common and important clinical issues encountered in caring for patients with ALL receiving standard chemotherapy, the identification of which we consider to be some of the cornerstones of successful ALL management.

Metabolic and Hematologic Complications

Patients with ALL may develop metabolic and hematologic derangements that often present as oncologic emergencies. These can be present at diagnosis or upon imitation of treatment. Knowledge of these entities is critical in the management of ALL patients.

Tumor Lysis Syndrome

Evaluation of a patient with newly diagnosed ALL should include laboratory studies to monitor for tumor lysis syndrome (TLS). TLS is defined by the metabolic derangements of hyperkalemia, hyperuricemia, hyperphosphatemia, and hypocalcemia. When cellular lysis occurs, the intracellular contents are released into the bloodstream overwhelming the metabolic pathways that normally maintain homeostasis. The clinical consequences of TLS can include acute renal failure secondary to uric acid or calcium phosphate deposition and myocardial electrical instability secondary to electrolyte derangements, which often need to be addressed emergently [1, 2]. Several classification systems exist to define the laboratory and clinical consequences of TLS [1–3]. Although models

A.R. Mato (✉)
Hematology and Medical Oncology, University of Pennsylvania Medical Center, Philadelphia, PA, USA
e-mail: amato@humed.com

A.S. Advani and H.M. Lazarus (eds.), *Adult Acute Lymphocytic Leukemia*, Contemporary Hematology,   97
DOI 10.1007/978-1-60761-707-5_8, © Springer Science+Business Media, LLC 2011

have been designed to risk stratify adult AML patients for the development of TLS, none exist to risk stratify patients with ALL receiving systemic chemotherapy [4–6]. Patients with aggressive lymphoid malignancies, including ALL and Burkitt's lymphoma, should be considered to be at the *highest risk* for developing TLS spontaneously, before treatment, or upon initiation of systemic chemotherapy (Table 8.1) [7]. Studies have reported its incidence to be as high as 24% in patients with ALL [8]. Presumed risk factors include preexisting renal insufficiency, elevated LDH, and bulky disease [7, 9, 10]. With respect to the management of a patient at risk for TLS, one must consider all of the following: (1) TLS prophylaxis, (2) early identification of clinical TLS, and (3) treatment of the TLS-related clinical consequences (Table 8.2).

TLS prevention is often accomplished with the combination of crystalloid (normal saline) administered intravenously at 1–3x maintenance doses, and the use of allopurinol (a xanthine oxidase inhibitor), which has been shown to be effective in preventing the development of uric acid nephropathy in several studies [11–13]. Urine alkalinization with sodium bicarbonate or acetazolamide is sometimes used to enhance excretion of uric acid [14–17]. Some centers do not recommended this practice for TLS prophylaxis as prospective data supporting its efficacy are lacking and there is a concern that alkalinized urine may facilitate the crystallization of calcium phosphate [7, 15]. Urine alkalinization should not be excluded if patients are receiving a methotrexate-containing regimen as this is critical to minimizing methotrexate toxicity. When using allopurinol for TLS prevention, it is important to adjust the dose for renal insufficiency. Since it does not treat existing hyperuricemia, it should be initiated as early as possible prior to the initiation of chemotherapy. Allopurinol can interfere with the metabolism of mercaptopurine and methotrexate, and the overlap of these medications during induction should be avoided [7]. More recently, recombinant uric oxidase (Rasburicase) has become available. It is superior to oral allopurinol in several studies in terms of the reduction/prevention of hyperuricemia and the prevention of renal insufficiency [18–22]. This agent, which is contraindicated in patients with G6PD deficiency, is approved for use in pediatric patients at high risk for TLS in a 5-day treatment schedule. The use of this agent in adult patients with ALL and the use of alternate regimens are less uniform and currently not FDA approved for this indication [23]. Due to its cost, its widespread administration to all adults with ALL is not

Table 8.1 Tumor lysis syndrome risk factors

- Burkitt's lymphoma
- WBC > 100,000/mcL
- Preexisting renal disease
- Preexisting cardiac arrhythmia
- Dehydration
- Evidence of TLS prior to initiation of cytotoxic chemotherapy
- Elevated serum LDH
- Bulky disease/renal infiltration/extramedullary disease

Table 8.2 Tumor lysis syndrome (TLS) in ALL: monitoring, prophylaxis, treatment options

	Monitoring	Prophylaxis	Treatment options
Tumor Lysis Syndrome	• TLS panel: serum K, Ca, creatinine, BUN, LDH, uric acid • Serial monitoring of TLS panels: 1–3 times daily • Telemetry monitoring • Careful monitoring of urine output	• Hydration with normal saline • Monitoring for fluid overload • Allopurinol or rasburicase	• Treat electrolyte abnormalities • Telemetry monitoring • Increase laboratory monitoring • Increase intravenous fluids • Consider renal consultation • Consider dialysis • Consider ICU transfer

feasible; we recommend considering its use in adult patients with Burkitt's lymphoma or patients with ALL with preexisting renal disease, known history of arrhythmia, or evidence of TLS prior to the initiation of systemic chemotherapy.

There are no evidence-based guidelines available to suggest how often one should optimally screen for TLS in patients with ALL receiving systemic chemotherapy. At our institution, "TLS panels" are checked between 1 and 3 times per day during the initiation of induction chemotherapy to assess for evidence of TLS and daily until the risk of TLS has resolved. The TLS laboratory panel consists of serum creatinine, potassium, phosphate, calcium, LDH, and uric acid level. When TLS is detected, a range of potential interventions are considered, including more aggressive monitoring (including more frequent laboratory evaluation, telemetry, and ICU transfer), additional intravenous fluids, rasburicase, treatment of electrolyte aberrations, cardiology consultation for management of arrhythmia, and nephrology consultation to address renal complications. Occasionally patients with TLS will require hemodialysis, and rarely a dialysis catheter will be placed preemptively in patients with spontaneous TLS prior to the initiation of systemic treatments.

Hyperleukocytosis

As many as 10–30% of patients with ALL present with hyperleukocytosis, or a white blood cell (WBC) count >100,000 cells/mm^3 [24]. The clinical significance of an elevation in WBC count can vary by leukemia subtype and patient population (child vs. adult, T-cell ALL vs. other subtype). It is believed that patients with hyperleukocytosis are at high risk for significant adverse events and potentially lethal complications. Intracerebral hemorrhage, DIC, hyperuricemia, hyperphosphotemia, hyperkalemia, hypocalcemia, and renal failure can occur, as can pulmonary leukostasis and respiratory failure. If leukostasis is not recognized early and dealt with effectively, the mortality rate can approach 20–40% [24, 25]. It also must be remembered that alternative explanations for organ dysfunction should be evaluated when considering this diagnosis. For example, mental status changes may be an early sign of sepsis warranting a thorough search for occult infection as an explanation for a change in mental status. Additional testing to consider when ruling out alternative diagnoses in patients considered to have leukostasis includes a complete blood count to assess for thrombocytopenia and bleeding risk; fibrinogen, aPTT and PT/INR to assess for coagulopathy; and an extended metabolic panel to assess for TLS, uremia, and metabolic acidoses.

The most common complications associated with leukostatis are pulmonary and neurologic. In patients with leukostasis, pulmonary symptoms are common, occurring in 23% of adult ALL patients with hyperleukocytosis in one series [24]. These can range from mild respiratory distress with minimal or no evidence of infiltrate on chest radiography, to severe hypoxemia and widespread alveolar or interstitial infiltrate on chest radiography [26]. It is important to keep in mind that pulse oximetry is the most accurate way to follow oxygenation in these patients as arterial blood gas sampling frequently demonstrates pseudohypoxemia (so-called "leukocyte larceny") due to oxygen consumption by the large number of blasts in the sample [27].

Neurologic symptoms can also vary widely, from mild confusion or somnolence to focal neurologic deficits to stupor and coma. In one reported series, 15.3% of patients with hyperleukocytosis presented with neurologic symptoms [24]. Patients presenting with complaints of headache, blurred vision, tinnitus, or gait instability should be considered to have neurologic complications of hyperleukocytosis (either leukostasis or intracerebral hemorrhage) until proven otherwise. Physical examination findings consistent with neurologic leukostasis include cranial nerve deficits, papilledema, retinal hemorrhages, and nuchal rigidity [28]. In addition to the more common pulmonary and neurologic presentations of leukostasis, patients may also rarely present with acute MI, priapism, bowel ischemia, renal vein thrombosis, and limb ischemia.

The prognosis of patients with ALL and hyperleukocytosis is thought to be directly related to the degree of leukocyte elevation. In adults, a leukocyte count at presentation >250,000 cells/mm³ or evidence of neurologic symptoms are poor prognostic indicators [29]. Development of leukostasis occurs in children most often with WBC counts >400,000 cells/mm³ [30]. As compared to AML, leukostasis is thought to be less common in ALL. Complications of hyperleukocytosis in ALL are more frequently related to the development of spontaneous tumor lysis syndrome or DIC as opposed to leukostasis.

The exact mechanism of damage by hyperleukocytosis continues to be an area of active research. Although hyperleukocytosis is often defined as WBC >100,000/mm³, patients can develop symptoms of leukostasis with WBC as low as 50,000/mm³. One hypothesis regarding the etiology of hyperleukocytosis is that a critical "leukocrit" (fractional volume of leukocytes) is reached, which results in increased blood viscosity, impaired blood flow, and the subsequent development of leukostasis [31]. Leukemic myeloblasts are theorized to initiate leukostasis more frequently than leukemic lymphoblasts because the MCV of myeloblasts are typically twice as large as the MCV of lymphoblasts [31]. More recent work has focused on cellular adhesion molecules and leukemic cell response to local cytokines in the pathophysiology of leukostasis. This is supported by the observation that patients can develop leukostasis with leukocyte counts as low as 50,000/mm³. Direct interactions between leukemic blasts and the endothelium may lead to leukocyte aggregation and formation of thrombi. Locally produced cytokines may attract leukemic blasts to the area resulting in increased viscosity, local stasis, and cellular damage resulting in thrombosis or hemorrhage [32]. Additionally, variation in expression of adhesion molecules between myeloblasts and lymphoblasts may also explain why patients with AML have higher rates of leukostasis [32]. Variations in endothelial cell surface expression of adhesion molecules may also explain why some areas, including the pulmonary and CNS vasculature, seem more prone to complications of leukostasis than others.

There are multiple risk factors reported for hyperleukocytosis in acute leukemia, including younger age, leukemic cell ploidy variants (<50 chromosomes), and certain subtypes of leukemia. Infants with either ALL or AML can frequently present with profound hyperleukocytosis, and children less than 1 year old present with this complication more frequently than any other patient population. A second peak in the incidence of hyperleukocytosis occurs in patients during the teenage years [24]. The presence of the Philadelphia chromosome, 11q23 rearrangements, mediastinal mass, male gender, and T-ALL are also reported to increase a patient's risk of developing hyperleukocytosis [24, 33–35].

The main goal of treatment for ALL patients with hyperleukocytosis is to reduce the leukocyte count rapidly and safely. Leukocytoreduction, or the reduction of blast cell number, can occur by administering hydroxyurea, initiation of induction chemotherapy, or use of leukapheresis. Hydroxyurea is a relatively well tolerated oral option for therapy that has demonstrated effectiveness in blast count reduction. Within 24–48 h, hydroxyurea given at doses of 50–100 mg/kg/day can reduce the circulating leukocyte count by up to 50–80% [24]. It can be administered immediately and continued until counts are in an acceptable range. Leukapheresis is another method of cytoreduction, although it is typically reserved for patients with leukocyte counts greater than 100,000 –200,000/mm³ [36]. Many centers do not perform leukapheresis in ALL unless the patient's leukocyte count is >250,000–300,000/mm³ or there is clear evidence of leukostasis, and it is less frequently used in children [37, 38]. It is exceedingly effective in reducing the circulating blasts by removing circulating WBCs and reinfusing lymphocyte-depleted plasma. A single session of leukapheresis can decrease the leukocyte count by 20–50% [36]. The use of this method, although effective in decreasing leukocyte count, remains somewhat controversial. Studies do not suggest a clear correlation between the degree of cytoreduction and reduction in mortality. There are not currently widely accepted guidelines available for leukapheresis, and there are no specific criteria for when to initiate or stop treatment [24]. Extracranial irradiation has been proposed as a treatment option for hyperleukocytosis to prevent development of intracerebral hemorrhage [38]. Doses of 400 cGy have been applied to the whole brain. Because of the significant morbidity associated with cerebral irradiation, and the lack of systemic effect of the treatment, it is not routinely used as part of the treatment regimen for hyperleukocytosis [39].

Disseminated Intravascular Coagulation (DIC)

Disseminated intravascular coagulation represents a disequilibrium in the balance between bleeding and thrombosis. DIC can complicate the course of diagnosis and treatment of patients with ALL. It can result in severe, life-threatening bleeding complications including GI bleeding, intracranial hemorrhage, diffuse alveolar hemorrhage, and diffuse mucosal bleeding. Alternatively, patients can manifest thrombotic complications, including mesenteric ischemia, ischemic limbs, or strokes due to embolic events. Still other patients develop both bleeding and thrombotic complications, rendering treatment especially difficult and uncertain.

The literature reports that approximately 10–20% of adult ALL patients have DIC at presentation and up to 30–40% may develop DIC while undergoing induction chemotherapy [40–43]. DIC in childhood ALL is thought to be less common and does not seem to be as clinically significant in terms of its morbidity and mortality, with an incidence of approximately 5% at diagnosis and 15% during induction [41, 42]. Some of the variability in reported incidence of DIC in ALL may be due to the various clinical and laboratory criteria used in the literature to define DIC. Most definitions include hypofibrinogenemia (fibrinogen <100–200 mg/dL), prolongation of the prothrombin time (PT), and activated partial thromboplastin (aPTT), and several also include elevated fibrinogen/ fibrin degradation products or fibrin split products (D-dimer). The presence of thrombocytopenia is sometimes used to define DIC; however, isolated thrombocytopenia is more often due to leukemic bone marrow infiltration and chemotherapy-related myelosuppression.

Predicting which patients will develop hemorrhage or thrombotic complications of DIC can be difficult, and risk factors for DIC in ALL vary in the literature. It is important to keep in mind that DIC may alternatively represent an early sign of severe sepsis in this patient population [44]. Its presence should prompt a search for occult infection. Rates of complications from DIC varied substantially between series and there is no consensus on specific risk factors that predispose patients to DIC-associated morbidity and mortality.

The pathogenesis of DIC in ALL is an area of ongoing investigation. Tissue factor and cancer procoagulant are thought to be involved in early stages of the initiation/activation of DIC [45]. Tissue factor can complex with factor VII to activate factors X and IX and initiate thrombus formation. Up to 30% of ALL blasts express cancer procoagulant, which is thought to directly activate factor X [45, 46]. L-asparaginase, which is widely used in the treatment of ALL, can increase the risk of DIC presumably by decreasing the production of antithrombin III and protein C, thereby increasing a patient's risk of thrombosis. It also induces hypofibrinogenemia and, therefore, hemorrhage by reducing the production of fibrinogen [47, 48].

In the majority of cases, treatment of DIC focuses on clotting factor replacement. Fresh frozen plasma (FFP) and cryoprecipitate are mainstays of therapy and are often used to replace clotting factors. FFP (typically 2–4 units per transfusion) and cryoprecipitate (typically 5–10 units per transfusion) are often coadministered to treat DIC. Successful factor replacement is measured by reversal of elevations of the aPTT and PT and repletion of fibrinogen to >100–150 mg/dL. In a series of adult patients with ALL with DIC, it was noted that fibrinogen levels <100 mg/dL were associated with a significantly higher rate of hemorrhage and thrombosis (38% vs. 4%). In addition, Sarris et al. suggest that the prophylactic administration of platelets, FFP, or cryoprecipitate to correct the laboratory manifestations of DIC may decrease the risk of common DIC-associated bleeding and thrombotic complications [43].

Cytopenias and Transfusion Support

Patients with ALL develop cytopenias as a result of the disease itself as well as the cytotoxic chemotherapy used for its treatment. In our practice, we maintain an active type and screen on our patients and alert the blood bank regarding patients who may require frequent transfusions. The American Red Cross has published transfusion support guidelines that are helpful for the selection of transfusion triggers in patients who carry an oncologic diagnosis [49]. For transfusion of platelets, we support the recommendation for prophylactic transfusion when platelets are ≤10,000/mm^3 for stable, afebrile, nonbleeding patients [50]. A higher platelet transfusion threshold (≤20,000/mm^3) should be considered in the setting of fever, active infection, hyperleukocytosis, liver dysfunction, coagulopathy, minor bleeding, and GI toxicity. In the setting of DIC, platelets should be transfused for a count ≤ 50,000/mm^3. For packed red blood cells (prbc), a conservative trigger for transfusion is generally recommended but the trigger for transfusion varies in the literature. In our practice, we use a trigger of Hb ≤ 8.0 g/dL for transfusion in asymptomatic patients. Randomized data from the critical care literature suggest no difference in 30-day mortality when comparing a conservative 7 g/dL trigger vs. 9 g/dL trigger for transfusion of PRBCs [51]. In the setting of hypoxia or symptomatic anemia, the trigger for transfusion of PRBCs is typically more liberal and based on symptoms and clinical comorbidities. Collaborating with the hospital blood bank is important in managing ALL patients since this patient population has special requirements for transfusion support and selection of appropriate blood products. Patients should receive leukoreduced or CMV-negative blood products that help to minimize the risk of leukocyte-associated viral infection, alloimmunization, and nonhemolytic transfusion reactions. Single donor platelets should be utilized in the setting platelet transfusion refractoriness. In the setting of confirmed alloimmunization to platelet transfusion, HLA antigen-matched platelets may help to support platelet counts. Patients with ALL who are considered to be candidates for allogeneic stem cell transplantation, those who are undergoing allogeneic or autologous stem cell transplantation, those who are receiving HLA-identical platelets, and those who are receiving blood products obtained from a relative should receive gamma-irradiated blood products to minimize the risk of rare, but often fatal, complication of transfusion-associated graft-versus-host disease [52, 53].

Infectious Complications

Among the many comorbidities associated with increased risk for sepsis, malignancy carries one of the highest associated risks for developing sepsis and sepsis-related mortality. As many as 10% of all cancer deaths (46,729 annual deaths) are attributable to sepsis [54–56]. Among oncology patients, those with a hematologic malignancy, particularly acute leukemia, are at the highest risk for developing a life-threatening infection, presumably because these patients have defects in their infection-fighting ability for multiple reasons (neutropenia on the basis of disease and its treatment as well as defects in both cellular and humoral immunity) [54]. Infections are the leading cause of death in patients with ALL and one cannot treat this disease without knowledge of preventing and treating both common and life-threatening infectious complications .

Febrile Neutropenia

This is a common problem encountered in the care of patients with ALL. This is considered to be an oncologic emergency because although the majority of patients do quite well when treated with empiric broad-spectrum antibiotics, a fraction of patients progress from febrile neutropenia to severe sepsis, septic shock, and death despite our best efforts [57]. It should be emphasized that most cases of febrile neutropenia meet the critical care definition of sepsis [44]. Excellent resources have been published by the IDSA and NCCN and are available online to guide antibiotic selection for patients with ALL and febrile neutropenia [58, 59]. Medical centers regularly assess antibiotic resistance patterns of common infections within their health system. This information should be incorporated into the decision making regarding the design of institution-specific treatment guidelines for patients with febrile neutropenia. At our institution, the divisions of hematology/oncology, infectious diseases, and critical care have produced a treatment algorithm for the management of hematologic malignancy patients with febrile neutropenia based on the susceptibility profiles of organisms at our institution (Fig. 8.1). Patients with neutropenic fever should be treated with broad-spectrum antibiotics that cover potential gram-negative organisms as they are most likely to be life threatening if present.

The prophylactic use of cytokines, G-CSF, and GM-CSF has been studied in patients with ALL receiving systemic chemotherapy thought to be at high risk for developing febrile neutropenia (sepsis). Although these studies consistently show a decrease in the duration of neutropenia, these agents have not been able to uniformly show a decrease in neutropenic fever episodes or improvements in disease free and overall survival [60–62]. Based on the absence of survival data, there is insufficient evidence to support the use of colony-stimulating factors following the administration of systemic chemotherapy in all patients with ALL. However, recent guidelines published by the

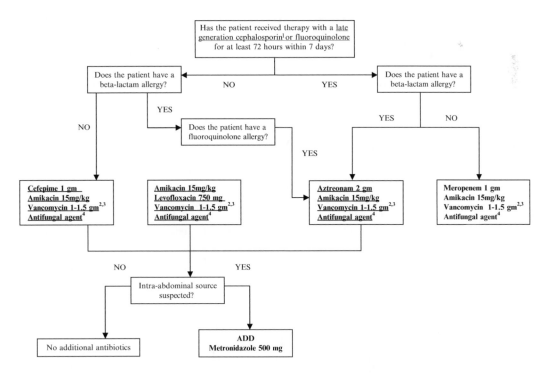

[1] 3rd or 4th gen cephalosporins = cefepime, ceftazidime, ceftriaxone
[2] Vancomycin dose: weight ≤ 70kg = 1 gm x 1, weight > 70kg = 1.5gm x 1
[3] Infuse vancomycin before antifungal agent, but after other antibiotics have been given
[4] Either liposomal amphotericin B 5 mg/kg x1 or caspofungin 70mg x 1

Fig. 8.1 Antibiotic choices for the neutropenic septic patient

NCCN regarding the use of myeloid growth factors in non-myeloid malignancies take a risk-adopted approach in recommending growth factors in the settings of neutropenic fever and neutropenia preventative strategies [63]. Such guidelines are useful in selecting patients who are likely to benefit from myeloid colony-stimulating factors

Sepsis

The early identification of sepsis in patients with ALL is critically important for allocating resources and implementing life-saving therapies. In patients with suspected infection, the early diagnosis of sepsis is dependent on the presence of vital signs and WBC abnormalities defined as the systemic inflammatory response syndrome (SIRS) criteria [44, 64]. The SIRS represents a host's inflammatory response to an infectious insult and is defined by the presence of two more of these criteria [64] (Table 8.3). Recent work from our center has evaluated the validity of SIRS criteria cut points as predictors for the development of severe sepsis in patients with hematologic malignancies [65]. We found that fever, tachycardia, and tachypnea are most predictive of an impending life-threatening infection in this patient population. Sensitivity, specificity, and likelihood ratios are now available for SIRS scores derived from hospitalized patients with an underlying hematologic malignancy [65] (Table 8.4). Other potential clinical and laboratory markers for the early identification of infection have been recently proposed; however, with the exception of procalcitonin, IL-6, and lactic acid, these largely remain untested in patients with malignancy [66–68].

Early and rapid fluid resuscitation guided by central venous pressure and oxygenation goals (early goal-directed therapy; EGDT) in patients with septic shock can reduce absolute mortality by 16% [69, 70]. In addition, the timeliness of the administration of appropriate antibiotics to patients with sepsis and hypotension is associated with graded reductions in mortality such that for every additional hour that antibiotic administration is delayed beyond the first, survival decreases by 7.6% [71]. The prompt administration (<1 h) of appropriate antibiotics to septic patients represents perhaps

Table 8.3 The systemic inflammatory response syndrome criteria[a]

Heart rate	>90 beats per minute
Respiratory rate	>20 breaths per minute or $PaCO_2$ < 32 torr
Temperature	>38.0°C or <36.0°C
White blood cell count	>12,000 cells/mcL, <4,000 cells/mcL, or >10% bands

[a] Two or more of the following conditions must be present to define SIRS. SIRS score is calculated by the summation of the number of SIRS criteria abnormalities present (range 0–4).

Table 8.4 Sensitivity, specificity, and likelihood-ratio estimates for SIRS score measured 24 h before septic shock event in hematologic malignancy patients

SIRS score	Sensitivity (95% CI)	Specificity (95% CI)	LR (+) (95% CI)	LR (−) (95% CI)
0	100	0	1	–
1	97 (96–99)	12 (8–16)	1.1 (1–1.2)	0.2 (.02–1.3)
2	76 (71–81)	59 (54–66)	1.9 (1.5–2.4)	0.4 (0.2–0.7)
3	35 (29–41)	91 (88–94)	3.9 (2.2–6.9)	0.7 (0.6–0.9)
4	7 (4–10)	99 (99–100)	7.1 (4.0–10.0)	0.94 (.87–1.0)

the single most important life-saving intervention the hematologist can employ prior to transfer of a patient to the ICU. These interventions have become the standard of care for sepsis management. Although limited data exist validating these approaches in patients with ALL, for patients that meet the various study inclusion criteria, we consider them to be the standard of care [72]. Additionally, these lifesaving interventions again underscore the importance of the early recognition of sepsis and the importance of care coordination among the hospital pharmacy, infectious disease specialist, ICU, and hematologist.

Invasive Fungal Infections

The combination of prolonged courses of corticosteroids and prolonged periods of neutropenia places patients with ALL at increased risk for invasive fungal infections (both candida and angioinvasive strains) [73]. In particular, *Aspergillus*, *Scedosporidium*, *Fusarium*, *Rhizopus*, and *Mucor* genii remain a significant cause of morbidity and mortality in this patient population. Because of their location (lung, liver, spleen) these infections are often treated based solely on radiographic evidence without a confirmatory culture. High resolution computerized tomography scans are more frequently being utilized to diagnose invasive fungal disease [73–75]. Although fluconazole is currently considered to be the standard of care for antifungal prophylaxis in patients at high risk for developing invasive fungal infections, it should not be used to treat a documented or suspected angioinvasive fungal infection. In the pediatric literature, it has been estimated that 13.6% of acute leukemia patients receiving fluconazole prophylaxis develop an invasive fungal infection [76, 77]. In addition, several fluconazole-resistant species of candida exist, and knowledge of resistance patterns should be used to shape antifungal choices in invasive/visceral candidal infections. Whereas amphotericin B was previously the only antifungal agent available to treat patients with invasive fungal infections, the last decade has seen a tremendous growth in research and development of novel classes of agents with antifungal properties.

We do now have randomized data favoring the use of voriconazole (vs. amphotericin B) in the treatment of documented invasive fungal infections [78]. This recommendation is supported by the IDSA [79]. Other "triazoles" such as posaconazole also have promising activity against invasive refractory fungal infections. However, it should be noted that voriconazole does not have activity in treating zygomycetes (rhizopus and mucor) infections, which should still be treated with traditional or liposomal amphotericin B formations. Voriconazole's classic toxicities are worth noting and include photopsia (patients should be prewarned about this), rash, and hepatitis. Liver function enzymes should be monitored serially. Voriconazole is a potent inducer of cytochrome (CY)P450 [73, 80]. The combination of this agent and sirolimus or ergot alkaloids can result in life-threatening complications. Blood concentrations of warfarin, tacrolimus, and cyclosporine may be increased when given in combination with voriconazole and should be monitored and adjusted carefully [73]. Triazole antifungal agents should not be given to patients who are receiving vincristine as they have been reported to exacerbate vincristine neurotoxicity [81–91]. A newer class of antifungals termed the echinocandins (glucan synthesis inhibitors) has promising activity in treating candida and aspergillus [92]. A major advantage of the echinocandins is their generally favorable side-effect profile; although unlike voriconazole, oral formulations are currently not available. These agents are presently used for the treatment of invasive fungal infections in the refractory setting or for patients who are intolerant to first-line agents such as voriconazole. An exciting area of clinical research involves testing novel combinations of echinocandins with liposomal formulations of amphotericin or triazoles to effect synergistic fungal cell death [93, 94]. In addition to medical therapies for invasive fungal infections, there may also be a limited role for surgical resection of fungal disease [95].

The lack of activity of fluconazole in treating aspergillus has raised the question whether this agent should be employed as the "antifungal" prophylactic agent of choice in patients with ALL undergoing systemic chemotherapy. Recent studies have addressed the role of newer antifungals as primary prophylactic agents in the management of high-risk leukemia patients in both transplant and non transplant treatment settings showing mixed results. In a prospective randomized trial of 200 patients with acute leukemia receiving systemic chemotherapy or HSCT, daily fluconazole was compared to itraconazole. There was no difference in the incidence of invasive fungal infections or mortality [96]. A recent study compared fluconazole, itraconazole, and posaconazole in 304 AML/MDS patients with expected prolonged neutropenia and found a 6% ARR of proven/probable invasive fungal infections in the posaconazole arm [97]. Patients receiving posaconazole were shown to have significantly longer overall survival ($p=0.04$) compared to the fluconazole and itraconazole arms. Recent data presented at the ASH 2007 annual meeting compared fluconazole with voriconazole prophylaxis in patients undergoing myeloablative HSCT and found no difference in the overall rate of invasive fungal infections or in fungal-free survival [98]. The rate of invasive aspergillus was, however, significantly lower in patients receiving voriconazole prophylaxis.

Herpes Family Viral Infections

Patients with ALL are at increased risk for the development of CMV, VZV, and HSV infections [99]. While the incidence, prevention, and treatment strategies are well described in patients with ALL undergoing allogeneic and unrelated stem cell transplantation [99, 100], more recently these herpes family viral infections are being recognized as a source of morbidity and mortality in hematologic malignancy patients receiving systemic chemotherapy [101, 102]. Adult ALL patients receiving chemotherapy are recommended to receive HSV prophylaxis with acyclovir. Without antiviral prophylaxis, the incidence of HSV reactivation can be as high as 60–80%. Alternatives to acyclovir include famcicylovir and valacyclovir. In the case of documented infection with HSV resistance, foscarnet or cidofovir can be tried under the guidance of an infectious disease specialist; however, these agents have significant toxicities. The use of antiviral agents for VZV prevention is not routinely recommended for all patients with ALL receiving systemic chemotherapy. The daily history and physical should include close inspection for early signs of HSV infection or VZV reactivation. Varicella zoster should be on the differential of a pneumonia that is unresponsive to antibiotics. Additionally, the initial history should question all newly diagnosed patients as to whether they have been previously diagnosed with chicken pox. In the case of a documented or suspect varicella infection in a hospitalized immunocompromised patient, great care must be taken to protect other such patients and previously unexposed health-care staff from exposure though infection control measures. A varicella-specific immunoglobin is available for use on a compassionate use basis. Consultation with hospital infection control would be warranted.

Respiratory Syncytial Virus (RSV)

Respiratory syncytial virus (RSV) is an underrecognized agent responsible for infection in ALL patients. In the Northern hemisphere, RSV is thought to be most infectious between the months of April and November. Its presentation may initially be subtle; however, it can be a significant source of morbidity and mortality especially when it progresses to the lower respiratory tract [103, 104]. RSV should be considered in patients who present with URI symptoms or patients with lower respiratory tract infections not responding to prescribed anti-infective therapies. Age ≥65 years, symptoms for >14 days prior to diagnosis, APACHE Score >15, presence of medical comorbidities, and progression to pneumonia are associated with increased mortality in patients with acute leukemia and RSV [103]. Aerosolized ribavirin monotherapy (a nucleoside analog), ribavirin + intravenous gamma globulin, and ribavirin + palivizumab (humanized monoclonal antibody against the RSV F glycoprotein) are available for treatment and prophylaxis of RSV [105–109]. They are often administered to immunocompromised patients with RSV pneumonia. A retrospective observational trial of 52 patients with RSV and acute leukemia at The MD Anderson Cancer Center noted that cough (87%), fever (85%), and coryza (62%) were the most common presenting symptoms in RSV infection [103]. Fewer patients with RSV pneumonia treated with ribavirin died at 30-day follow-up as compared to those with RSV pneumonia who did not receive treatment (1/16 patients vs. 4/11 patients, $p = .01$), suggesting a potential benefit to treatment of RSV pneumonia in this patient population [103]. Although randomized clinical trials have not been performed documenting a mortality benefit to treating patients with acute leukemia diagnosed with RSV, prompt treatment of RSV-documented lower respiratory tract infections should be discussed with the infectious disease consultant.

Pneumocystis jiroveci

Pneumocystis jiroveci is an opportunistic bacterial infection that can result in life-threatening pulmonary infections in patients with immune dysregulation. In ALL, the risk of *Pneumocystis jiroveci* pneumonia is estimated to be 5–16% depending on whether the patient is adult vs. pediatric and whether their treatment includes HSCT and prolonged corticosteroids. Bactrim (TMP/SMX), dapsone, pentamidine, and atovaquone are available agents for *Pneumocystis jiroveci* prophylaxis – each with different dosing and safety issues. In the pediatric literature, bactrim (TMP/SMX) is generally considered to be the first-line prophylactic agent; however, pentamidine and atovaquone have also been used in the second-line setting in bactrim-intolerant patients [110, 111]. In adult ALL patients receiving systemic chemotherapy and corticosteroids, *Pneumocystis jiroveci* prophylaxis should be considered.

Issues Related to Specific Antileukemic Agents

Conventional therapies employed in the treatment of ALL have classic toxicities that one should monitor as a component of the generalized care of the leukemia patient. Vincristine, derived from the periwinkle plant, can be associated with permanent and debilitating neurotoxic complications that need to be closely monitored for, since if they are detected early, they may be reversible. Because of the concern of constipation and obstruction if not treated, patients receiving vincristine should be monitored closely for regular bowel movements and an aggressive bowel regiment should be used whenever needed. As patients with ALL often receive multiple doses of vincristine over a period of several years, assessment of peripheral neuropathy should be done prior to each dose. Since patients with ALL frequently receive concomitant corticosteroids along with vincristine, it can be quite difficult to discern neuropathy related to vincristine administration from steroid myopathy [112, 113]. Because both agents are critical to treatment success, the clinician interviewing and examining ALL patients with suspected neurotoxic vs. myotoxic [114, 115] effects must be astute at the neurological examination. DeAngelis et al. review several differences one can detect on physical examination between vincristine toxicity (distal weakness, typically symmetric, both upper and lower extremities) and corticosteroid toxicity (proximal weakness, difficult to go from sitting to standing position) [112]. Making the distinction between toxicities from these agents is critical in guiding the clinician in making dose modifications. In general, vincristine should not be dose reduced unless a patient develops ≥ grade 3 neuropathy thought to be secondary to vincristine. Several strategies have been employed to minimize vinca-related neurotoxicities, including capping the IVP dose at 2 mg, continuous infusion strategies, coadministration of neuroprotectants, and liposomal formulations. At this time, randomized data are lacking to suggest an optimal approach to maximize efficacy and minimize toxicity [112, 116–118]. The literature also suggests that the combination of vincristine and myeloid colony-stimulating factors may exacerbate vincristine toxicity, and as noted earlier, the concomitant administration of vincristine and triazole antifungal agents can exacerbate vincristine toxicity [119].

In addition to steroid myopathy, corticosteroid administration can be associated with other serious toxicities. As might be expected, many patients develop glucose intolerance while on steroids requiring the use of insulin during that time. Steroid use may be associated with mucosal gastrointestinal injuries. Randomized data support the addition of either an H2-receptor blocker or proton pump inhibitor to a patient's medication regimen while receiving steroids to minimize GI toxicities such as upper tract ulceration [120, 121]. The risk of avascular necrosis (AVN) has been the subject of much interest. The occurrence of AVN may be related to choice of corticosteroid (dexamethasone vs. prednisone), body mass index, male sex, age of the patient (pediatric), and cumulative steroid dose [122–128]. Corticosteroids may also be associated with neuropsychiatric symptoms such as acute psychosis, mania, and depression [113, 123], and occasionally these require the use of antipsychotic medications and/or consultation with a psychiatrist in order to manage the patient during the obligate period of steroid treatment.

Typically ALL protocols call for corticosteroid administration for a period of weeks during induction with an abrupt end to steroid exposure (versus tapering schedule). This approach may place patients at risk for corticosteroid withdrawal symptoms. Clinicians caring for such patients should consider adrenal insufficiency on the differential diagnosis following an abrupt cessation of glucocorticoid exposure if they present with vague symptoms/signs such as lethargy, hypotension, abdominal pain, electrolyte abnormalities, or skin problems. Steroid withdrawal syndrome may be particularly prevalent when a dexamethasone-containing protocol is used [129].

Conclusions

The care of the patient with ALL is often very complicated. All patients have cytopenias at some point in their course, which need to be addressed. The treatment regimens used are very involved and have numerable toxicities. ALL patients may present with or develop tumor lysis syndrome, DIC, neutropenic fever, sepsis, or symptoms of hyperleukocytosis, which require emergent intervention. During treatment, attention must be paid to all of the organ systems in order to identify any toxicities seen as a result of the disease or its treatment. Some prophylactic or preemptive measures can be employed (Tables 8.2 and 8.5). Unexpected complications are not unusual. Care of the patient with ALL often requires the input and advice from other medicine subspecialists, social workers, nurses, clergy, and house staff. With a meticulous and concerted effort, we can provide the patient with the best chance of a successful outcome.

Table 8.5 Supportive care strategies in ALL

	Monitoring	Prophylaxis	Treatment
DIC	PT/aPTT/Platelet count/Fibrinogen/D-Dimer 1–3 times daily during infection. Monitor closely for bleeding/thrombotic complications. Patients receiving L-asparaginase at increased risk.	None recommended.	Use of FFP, Cryoprecipitate, platelet transfusion to correct laboratory DIC (elevated PT/aPTT/depressed Fibrinogen).
Febrile neutropenia Sepsis	Frequent assessment of vital signs/urine output/organ functions as indicators of underlying infectious process. Detailed evaluation for infectious source (careful history, physical examination, blood cultures, urine culture/analysis, chest x ray, additional images/investigations as warranted). Avoid antipyretic medications in patients who are neutropenic.	Bacterial: None recommended. HSV: Acyclovir, famcyclovir, valacyclovir. Fungal: Fluconazole. Consider posaconazole or other "triazoles" in high-risk patients. Pneumocystis jiroveci: Bactrim. Alternatives include pentamidine or atovaquone.	Treatment with empiric antibiotics according to IDSA treatment guidelines. Emphasis on early gram-negative empiric coverage. Consider infectious disease consultation. Prompt administration of antibiotics (<1 h). Removal of invasive devices/catheters in the setting of hemodynamic instability. ICU monitoring/critical care consultation with any evidence of hemodynamic instability.
Upper GI toxicity	Careful daily history and physical examination. Patients receiving corticosteroids or with mucosal damage at increased risk.	Avoid NSAIDs/aspirin containing regimens. Daily prophylaxis with H2 blocker or proton pump inhibitor.	GI consultation. Nutrition consultation. Treatment with H2 blocker or proton pump inhibitor (PO/IV formulations available). Careful monitoring of Hb/platelet count if GIB suspected.

References

1. Cairo, M.S., et al., *Tumour lysis syndrome: new therapeutic strategies and classification.* British Journal of Haematology, 2004. **127**(1): p. 3–11.
2. Razis, E., et al., *Incidence and treatment of tumor lysis syndrome in patients with acute leukemia.* Acta Haematologica, 1994. **91**(4): p. 171–4.
3. Hande, K.R. and G.C. Garrow, *Acute tumor lysis syndrome in patients with high-grade non-Hodgkin's lymphoma.* American Journal of Medicine, 1993. **94**(2): p. 133–139.
4. Mato, A.R., et al., *A predictive model for the detection of tumor lysis syndrome during AML induction therapy. [see comment].* Leukemia & Lymphoma, 2006. **47**(5): p. 877–83.
5. Montesinos, P., et al., *Tumor lysis syndrome in patients with acute myeloid leukemia: identification of risk factors and development of a predictive model.* Haematologica-The Hematology Journal. **93**(1): p. 67–74.
6. Seftel, M.D., et al., *Fulminant tumour lysis syndrome in acute myelogenous leukaemia with inv(16)(p13;q22).* European Journal of Haematology. **69**(4): p. 193–199.
7. Coiffier, B., et al., *Guidelines for the management of pediatric and adult tumor lysis syndrome: an evidence-based review.* Journal of Clinical Oncology, 2008. **26**(16): p. 2767–78.
8. Woessmann, W., et al., *Incidence of tumor lysis syndrome in children with advanced stage Burkitt's lymphoma/leukemia before and after introduction of prophylactic use of urate oxidase.* Annals of Hematology. **82**(3): p. 160–165.
9. Arrambide, K. and R.D. Toto, *Tumor lysis syndrome.* Seminars in Nephrology, 1993. **13**(3): p. 273–80.
10. Chasty, R.C. and J.A. Liu-Yin, *Acute tumour lysis syndrome.* British Journal of Hospital Medicine, 1993. **49**(7): p. 488–92.
11. DeConti, R.C. and P. Calabresi, *Use of allopurinol for prevention and control of hyperuricemia in patients with neoplastic disease.* New England Journal of Medicine, 1966. **274**(9): p. 481–6.
12. Feusner, J. and M.S. Farber, *Role of intravenous allopurinol in the management of acute tumor lysis syndrome.* Seminars in Oncology, 2001. **28**(2 Suppl 5): p. 13–18.
13. Smalley, R.V., et al., *Allopurinol: Intravenous Use for Prevention and Treatment of Hyperuricemia.* J Clin Oncol, 2000. **18**(8): p. 1758–1763.
14. Chantada, G.L. and F. Sackmann-Muriel, *Letter to the editor: Alkalinization and tumor lysis syndrome.* Medical & Pediatric Oncology, 1999. **32**(2): p. 156.
15. Ten Harkel, A.D.J., et al., *Topic topic: Alkalinization and the tumor lysis syndrome.* Medical & Pediatric Oncology, 1998. **31**(1): p. 27–28.
16. Aviles, A., *Acute tumor lysis syndrome and alkali therapy.[comment].* American Journal of Medicine, 1995. **98**(4): p. 417–8.
17. Koduri, P.R., *Alkali therapy, hyperphosphatemia, and acute tumor lysis syndrome.* Medical & Pediatric Oncology, 1996. **26**(1): p. 73.
18. Bosly, A., et al., *Rasburicase (recombinant urate oxidase) for the management of hyperuricemia in patients with cancer: report of an international compassionate use study.* Cancer, 2003. **98**(5): p. 1048–54.
19. Goldman, S.C., et al., *A randomized comparison between rasburicase and allopurinol in children with lymphoma or leukemia at high risk for tumor lysis.* Blood, 2001. **97**(10): p. 2998–3003.
20. Jeha, S., et al., *Efficacy and safety of rasburicase, a recombinant urate oxidase (Elitek), in the management of malignancy-associated hyperuricemia in pediatric and adult patients: final results of a multicenter compassionate use trial.* Leukemia, 2005. **19**(1): p. 34–8.
21. Pui, C.H., et al., *Urate oxidase in prevention and treatment of hyperuricemia associated with lymphoid malignancies.* Leukemia, 1997. **11**(11): p. 1813–1816.
22. Pui, C.-H., et al., *Recombinant urate oxidase for the prophylaxis or treatment of hyperuricemia in patients with leukemia or lymphoma.* Journal of Clinical Oncology, 2001. **19**(3): p. 697–704.
23. Trifilio, S., et al., *Low-Dose Recombinante Urate Oxidase (Rasburicase) Is Effective in Treating Hyperuricemia in Patients with Hematologic Malignancies.* Blood (ASH Annual Meeting Abstracts), 2005. **106**(11): p. 3123-.
24. Porcu, P., et al., *Hyperleukocytic leukemias and leukostasis: a review of pathophysiology, clinical presentation and management.* Leukemia & Lymphoma, 2000. **39**(1–2): p. 1–18.
25. van Buchem, M.A., et al., *Leucostasis, an underestimated cause of death in leukaemia.* Blut, 1988. **56**(1): p. 39–44.
26. van Buchem, M.A., et al., *Pulmonary leukostasis: radiologic-pathologic study.* Radiology, 1987. **165**(3): p. 739–741.
27. Gartrell, K. and W. Rosenstrauch, *Hypoxaemia in patients with hyperleukocytosis: true or spurious, and clinical implications.* Leukemia research, 1993. **17**(11): p. 915–919.
28. Karesh, J.W., et al., *A prospective ophthalmic evaluation of patients with acute myeloid leukemia: correlation of ocular and hematologic findings.* Journal of Clinical Oncology, 1989. **7**(10): p. 1528–1532.
29. Flasshove, M., et al., *Pulmonary and cerebral irradiation for hyperleukocytosis in acute myelomonocytic leukemia.* Leukemia, 1994. **8**(10): p. 1792.

30. Lowe, E.J., et al., *Early complications in children with acute lymphoblastic leukemia presenting with hyperleu-kocytosis.* Pediatric Blood & Cancer, 2005. **45**(1): p. 10–15.
31. Lightman, M.A., *Rheology of leukocytes, leukocyte suspensions, and blood in leukemia. Possible relationship to clinical manifestations.* Journal of Clinical Investigation, 1973. **52**(2): p. 350–358.
32. Porcu, P., et al., *Leukocytoreduction for acute leukemia.[see comment].* Therapeutic Apheresis, 2002. **6**(1): p. 15–23.
33. Eguiguren, J.M., et al., *Complications and outcome in childhood acute lymphoblastic leukemia with hyperleuko-cytosis.* Blood, 1992. **79**(4): p. 871–875.
34. Harousseau, J.L., et al., *High risk acute lymphocytic leukemia: a study of 141 cases with initial white blood cell counts over 100,000/cu mm.* Cancer, 1980. **46**(9): p. 1996–2003.
35. Hoelzer, D., et al., *Prognostic factors in a multicenter study for treatment of acute lymphoblastic leukemia in adults.* Blood, 1988. **71**(1): p. 123–131.
36. Majhail, N.S. and A.E. Lichtin, *Acute leukemia with a very high leukocyte count: confronting a medical emer-gency.* Cleveland Clinic Journal of Medicine, 2004. **71**(8): p. 633–637.
37. Basade, M., et al., *Rapid cytoreduction in childhood leukemic hyperleukocytosis by conservative therapy.* Medical & Pediatric Oncology, 1995. **25**(3): p. 204–207.
38. Nelson, S.C., et al., *Management of leukemic hyperleukocytosis with hydration, urinary alkalinization, and allopurinol. Are cranial irradiation and invasive cytoreduction necessary?* American Journal of Pediatric Hematology/Oncology, 1993. **15**(3): p. 351–355.
39. Butler, R.W., et al., *Neuropsychologic effects of cranial irradiation, intrathecal methotrexate, and systemic methotrexate in childhood cancer.* Journal of Clinical Oncology, 1994. **12**(12): p. 2621–2629.
40. Sarris, A.H., et al., *High incidence of disseminated intravascular coagulation during remission induction of adult patients with acute lymphoblastic leukemia.* Blood, 1992. **79**(5): p. 1305–1310.
41. Higuchi, T., et al., *Disseminated intravascular coagulation complicating acute lymphoblastic leukemia: a study of childhood and adult cases.* Leukemia & Lymphoma, 2005. **46**(8): p. 1169–1176.
42. Higuchi, T., et al., *Disseminated intravascular coagulation in acute lymphoblastic leukemia at presentation and in early phase of remission induction therapy.* Annals of Hematology, 1998. **76**(6): p. 263–269.
43. Sarris, A., et al., *Disseminated intravascular coagulation in adult acute lymphoblastic leukemia: frequent com-plications with fibrinogen levels less than 100 mg/dl.* Leukemia & Lymphoma, 1996. **21**(1–2): p. 85–92.
44. Levy, M.M., et al., *2001 SCCM/ESICM/ACCP/ATS/SIS International Sepsis Definitions Conference.* Intensive care medicine, 2003. **29**(4): p. 530–538.
45. Barbui, T. and A. Falanga, *Disseminated intravascular coagulation in acute leukemia.* Seminars in Thrombosis & Hemostasis, 2001. **27**(6): p. 593–604.
46. Alessio, M.G., et al., *Cancer procoagulant in acute lymphoblastic leukemia.* European Journal of Haematology, 1990. **45**(2): p. 78–81.
47. Alberts, S.R., et al., *Thrombosis related to the use of L-asparaginase in adults with acute lymphoblastic leukemia: a need to consider coagulation monitoring and clotting factor replacement.* Leukemia & Lymphoma, 1999. **32**(5–6): p. 489–496.
48. Beinart, G. and L. Damon, *Thrombosis associated with L-asparaginase therapy and low fibrinogen levels in adult acute lymphoblastic leukemia.* American Journal of Hematology, 2004. **77**(4): p. 331–335.
49. *Practice Guidelines For Transfusion* American Red Cross, 2007.
50. Finazzi, G., *Prophylactic platelet transfusion in acute leukemia: which threshold should be used.[comment].* Haematologica, 1998. **83**(11): p. 961–2.
51. Hebert, P.C., et al., *A multicenter, randomized, controlled clinical trial of transfusion requirements in critical care. Transfusion Requirements in Critical Care Investigators, Canadian Critical Care Trials Group.[see com-ment][erratum appears in N Engl J Med 1999 Apr 1;340(13):1056].* New England Journal of Medicine, 1999. **340**(6): p. 409–17.
52. Anonymous, *Guidelines on gamma irradiation of blood components for the prevention of transfusion-associated graft-versus-host disease. BCSH Blood Transfusion Task Force.[see comment].* Transfusion Medicine, 1996. **6**(3): p. 261–71.
53. Dwyre, D.M. and P.V. Holland, *Transfusion-associated graft-versus-host disease.* Vox Sanguinis, 2008. **95**(2): p. 85–93.
54. Williams, M.D., et al., *Hospitalized cancer patients with severe sepsis: analysis of incidence, mortality, and associated costs of care.* Critical care (London, England), 2004. **8**(5): p. R291–8.
55. Angus, D.C., et al., *Epidemiology of severe sepsis in the United States: analysis of incidence, outcome, and associated costs of care.* Critical care medicine, 2001. **29**(7): p. 1303–1310.
56. Danai, P.A., et al., *The epidemiology of sepsis in patients with malignancy.* Chest, 2006. **129**(6): p. 1432–1440.
57. Hamalainen, S., et al., *Neutropenic fever and severe sepsis in adult acute myeloid leukemia (AML) patients receiving intensive chemotherapy: Causes and consequences.[see comment].* Leukemia & lymphoma, 2008. **49**(3): p. 495–501.

58. *http://www.idsociety.org/Content.aspx?id=9088*
59. *http://nccn.org/professionals/physician_gls/PDF/infections.pdf.*
60. Ottmann, O.G., et al., *Concomitant granulocyte colony-stimulating factor and induction chemoradiotherapy in adult acute lymphoblastic leukemia: a randomized phase III trial.* Blood, 1995. **86**(2): p. 444–50.
61. Larson, R.A., et al., *A randomized controlled trial of filgrastim during remission induction and consolidation chemotherapy for adults with acute lymphoblastic leukemia: CALGB study 9111.* Blood, 1998. **92**(5): p. 1556–64.
62. Geissler, K., et al., *Granulocyte colony-stimulating factor as an adjunct to induction chemotherapy for adult acute lymphoblastic leukemia–a randomized phase-III study.* Blood, 1997. **90**(2): p. 590–6.
63. *http://nccn.org/professionals/physician_gls/PDF/myeloid_growth.pdf.*
64. *American College of Chest Physicians/Society of Critical Care Medicine Consensus Conference: definitions for sepsis and organ failure and guidelines for the use of innovative therapies in sepsis.[see comment].* Critical care medicine, 1992. **20**(6): p. 864–874.
65. Mato, A., et al., *Systemic Inflammatory Response Syndrome (SIRS) as Predictor of Severe Sepsis (SS) in Hospitalized Patients (pts) with Hematologic Malignancies.* Blood (ASH Annual Meeting Abstracts), 2007. **110**(11): p. 633.
66. von Lilienfeld-Toal, M., et al., *Markers of bacteremia in febrile neutropenic patients with hematological malignancies: procalcitonin and IL-6 are more reliable than C-reactive protein.* European Journal of Clinical Microbiology & Infectious Diseases, 2004. **23**(7): p. 539–44.
67. Mato, A.R., et al., *Serum Lactic Acid (LA) as a Predictor of Septic Shock in Patients with Hematologic Malignancies (HM) Who Develop Febrile Neutropenia.* Blood (ASH Annual Meeting Abstracts), 2008. **112**(11): p. 666.
68. Nomura, S., et al., *Relationship between platelet activation and cytokines in systemic inflammatory response syndrome patients with hematological malignancies.* Thrombosis Research, 1999. **95**(5): p. 205–13.
69. Rivers, E.P., et al., *Early and innovative interventions for severe sepsis and septic shock: taking advantage of a window of opportunity.* CMAJ Canadian Medical Association Journal, 2005. **173**(9): p. 1054–1065.
70. Rivers, E., et al., *Early goal-directed therapy in the treatment of severe sepsis and septic shock.* New England Journal of Medicine, 2001. **345**(19): p. 1368–1377.
71. Kumar, A., et al., *Duration of hypotension before initiation of effective antimicrobial therapy is the critical determinant of survival in human septic shock.* Critical care medicine, 2006. **34**(6): p. 1589–1596.
72. Pastores, S.M., et al., *A safety evaluation of drotrecogin alfa (activated) in hematopoietic stem cell transplant patients with severe sepsis: lessons in clinical research.* Bone marrow transplantation, 2005. **36**(8): p. 721–724.
73. Kauffman, C.A. and C.A. Kauffman, *Fungal infections.* Proceedings of the American Thoracic Society, 2006. **3**(1): p. 35–40.
74. Caillot, D., et al., *Increasing volume and changing characteristics of invasive pulmonary aspergillosis on sequential thoracic computed tomography scans in patients with neutropenia.* Journal of Clinical Oncology, 2001. **19**(1): p. 253–9.
75. Caillot, D., et al., *Improved management of invasive pulmonary aspergillosis in neutropenic patients using early thoracic computed tomographic scan and surgery.* Journal of Clinical Oncology, 1997. **15**(1): p. 139–47.
76. Ribeiro, P., et al., *Candidemia in acute leukemia patients.* Supportive Care in Cancer, 1997. **5**(3): p. 249–51.
77. Rosen, G.P., et al., *Invasive fungal infections in pediatric oncology patients: 11-year experience at a single institution.* Journal of Pediatric Hematology/Oncology, 2005. **27**(3): p. 135–40.
78. Herbrecht, R., et al., *Voriconazole versus amphotericin B for primary therapy of invasive aspergillosis.[see comment].* New England Journal of Medicine, 2002. **347**(6): p. 408–15.
79. *http://www.idsociety.org/content.aspx?id=9200#aspe.*
80. Johnson, L.B., et al., *Voriconazole: a new triazole antifungal agent.* Clinical Infectious Diseases, 2003. **36**(5): p. 630–7.
81. Ariffin, H., et al., *Severe vincristine neurotoxicity with concomitant use of itraconazole.* Journal of Paediatrics & Child Health, 2003. **39**(8): p. 638–9.
82. Bermudez, M., et al., *Itraconazole-related increased vincristine neurotoxicity: case report and review of literature.* Journal of Pediatric Hematology/Oncology, 2005. **27**(7): p. 389–92.
83. Bohme, A., A. Ganser, and D. Hoelzer, *Aggravation of vincristine-induced neurotoxicity by itraconazole in the treatment of adult ALL.* Annals of Hematology, 1995. **71**(6): p. 311–2.
84. Chen, S., et al., *Itraconazole-enhanced vindesine neurotoxicity in adult acute lymphoblastic leukaemia.* American Journal of Hematology, 2007. **82**(10): p. 942.
85. Gillies, J., et al., *Severe vincristine toxicity in combination with itraconazole.* Clinical & Laboratory Haematology, 1998. **20**(2): p. 123–4.
86. Jeng, M.R. and J. Feusner, *Itraconazole-enhanced vincristine neurotoxicity in a child with acute lymphoblastic leukemia.* Pediatric Hematology & Oncology, 2001. **18**(2): p. 137–42.
87. Kamaluddin, M., et al., *Potentiation of vincristine toxicity by itraconazole in children with lymphoid malignancies.* Acta Paediatrica, 2001. **90**(10): p. 1204–7.

88. Mantadakis, E., et al., *Possible increase of the neurotoxicity of vincristine by the concurrent use of posaconazole in a young adult with leukemia.* Journal of Pediatric Hematology/Oncology, 2007. **29**(2): p. 130.
89. Sathiapalan, R.K., et al., *Vincristine-itraconazole interaction: cause for increasing concern.* Journal of Pediatric Hematology/Oncology, 2002. **24**(7): p. 591.
90. Sathiapalan, R.K. and H. El-Solh, *Enhanced vincristine neurotoxicity from drug interactions: case report and review of literature.* Pediatric Hematology & Oncology, 2001. **18**(8): p. 543–6.
91. Takahashi, N., et al., *Itraconazole oral solution enhanced vincristine neurotoxicity in five patients with malignant lymphoma.* Internal Medicine, 2008. **47**(7): p. 651–3.
92. Maertens, J., et al., *Efficacy and safety of caspofungin for treatment of invasive aspergillosis in patients refractory to or intolerant of conventional antifungal therapy.* Clinical Infectious Diseases, 2004. **39**(11): p. 1563–71.
93. Aliff, T.B., et al., *Refractory Aspergillus pneumonia in patients with acute leukemia: successful therapy with combination caspofungin and liposomal amphotericin.* Cancer, 2003. **97**(4): p. 1025–32.
94. Marr, K.A., et al., *Combination antifungal therapy for invasive aspergillosis.[see comment].* Clinical Infectious Diseases, 2004. **39**(6): p. 797–802.
95. Ali, R., et al., *Invasive pulmonary aspergillosis: role of early diagnosis and surgical treatment in patients with acute leukemia.* Annals of Clinical Microbiology & Antimicrobials, 2006. **5**: p. 17.
96. Oren, I., et al., *A prospective randomized trial of itraconazole vs fluconazole for the prevention of fungal infections in patients with acute leukemia and hematopoietic stem cell transplant recipients.* Bone marrow transplantation, 2006. **38**(2): p. 127–34.
97. Cornely, O.A., et al., *Posaconazole vs. fluconazole or itraconazole prophylaxis in patients with neutropenia.[see comment].* New England Journal of Medicine, 2007. **356**(4): p. 348–59.
98. Wingard, J.R., et al., *Results of a Randomized, Double-Blind Trial of Fluconazole (FLU) vs. Voriconazole (VORI) for the Prevention of Invasive Fungal Infections (IFI) in 600 Allogeneic Blood and Marrow Transplant (BMT) Patients.* Blood (ASH Annual Meeting Abstracts), 2007. **110**(11): p. 163-.
99. Wingard, J.R., *Viral infections in leukemia and bone marrow transplant patients.* Leukemia & lymphoma, 1993. **11 Suppl 2**: p. 115–25.
100. Anaissie, E.J., et al., *The natural history of respiratory syncytial virus infection in cancer and transplant patients: implications for management.* Blood, 2004. **103**(5): p. 1611–7.
101. Bustamante, C.I. and J.C. Wade, *Herpes simplex virus infection in the immunocompromised cancer patient.* Journal of Clinical Oncology, 1991. **9**(10): p. 1903–15.
102. Reusser, P., *Current concepts and challenges in the prevention and treatment of viral infections in immunocompromised cancer patients.* Supportive Care in Cancer, 1998. **6**(1): p. 39–45.
103. Torres, H.A., et al., *Characteristics and outcome of respiratory syncytial virus infection in patients with leukemia.* Haematologica, 2007. **92**(9): p. 1216–23.
104. Whimbey, E., et al., *Respiratory syncytial virus pneumonia in hospitalized adult patients with leukemia.* Clinical Infectious Diseases, 1995. **21**(2): p. 376–9.
105. Boeckh, M., et al., *Randomized controlled multicenter trial of aerosolized ribavirin for respiratory syncytial virus upper respiratory tract infection in hematopoietic cell transplant recipients.* Clinical Infectious Diseases, 2007. **44**(2): p. 245–9.
106. Ghosh, S., et al., *Respiratory syncytial virus upper respiratory tract illnesses in adult blood and marrow transplant recipients: combination therapy with aerosolized ribavirin and intravenous immunoglobulin.* Bone marrow transplantation, 2000. **25**(7): p. 751–5.
107. Ghosh, S., et al., *Respiratory syncytial virus infections in autologous blood and marrow transplant recipients with breast cancer: combination therapy with aerosolized ribavirin and parenteral immunoglobulins.* Bone marrow transplantation, 2001. **28**(3): p. 271–5.
108. Whimbey, E., et al., *Combination therapy with aerosolized ribavirin and intravenous immunoglobulin for respiratory syncytial virus disease in adult bone marrow transplant recipients.* Bone marrow transplantation, 1995. **16**(3): p. 393–9.
109. Boeckh, M., et al., *Phase 1 evaluation of the respiratory syncytial virus-specific monoclonal antibody palivizumab in recipients of hematopoietic stem cell transplants.* Journal of Infectious Diseases, 2001. **184**(3): p. 350–4.
110. Madden, R.M., et al., *Prophylaxis of Pneumocystis carinii pneumonia with atovaquone in children with leukemia.[see comment].* Cancer, 2007. **109**(8): p. 1654–8.
111. Weinthal, J., et al., *Successful Pneumocystis carinii pneumonia prophylaxis using aerosolized pentamidine in children with acute leukemia.[see comment].* Journal of Clinical Oncology, 1994. **12**(1): p. 136–40.
112. DeAngelis, L.M., et al., *Evolution of Neuropathy and Myopathy During Intensive Vincristine/Corticosteroid Chemotherapy for Non - Hodgkin's Lymphoma.* Cancer, 1991. **67**: p. 2241–2246.
113. Plotkin, S.R. and P.Y. Wen, *Neurologic complications of cancer therapy.* Neurologic Clinics of North America, 2003. **21**: p. 279–318.
114. Garewal, H.S. and W.S. Dalton, *Metoclopramide in vincristine-induced ileus.* Cancer Treatment Reports, 1985. **69**(11): p. 1309–11.

115. Harris, A.C. and J.M. Jackson, *Lactulose in vincristine-induced constipation.* Medical Journal of Australia, 1977. **2**(17): p. 573–4.
116. Bedikian, A., et al., *A pilot study with vincristine sulfate liposome infusion in patients with metastatic melanoma.* Melanoma Research, 2008. **18**(6): p. 400–404.
117. Gelmon, K.A., et al., *Phase I Study of Liposomal Vincristine.* Journal of Clinical Oncology, 1999. **17**: p. 697–705.
118. Jackson, D.V., et al., *Phase II trial of vincristine infusion in acute leukemia.* Cancer Chemotherapy and Pharmacotherapy, 1985. **14**: p. 26–27–29.
119. Weintraub, M., et al., *Severe atypical neuropathy associated with administration of hematopoietic colony-stimulating factors and vincristine.* Journal of Clinical Oncology, 1996. **14**(3): p. 935–40.
120. Brown, G.J.E. and N.D. Yeomans, *Prevention of the Gastrointestinal Adverse Effects of Nonsteroidal Anti-Inflammatory Drugs The Role of Proton Pump Inhibitors.* Drug Safety, 1999. **21**(6): p. 503–512.
121. Sartori, S., et al., *Randomized Trial of Omeprazole or Ranitidine Versus Placebo in the Prevention of Chemotherapy-Induced Gastroduodenal Injury.* J Clin Oncol, 2000. **18**(3): p. 463-.
122. Bostrom, B.C., et al., *Dexamethasone versus prednisone and daily oral versus weekly intravenous mercaptopurine for patients with standard-risk acute lymphoblastic leukemia: a report from the Children's Cancer Group.* Blood, 2003. **101**(10): p. 3809–3817.
123. C. D. Mitchell, S.M.R.S.E.K.J.L.A.V.T.O.B.E., *Benefit of dexamethasone compared with prednisolone for childhood acute lymphoblastic leukaemia: results of the UK Medical Research Council ALL97 randomized trial.* British Journal of Haematology, 2005. **129**(6): p. 734–745.
124. Fink, J.C., et al., *Avascular Necrosis Following Bone Marrow Transplantation: A Case-Control Study.* Bone, 1998. **22**(1): p. 67–71.
125. Gaynon, P.S.L., R.H., *The Use of Glucocorticoids in Acute Lymphoblastic Leukemia of Childhood.* Journal of Pediatric Hematology/Oncology, 1995. **17**(1): p. 1–12.
126. Niinimaki, R.A., et al., *High Body Mass Index Increases the Risk for Osteonecrosis in Children With Acute Lymphoblastic Leukemia.* Journal of Clinical Oncology, 2007. **25**(12): p. 1498–1504.
127. Patel, B., et al., *High incidence of avascular necrosis in adolescents with acute lymphoblastic leukaemia: a UKALL XII analysis.* Leukemia, 2008. **22**: p. 308–312.
128. Strauss, A.J., et al., *Bony Morbidity in Children Treated for Acute Lymphoblastic Leukemia.* J Clin Oncol, 2001. **19**(12): p. 3066–3072.
129. Saracco, P.B., N.; Farinasso, L.; Einaudi, S.; Barisone, E.; Altare, F.; Pastore,G., *Steroid Withdrawal Syndrome During Steroid Tapering in Childhood Acute Lymphoblastic Leukemia; A Controlled Study Comparing Prednisone Versus Dexamethason in Induction Phase.* J Pediatr Hematol Oncol, 2005. **27**(3): p. 141–144.

Chapter 9
Treatment of Acute Lymphoblastic Leukemia in Middle-Age and Older Adults

Vaishalee P. Kenkre and Richard A. Larson

Introduction

Acute lymphoblastic leukemia (ALL) is the most common malignant disease in children, with the peak incidence between 3 and 5 years of age. In contrast, ALL is uncommon in adults and accounts for only about 20% of adult acute leukemia. Adults have a less favorable prognosis, with long-term disease-free survival (DFS) of 25–50% [1, 2]. Clinical presentation of ALL is covered in detail in other chapters, but both clinical and biological characteristics weigh heavily on determining treatment strategies, so will be mentioned here as well.

ALL presents with varying degrees of neutropenia, anemia, and thrombocytopenia. Leukocytosis is most common, but symptomatic leukostasis is rare in ALL. Nevertheless, a high white blood cell (WBC) count is an independent predictor of poor outcome. Central nervous system (CNS) involvement by ALL occurs in about 5–10% of adult cases during the course of their disease, but neurologic symptoms are uncommon at diagnosis. Two important subgroups of childhood ALL associated with favorable outcomes, i.e., hyperdiploid ALL with greater than 50 chromosomes, and ALL with the *TEL/AML1* fusion gene, are rarely seen in adults. Instead, the single largest subgroup of adult patients with ALL are those with the BCR-ABL fusion gene, resulting from t(9;22), the so called Philadelphia chromosome-positive (Ph+) ALL. This makes up 25–30% of ALL in middle-aged adults and is even more common in older adults. Other unfavorable karyotypes include trisomy 8 (+8) and monosomy 7 (−7). Other genetic abnormalities characteristic of T-cell and Burkitt (mature B-cell) ALL are detailed in other chapters. Thus, the primary determinants of outcome for adults are age (and associated co-morbidities), WBC count, and genetic characteristics of their ALL.

The aims of modern ALL treatment regimens are the rapid restoration of bone marrow function by use of multiple cytotoxic chemotherapy drugs in combinations with acceptable toxicities to prevent the emergence of resistant subclones, the use of adequate prophylactic treatment of sanctuary sites, such as the CNS, and post-remission continuation therapies to eliminate minimal (undetectable)

Supported in part by grants from the National Institutes of Health CA-14599, CA-31946, CA-41287, and CA-33601.

R.A. Larson (✉)
Department of Medicine and Cancer Research Center, University of Chicago,
Chicago, IL 60637, USA
and
Section of Hematology/Oncology, University of Chicago, MC-2115, 5841 S. Maryland Avenue,
Chicago, IL 60637, USA
e-mail: rlarson@medicine.bsd.uchicago.edu

residual disease. Long-term survival is achieved only via induction of a complete remission (CR). Post-remission therapy has traditionally been categorized as intensification or consolidation treatment followed by prolonged maintenance or continuation therapy. The use of hematopoietic cell transplantation (HCT) as post-remission therapy is discussed elsewhere. Typically, the total duration of anti-ALL chemotherapy is 2–3 years.

Current remission induction programs achieve CR in 70–80% of middle-aged patients with unfavorable cytogenetics and 90% in those with a normal karyotype or T-ALL. Vincristine, a corticosteroid (prednisone or dexamethasone), and an anthracycline comprise the principal agents in most remission induction regimens. Other agents, such as cyclophosphamide, cytarabine, methotrexate, and asparaginase, act through various and different biochemical mechanisms, and are often included to destroy leukemia cells before they develop drug resistance. Purine antimetabolites such as mercaptopurine and thioguanine have proven effectiveness and allow continuous exposure to these orally bioavailable agents.

The following is a brief review of recent clinical trial data on treatment and outcomes of middle-aged adults with ALL, which is based on the aforementioned principles. Then, we address the special challenges involving treatment of ALL among older patients (>60 years).

Recent Clinical Trials

The Cancer and Leukemia Group B (CALGB) has completed a series of prospective clinical trials evaluating a 5-drug induction regimen with intensive consolidation based in part on the pediatric Berlin-Frankfurt-Muenster regimen [3]. In CALGB study 8811, 197 patients (median age, 32 years; range, 16–80) received cyclophosphamide, daunorubicin, vincristine, prednisone, and L-asparaginase for induction. Those in CR received a total of 24 months of multi-agent consolidation, CNS prophylaxis with cranial radiation therapy (RT), late intensification, and maintenance therapy. After induction, 85% achieved a CR, 7% had refractory disease, and 9% had died. The CR rate varied by age: 94% for < 30 years, 85% for 30–59 years, 39% for 60+ years. Only a small number of patients, mostly those with Ph+ ALL, underwent allogeneic HCT in first complete remission (CR1). After a median follow-up of 43 months, median overall survival (OS) was 36 months, and median remission duration 29 months. Again, the outcomes varied by age; estimated 3 year OS by age group was 69% (<30 years), 39% (30–59 years), and 17% (60+ years). Favorable pretreatment characteristics included younger age, presence of a mediastinal mass, WBC count < 30,000/μL, T cell immunophenotype, and Ph negative disease. The co-expression of myeloid antigens on ALL blasts did not affect the outcome.

Subsequent clinical trials by the CALGB attempted to improve upon these results. CALGB 9111 was a randomized, placebo-controlled trial evaluating filgrastim (G-CSF) during the same remission and consolidation therapy [4]. Despite a significantly shorter time to recovery of neutrophils, there was no overall benefit from daily administration of G-CSF in terms of OS and DFS. However, the CR rate was higher among patients older than 60 years who received G-CSF, and concomitantly, their induction death rate was lower. A small phase II study, CALGB 9311, showed no benefit to the addition of anti-B4 blocked ricin, an anti-CD19 monoclonal immunotoxin, to a standard chemotherapy regimen [5]. However, patients with T-ALL were enrolled onto a separate arm of that trial and seemed to benefit from receiving one course high-dose cytarabine (HiDAC) as part of their consolidation therapy. CALGB 9511 was a Phase 2 study that substituted pegylated-asparaginase for conventional native *E. coli* asparaginase during induction and consolidation [6]. Patients with the greatest degree of asparagine depletion had the best outcomes for both DFS and OS.

More recent CALGB studies (19802 and 10102) have intensified both induction and consolidation regimens by increasing the dose of daunorubicin in both younger and older adults in an attempt to overcome the rapid emergence of multi-drug resistance mediated by the P-glycoprotein-mediated drug efflux mechanism [7]. At the same time, consolidation courses of high dose intravenous (IV) and oral methotrexate were evaluated in addition to high dose cytarabine (HiDAC). Extensive intrathecal plus high-dose systemic chemotherapy was used for CNS prophylaxis in lieu of cranial or craniospinal irradiation, and the CNS disease recurrence rate was only 4%. In CALGB 10,102, patients with >20% expression of CD52 on their ALL blasts were also given the anti-CD52 monoclonal antibody alemtuzumab (12 doses over 4 weeks) as post-remission therapy. CD52 is expressed on about two-thirds of adult ALL cases, and interestingly, on almost all cases of Ph+ ALL [8]. All of the interventions described above were proven feasible in these multi-center studies, but none appeared to offer an important breakthrough.

Investigators at the MD Anderson Cancer Center have continued to refine the hyperCVAD regimen (hyperfractionated cyclophosphamide plus vincristine, doxorubicin, and dexamethasone) [9]. One recent analysis reported on 288 patients (median age, 40 years; range, 15–92). Twenty percent were over 60 years old. The treatment regimen had 8 total cycles; cycles 1, 3, 5, and 7 were hyperCVAD, while cycles 2, 4, 6, and 8 consisted of 3 day courses of high-dose methotrexate and cytarabine. Overall, 92% of patients achieved a CR; 14 patients (5%) had induction deaths. After a median follow up time of 63 months, the median OS was 32 months. The 5 year survival rate was 38% and the 5 year continuous CR rate was 38%. The hyperCVAD regimen was less effective among patients >60 years. The CR rate for older patients was 80%, mostly due to higher induction mortality; the 5 year survival was 17%, and 5 year continuous CR rate was 27%. Survival and remission duration were considerably better with hyperCVAD compared to their own historical results with VAD [10]. The CR rate did not vary according to WBC count or cytogenetics. Factors associated with shorter survival included older age, Ph+ ALL, leukocytosis, thrombocytopenia, poor performance status, and hepatomegaly. CR duration was shorter for age >45 years, leukocytosis >50,000/µL, poor performance status, Ph+ ALL, FAB L2 morphology, the need for more than one course to achieve CR, and bone marrow lymphoblasts > 5% on day 14. As yet, similar results with hyperCVAD have not been reported from other centers or groups.

British and American investigators have recently reported results from the MRC UKALL XII/ECOG E2993 study that enrolled 1929 newly diagnosed adults (age range, 15–64 years). Initial analysis of the patient group revealed that patients who failed to achieve CR after induction had an OS rate of 5% compared with 45% for patients who achieved CR [11]. Thus, these data emphasize that achieving CR with induction therapy is crucial for long-term survival in adult patients with ALL. Factors at diagnosis that were predictive of OS and DFS were age, WBC count, and immunophenotype, confirming most previously published reports of independent prognostic factors in ALL. A subset analysis of patients with CNS involvement at diagnosis (present in 5% of the 1,508 patients) reported 5 year OS of 29% compared with 38% for those without CNS ALL [12].

The most recent analysis from this study evaluated the role of HCT in CR1 [13]. After achieving a CR, patients <55 years old with a matched sibling donor were assigned to receive an allogeneic HCT, while those without a donor were randomized to receive either an autologous HCT or a consolidation and maintenance chemotherapy regimen. High risk patients were defined by age >35 years or high WBC count at presentation (>30,000/µL for B-lineage ALL and >100,000/µL for T-ALL). A detailed analysis of the Ph+ ALL patients was reported separately. The CR rate for the 1,646 non-Ph+ patients was 90%. After a median follow up of 4 years and 11 months, the 5 year OS was 39% overall and 43% for the non-Ph+ ALL cases. A donor/no-donor comparison was reported. Among the 1,646 patients who had non-Ph+ ALL, the 5 year OS was 53% for those who had a donor compared with 45% with no donor; subset analyses are shown in Table 9.1. Autologous HCT was well tolerated, and there was no difference in non-relapse mortality between the chemotherapy and the autologous HCT arms. Patients who received autologous HCT had inferior EFS (32% vs 41%, $p=0.02$) and OS (37% vs 46%, $p=0.03$) compared with the chemotherapy group. One possible explanation may be the lack of maintenance therapy on the autologous HCT arm. Comparing 5 year OS in patients treated with allogeneic HCT versus only chemotherapy, the high-risk

Table 9.1 Treatment outcomes for young, middle-age, and older adults with ALL

Research group	Age group (years)	No. of patients	Complete remission (%)	Leukemia-free survival		Overall survival	
				Median (months)	3-years (%)	Median (months)	3-years (%)
Cancer and Leukemia Group B (CALGB) [3–7]							
	<30	360	89	31	48	62	59
	30–59	502	81	21	39	22	39
	≥60	197	61	12	20	10	15
Hospital Edouard Herriot, Lyon [16]							
	<35	192	84	16	35	24	39
	35–60	118	85	15	31	18	34
	>60	66	58	8	11	6	11
MD Anderson Cancer Center, Houston [9]							
	<40	147	95	NR	NR	NR	51 (5 year)
	40–59	82	94	NR	NR	NR	30 (5 year)
	≥60	59	80	NR	NR	NR	17 (5 yvear)
ECOG/MRC UKALL [11]							
	15–59	1521	91	NR	41 (5 year)	NR	38 (5 year)
	Ph pos	293	83	NR	28 (5 year)	NR	25 (5 year)
	Ph neg	1153	93	NR	44 (5 year)	NR	41 (5 year)
	<30[a]	535	NR	NR	NR	NR	45 (5 year)
	30–39[a]	217	NR	NR	NR	NR	34 (5 year)
	40–59[a]	271	NR	NR	NR	NR	15–23 (5 year)

NR not reported

[a]Only Ph negative ALL cases are included here

ALL population did not demonstrate any advantage from allogeneic HCT, due in large part to high transplant-related mortality (TRM). Unless TRM can be reduced, allogeneic HCT is not recommended for middle-age ALL patients in CR1 unless high-risk cytogenetic features, such as Ph+, t(4, 11), +8, or −7, are present.

Among the standard-risk group, however, 5 year survival was 63% vs 52% for the donor/no donor comparison, respectively. The authors concluded that standard risk ALL patients should undergo allogeneic HCT in CR1 if the patient had a matched sibling donor. Others have commented, however, that the patients who received chemotherapy only, i.e., the comparator group, did less well in this study than in several other large multicenter studies using similar or more intensive chemotherapy. The patients receiving allogeneic HCT were young with a median age in the early 1930s. The results using pediatric therapeutic regimens in this age group appear equivalent to allogeneic HCT. In summary, these appear to be equally valid treatment modalities for younger adults in CR1 [14]. Since it is uncommon to rescue a patient who relapses after an allogeneic HCT, many would prefer to cure patients with chemotherapy during CR1, if possible, and reserve allogeneic HCT in CR2 for those who relapse. In the future, further risk stratification using assessments of minimal residual disease and/or gene expression profiling may identify better which standard risk patients are at higher risk for relapse after conventional chemotherapy and may benefit from allogeneic HCT in CR1.

ALL in Older Adults

Available data on ALL in older patients are relatively scarce. One population based registry reported that 31% of all cases occurred in patients 60 years or older [15]. The age-specific annual incidence in the USA is only 0.4 to 0.6 cases per 100,000 individuals between 25 and 50 years old. However,

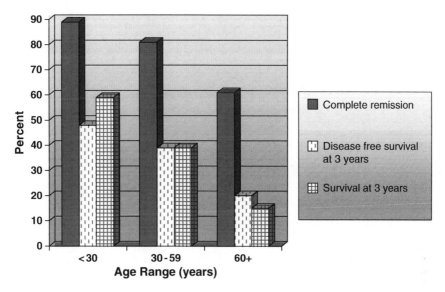

Fig. 9.1 Treatment outcome by age cohort (CALGB studies with 1059 ALL patients by intention to treat, 1988–2008)

the incidence rises steadily during the older decades and is two- to threefold higher above the age of 60 years (0.9–1.6 cases per 100,000). Older patients with ALL clearly do not fare as well as children or younger adults receiving standard treatment (Fig. 9.1). This is likely due to co-existing medical disorders as well as fundamental biological differences in the disease.

There is considerable evidence that the clinical and biological characteristics of the disease change dramatically between childhood, the middle adult years, and older age groups. For example, the ratio of males to females declines from 1.75 in younger adults to 0.97 in older adults. Comparative data on clinical characteristics are available from large treatment centers, although these are not free of referral bias. Sixty-nine patients between 60 and 89 years old (median, 68) were evaluated at the Edouard Herriot Hospital in Lyon, France, between 1980 and 1998, and were compared with 309 younger adults 15–59 years old (median, 29) [16]. Of note, 14% of the older adults had previously had a malignant disease compared with 3% of the younger patients. The older adults were less likely to have peripheral lymphadenopathy (21% vs 51%) or a mediastinal mass (1% vs 14%) or splenomegaly (26% vs 45%), but there were no differences in hepatomegaly or central nervous system involvement. Weight loss was slightly more common among older patients, but fever, infection, and bleeding were less common.

Modest differences were noted in presenting blood counts. The median WBC count was 8,400/μL (range, 500–520,000/μL) among the older patients compared with 13,200/μL (range, 500–1,440,000/μL) among the younger adults ($p=0.05$). There were no differences in the initial median hemoglobin levels (9.7 g/dL vs 10.1 g/dL) or platelet counts (47,000/μL vs 55,000/μL). Pretreatment data from 909 adults enrolled on multicenter clinical trials by the CALGB between 1988 and 2005 show similar trends (Table 9.2).

The most significant age-related differences in the Lyon series were noted in the immunophenotype and karyotype results. Lymphoblasts were of B-cell lineage in 89% of the older patients compared with 66% of the younger adults ($p=0.0004$). Conversely, T-cell ALL was present in only 8% of older patients compared with 29% of the younger patients ($p=0.0007$). Myeloid antigens were co-expressed by 19% of the older adult cases compared with 11% of the younger cases; lymphoblasts from 69% of older ALL patients also expressed CD34.

Table 9.2 Pretreatment characteristics by age cohort for 909 adults with newly diagnosed ALL enrolled on Cancer and Leukemia Group B studies between 1988 and 2005

Feature		Age group at diagnosis (years)		
		16–29	30–59	≥60
No. of patients		318	425	166
Median age (years)		22	43	66
Gender	Male (%)	69	55	51
Race/ethnic group	White (%)	73	83	88
	Black (%)	10	8	8
	Hispanic (%)	13	6	2
History of other cancer (%)		0	3	13
Infection	Fever (%)	50	44	34
	Pneumonia (%)	9	11	20
	Septicemia (%)	6	2	7
	Skin/mucosa (%)	12	10	13
Lymphadenopathy (%)		41	28	17
Splenomegaly (%)		32	23	12
Hepatomegaly (%)		18	17	11
Mediastinal mass (%)		12	9	1
CNS leukemia (%)		1	2	1
Median blood counts	Hemoglobin (g/dL)	9.6	9.5	9.8
	Platelets (/uL)	56,000	53,000	45,000
	Leukocytes (/uL)	13,800	12,500	7,600
	Blasts (%)	57	42	36
	Neutrophils (%)	8	13	12
Median marrow cellularity (%)		100	95	95
Median marrow blasts (%)		90	88	90

A similar analysis has been reported by the German Multicenter ALL Study Group (GMALL), although the older age group was truncated at 65 years old [17]. Between 1984 and 1999, 342 patients (12%) from 55 to 65 years old were enrolled on one of 4 prospective clinical trials and were compared with 2,463 patients (88%), ages 15–54 years. The older patients less frequently had peripheral lymph node involvement, mediastinal tumor, or splenomegaly. A common or pre-B immunophenotype was more frequent among older patients (75% vs 59%; $p = 0.001$) whereas T-cell ALL was less frequent (3% vs 14%), and the frequencies of null plus pro-B ALL were similar (13% vs 12%). Among T-ALL cases, mature T-ALL (2% vs 7%) and thymic T-ALL (3% vs 14%) occurred less commonly in older patients. In a recent multicenter series of older ALL patients from Poland, no remarkable differences in pretreatment characteristics were reported between 64 patients 60–69 years old and 23 patients 70 years and older [18].

Cytogenetic abnormalities characterize the biological heterogeneity of ALL and provide a strong and independent prognostic factor for treatment outcome [19]. The presence of the *BCR/ABL* fusion gene (Ph+ ALL) has had a dramatic negative impact on the outcomes of older patients (Table 9.3), and the admixture of these patients into various series must be taken into account when evaluating the efficacy of different treatment regimens. The recent development of specific tyrosine kinase inhibitors (imatinib, dasatinib, nilotinib) appears to be changing this previously grim prognosis.

The incidence of Ph+ ALL, a subset that is resistant to conventional chemotherapy, clearly increases with age [20]. Clonal chromosomal abnormalities were found at diagnosis in 378 of 443 adults (85%) by the Groupe Francais de Cytogenetique Hematologique; 60 (13%) were older than 60 years (range, 60–84) [21]. In this series, 18% of those less than 40 years old and 46% of those 40–60 years old were Ph+ compared with 35% of those older than 60 years. Among 276 patients (ages 16–83) with centrally reviewed karyotypes enrolled on a prospective study by the CALGB,

Table 9.3 Outcomes for older adults (≥60 years) with ALL with or without the Philadelphia chromosome or *BCR/ABL* fusion gene enrolled on CALGB clinical trials

Genetic subgroup	Age		CR		DFS		OS		DFS at 3 years		OS at 3 years	
	N	Median years (range)	N	% (95% CI)	N	Median months (95% CI)	N	Median months (95% CI)	N	% (95% CI)	N	% (95% CI)
Ph neg	79	68 (60–83)	79	58 (47–69)	46	13 (8–21)	79	7 (3–12)	46	27 (15–41)	79	16 (9–25)
Ph pos	45	67 (60–80)	45	62 (47–76)	28	12 (7–15)	45	11 (7–15)	28	5 (0–19)	45	4 (0–16)
Total	124	67 (60–83)	124	60 (51–68)	74	13 (10–17)	124	9 (5–12)	74	20 (11–30)	124	12 (7–19)

Ph neg denotes cases where neither the t(9;22) nor *BCR/ABL* was detected

Ph pos denotes cases where either t(9;22) or *BCR/ABL* were detected

CR complete remission, DFS disease-free survival, OS overall survival, 95% CI 95% confidence interval. Almost all of these patients were treated prior to the development of specific BCR/ABL tyrosine kinase inhibitors

76% had a clonal abnormality; 28% overall and 33% of those older than 60 years had a t(9;22) [22]. In a recent report from the Southwest Oncology Group, the frequency of Ph+ ALL increased from 6% in those less than 25 years old to 14% for those 25–35 years old, 33% for those 36–55 years old, and 53% for patients older than 56 years [23]. In the large GMALL series described above, among those with common or pre-B ALL, the incidence of Ph+ or *BCR/ABL*+ ALL was significantly higher among adults older than 55 years than younger adults (54% vs 37%; $p=0.001$) [17]. In the French series from Lyon, the Ph chromosome or *BCR/ABL* fusion gene was detected in 24% of older patients and 19% of young patients [16]. In contrast, a rearrangement of chromosome 11q23 was observed in only 2% of older and 5% of younger patients (X^2 statistic, $p=0.001$).

Clinical Trial Data

There are minimal clinical data on treatment outcomes for ALL in older patients. Many clinical trials have excluded patients >55–60 years old. Overall, it is estimated that 54% of patients with leukemia in the USA are greater than 65 years of age. However, only approximately 19% of patients enrolled on CALGB trials have been 60 years or older, and 22% of those on MD Anderson Cancer Center frontline ALL studies [24]. Similarly, only 4–15% patients enrolled each year on the nationwide MRC UKALL X and XA studies in the UK were >60 years old 25]. Thus, older patients are clearly underrepresented in prospective ALL clinical trials. Comparative outcome data by age group (with the exception of the MRC UKALL/ECOG study which did not enroll patients above 60 years), from the aforementioned studies as well as data from Edouard Herriot Hospital in Lyon, France, are shown in Table 9.1.

The GMALL Study Group reported on a pilot study for patients older than 65 years, in which it was shown that favorable factors for achievement of CR were pro-B ALL or T-ALL, Ph-negative disease, and WBC < 30,000/μL [26]. The CR rate was 74% for patients without any of these risk factors. However, 52% of patients had one or more of these risk factors, and they had a CR rate of only 19% ($p=0.001$). Survival was also significantly better for the group with no risk factors (median, 17 months compared to 6 months, $p=0.002$). Recently updated to include 94 patients, the CR rate overall was 48%, but survival was less than 10% at 5 years [27].

Both Hoelzer and Pagano et al. have recently reviewed the literature describing the outcomes of older ALL patients reported between 1990 and 2004 [(28, 29]. Taken altogether, the weighted mean CR rate was 56% for the 519 patients older than 60 years who received intensive chemotherapy on a prospective trial; 23% of patients had early deaths, and 30% had chemotherapy-resistant disease. The median remission duration was 9 months, and the median OS was 7 months.

Palliative chemotherapy approaches are sometimes recommended to older patients because of poor performance status or the presence of co-morbid disorders such as diabetes, cardiac disease, or renal insufficiency. In a report from the Instituto di Demeitotica Medica in Rome, 37 (31%) of 119 patients, newly diagnosed with ALL between 1986 and 1998, were older than 65 years; 25 received intensive chemotherapy and 12 received only vincristine and steroids [30]. A CR was achieved in 80% of the intensively treated older patients and their median survival was 14 months (range, 2–82). Among the patients managed with palliative treatment, 42% had a CR; the median survival for all 12 patients was only 2.6 months (range, 0.3–19).

Similar results were reported when practice patterns in the northern region of England were surveyed [31]. Among 62 consecutive, newly diagnosed ALL patients older than 60 years, 28 (median age, 67 years; range, 60–80) received "curative" therapy, 25 (median age, 74) received palliative therapy, and 9 (median age, 83) received no treatment. A CR was achieved in 10 (36%) of the intensively treated group and 4 (16%) of the palliative therapy group. The median survival for each treatment group was only 3 months, although several patients survived longer than 3 years after intensive therapy.

Co-morbidities and Complications

Co-morbid conditions, interactions with multiple other medications, nutritional status, and adherence to complex treatment regimens all influence the pharmacokinetic profile in older adults. There is little evidence that drug absorption is affected by the chronological age of the patient. However, the volume of distribution of a drug may be less than in younger adults due to different proportions of body fat to lean body mass, hydration status, and plasma protein levels. Hepatic blood flow and renal clearance may be diminished in older patients. However, older adults with normal calculated renal function appear to tolerate chemotherapy drugs and have similar toxicity profiles as younger adults.

Nevertheless, the pharmacodynamic effects of particular drugs may be greater in older individuals. The number of hematopoietic stem cells declines with age; thus, the neutrophil nadir may be lower and recovery from myelotoxic chemotherapy more prolonged in older adults [32]. Mucositis appears more frequent and more severe in older patients, and the consequences with regard to pain, diminished nutrition, and infection may be graver. Pain may respond to considerably lower doses of analgesics in older patients. Delirium during treatment is under-recognized and misdiagnosed. It must be treated promptly by removing the causative factors or with psychotropic medications such as haloperidol. Interestingly, nausea and vomiting after chemotherapy have been reported to be less common in older adults.

Specific leukemia drugs have well known toxicities that require special attention in older patients. Vincristine may cause severe constipation, and thus laxatives should be used prophylactically. Corticosteroids can exacerbate diabetes, and hyperglycemia may lead to infection and fluid and electrolyte abnormalities. L-asparaginase causes cognitive impairment leading to encephalopathy more often in older adults than in children. The appearance of somnolence and confusion in such cases can be mistakenly attributed to depression or viral encephalitis. Discontinuation of the enzyme and prompt refeeding or infusion of amino acid solutions containing glutamine can yield a dramatic improvement in mental status. Discontinuation of extraneous medications that many older adults take for chronic but mild disorders can prevent serious drug interactions during chemotherapy.

Among randomized clinical trials testing the use of hematopoietic growth factors during chemotherapy for ALL, older patients have enjoyed the most measureable benefits. In a CALGB study of 185 ALL patients who were randomly assigned to receive either G-CSF or a placebo during induction and consolidation therapy, 36 were 60 years or older. [4] For these older patients, the time to recovery of >1,000 neutrophils/μL during remission induction was shortened from 29 days in the placebo group to 16 days in the G-CSF group ($p < 0.001$). The corresponding CR rates were 69% in the placebo group and 85% in the G-CSF group, and the induction death rate fell from 31% to 5% with G-CSF support. Older patients who received placebo had a median time to platelet recovery >50,000/μL of 26 days, whereas the older patients who received G-CSF had a median of 17 days to platelet recovery. It has become routine practice within the CALGB to use G-CSF during treatment of ALL in older adults.

Approaches to minimize toxicity will be crucial for future successes in treatment of elderly patients with ALL. One method by which to achieve this may be treatment with lower doses of chemotherapy for longer duration, a phenomenon seen more commonly in treatment of pediatric ALL patients. A recent retrospective analysis at MD Anderson Cancer Center compared 122 older patients who received hyper-CVAD to 34 older patients who received less intensive regimens and 409 younger patients who received hyper-CVAD [33]. CR rates were 84%, 59%, and 92%, respectively. While the older patients treated with hyper-CVAD showed a lower incidence of disease resistance during induction (5% vs 27%), they showed a higher rate of death in CR (34% vs 15%). Therefore, while the overall benefit:risk ratio was favorable, clearly new low intensity regimens and agents will further improve the results of elderly ALL patients.

Alternatively, delivering higher doses of chemotherapy more safely to avoid toxicity may be employed. Some preliminary data exist on administering standard ALL chemotherapy agents in the liposomal form. A Phase 2 study showed that high dose daunorubicin in a liposomal form administered to elderly ALL patients improved CR, EFS, and OS without increasing toxicity [34]. Similarly, liposomal vincristine administered to relapsed ALL patients also showed good efficacy with minimal toxicity in a recent Phase 2 study [35]. Further studies with liposomal forms of these standard chemotherapy agents may allow delivery of higher doses with minimal toxicity, which would be advantageous in any, but specifically in the elderly, population.

Options that steer away from conventional chemotherapy may also hold promise for the older patient population, due to novel mechanisms of action and the potential for lesser toxicity. Given that a large percentage of older patients have Ph+ ALL, tyrosine kinase inhibitors that target this mutated enzyme are an important option in this age group. Recent data show evidence in favor of incorporating imatinib into induction and post-remission therapy for patients [36]. Additionally, other second generation ABL kinase inhibitors are currently in Phase 2 trials, either as single agents or in combinations [37].

Rituximab, which binds to CD20 (a marker expressed on more than 20% of lymphoblasts in about half of common or pre-B ALL cases), has been incorporated into frontline hyper-CVAD therapy for CD20+ ALL [38]. The antigen CD52 is expressed on normal and malignant lymphocytes and is the target for alemtuzumab. Approved for the treatment of B-cell chronic lymphocytic leukemia, this antibody has also shown single-agent activity in a small number of patients with refractory ALL. It is currently being tested in both young and older adults with CD52+ ALL in first remission by the CALGB [8]. Approximately 69% of ALL cases have been shown to express CD52 on >10% of the blasts. A dose-escalation pilot study has demonstrated the safety of administering 30 mg subcutaneously 3 times per week for 4 weeks between courses of intensive chemotherapy at a time when minimal residual disease is likely to be present. Whether this intervention improves outcomes remains to be determined. Clofarabine and nelarabine are both active and approved agents in relapsed ALL, but there is limited experience reported using these novel drugs in older patients.

Summary

For adults with newly diagnosed ALL, careful diagnostic studies are essential for risk stratification. The goal of treatment is to achieve CR quickly in order to avoid the emergence of resistant subclones, to adequately prophylax sanctuary sites, and then to maintain remission through the use of consolidation and maintenance therapies to eliminate minimal residual disease. The appropriate role for allogeneic HCT in CR1 for standard risk patients remains controversial, but this is an important treatment option for high-risk patients. While there has been increasing success in treating younger and middle-aged adults with ALL, older patients have considerably inferior outcomes and are candidates for novel agents, including monoclonal antibodies, such as rituximab, epratuzumab, or alemtuzumab; liposomal vincristine; and various targeted agents. These will be further detailed in subsequent chapters.

Acknowledgments We thank Ben L. Stanford, MS in the CALGB Statistical Center at Duke University for his analysis of the CALGB data.

References

1. Jabbour, E. J., Faderl, S., & Kantarjian, H. M. (2005). Adult acute lymphoblastic leukemia. *Mayo Clinic Proceedings, 80*(11), 1517–1527.
2. Pui, C. H., & Evans, W. E. (2006). Treatment of adult lymphoblastic leukemia. *The New England Journal of Medicine, 354*(2), 166–178.
3. Larson, R. A., Dodge, R. K., Burns, P., et al. (1995). A five-drug remission induction regimen with intensive consolidation for adults with acute lymphoblastic leukemia: Cancer and Leukemia Group B study 8811. *Blood, 85*(8), 2025–2037.

4. Larson, R. A., Dodge, R. K., Linker, C. A., et al. (1998). A randomized controlled trial of filgrastim during remission induction and consolidation chemotherapy for adults with acute lymphoblastic leukemia: CALGB Study 9111. *Blood, 92*(5), 1556–1564.
5. Szatrowski, T. P., Dodge, R. K., Reynolds, C., et al. (2002). Lineage specific treatment of adult patients with acute lymphoblastic leukemia in first remission with anti-B4-blocked ricin or high-dose cytarabine: CALGB Study 9311. *Cancer, 97*, 1471–1480.
6. Wetzler, M., Sanford, B. L., Kurtzberg, J., et al. (2007). Effective asparagine depletion with pegylated asparaginase results in improved outcomes in adult acute lymphoblastic leukemia: Cancer and Leukemia Group B Study 9511. *Blood, 109*, 4164–4167.
7. Stock, W., Yu, D., Johnson, J., et al. (2003). Intensified daunorubicin during induction and post remission therapy for adults with acute lymphoblastic leukemia (ALL), results of CALGB 19802 [abstract]. *Blood, 102*, 379a.
8. Lozanski, G., Sanford, B., Mrozek, K., et al. (2007). Quantitative measurement of CD52 expression and alemtuzumab binding in adult acute lymphoblastic leukemia (ALL): Correlation with immunophenotype and cytogenetics in patients enrolled on a phase I/II trial from the Cancer and Leukemia Group B (CALGB 10102) [abstract]. *Blood, 110*, 2386.
9. Kantarjian, H., Thomas, D., O'Brien, S., et al. (2004). Long-term follow-up results of hyperfractionated cyclophosphamide, vincristine, doxorubicin, and dexamethasone (Hyper-CVAD), a dose-intensive regimen, in adult acute lymphocytic leukemia. *Cancer, 101*(12), 2788–2801.
10. Kantarjian, H. M., Walters, R. S., Keating, M. J., et al. (1990). Results of the vincristine, doxorubicin, and dexamethasone regimen in adults with standard- and high-risk acute lymphocytic leukemia. *Journal of Clinical Oncology, 8*(6), 994–1004.
11. Rowe, J. M., Buck, G., Burnett, A. K., et al. (2005). Induction therapy for adults with acute lymphoblastic leukemia: Results of more than 1500 patients from the international ALL trial: MRC UKALLXII/ECOG E2993. *Blood, 106*, 3760–3767.
12. Lazarus, H. M., Richards, S. M., Chopra, R., et al. (2006). Central nervous system involvement in adult acute lymphoblastic leukemia at diagnosis: Results from the international ALL trial MRC UKALL XII/ECOG E2993. *Blood, 108*, 465–472.
13. Goldstone, A. H., Richards, S. M., Lazarus, H. M., et al. (2008). In adults with standard-risk acute lymphoblastic leukemia, the greatest benefit is achieved from a matched sibling allogeneic transplantation in first complete remission, and an autologous transplantation is less effective than conventional consolidation/maintenance chemotherapy in all patients: Final results of the International ALL Trial (MRC UKALL XII/ECOG E2993). *Blood, 111*(4), 1827–1833.
14. Hahn, T., Wall, D., Camitta, B., et al. (2006). The role of cytotoxic therapy with hematopoietic stem cell transplantation in the therapy of acute lymphoblastic leukemia in adults: An evidence-based review. *Biology of Blood and Marrow Transplantation, 12*(1), 1–30.
15. National Cancer Institute, Surveillance, Epidemiology, and End Results Program, www.seer.cancer.gov
16. Thomas, X., Olteanu, N., Charrin, C., et al. (2001). Acute lymphoblastic leukemia in the elderly: The Edouard Herriot Hospital experience. *American Journal of Hematology, 67*(2), 73–83.
17. Gökbuget, N., Hoelzer, D., Arnold, R., et al. (2001). Subtypes and treatment outcome in adult acute lymphoblastic leukemia less than or greater than 55 years. *The Hematology Journal, 1*(Suppl 1), 186.
18. Robak, T., Szmigielska-Kaplon, A., Wrzesien-Kus, A., et al. (2004). Acute lymphoblastic leukemia in elderly: The Polish Adult Leukemia Group experience. *Annals of Hematology, 83*, 225–231.
19. Mrozek, K., Heerema, N. A., & Bloomfield, C. D. (2004). Cytogenetics in acute leukemia. *Blood Reviews, 18*, 115–136.
20. Secker-Walker, L. M., Prentice, H. G., Durrant, J., et al. (1997). Cytogenetics adds independent prognostic information in adults with acute lymphoblastic leukaemia on MRC trial UKALL XA. MRC Adult Leukaemia Working Party. *British Journal Haematology, 96*(3), 601–10.
21. Groupe Francais de Cytogenetique Hematologique. (1996). Cytogenetic abnormalities in adult acute lymphoblastic leukemia: Correlations with hematologic findings and outcome. *Blood, 87*, 3135–3142.
22. Wetzler, M., Dodge, R. K., Mrozek, K., et al. (1999). Prospective karyotype analysis in adult acute lymphoblastic leukemia. The Cancer and Leukemia Group B experience. *Blood, 93*, 3983–3993.
23. Appelbaum, F. R. (2005). Impact of age on the biology of acute leukemia. In M. C. Perry (Ed.), *American Society of Clinical Oncology educational book* (pp. 528–532). Alexandra, VA: ASCO.
24. Kantarjian, H. M., O'Brien, S., Smith, T. L., et al. (2000). Results of treatment with hyper-CVAD, a dose-intensive regimen, in adult acute lymphocytic leukemia. *Journal of Clinical Oncology, 18*(3), 547–561.
25. Chessells, J. M., Hall, E., Prentice, H. G., et al. (1998). The impact of age on outcome in lymphoblastic leukaemia; MRC UKALL X and XA compared: A report from the MRC Paediatric and Adult Working Parties. *Leukemia, 12*(4), 463–73.
26. Gökbuget, N., de Wit, M., Gerhardt, A., et al. (2000). Results of a shortened, dose reduced treatment protocol in elderly patients with acute lymphoblastic leukemia [abstract]. *Blood, 96*(Suppl 1), 718a. abstr 3104.

27. Hoelzer D, Gökbuget N, Beck J, et al. Subtype adjusted therapy improves outcome of elderly patients with acute lymphoblastic leukemia [abstract]. Blood 2004; 104 (Suppl 1): abstr 2732.

28. Hoelzer, D., & Gökbuget, N. (2005). Treatment of elderly patients with acute lymphoblastic leukemia. In M. C. Perry (Ed.), *American Society of Clinical Oncology educational book* (pp. 533–539). Alexandria, VA: ASCO.

29. Pagano, L., Mele, L., Trape, G., & Leone, G. (2004). The treatment of acute lymphoblastic leukaemia in the elderly. *Leukemia & Lymphoma, 45*, 117–123.

30. Pagano, L., Mele, L., Casorelli, I., et al. (2000). Acute lymphoblastic leukemia in the elderly. A twelve-year retrospective, single center study. *Haematologica, 85*, 1327–1329.

31. Taylor, P. R. A., Reid, M. M., & Proctor, S. J. (1994). Acute lymphoblastic leukaemia in the elderly. *Leukemia & Lymphoma, 13*, 373–380.

32. Lipschitz, D. A. (1995). Age-related declines in hematopoietic reserve capacity. *Seminars in Oncology, 22*(Suppl 1), 3–5.

33. O'Brien S, Thomas DA, Ravandi F, et al. Results of the hyperfractionated cyclophosphamide, vincristine, doxorubicin, and dexamethasone regimen in elderly patients with acute lymphocytic leukemia. Cancer 2008 (Epub ahead of print)

34. Offidani, M., Corvatta, L., Malerba, L., et al. (2005). Comparison of two regimens for the treatment of elderly patients with acute lymphoblastic leukaemia (ALL). *Leukemia & Lymphoma, 46*(2), 233–238.

35. Thomas, D. A., Sarris, A. H., Cortes, J., et al. (2006). Phase II study of sphingosomal vincristine in patients with recurrent or refractory adult acute lymphocytic leukemia. *Cancer, 106*, 120–127.

36. Ottmann, O. G., Wassmann, B., Pfeifer, H., et al. (2007). Imatinib compared with chemotherapy as front-line treatment of elderly patients with Philadelphia chromosome-positive acute lymphoblastic leukemia (Ph+ALL). *Cancer, 109*(10), 2068–2076.

37. Foa R, Vignetti M, Vitale A, et al. Dasatinib as front-line monotherapy for the induction treatment of adult and elderly Ph+ acute lymphoblastic leukemia (ALL) patients: Interim analysis of the GIMEMA prospective study LAL1205 [abstract]. Blood 2007; 110(11): abstr 7.

38. Thomas, D. A., Faderl, S., O'Brien, S., et al. (2006). Chemoimmunotherapy with hyper-CVAD plus rituximab for the treatment of adult Burkitt and Burkitt-type lymphoma or acute lymphoblastic leukemia. *Cancer, 106*(7), 1569–1580.

Chapter 10
Pharmacology of Acute Lymphoblastic Leukemia Therapy

Paul M. Barr, Richard J. Creger, and Nathan A. Berger

Introduction

In 1948, Farber and colleagues demonstrated that the administration of the folate analog aminopterin led to transient remissions in acute lymphoblastic leukemia (ALL) ushering in the modern era of chemotherapy and laying the foundation for the treatment of ALL [1]. With the development of additional active agents, including microtubule active agents, purine analogs, and glucocorticosteroids, there soon developed the rational basis for combination chemotherapy using multiple agents with different mechanisms of action to produce additive or synergistic antileukemic effects without compounding toxicity [2–4]. Another important strategic development in the treatment of ALL was the realization that while combination chemotherapy could result in the disappearance of all clinical and laboratory evidence of disease [4, 5], this so-called complete remission was soon followed by disease relapse indicating the persistence of leukemic cells. The continuation of chemotherapy beyond remission induction was necessary to induce long-term disease free survival and ultimately cures. In some cases, residual leukemic cells harbored in protected sanctuaries, such as the testes or central nervous system (CNS), are not affected by chemotherapy leading to recurrence at later times [6]. The latter problem requires therapies capable of penetrating these sanctuaries and eliminating residual leukemic cells [7, 8]. For the following 3 decades, cure in adult patients remained elusive despite encouraging responses. However, once treatment regimens were based on lessons learned from the pediatric combinations, survival rates in adult ALL improved to 30–40%. Now with development of increasingly targeted therapeutics and the understanding of which patient subsets should receive these agents, further advances in outcomes seems within reach.

A basic understanding of the clinical pharmacology behind the agents used in the standard treatment of ALL is important to prevent undue toxicity as many of the traditional cytotoxic agents have a narrow window between clinical efficacy and toxicity. Further, the rational combination of agents with synergistic mechanisms of action and nonoverlapping toxicities allows for the most effective treatment and prevents selecting out resistant clones. In theory, scheduling the administration of agents based on their cell cycle specificity and pharmacokinetic behavior while taking into account potential drug interactions and patient tolerance will lead to improved outcomes. Additionally, the use of hematopoietic growth factors to minimize hematologic toxicity and cytopenias, allow for maintaining dose intensity to achieve maximum ALL cell kill [2].

P.M. Barr (✉)
Department of Medicine, Case Comprehensive Cancer Center, Center for Science, Health and Society,
Case Western Reserve University School of Medicine and University Hospitals Case Medical Center,
11100 Euclid Ave, Cleveland, OH 44106, USA
e-mail: paul.barr@uhhospitals.org

A.S. Advani and H.M. Lazarus (eds.), *Adult Acute Lymphocytic Leukemia*, Contemporary Hematology,   127
DOI 10.1007/978-1-60761-707-5_10, © Springer Science+Business Media, LLC 2011

Glucocorticoids

For nearly 60 years, glucocorticoids have been used to treat ALL. Their integral role in treatment protocols has been demonstrated by inferior outcomes with their omission from induction therapy. The prognostic significance of response to initial steroid monotherapy supports this as well [9].

Mechanism of Action

Glucocorticosteroids bind to the glucocorticoid receptor resulting in translocation to the nucleus. This induces the transcription and translation of a variety of genes and in some cases ultimately activates the caspase cascade leading to cellular apoptosis [10].

Clinical Pharmacology and Pharmacokinetics

Studies done using orally administered prednisone in the setting of nonmalignant disease demonstrated peak plasma levels at 2 h with a $t_{1/2}$ of 2 h as well [11]. Metabolism is hepatic for the most part with the elimination of prednisone appearing to inversely correlate with age [12]. Intravenous dexamethasone appears to have a longer and more variable half-life of 2–9 h [13]. In an evaluation of dexamethasone in the setting of ALL, marked variability in clearance was demonstrated [14]. The variability may in part be related to significant serum protein binding or more likely, induction of the cytochrome P450 (CYP450) enzymes increasing drug clearance. Despite a variety of dosing schedules used in treatment protocols, it is clear that the efficacy of glucocorticoids relates to the duration of exposure rather than peak plasma levels [15]. Prednisone does cross the blood-brain barrier, achieving peak cerebrospinal fluid (CSF) levels after 6 h at roughly 1/3 of the level achieved in the plasma [16]. Dexamethasone enters the CNS in higher levels potentially related to higher serum free-drug levels. After systemic administration, dexamethasone demonstrated a CSF $t_{1/2}$ of 4 h compared to 3 h after prednisone[17]. This, in combination with clinical data demonstrating a decrease in CNS relapses and improved event-free survival, support the use of dexamethasone over prednisone as part of induction therapy [18].

Adverse Effects

The toxicity of glucocorticoids has been well described. While myelosuppression or gastrointestinal effects do not occur, insomnia, anxiety, palpitations, dyspepsia, proximal myopathy, and hyperglycemia occur commonly with the dosing schedules used in treating ALL. Prolonged exposure can put patients at risk for osteoporosis, Cushing syndrome, avascular necrosis, proximal myopathy, hypertension, glaucoma, and cataracts. Immunosuppression is also significant, predisposing patients to opportunistic infections, most notably *Pneumocystis carinii* pneumonia [19].

Drug Interactions

Glucocorticoids cause the induction of multiple CYP450 enzymes in the liver [20]. As such, drug interactions may occur with any inducer or inhibitor, especially of CYP3A4. In addition, pretreatment with asparaginase prior to glucocorticoid use may alter steroid pharmacokinetics likely related to the reduction in serum protein levels [14].

Methotrexate

Mechanism of Action

The antimetabolites are the most commonly used agents in the treatment of ALL as their efficacy depends on rapid cell cycling. Given the inhibition of DNA synthesis, they have their greatest cytotoxic effect during the S-phase of the cell cycle. Methotrexate, (MTX) is an antifolate antimetabolite which inhibits dihydrofolate reductase (DHFR) causing the depletion of reduced folates, essential cofactors involved in the synthesis of thymidylate and purines. In addition, the polyglutamation of MTX in lymphoblasts likely leads to the direct inhibition of folate-dependent enzymes responsible for purine and thymidylate synthesis [21]. The result is the inhibition of DNA synthesis and cell replication leading to apoptosis.

Clinical Pharmacology and Pharmacokinetics

Small doses of MTX are efficiently absorbed from the gastrointestinal tract. However, absorption of doses higher than 20 mg/m^2 may be unreliable necessitating intravenous administration [22, 23]. MTX is transported across the cell membrane primarily by the reduced-folate carrier system [24]. The naturally occurring process of intracellular polyglutamation renders MTX a more potent but reversible inhibitor of DHFR [25]. In ALL, cytotoxicity appears to be due primarily to the duration of drug exposure. The efficacy of MTX relates to the rapid doubling time of lymphoblast growth as the cells enter the S-phase of DNA synthesis. The concentration of reduced folates further determines the effect of MTX. When administered as part of high-dose regimens, during the first 12–24 h, the half-life is 2–3 h predominately determined by the rate of renal excretion. As such, patients with renal impairment should not receive MTX due to prolonged elimination and subsequent severe hematologic and gastrointestinal toxicity [26]. After 24 h, the terminal half-life lengthens to 8–10 h. As third-space fluids can act as a reservoir for the drug, MTX should not be used in patients with pleural effusion, ascites, or peripheral edema. MTX is metabolized in the liver but this appears to contribute minimally to the pharmacokinetics under normal circumstances. As a result, dose adjustments for hepatic dysfunction are not required.

As higher MTX serum concentrations have predicted for a lower risk of relapse, current use in induction therapy has evolved to administering high doses of the drug in conjunction with measures to prevent toxicity [27]. Further, higher doses and prolonged infusions penetrate sanctuary sites such as the CNS. Due to the potential morbidity and mortality associated with high dose infusions, this should only be performed in centers who have trained nursing and the ability to reliably measure serum levels [28]. Patients typically receiving intravenous sodium bicarbonate to maintain urine alkalinity thus preventing renal tubular precipitation as MTX has limited solubility below a pH of 7. Intensive intravenous hydration is given to promote adequate renal blood flow and filtration. Following a 6–36 h infusion of MTX doses ranging from 1 to 8 g/m^2, 5-formyltetrahydrofolate, or leucovorin, is administered repleting intracellular folate pools thus preventing MTX-induced cellular toxicity. Doses 10–15 mg/m^2 are administered every 6 h starting 18–36 h after the MTX dose and continued until the serum level is <0.05 μM [29]. Doses are typically increased to 50–200 mg/m^2 when plasma concentrations >5 μM at 24 h, >1 μM at 48 h or >0.5 μM at 72 h after administration.

Intrathecal administration of MTX is frequently used in ALL protocols. Distribution is typically unequal throughout the CSF and absorption into the brain parenchyma is minimal. A dose of 12 mg displays a terminal half-life of 7–16 h with prolonged disappearance in the elderly and those with meningeal disease [30].

Adverse Effects

Hematologic and gastrointestinal toxicities are most commonly observed side effects. Prolonged exposure in particular can lead to significant mucositis and myelosuppression. Less frequent effects include rash, pneumonitis, hepatitis, and renal failure. In the setting of MTX-induced nephrotoxicity, hemodialysis using a high-flux dialyzer may be effective in significant MTX clearance [31]. The use of carboxypeptidase G, a pseudomonal enzyme which converts MTX to its inactive metabolites, has also been effective in rescuing patients after MTX-induced nephrotoxicity [32, 33].

Intrathecal use can be accompanied by acute arachnoiditis. A more subacute syndrome consisting of paralysis, seizures, and coma is rarely observed. Repeated use and in combination with cranial irradiation, can lead to a chronic demyelinating encephalopathy predominately described in children. Neither leucovorin nor carboxypeptidase G is effective in preventing these effects given their poor CNS penetration [28].

Drug Interactions

MTX is synergistic with other classes of antimetabolites such as purine synthesis inhibitors and pyrimidine analogues. L-Asparaginase prevents cellular entry into the S-phase of the cell cycle, therefore antagonizing the effects of MTX. The two are not used concurrently for this reason. Excretion is inhibited by weak acids such as ciprofloxacin [34], the penicillins, and probenecid [35]. The cephalosporins enhance the renal excretion [36]. Nephrotoxic agents and agents diminishing renal blood flow such as NSAIDS should not be used concurrently with high-dose MTX [37].

6-Mercaptopurine and 6-Thioguanine

Mechanism of Action

The guanine analogs used in ALL therapy include 6-mercaptopurine (6-MP) and 6-thioguanine (6-TG). They are structurally related to hypoxanthine and guanine respectively, each with a thiol group substituted for the 6-oxo or 6-hydroxy group. 6-MP is converted by hypoxanthine-guanine phosphoribosyl transferase (HGPRT) to 6-thioinosine monophosphate which directly inhibits purine synthesis and subsequently to deoxy-6-thioguanosine triphosphate which is incorporated into DNA and RNA. Its cytotoxicity is therefore specific to the S-phase of the cell cycle. 6-TP is similarly activated by HGPRT to 6-thioguanylic acid and incorporated into DNA and RNA [38]. In both cases, the degree of DNA incorporation appears to correlate with cytotoxicity [34, 35].

Clinical Pharmacology and Pharmacokinetics

6-MP and 6-TG are administered orally at doses of 50–100 mg/m^2 per day and have variable bioavailability [39, 40]. It has been suggested that children who attain higher systemic exposure to 6-MP have better outcomes [41, 42]. Both parent drugs exhibit a half-life to 50–100 min while the active metabolites have a half-life of several days [43]. 6-MP is metabolized by xanthine oxidase (XO) to its inactive metabolite, 6-thiouric acid, the primary metabolite in plasma and urine. High concentrations of XO exist in the liver and mucosa of the small intestine accounting for its variable bioavailability. 6-TG is not metabolized by XO and is not subject to the same first-pass effects. 6-MP is also inactivated through S-methylation by thiopurine methyltransferase (TPMT) to a second metabolite, 6-methylmercaptopurine. 6-TG is also catabolized by TPMT to 6-methylthiopurine. This is the primary inactivation pathway in hematopoietic cells.

Adverse Effects

The primary side effect of the guanine analogs is myelosuppression. Inherited TMPT deficiencies can lead to increase myelosuppression from guanine analogs. It is estimated that 0.3% and 10% of Caucasians have nearly absent and intermediate enzyme activity, respectively [44]. Further, higher levels of TPMT activity may correlate with worse outcomes [45]. In addition, mild gastrointestinal toxicity is frequent. Rarely, hepatotoxicity and pancreatitis have been observed.

Drug Interactions

Allopurinol and MTX are inhibitors of XO. As allopurinol is a strong inhibitor, it dramatically increases the bioavailability of 6-MP [46]. With concominant use, a 75% dose reduction of 6-MP is recommended. MTX administered concomitantly with 6-MP results in clinically insignificant increase in the bioavailability of 6-MP as it is a weak inhibitor of XO [39]. 6-MP also inhibits the anticoagulant effect of warfarin [47].

Cytarabine

Mechanism of Action

From the pyrimidine analog class of antimetabolites, cytosine arabinoside, or ara-C is an arabinose nucleoside originally isolated from the sponge *Cryptothethya crypta* [48] originally demonstrating activity in children with relapsed ALL [49, 50]. It acts as an analog of deoxycytidine inhibiting DNA polymerase α and thus inhibiting DNA synthesis. However, its incorporation into DNA and the termination of chain elongation likely account for the majority of its cytotoxicity [51]. With the primary effect on DNA synthesis, ara-C is also an S-phase specific agent.

Clinical Pharmacology and Pharmacokinetics

Typically administered as an intravenous bolus or by continuous infusion, ara-C enters the cell by means of various transporters as well as by passive diffusion [52, 53]. It is activated to ara-C triphosphate in the tumor cell and ultimately inactivated via deamination in the liver, plasma, granulocytes, and gastrointestinal tract by cytidine deaminase and deoxycytidylate deaminase to ara-U. Given the presence of cytosine deaminase in the gastrointestinal mucosa, intravenous administration is preferred to the oral route. Likewise, the presence of cytosine deaminase in the plasma leads to a short half life of 7–20 min. When high doses are administered (2–3 g/m^2), a longer terminal half-life of 30–150 min is observed [54, 55]. After systemic administration, it crosses the blood-brain barrier achieving levels of 20–40% of that in the plasma.

As with MTX, ara-C can be administered by intrathecal injection as well. Very low levels of cytosine deaminase exist in the CSF. Elimination with CSF bulk flow explains the longer terminal half-life of 3.4 h [56]. A liposomal formulation of cytarabine has also been used and demonstrates a half-life 40–50 times longer than that of standard cytarabine [57, 58].

Adverse Effects

Toxicity is predominately determined by duration of exposure to ara-C, but peak levels contribute as well. Myelosuppression and gastrointestinal effects are most commonly observed and are more severe with prolonged administration. Hepatotoxicity, noncardiogenic pulmonary edema, cholestasis, pancreatitis, and neutrophilic eccrine hydradenitits, a rare febrile cutaneous reaction, can also occur [59–61]. Cerebral and cerebellar toxicity appears more common with higher doses and is also related to age and renal dysfunction [62]. It typically manifests as gait instability, dysgraphia, slurred speech, and coma and may not resolve in a significant number of patients. Intrathecal administration can be associated with a chemical arachnoiditis much like MTX, while rarely causing severe brainstem dysfunction [63].

Drug Interactions

Cytarabine has synergistic activity with a number of other agents. As it blocks DNA repair, the activity of alkylating agents is enhanced. MTX and fludarabine increase the conversion of ara-C to its active form, ara-CTP [64, 65]. Like fludarabine, the other purine anti-metabolites, 6-mercaptopurine and 6-thioguanine also enhance the cytotoxicity of ara-C [66, 67].

Anthracyclines

Mechanism of Action

Despite being discovered more than 4 decades ago, daunorubicin continues to be an important component of standard ALL regimens [68]. Other anthracyclines including doxorubicin, mitoxantrone, and idarubicin have demonstrated activity as well. Unlike the antimetabolites, their cytotoxic effects appear to be nonspecific to the cell cycle phase. The primary cytotoxic effect of anthracylines is mediated by its binding to topoisomerase II, formation of a stable drug-topoisomerase II-DNA complex leading to DNA double-strand breaks and apotoposis [66]. Other cytotoxic effects include DNA intercalation, free radical formation, and effects on cell signaling pathways have been proposed [69].

Clinical Pharmacology and Pharmacokinetics

Daunorubicin is typically administered in weekly intravenous boluses during induction, intensification, or consolidation. It enters the cell by passive diffusion, rapidly binds DNA, and is stored in several cellular compartments [70]. After bolus administration, an initial half-life ($t_{1/2\alpha}$) of 40 min is followed by a secondary half-life ($t_{1/2\beta}$) of the primary metabolite, daunorubicinol [71], of 20–50 h. This reflects the efficient cellular uptake followed by the drug's release back into the circulation and the resultant prolonged systemic exposure. As such, the cytotoxicity of anthracyclines is related to its area under the curve rather than peak drug levels. Occurring in the liver, drug activation occurs via one-electron reduction, also leading to the formation of oxygen radicals. Drug inactivation likely occurs via two-electron reduction to 7-deoxyaglycone. Anthracyclines are primarily eliminated through biliary excretion. As such, doses should be reduced in patients with moderate to severe hepatic dysfunction. Except in the case of idarubicin, only a minor component of the dose is excreted in the urine.

Adverse Effects

Myelosuppression is the most common and dose-limiting toxicity with daunorubicin. The nadir occurs at 7–10 days after administration. Mucositis is common and follows the same time course. Alopecia is common as well. Drug extravasation can cause tissue necrosis, however this effect can be neutralized by prompt tissue infiltration with dexrazoxane [70]. Cardiac toxicity can manifest acutely as arrhythmias, conduction abnormalities, or pericarditis as well as heart failure in the sub-acute setting. The one-electron reduction of anthracyclines is largely responsible for its cardiac toxicity [72]. Free-radical generation is believed to originate from the formation of anthracycline–iron complexes. When doxorubicin was preceded by dexrazoxane, an iron chelator, a diminution in anthracycline-related cardiac toxicity has been demonstrated [73, 74]. Unlike the efficacy of anthra-cyclines, cardiac toxicity appears to be related to peak drug levels leading to infusional protocols in other disease states [75]. Furthermore, heart failure is more common in patients who have preexist-ing risks for cardiac dysfunction [76–78]. The risk of cardiac toxicity likely does not exceed 5% with cumulative daunorubicin doses of 900–1000 mg/m². Finally, secondary malignancies including acute myelogenous leukemia have been reported after anthracycline exposure. The typical time course is 1–4 years after therapy, shorter than that reported for alkylator-induced leukemia and without the preceding myelodysplasia. Cytogenetic abnormalities involving the mixed lineage leu-kemia or MLL gene at the locus 11q23 are classically observed.

Drug Interactions

Few interactions with daunorubicin have been reported. However, radiation recall can occur. Most notably, cardiac toxicity can occur at lower-than-expected anthracycline doses if the patient has previously received mantle irradiation.

Vincristine

Mechanism of Action

The only antimicrotubule agent used in the routine treatment of ALL is the vinca alkaloid, vincristine. The chemical structure consists of a dihydroindole nucleus, the major alkaloid in the periwinkle plant, linked to an indole nucleus. Its cytotoxicity relates to the disruption of microtubule assembly and architecture, therefore disabling the mitotic spindle apparatus and blocking mitosis or M-Phase at the metaphase/anaphase transition [79].

Clinical Pharmacology and Pharmacokinetics

The primary determinant for the cytoxicity is the ability to achieve plasma concentration above a threshold level. Vincristine is therefore typically administered as a rapid intravenous bolus. It exhibits a wide volume of distribution and rapid cellular uptake. Large intra-patient and inter-patient variability in distribution half-life, elimination half-life, total body clearance, and volume of distribution at steady state have been demonstrated in children after repetitive dosing [80]. Reported elimination half-lives in adults have ranged from 155 to 5100 min [81]. Despite the variability, its clearance from the tissue compartment may take several days. It is widely distributed in the body, but minimal CSF penetration is achieved, with concentrations being 20–30 times lower than in plasma [82]. Vincristine is metabolized in the liver and predominately excreted in the bile and feces. Despite the absence of firm guidelines, a 50% dose reduction is usually employed for total bilirubin levels between 1.5 and 3.0 mg/dL.

Adverse Effects

Neurotoxicity is the principal toxicity of vincristine typically characterized by a peripheral symmetric mixed sensory motor and autonomic neuropathy [83]. Typically, the distal extremities are affected first and progressive symptoms are observed with continued exposure to the drug. This has led to the practice of capping the total dose at each administration to 2.0 mg. However, cumulative dose may predict for neurologic effects more predictably than peak concentrations [84]. Despite the evaluation of several agents, the only way to decrease neuropathic effects is dose reduction or drug discontinuation. Gastrointestinal toxicities, including constipation and ileus are believed to be related to autonomic nerve dysfunction. They are typically dose related and can be quite severe. Autonomic dysfunction also accounts for cardiovascular effects including hypertension and hypotension as well as genitourinary effects including incontinence and urinary retention. Myelosuppression can also be observed, predominately neutropenia. Syndrome of inappropriate antidiuretic hormone production has been reported as well.

Drug Interactions

The hepatic cytochrome P-450 3A (CYP3A) plays a role in vincristine metabolism [81]. As such, CYP3A inhibitors like intraconazole and cyclosporine can inhibit biotransformation and increase the toxicity of vincristine. Inducers, such as phenytoin and carbamazepine, may enhance clearance. L-Asparaginase may also reduce the hepatic clearance of vincristine. For this reason, the administration of the two is typically separated by 24 h.

Cyclophosphamide

Mechanism of Action

The alkylating agents are a diverse group of antitumor drugs that act through the binding of alkyl groups to DNA forming interstand cross-links leading to cell cycle arrest and apoptosis. Like anthracyclines, alkylating agents do not require that cells be in a specific phase of cycle. Cyclophosphamide is a nitrogen mustard alkylator requiring metabolic transformation to its active form

Clinical Pharmacology and Pharmacokinetics

It is unclear whether active uptake or passive diffusion is the predominant route for cellular uptake as it is not clear whether the parent compound or metabolites are the critical compounds for transport. Cyclophosphamide must undergo a complex series of activation reactions to produce alkylating compounds and degradation reactions to be eliminated. Hepatic CYP450 enzymes, in particular the 3A4 subtype, metabolize the parent compound to ultimately generate phosphoramide mustard, an active alkylator [85]. Significant variations in metabolism among patients exist due to differences in the expression of individual CYP450 enzymes [86]. While cyclophosphamide has excellent oral bioavailability [87], it is typically administered by the intravenous route given the need for higher doses in ALL. There is considerable variation in the drug's pharmacokinetics as well. Its half-life has varied between 1.1 and 16.8 h, with a clearance between 1.2 and 10.61 h [88], while the metabolites, phosphoramide mustard, nornitrogen mustard, and aldophosphamide exhibit a plasma $t_{1/2}$ ranging between 1.5 and 8.7 h [87, 89]. Based on this, cyclophosphamide was originally administered as single-dose intermittent therapy. Six 12-hourly doses, each at 3 g/m^2 has demonstrated to be highly effective when used in combination therapy [90]. Elimination is primarily through urinary excretion of inactive oxidation products. Dose reductions in patients with renal failure have been suggested based on prolonged metabolite excretion [91].

Adverse Effects

The acute toxicity of cyclophosphamide is similar to other DNA damaging agents. Myelosuppression is dose-limiting with the majority of alkylating agents with a lesser effect observed on megakaryocytes with cyclophosphamide. Other frequent effects, include nausea and vomiting, alopecia, and renal and bladder toxicity. Acrolein, a metabolite of cyclophosphamide, causes irritation of the bladder mucosa [91]. High-dose administration demonstrates prolonged delays in excretion and therefore requires 2-mercaptoethane sulfonate (MESNA) uroprotection to prevent cystitis. Fertility can be affected as well with aspermia being well demonstrated [92]. Sperm banking should be offered appropriately. Amenorrhea and ovarian failure may result from cyclophosphamide as well [93, 94]. Delayed toxicity after cyclophosphamide therapy has been described. While repeated high doses of cyclophosphamide can be given without any obvious progressive cytopenias, second malignancies can occur. Acute myelogenous leukemia after 2–10 years, preceded by myelodysplasia has been observed after alkylating agent use in malignant and nonmalignant diseases [95]. Solid tumors occur less often, but also appear directly related to alkylator use [95]. Cardiotoxicity is related to individual doses when used as part of stem cell mobilization and bone marrow transplantation [96]. It is not typically seen in patients receiving routine ALL therapy.

Drug Interactions

Given the reliance on the CVP450 enzymes for activation, potential drug interactions exist. P450 induction may increase metabolism while suppression significantly increases the half-life as demonstrated by the effects of phenobarbital and allopurinol, respectively [88, 97].

Asparaginase

Mechanism of Action

L-Asparagine is an amino acid required by malignant lymphoblasts for protein synthesis and cellular growth given their inability for its de novo synthesis. L-Asparaginase catalyzes the hydrolysis of asparagine thus depleting the circulating pools [98, 99]. Traditional asparaginase is purified from *Escherichia coli*, while a longer acting formulation, pegasparaginase is produced by the attachment of polyethylene glycol to the bacterial enzyme [100].

Clinical Pharmacology and Pharmacokinetics

Asparaginase can be administered subcutaneously, intramuscularly, or intravenously with the IV route leading to 50% higher blood levels. It is administered in doses of 6,000–10,000 IU as an intravenous bolus given at variable daily schedules. PEG-asparaginase is typically given at 2500 IU/m^2 every 1–2 weeks. The primary half-life is 30 h for asparaginase while the polyethylene glycol conjugation extends the half-life to 6 days [98, 101]. While asparaginase penetration into the CSF is poor, asparagine depletion in this sanctuary site has been demonstrated with systemic PEG-asparaginase administration [99]. Metabolic degradation of the enzyme is responsible for the drug's elimination.

Adverse Effects

Given the constitutive activity of L-asparagine synthetase in normal tissues and the ability to synthesize asparagine, toxicity is modest. Hypersensitivity reactions can develop to asparginase and can vary in severity from urticaria to anaphylaxis. As a result, pretreatment skin testing has been recommended. In addition, less immunogenicity has been demonstrated with intravenous administration. The other side effects relate to the inability of protein synthesis to occur in normal tissues.

Decreased anticoagulant or clotting factor production can initially lead to thromboses [100] or bleeding with prolonged administration [102, 103]. Hyperglycemia may result from impaired insulin production. Acute pancreatitis has been observed in a significant number of patients. The absence of myelosuppression or gastrointestinal toxicity has allowed its use in combination with other agents active in ALL. CNS toxicity including thrombosis and acute encephalopathy possibly related to elevated ammonia levels have been described [104, 105]. Caution should be used in the setting of hepatic dysfunction given the possibility of potentiating a bleeding diathesis.

Drug Interactions

As mentioned above, asparaginase antagonizes the effects of systemic MTX by preventing cell cycle progression into the S-phase. This effect has been used to partially "rescue" patients from MTX-induced toxicity [106]. No other clinically relevant drug interactions have been described.

Nelarabine, Clofarabine, and Forodesine

Mechanism of Action

Three novel purine nucleoside analogs have demonstrated promising activity in relapsed or refractory ALL. Nelarabine or 2 amino-9-β-D-arabino-6-methoxy-9H-guanine is demethoxylated to produce ara-G and subsequently converted to its corresponding arabinosylguanine nucleoside triphosphate (ara-GTP) inside the cell. It is incorporated into DNA during the S-phase, resulting in inhibition of DNA synthesis and cellular death. Clofarabine, or 2-chloro-2-fluoro-deoxy-9-β-D-arabinofuranosyladenine, is a synthetic analog of adenosine. The triphosphate form inhibits DNA polymerases thus inhibiting DNA repair and synthesis as well as ribonucleotide reductase thus depleting deoxynucleotide triphosphate pools [107]. Forodesine is a purine nucleoside phosphorylase inhibitor that results in an absence 2′-deoxyguanosine phosphorolysis, intracellular accumulation of deoxyguanosine triphosphate (dGTP), and T lymphocyte specific apoptosis [108].

Clinical Pharmacology and Pharmacokinetics

The three agents are administered by intravenous bolus for 5 consecutive days on 21–28 day cycles. After nelarabine administration at relatively low doses, cytotoxic intracellular concentrations of ara-GTP are obtained. Despite a $t_{1/2}$ of only 14 min for the parent drug, ara-G demonstrates a half-life of 3 h [109, 110]. Drug levels appear to vary widely between patients and may correlate with response [111]. Forty mg/m^2/day for 5 consecutive days has been demonstrated as the maximum tolerated dose for clofarabine [112]. Also similar to nelarabine, the triphosphate nucleotide is the active cellular cytotoxic metabolite. Despite a short and variable $t_{1/2}$, when administered at the 40 mg/m^2/day, DNA synthesis was inhibited for greater than 24 h [113]. Few pharmacologic investigations using forodesine exist. It appears to have a median $t_{1/2}$ of 11 h. While a maximum tolerated dose has not been demonstrated, increasing the dose beyond 60 mg/m^2 did not appear to increase intracellular dGTP further [114]. Despite a paucity of evidence, the major route of elimination for the three agents appears to be renal.

Adverse Effects

All three agents cause myelosuppression. This is most significant with clofarabine as 81% of patients experience febrile neutropenia [115]. However, hepatotoxicity is dose-limiting with 40% of patients experiencing transient grade 3/4 transaminase or bilirubin elevation [112, 115]. Less common effects include skin rashes, palmoplantar erythrodyesthesia, mucositis, nausea, vomiting, and headache. Neurotoxicity is the most common event reported in phase I and II studies with nelarabine and is dose-limiting [116]. Neurotoxicity in the form of peripheral neuropathy and orthostasis has been reported with forodesine. Mild gastrointestinal effects, fatigue, and headache have been reported with the three agents as well.

Drug Interactions

To date, no drug interactions have been reported with these three new agents.

Imatinib, Nilotinib, Dasatinib

Mechanism of Action

Imatinib, nilotinib, and dasatinib are all tyrosine kinase inhibitors, representative of a new generation of agents based on structural biologic investigations, targeted at inhibition of specific enzymes important in the signal transduction pathways that enhance proliferation of the malignant cells [117–120]. Imatinib, the first agent in this series to reach clinical application was developed for the treatment of chronic myelogenous leukemia (CML) to inhibit the protein tyrosine kinase activity of the Philadelphia chromosome fusion protein, bcr-abl oncogene [117, 119]. Highly selective, imatinib competes with ATP binding to the bcr-abl kinase and thereby inhibits its tyrosine kinase activity, blocking phosphorylation of downstream proteins, resulting in inhibition of proliferation and induction of apoptosis [117, 120]. Imatinib is highly successful in inducing complete and sustained remission of CML, however point mutations in the bcr-abl kinase result in development of resistance and disease progression may occur leading to blast crisis and/or bcr-abl positive ALL [121].

Bcr-abl positive ALL may occur also in the apparent absence of preceding clinical CML. Although occurrence of the bcr-abl fusion protein is sufficient to cause CML, progression to ALL is characterized by activation of other tyrosine kinase oncogenes including several src family kinases [122]. Based on structural biology principles, nilotinib was designed to bind and inhibit the bcr-abl kinase with higher affinity and more selectivity than imatinib [123, 124]. It is effective at inhibiting most mutant forms of bcr-abl that have developed resistance to imatinib. Dasatinib, which has a molecular structure that is different from that of the other two agents, was originally identified as a src kinase inhibitor [120]. It has higher affinity than imatinib for bcr-abl kinase but less selectivity [125, 126]. Thus, all three agents inhibit bcr-abl kinase and have efficacy in bcr-abl positive ALL [127–131]. Dasatinib has a theoretical advantage of inhibiting a broader spectrum of tyrosine kinases that may also be involved in bcr-abl positive ALL. Moreover, it is the only tyrosine kinase inhibitor with FDA approval for treating bcr-abl positive ALL [122].

Clinical Pharmacology and Pharmacokinetics

These three tyrosine kinase inhibitors are all well absorbed after oral administration [132–134]. Imatinib reaches peak blood levels in 2–4 h, is eliminated with a half-life of 18 h and its major metabolite, which is also biologically active, has a half-life of 40 h [132]. Nilotinib reaches peak levels in 3 h and is eliminated with a half-life of 17 h [133]. Dasatinib reaches maximum levels between 30 min and 6 h following oral administration and is eliminated with a half life of 3–5 h [134]. In accordance with these pharmacokinetics, all agents are administered orally. Imatinib and dasatinib are given orally usually as a once daily dose or split into twice daily doses whereas nilotinib is routinely given orally on a twice daily schedule [132–134]. Imatinib and nilotinib bind the P-glycoprotein associated with multidrug resistance, which may contribute to clinical resistance to these agents [135]. Conversely, their P-glycoprotein binding capacity may be useful to bind the transport protein and overcome drug resistance [136]. Dasatinib is more effective than imatinib for treatment of CNS ALL, probably associated with its better CNS penetration [137, 138]. All three agents are extensively metabolized by the CYPP450 enzyme 3A4 [132–134]. Elevated concentrations of these agents are associated with use of CYP3A4 inhibitors, whereas drug clearance increases when used in association with CYP3A4 inducers. Likewise, these tyrosine kinase inhibitors are likely to increase blood concentrations of other agents metabolized by CYP3A4.

Adverse Effects

Adverse reactions occurring with imatinib and dasatinib include edema, usually periorbital or lower limb, nausea and vomiting, muscle cramps, diarrhea, rash and other skin disorders, as well as hematologic cytopenias particularly neutropenia and thrombocytopenia [127, 128, 132, 134]. Dasatinib also causes platelet dysfunction and has been associated with bleeding, particularly epistaxsis and gastrointestinal bleeding [134]. In addition to the above adverse effects, nilotinib has been associated with prolonged cardiac ventricular repolarization as demonstrated by prolonged QT intervals on ECG and sudden death [128]. Nilotinib should not be used in patients with hypokalemia, hypomagnesium, or prolonged QT intervals [127, 133].

Drug Interactions

Dosage adjustments should be made in the presence of decreased hepatic function. Dose adjustments need also be considered when any of these three agents are used with CYP3A4 inhibitors such as ketoconazole, itraconazole, erythromycin, or clarithromycin [132–134]. Increased dosage may be necessary to maintain plasma levels when used in association with CYP3A4 inducers such as dexamethasone, phenytoin, phenobarbital, rifampicin, Saint-John's-wort, or grapefruit juice. Imatinib inhibits acetaminophen-0 glucuronidation resulting in increased exposure to acetaminophen possibly leading to severe hepatotoxicity [139]. The latter should be avoided when these tyrosine kinase inhibitors are being used. Dasatinib uptake from the gastrointestinal track is enhanced by an acidic pH. Utilization of antacids or H2 blockers/protein pump inhibitors may reduce uptake and limit exposure to the tyrosine kinase inhibitors. If antacids are needed, they should be given 2 h before or after administration of dasatinib [134].

References

1. Farber, S., et al. (1948). Temporary remissions in acute leukemia in children produced by folic acid antagonist, 4-aminopteroylglutamic acid (aminopterin). *The New England Journal of Medicine, 238*(787), 787–793.
2. Frei, E., 3rd. (1985). Curative cancer chemotherapy. *Cancer Research, 45*(12 Pt 1), 6523–6537.
3. Chabner, B. A., et al. (1984). Cancer chemotherapy. Progress and expectations. *Cancer, 54*(11 Suppl), 2599–2608.
4. Freireich, E., Karon, M., & Frei, I. E. (1964). Quadruple combination therapy (VAMP) for acute lymphocytic leukemia of childhood. *Proceedings of the American Association for Cancer Research, 5*, 20.
5. Rivera, G., et al. (1976). Recurrent childhood lymphocytic leukemia following cessation of therapy: Treatment and response. *Cancer, 37*(4), 1679–1686.
6. Evans, A. E., Gilbert, E. S., & Zandstra, R. (1970). The increasing incidence of central nervous system leukemia in children. (Children's Cancer Study Group A). *Cancer, 26*(2), 404–409.
7. Holland, J. F. (1983). Karnofsky Memorial Lecture. Breaking the cure barrier. *Journal of Clinical Oncology, 1*(2), 75–90.
8. Aur, R. J., et al. (1972). A comparative study of central nervous system irradiation and intensive chemotherapy early in remission of childhood acute lymphocytic leukemia. *Cancer, 29*(2), 381–391.
9. Gaynon, P. S., & Carrel, A. L. (1999). Glucocorticosteroid therapy in childhood acute lymphoblastic leukemia. *Advances in Experimental Medicine and Biology, 457*, 593–605.
10. Distelhorst, C. W. (2002). Recent insights into the mechanism of glucocorticosteroid-induced apoptosis. *Cell Death and Differentiation, 9*(1), 6–19.
11. Green, O. C., et al. (1978). Plasma levels, half-life values, and correlation with physiologic assays for growth and immunity. *Journal de Pediatria, 93*(2), 299–303.
12. Hill, M. R., et al. (1990). Monitoring glucocorticoid therapy: A pharmacokinetic approach. *Clinical Pharmacology and Therapeutics, 48*(4), 390–398.
13. Richter, O., et al. (1983). Pharmacokinetics of dexamethasone in children. *Pediatric Pharmacology (New York), 3*(3–4), 329–337.
14. Yang, L., et al. (2008). Asparaginase may influence dexamethasone pharmacokinetics in acute lymphoblastic leukemia. *Journal of Clinical Oncology, 26*(12), 1932–1939.
15. Leikin, S. L., et al. (1968). Varying prednisone dosage in remission induction of previously untreated childhood leukemia. *Cancer, 21*(3), 346–351.
16. Bannwarth, B., et al. (1997). Prednisolone concentrations in cerebrospinal fluid after oral prednisone. Preliminary data. *Revue du Rhumatisme. English Edition, 64*(5), 301–304.
17. Balis, F. M., et al. (1987). Differences in cerebrospinal fluid penetration of corticosteroids: Possible relationship to the prevention of meningeal leukemia. *Journal of Clinical Oncology, 5*(2), 202–207.
18. Bostrom, B. C., et al. (2003). Dexamethasone versus prednisone and daily oral versus weekly intravenous mercaptopurine for patients with standard-risk acute lymphoblastic leukemia: A report from the Children's Cancer Group. *Blood, 101*(10), 3809–3817.
19. Dale, D. C., & Petersdorf, R. G. (1973). Corticosteroids and infectious diseases. *The Medical Clinics of North America, 57*(5), 1277–1287.
20. Jugert, F. K., et al. (1994). Multiple cytochrome P450 isozymes in murine skin: Induction of P450 1A, 2B, 2E, and 3A by dexamethasone. *Journal of Investigative Dermatology, 102*(6), 970–975.
21. Chabner, B., & Longo, D. L. (2006). *Cancer chemotherapy and biotherapy* (4th ed., pp. 91–124). Philadelphia: Lippincott Williams & Wilkins.
22. Balis, F. M., Savitch, J. L., & Bleyer, W. A. (1983). Pharmacokinetics of oral methotrexate in children. *Cancer Research, 43*(5), 2342–2345.
23. Stuart, J. F., et al. (1979). Bioavailability of methotrexate: Implications for clinical use. *Cancer Chemotherapy and Pharmacology, 3*(4), 239–241.
24. Price, E. M., & Freisheim, J. H. (1987). Photoaffinity analogues of methotrexate as folate antagonist binding probes. 2. Transport studies, photoaffinity labeling, and identification of the membrane carrier protein for methotrexate from murine L1210 cells. *Biochemistry, 26*(15), 4757–4763.
25. Allegra, C. J., et al. (1987). Evidence for direct inhibition of de novo purine synthesis in human MCF-7 breast cells as a principal mode of metabolic inhibition by methotrexate. *The Journal of Biological Chemistry, 262*(28), 13520–13526.
26. Stoller, R. G., et al. (1977). Use of plasma pharmacokinetics to predict and prevent methotrexate toxicity. *The New England Journal of Medicine, 297*(12), 630–634.
27. Evans, W. E., et al. (1986). Clinical pharmacodynamics of high-dose methotrexate in acute lymphocytic leukemia. Identification of a relation between concentration and effect. *The New England Journal of Medicine, 314*(8), 471–477.

28. Von Hoff, D. D., et al. (1977). Incidence of drug-related deaths secondary to high-dose methotrexate and citrovorum factor administration. *Cancer Treatment Reports, 61*(4), 745–748.
29. Ackland, S. P., & Schilsky, R. L. (1987). High-dose methotrexate: A critical reappraisal. *Journal of Clinical Oncology, 5*(12), 2017–2031.
30. Blaney, S. M., Balis, F. M., & Poplack, D. G. (1991). Current pharmacological treatment approaches to central nervous system leukaemia. *Drugs, 41*(5), 702–716.
31. Susan, M. W., et al. (1996). Effective clearance of methotrexate using high-flux hemodialysis membranes. *American Journal of Kidney Diseases: The Official Journal of the National Kidney Foundation, 28*(6), 846–854.
32. Widemann, B. C., et al. (1997). Carboxypeptidase-G2, thymidine, and leucovorin rescue in cancer patients with methotrexate-induced renal dysfunction. *Journal of Clinical Oncology, 15*(5), 2125–2134.
33. Buchen, S., et al. (2005). Carboxypeptidase G2 rescue in patients with methotrexate intoxication and renal failure. *British Journal of Cancer, 92*(3), 480–487.
34. Dalle, J. H., et al. (2002). Interaction between methotrexate and ciprofloxacin. *Journal of Pediatric Hematology/ Oncology, 24*(4), 321–322.
35. Iven, H., & Brasch, H. (1988). The effects of antibiotics and uricosuric drugs on the renal elimination of methotrexate and 7-hydroxymethotrexate in rabbits. *Cancer Chemotherapy and Pharmacology, 21*(4), 337–342.
36. Iven, H., & Brasch, H. (1990). Cephalosporins increase the renal clearance of methotrexate and 7-hydroxymethotrexate in rabbits. *Cancer Chemotherapy and Pharmacology, 26*(2), 139–143.
37. Thyss, A., et al. (1986). Clinical and pharmacokinetic evidence of a life-threatening interaction between methotrexate and ketoprofen. *Lancet, 1*(8475), 256–258.
38. Chabner, B., & Longo, D. L. (2006). *Cancer chemotherapy and biotherapy* (4th ed., pp. 212–228). Philadelphia: Lippincott Williams & Wilkins.
39. Balis, F. M., et al. (1987). The effect of methotrexate on the bioavailability of oral 6-mercaptopurine. *Clinical Pharmacology and Therapeutics, 41*(4), 384–387.
40. LePage, G. A., & Whitecar, J. P., Jr. (1971). Pharmacology of 6-thioguanine in man. *Cancer Research, 31*(11), 1627–1631.
41. Koren, G., et al. (1990). Systemic exposure to mercaptopurine as a prognostic factor in acute lymphocytic leukemia in children. *The New England Journal of Medicine, 323*(1), 17–21.
42. Lennard, L., & Lilleyman, J. S. (1989). Variable mercaptopurine metabolism and treatment outcome in childhood lymphoblastic leukemia. *Journal of Clinical Oncology, 7*(12), 1816–1823.
43. Chan, G. L., et al. (1990). Azathioprine metabolism: Pharmacokinetics of 6-mercaptopurine, 6-thiouric acid and 6-thioguanine nucleotides in renal transplant patients. *Journal of Clinical Pharmacology, 30*(4), 358–363.
44. Lennard, L., Van Loon, J. A., & Weinshilboum, R. M. (1989). Pharmacogenetics of acute azathioprine toxicity: Relationship to thiopurine methyltransferase genetic polymorphism. *Clinical Pharmacology and Therapeutics, 46*(2), 149–154.
45. Lennard, L., et al. (1990). Genetic variation in response to 6-mercaptopurine for childhood acute lymphoblastic leukaemia. *Lancet, 336*(8709), 225–229.
46. Zimm, S., et al. (1983). Inhibition of first-pass metabolism in cancer chemotherapy: Interaction of 6-mercaptopurine and allopurinol. *Clinical Pharmacology and Therapeutics, 34*(6), 810–817.
47. Singleton, J. D., & Conyers, L. (1992). Warfarin and azathioprine: An important drug interaction. *The American Journal of Medicine, 92*(2), 217.
48. Roberts, W. K., & Dekker, C. A. (1967). A convenient synthesis of arabinosylcytosine (cytosine arabinoside). *The Journal of Organic Chemistry, 32*(3), 816–817.
49. Howard, J. P., Albo, V., & Newton, W. A., Jr. (1968). Cytosine arabinoside. Results of a cooperative study in acute childhood leukemia. *Cancer, 21*(3), 341–345.
50. Ellison, R. R., et al. (1968). Arabinosyl cytosine: A useful agent in the treatment of acute leukemia in adults. *Blood, 32*(4), 507–523.
51. Kufe, D. W., et al. (1980). Correlation of cytotoxicity with incorporation of ara-C into DNA. *The Journal of Biological Chemistry, 255*(19), 8997–9000.
52. Jamieson, G. P., Snook, M. B., & Wiley, J. S. (1990). Saturation of intracellular cytosine arabinoside triphosphate accumulation in human leukemic blast cells. *Leukemia Research, 14*(5), 475–479.
53. Wiley, J. S., et al. (1982). Cytosine arabinoside influx and nucleoside transport sites in acute leukemia. *Journal of Clinical Investigation, 69*(2), 479–489.
54. Slevin, M. L., et al. (1983). Effect of dose and schedule on pharmacokinetics of high-dose cytosine arabinoside in plasma and cerebrospinal fluid. *Journal of Clinical Oncology, 1*(9), 546–551.
55. Breithaupt, H., et al. (1982). Clinical results and pharmacokinetics of high-dose cytosine arabinoside (HD ARA-C). *Cancer, 50*(7), 1248–1257.
56. Ho, D. H., & Frei, E., III. (1971). Clinical pharmacology of 1-beta-D-arabinofuranosyl cytosine. *Clinical Pharmacology and Therapeutics, 12*(6), 944–954.

57. Chamberlain, M. C., et al. (1995). Pharmacokinetics of intralumbar DTC-101 for the treatment of leptomeningeal metastases. *Archives of Neurology, 52*(9), 912–917.
58. Kim, S., et al. (1993). Extended CSF cytarabine exposure following intrathecal administration of DTC 101. *Journal of Clinical Oncology, 11*(11), 2186–2193.
59. Andersson, B. S., et al. (1990). Fatal pulmonary failure complicating high-dose cytosine arabinoside therapy in acute leukemia. *Cancer, 65*(5), 1079–1084.
60. George, C. B., et al. (1984). Hepatic dysfunction and jaundice following high-dose cytosine arabinoside. *Cancer, 54*(11), 2360–2362.
61. Flynn, T. C., et al. (1984). Neutrophilic eccrine hidradenitis: A distinctive rash associated with cytarabine therapy and acute leukemia. *Journal of the American Academy of Dermatology, 11*(4 Pt 1), 584–590.
62. Rubin, E. H., et al. (1992). Risk factors for high-dose cytarabine neurotoxicity: An analysis of a cancer and leukemia group B trial in patients with acute myeloid leukemia. *Journal of Clinical Oncology, 10*(6), 948–953.
63. Kleinschmidt-DeMasters, B. K., & Yeh, M. (1992). "Locked-in syndrome" after intrathecal cytosine arabinoside therapy for malignant immunoblastic lymphoma. *Cancer, 70*(10), 2504–2507.
64. Gandhi, V., et al. (1997). Minimum dose of fludarabine for the maximal modulation of 1-beta-D-arabinofurano-sylcytosine triphosphate in human leukemia blasts during therapy. *Clinical Cancer Research, 3*(9), 1539–1545.
65. Cadman, E., & Eiferman, F. (1979). Mechanism of synergistic cell killing when methotrexate precedes cytosine arabinoside: Study of L1210 and human leukemic cells. *Journal of Clinical Investigation, 64*(3), 788–797.
66. Fu, C. H., et al. (2001). Reversal of cytosine arabinoside (ara-C) resistance by the synergistic combination of 6-thioguanine plus ara-C plus PEG-asparaginase (TGAP) in human leukemia lines lacking or expressing p53 protein. *Cancer Chemotherapy and Pharmacology, 48*(2), 123–133.
67. Nandy, P., Periclou, A. P., & Avramis, V. I. (1998). The synergism of 6-mercaptopurine plus cytosine arabinoside followed by PEG-asparaginase in human leukemia cell lines (CCRF/CEM/0 and (CCRF/CEM/ara-C/7A) is due to increased cellular apoptosis. *Anticancer Research, 18*(2A), 727–737.
68. Dimarco, A., et al. (1964). Daunomycin: A new antibiotic with antitumor activity. *Cancer Chemotherapy Reports, 38*, 31–38.
69. Estlin, E. J., et al. (2000). The clinical and cellular pharmacology of vincristine, corticosteroids, L-asparaginase, anthracyclines and cyclophosphamide in relation to childhood acute lymphoblastic leukaemia. *British Journal Haematology, 110*(4), 780–790.
70. Johnson, B. A., Cheang, M. S., & Goldenberg, G. J. (1986). Comparison of adriamycin uptake in chick embryo heart and liver cells an murine L5178Y lymphoblasts in vitro: Role of drug uptake in cardiotoxicity. *Cancer Research, 46*(1), 218–223.
71. Huffman, D. H., & Bachur, N. R. (1972). Daunorubicin metabolism in acute myelocytic leukemia. *Blood, 39*(5), 637–643.
72. Doroshow, J. H., Locker, G. Y., & Myers, C. E. (1980). Enzymatic defenses of the mouse heart against reactive oxygen metabolites: Alterations produced by doxorubicin. *Journal of Clinical Investigation, 65*(1), 128–135.
73. Swain, S. M., et al. (1997). Cardioprotection with dexrazoxane for doxorubicin-containing therapy in advanced breast cancer. *Journal of Clinical Oncology, 15*(4), 1318–1332.
74. Speyer, J. L., et al. (1988). Protective effect of the bispiperazinedione ICRF-187 against doxorubicin-induced cardiac toxicity in women with advanced breast cancer. *The New England Journal of Medicine, 319*(12), 745–752.
75. Legha, S. S., et al. (1982). Reduction of doxorubicin cardiotoxicity by prolonged continuous intravenous infusion. *Annals of Internal Medicine, 96*(2), 133–139.
76. Lipshultz, S. E., et al. (1991). Late cardiac effects of doxorubicin therapy for acute lymphoblastic leukemia in childhood. *The New England Journal of Medicine, 324*(12), 808–815.
77. Alexander, J., et al. (1979). Serial assessment of doxorubicin cardiotoxicity with quantitative radionuclide angio-cardiography. *The New England Journal of Medicine, 300*(6), 278–283.
78. Von Hoff, D. D., et al. (1977). Daunomycin-induced cardiotoxicity in children and adults. A review of 110 cases. *The American Journal of Medicine, 62*(2), 200–208.
79. Rowinsky, E. K. (2006). Antimicrotubule Agents. In B. A. Chabner & D. L. Longo (Eds.), *Cancer chemotherapy and biotherapy: Principles and practice* (4th ed., pp. 237–282). Philadelphia: Lippincott Williams & Wilkins.
80. Gidding, C. E., et al. (1999). Vincristine pharmacokinetics after repetitive dosing in children. *Cancer Chemotherapy and Pharmacology, 44*(3), 203–209.
81. Gidding, C. E., et al. (1999). Vincristine revisited. *Critical Reviews in Oncology/Hematology, 29*(3), 267–287.
82. Jackson, D. V., Jr., et al. (1981). Pharmacokinetics of vincristine infusion. *Cancer Treatment Reports, 65*(11–12), 1043–1048.
83. Quasthoff, S., & Hartung, H. P. (2002). Chemotherapy-induced peripheral neuropathy. *Journal of Neurology, 249*(1), 9–17.
84. Peltier, A. C., & Russell, J. W. (2002). Recent advances in drug-induced neuropathies. *Current Opinion in Neurology, 15*(5), 633–638.

85. Colvin, M., Padgett, C. A., & Fenselau, C. (1973). A biologically active metabolite of cyclophosphamide. *Cancer Research, 33*(4), 915–918.
86. Yule, S. M., et al. (1995). Cyclophosphamide metabolism in children. *Cancer Research, 55*(4), 803–809.
87. Struck, R. F., et al. (1987). Plasma pharmacokinetics of cyclophosphamide and its cytotoxic metabolites after intravenous versus oral administration in a randomized, crossover trial. *Cancer Research, 47*(10), 2723–2726.
88. Yule, S. M., et al. (1996). Cyclophosphamide pharmacokinetics in children. *British Journal of Clinical Pharmacology, 41*(1), 13–19.
89. Tew, K. D., Colvin, O. M., & Jones, R. B. (2006). Clinical and high-dose alkylating agents. In B. A. Chabner & D. L. Longo (Eds.), *Cancer chemotherapy and biotherapy: Principles and practice* (4th ed., pp. 283–309). Philadelphia: Lippincott Williams & Wilkins.
90. Murphy, S. B., et al. (1986). Results of treatment of advanced-stage Burkitt's lymphoma and B cell (SIg+) acute lymphoblastic leukemia with high-dose fractionated cyclophosphamide and coordinated high-dose methotrexate and cytarabine. *Journal of Clinical Oncology, 4*(12), 1732–1739.
91. Mouridsen, H. T., & Jacobsen, E. (1975). Pharmacokinetics of cyclophosphamide in renal failure. *Acta Pharmacologica et Toxicologica, 36*(Suppl 5), 409–414.
92. Miller, D. G. (1971). Alkylating agents and human spermatogenesis. *Journal of the American Medical Association, 217*(12), 1662–1665.
93. Kumar, R., et al. (1972). Cyclophosphamide and reproductive function. *Lancet, 1*(7762), 1212–1214.
94. Miller, J. J., 3rd, Williams, G. F., and Leissring, J. C. (1971). Multiple late complications of therapy with cyclophosphamide, including ovarian destruction. *The American Journal of Medicine, 50*(4), 530–535.
95. Tucker, M. A., et al. (1988). Risk of second cancers after treatment for Hodgkin's disease. *The New England Journal of Medicine, 318*(2), 76–81.
96. Goldberg, M. A., et al. (1986). Cyclophosphamide cardiotoxicity: An analysis of dosing as a risk factor. *Blood, 68*(5), 1114–1118.
97. Jao, J. Y., Jusko, W. J., & Cohen, J. L. (1972). Phenobarbital effects on cyclophosphamide pharmacokinetics in man. *Cancer Research, 32*(12), 2761–2764.
98. Ho, D. H., et al. (1986). Clinical pharmacology of polyethylene glycol-L-asparaginase. *Drug Metabolism and Disposition, 14*(3), 349–352.
99. Hawkins, D. S., et al. (2004). Asparaginase pharmacokinetics after intensive polyethylene glycol-conjugated L-asparaginase therapy for children with relapsed acute lymphoblastic leukemia. *Clinical Cancer Research, 10*(16), 5335–5341.
100. Semeraro, N., et al. (1990). Unbalanced coagulation-fibrinolysis potential during L-asparaginase therapy in children with acute lymphoblastic leukaemia. *Thrombosis and Haemostasis, 64*(1), 38–40.
101. Asselin, B. L., et al. (1993). Comparative pharmacokinetic studies of three asparaginase preparations. *Journal of Clinical Oncology, 11*(9), 1780–1786.
102. Ramsay, N. K., et al. (1977). The effect of L-asparaginase of plasma coagulation factors in acute lymphoblastic leukemia. *Cancer, 40*(4), 1398–1401.
103. Gralnick, H. R., & Henderson, E. (1971). Hypofibrinogenemia and coagulation factor deficiencies with L-asparaginase treatment. *Cancer, 27*(6), 1313–1320.
104. Bushara, K. O., & Rust, R. S. (1997). Reversible MRI lesions due to pegaspargase treatment of non-Hodgkin's lymphoma. *Pediatric Neurology, 17*(2), 185–187.
105. Leonard, J. V., & Kay, J. D. (1986). Acute encephalopathy and hyperammonaemia complicating treatment of acute lymphoblastic leukaemia with asparaginase. *Lancet, 1*(8473), 162–163.
106. Harris, R. E., et al. (1980). Methotrexate/L-asparaginase combination chemotherapy for patients with acute leukemia in relapse: A study of 36 children. *Cancer, 46*(9), 2004–2008.
107. Xie, K. C., & Plunkett, W. (1996). Deoxynucleotide pool depletion and sustained inhibition of ribonucleotide reductase and DNA synthesis after treatment of human lymphoblastoid cells with 2-chloro-9-(2-deoxy-2-fluoro-beta-D-arabinofuranosyl) adenine. *Cancer Research, 56*(13), 3030–3037.
108. Bantia, S., et al. (2001). Purine nucleoside phosphorylase inhibitor BCX-1777 (Immucillin-H)–a novel potent and orally active immunosuppressive agent. *International Immunopharmacology, 1*(6), 1199–1210.
109. Kisor, D. F., et al. (2000). Pharmacokinetics of nelarabine and 9-beta-D-arabinofuranosyl guanine in pediatric and adult patients during a phase I study of nelarabine for the treatment of refractory hematologic malignancies. *Journal of Clinical Oncology, 18*(5), 995–1003.
110. Gandhi, V., et al. (1998). Compound GW506U78 in refractory hematologic malignancies: Relationship between cellular pharmacokinetics and clinical response. *Journal of Clinical Oncology, 16*(11), 3607–3615.
111. Kisor, D. F. (2005). Nelarabine: A nucleoside analog with efficacy in T-cell and other leukemias. *The Annals of Pharmacotherapy, 39*(6), 1056–1063.
112. Kantarjian, H. M., et al. (2003). Phase I clinical and pharmacology study of clofarabine in patients with solid and hematologic cancers. *Journal of Clinical Oncology, 21*(6), 1167–1173.

113. Gandhi, V., et al. (2003). Pharmacokinetics and pharmacodynamics of plasma clofarabine and cellular clofarabine triphosphate in patients with acute leukemias. *Clinical Cancer Research, 9*(17), 6335–6342.
114. Gandhi, V., et al. (2005). A proof-of-principle pharmacokinetic, pharmacodynamic, and clinical study with purine nucleoside phosphorylase inhibitor immucillin-H (BCX-1777, forodesine). *Blood, 106*(13), 4253–4260.
115. Kantarjian, H., et al. (2003). Phase 2 clinical and pharmacologic study of clofarabine in patients with refractory or relapsed acute leukemia. *Blood, 102*(7), 2379–2386.
116. Larson, R. A. (2007). Three new drugs for acute lymphoblastic leukemia: Nelarabine, clofarabine, and forodesine. *Seminars in Oncology, 34*(6 Suppl 5), S13–S20.
117. Schiffer, C. A. (2007). BCR-ABL tyrosine kinase inhibitors for chronic myelogenous leukemia. *The New England Journal of Medicine, 357*(3), 258–265.
118. O'Hare, T., et al. (2005). In vitro activity of Bcr-Abl inhibitors AMN107 and BMS-354825 against clinically relevant imatinib-resistant Abl kinase domain mutants. *Cancer Research, 65*(11), 4500–4505.
119. Druker, B. J., et al. (2001). Efficacy and safety of a specific inhibitor of the BCR-ABL tyrosine kinase in chronic myeloid leukemia. *The New England Journal of Medicine, 344*(14), 1031–1037.
120. Druker, B. J., et al. (1996). Effects of a selective inhibitor of the Abl tyrosine kinase on the growth of Bcr-Abl positive cells. *Natural Medicines, 2*(5), 561–566.
121. Druker, B. J. (2006). Circumventing resistance to kinase-inhibitor therapy. *The New England Journal of Medicine, 354*(24), 2594–2596.
122. Hu, Y., et al. (2006). Targeting multiple kinase pathways in leukemic progenitors and stem cells is essential for improved treatment of Ph+ leukemia in mice. *Proceedings of the National Academy of Sciences of the United States of America, 103*(45), 16870–16875.
123. Deininger, M. W. (2008). Nilotinib. *Clinical Cancer Research, 14*(13), 4027–4031.
124. Golemovic, M., et al. (2005). AMN107, a novel aminopyrimidine inhibitor of Bcr-Abl, has in vitro activity against imatinib-resistant chronic myeloid leukemia. *Clinical Cancer Research, 11*(13), 4941–4947.
125. Keam, S. J. (2008). Dasatinib: In chronic myeloid leukemia and Philadelphia chromosome-positive acute lymphoblastic leukemia. *BioDrugs, 22*(1), 59–69.
126. Steinberg, M. (2007). Dasatinib: A tyrosine kinase inhibitor for the treatment of chronic myelogenous leukemia and philadelphia chromosome-positive acute lymphoblastic leukemia. *Clinical Therapeutics, 29*(11), 2289–2308.
127. Hazarika, M., et al. (2008). Tasigna for chronic and accelerated phase Philadelphia chromosome–positive chronic myelogenous leukemia resistant to or intolerant of imatinib. *Clinical Cancer Research, 14*(17), 5325–5331.
128. Brave, M., et al. (2008). Sprycel for chronic myeloid leukemia and Philadelphia chromosome-positive acute lymphoblastic leukemia resistant to or intolerant of imatinib mesylate. *Clinical Cancer Research, 14*(2), 352–359.
129. Talpaz, M., et al. (2006). Dasatinib in imatinib-resistant Philadelphia chromosome-positive leukemias. *The New England Journal of Medicine, 354*(24), 2531–2541.
130. Kantarjian, H., et al. (2006). Nilotinib in imatinib-resistant CML and Philadelphia chromosome-positive ALL. *The New England Journal of Medicine, 354*(24), 2542–2551.
131. Kantarjian, H. M., et al. (2002). Imatinib mesylate (STI571) therapy for Philadelphia chromosome-positive chronic myelogenous leukemia in blast phase. *Blood, 99*(10), 3547–3553.
132. Prescribing Information. Gleevec (imatinib mesylate). Novartis Pharmaceuticals Corporation [cited; Available from: www.FDA.gov/cder/foi].
133. Prescribing Information. Tasigna (nilotinib). Novartis Pharmaceuticals Corporation [cited; Available from: www.fda.gov/cder/foi].
134. Prescribing Information: Sprycell (Dasatinib). Micromedix [cited; Available from: www.fda/gov/cder/foi/label/2006/021986LbL.pdr].
135. Brendel, C., et al. (2007). Imatinib mesylate and nilotinib (AMN107) exhibit high-affinity interaction with ABCG2 on primitive hematopoietic stem cells. *Leukemia, 21*(6), 1267–1275.
136. Hamada, A., et al. (2003). Interaction of imatinib mesilate with human P-glycoprotein. *The Journal of Pharmacology and Experimental Therapeutics, 307*(2), 824–828.
137. Porkka, K., et al. (2008). Dasatinib crosses the blood-brain barrier and is an efficient therapy for central nervous system Philadelphia chromosome-positive leukemia. *Blood, 112*(4), 1005–1012.
138. Bujassoum, S., Rifkind, J., & Lipton, J. H. (2004). Isolated central nervous system relapse in lymphoid blast crisis chronic myeloid leukemia and acute lymphoblastic leukemia in patients on imatinib therapy. *Leukaemia & Lymphoma, 45*(2), 401–403.
139. Ridruejo, E., et al. (2007). Imatinib-induced fatal acute liver failure. *World Journal of Gastroenterology, 13*(48), 6608–6611.

Chapter 11
Assessment of Response to Treatment

Christopher P. Fox and A.K. McMillan

Introduction

Modest but significant improvements in the outcome of adults with acute lymphoblastic leukemia (ALL) have been achieved over the past 3 decades, exemplified by the outcomes of consecutive cohorts of patients treated in UK Medical Research Council trials (MRCUKALL Xa and MRCUKALL XII/ECOG2993) [1, 2]. This has been achieved largely through the development and intensification of multiagent, multi-cycle chemotherapy protocols, with concomitant improvements in supportive care. However, in spite of this progress and the achievement of complete hematologic remission (CHR) in 80–90% of cases, approximately two-thirds of adults younger than 60 years and greater than 90% of those over 60 years remain destined to die of their disease [3]. A plateau in survival has been observed as the further anticipated benefits of more intensive regimens and allogeneic stem cell transplantation (SCT) are frequently, at least in part, offset by a greater treatment-related mortality. At relapse, only a minority of patients respond to salvage therapy and achieve long-term survival [2, 4]. Of particular note is that up to 50% of "standard risk" patients treated with standard chemotherapy protocols will experience relapse [5]. There is therefore an urgent need to rationally tailor first-line therapy on an individual basis according the perceived relapse risk. It is now clear that response assessment is of central importance to this aspiration.

Traditional models of risk stratification have been predominantly based upon clinical and laboratory data collected at diagnosis [6, 7] which can lack prognostic precision for individual patients. More recent clinical studies have attempted to further refine risk stratification by analyzing diagnostic immunophenotypic, cytogenetic and molecular data to better identify those patients at highest risk of relapse. Many of these risk-assessment variables are proximate, surrogate markers for underlying biological factors of the patient, the leukemic cell and its microenvironment. The importance of many of these factors is dependent on the schedule of therapy delivered and consequently prognostic impact may be lost as therapies are further optimized, emphasizing the importance of a more dynamic approach to risk assessment. Intuitively, an individual's response to therapy (however assessed) has prognostic value as it directly reflects the inherent sensitivity of the leukemic blasts to therapy. In principle, this provides an opportunity to apply risk-adapted therapeutic protocols, including early intensification of anti-leukemic therapy for individuals deemed to be at highest risk of relapse [8]. Increasingly sensitive techniques to assess response to therapy have become widely available and detailed studies of these factors in both pediatric and adult trials has established their

C.P. Fox (✉)
University of Birmingham, Birmingham, UK
e-mail: C.P.Fox@bham.ac.uk

A.S. Advani and H.M. Lazarus (eds.), *Adult Acute Lymphocytic Leukemia*, Contemporary Hematology, 145
DOI 10.1007/978-1-60761-707-5_11, © Springer Science+Business Media, LLC 2011

significance in providing the clinician with powerful prognostic data [5, 9–16]. There remains, however, some uncertainty as to how this response data should be interpreted and applied to an individual with ALL. To date, differences in treatment protocols, trial design, methodology, and sensitivity of techniques for response assessment have somewhat restricted the widespread application of this important data for risk-adapted therapy in adult ALL.

The utility of the available approaches for assessing response to treatment will be examined.

Clinical Response Assessment

This approach undoubtedly has its limitations, particularly in the era of highly sensitive molecular techniques, but nonetheless remains a valuable tool for response assessment at the bedside in the early days of therapy. It is noteworthy to observe that clinical evidence of lymphadenopathy, hepatomegaly or splenomegaly is reported at diagnosis in 30–60% of adult patients with ALL (CALGB, MRC, GIMEMA, GMALL trials). Prompt clinical responses are anticipated with modern treatment protocols and can be reassuring for both the clinician and patient in the early days of induction therapy, particularly for those individuals with no immediately measurable laboratory parameter; for example, those with a low peripheral-blood blast count at presentation. Extramedullary disease may also provide an early clinical opportunity to assess response, for example, skin, liver, or testes involvement. Although unusual (<10% of relapsed cases [2]), the occurrence of isolated extramedullary relapse (during or after therapy) is well recognized and, importantly, is often accompanied by "negative" minimal residual disease (MRD) status in the bone marrow [14, 17]

Hematologic/Morphologic

The observation that initial response to therapy was a key determinant of outcome in ALL has been recognized for over 30 years. The prognostic power of response to induction chemotherapy was initially observed in pediatric studies [18–20] and subsequently in adult ALL [6, 21, 22]. An early multicentre study in Germany reported a 3-year relapse-free survival of 49 months for those patients who achieved morphologic complete remission (CR) by 4 weeks of induction therapy, significantly superior to a median survival of 29 months experienced by late remitters [22].

These findings were supported by a US study [23] that employed a similar induction regimen but with higher doses of anthracycline and demonstrated that of the small number of patients in whom CR was achieved after 4 weeks, none remained alive and disease-free at 5 years. A larger study from the CALGB [24], however, was unable to corroborate these findings. This group used a five drug induction regimen including cyclophosphamide, asparaginase and anthracycline, and reported a lower CR rate at 30 days (74%); but no statistically significant difference in remission duration or survival when comparing "early remitters" (<30 days) with "late remitters" (>30 days). These apparently disconcordant observations exemplify that response data must be interpreted in the context of the treatment protocol delivered. This is a key consideration when correlating MRD data with response and survival.

The clinical importance of the kinetics of leukemic blast clearance was further explored by evaluation at earlier time points during induction therapy. It became clear that rapidity of response in the early days of induction was a crucial predictor of outcome, in both pediatric [25, 26] and adult ALL studies [27] whereupon an excess of BM blasts on day 15 (>5%) was associated with a significantly worse overall and disease-free survival ($p < 0.0001$ and 0.02, respectively).

Persistent disease at 7 days is thought to represent primary resistance to corticosteroids [28], now understood to be associated with increased expression of the anti-apoptotic gene *MCL1* [29]. In adult ALL, blast clearance from the peripheral blood following 1 week of prednisolone monotherapy, prior to standard induction therapy, was highly predictive of achievement of CR at 39 days, remission duration, and overall survival [30]. Although the day 8 response to prednisolone is a robust and well-established parameter for risk assessment, it is only able to identify a limited number of patients at high risk of relapse, and does provide information about the relative reduction in leukemic burden for an individual. The molecular and genetic determinants of blast susceptibility to treatment are now beginning to be unraveled. A recent study analyzed gene expression of lymphoblasts and correlated this with reduction of circulating leukemia cells after treatment and long-term disease-free survival. Response to therapy was significantly associated with genes involved in proliferation, apoptosis, and DNA repair [31]. Further detailed studies of gene expression and levels of MRD have identified several key genes that are commonly associated with treatment response and drug resistance [32].

Central Nervous System Involvement

Many protocols do not mandate that a lumbar puncture (LP) is performed at diagnosis unless clinically indicated, but this assessment is often undertaken early in induction therapy. Central nervous system (CNS) involvement with ALL occurred in 5% of the 1,508 patients studied in the MRC UKALL XII/ECOG E2993 trial [33], of whom 21 (27%) did not have clinical manifestations but were subsequently diagnosed with the first scheduled LP. In this study, if CNS leukemia was detected, intrathecal therapy was undertaken thrice weekly until blasts were cleared from the spinal fluid. Response assessment of CNS leukemia following therapy is routinely performed by morphological evaluation of cerebrospinal fluid (CSF) cytospin preparations. However, it is now recognized that morphological assessment alone can fail to demonstrate lymphoblasts in a significant proportion of patients in whom meningeal involvement is present [34–36]. Small studies have shown the value of increased sensitivity (to 1% of total CSF cells) of detection of leukemic cells in CSF at diagnosis, by both multi-color flow cytometry and IgH PCR [37–39]. Isolated relapse within the central nervous system occurs in approximately 4% of adults with ALL [2]; but in practice this will rarely be detected during follow-up in the absence of clinical manifestations. In principle, detection of MRD in the CSF by sensitive techniques would allow augmentation of CNS-directed therapy in an attempt to further reduce the CNS relapse risk. Employing these techniques to enhance the sensitivity of detecting CNS leukemia following treatment is not yet routine and would require prospective validation of their clinical utility and impact on outcome before being incorporated into standard protocols [40].

In the context of response assessment of CNS disease, it is important to note data derived from large pediatric studies, demonstrating that those patients who experience a traumatic lumbar puncture (≥10 erythrocytes/μL) with blasts in the CSF at diagnosis, have an inferior disease-free survival compared to those having an atraumatic procedure [41–43]. Identification of these patients allows intensification of therapy to reduce the risk of CNS relapse and may overcome the adverse effect on outcome [44]. It is not entirely clear why such patients have an inferior outcome, but this may be explained by the introduction of blasts into the CNS from the circulating blood and/or relate to impaired distribution of intrathecal chemotherapy through the CNS due to hematoma formation. There are currently no data available to corroborate this association in adults with ALL, but, nonetheless, it remains an important observation and may warrant intensification of therapy for those at risk [45].

Minimal Residual Disease

Chapter 4 (refer to the MRD chapter) has addressed the molecular basis and methodological details underpinning MRD monitoring. We shall now focus on the available clinical data and its utility for clinical decision-making.

Definitions of Response

Traditionally, CR has been defined by less than 5% (i.e., a $10^{-1.3}$ reduction) blast cells in a regenerating BM aspirate, with peripheral blood neutrophil and platelet counts of greater than $1.5 \times 10^9/L$ and $100 \times 10^9/L$, respectively. This definition is far from stringent and its origins may be, at least in part, explained by the difficulties encountered when attempting to distinguish lymphoblasts from regenerating hematopoietic precursors by morphologic criteria alone. Its limitations are further emphasized when it is considered that at diagnosis the leukemic burden for an individual is in the order of 10^{12} blasts and thus at time of morphological remission, there may still be as many as 10^{10} residual leukemic cells present [46]. Traditionally, such patients have been treated on identical protocols to those achieving more significant log reductions in the leukemic burden [1, 7, 8, 25, 31].

In practical terms, MRD can be defined as the lowest level of disease detectable in patients deemed to be in complete morphological remission, by the most sensitive methods available at the time of assessment. The evolution of molecular genetics techniques has allowed increasingly sensitive detection of malignant clones. Applying standard cytogenetic methodology approximately 80% of adults with ALL are found to have an abnormal cytogenetic clone at baseline [7], the identification of which can play a key role in diagnosis, initial risk stratification and prognostication. (refer to the Chap. 5). Although fluorescence in situ hybridization (FISH) can provide superior sensitivity and specificity to conventional metaphase banding for the detection of chromosomal translocations, both methodologies lack the sensitivity required to serve as meaningful MRD techniques.

Improved understanding of the unique molecular characteristics of leukemic blasts has resulted in the ability to detect MRD in the vast majority of patients. This is most commonly achieved either by multi-color flow cytometry to detect a leukemia-associated phenotype, or by amplifying transcripts using polymerase chain reaction (PCR) to detect rearrangements of antigen-receptor genes. Both methods provide a level of sensitivity at least 100-fold greater than that of morphological assessment alone. The benefits afforded by such sensitive applications are clear but clinicians should also be aware of the potential disadvantages (Table 11.1). Of note is the potential for false-positive results with PCR due to its inherent ability to amplify nanogram quantities of contaminating DNA. Alternatively, the positive PCR signal may be amplified from irreversibly damaged or dying cells or from leukemic progenitors without proliferative capacity. Although less sensitive and less widely standardized than PCR, flow cytometry is more rapid, generally less expensive and provides informative results in a higher percentage of patients than molecular methods. In common with PCR assessment, flow cytometry can also be limited by clonal evolution of the leukemic blast.

Table 11.1 Comparison of available methods for response assessment

Method	Sensitivity	Advantages	Disadvantages
Clinical	Low (subjective/ qualitative)	Early reassurance for patient	Crude
			Limited role
Hematological/ morphological	$10^{-1} \rightarrow 10^{-2}$	Rapid, inexpensive	Insensitive
			Inter-observer variation
Cytogenetics (metaphase banding/ FISH)	10^{-2}	Allows follow-up and relative quantitation of leukemic clone	Insufficient sensitivity
			May detect irrelevant clone
Flow cytometry	$10^{-4} \rightarrow 10^{-5}$	Rapid	Labor-intensive
		Quantitative	Phenotypic/clonal
		Reproducible	evolution
RT-PCR	10^{-4} (quantitative)	Highly sensitive	False positives
	$10^{-5} \rightarrow 10^{-6}$ (qualitative)	Quantitative	Requires synthesis of patient-specific primers
			Ongoing target gene mutations (e.g., IgH)

Role of Imatinib Post Allogeneic Stem Cell Transplantation

Radich et al. [33, 74] previously demonstrated that persistent PCR-positivity for *BCR-ABL* transcripts after allogeneic SCT was associated with an increased risk of disease recurrence. Postallogeneic SCT maintenance strategies have therefore been explored. Wassmann et al. [75] investigated the use of single agent imatinib in the posttransplant setting after detection of *BCR-ABL* transcripts by PCR. Standard dose imatinib (400 mg with dose escalation to 600 or 800 mg if persistence of disease) resulted in eradication of molecular disease in 52% of the 27 patients treated. Notably, failure to achieve molecular CR within the first 6 weeks of therapy heralded overt leukemia relapse despite additional manipulations (e.g., donor lymphocyte infusions); 12 of 13 (92%) patients relapsed within a median of 3 months. The DFS rates were 91 and 54% at 12 and 24 months, respectively, if molecular CR was achieved after imatinib therapy, compared with 8% at 12 months if it was not.

Using imatinib in the post transplant setting in a prophylactic manner, immediately after engraftment and prior to the detection of *BCR-ABL* transcripts by PCR, may further improve outcome by preventing resurgence of the leukemia clone. Two small series have shown the feasibility of this approach, with transient elevations in hepatic transaminases usually responding to dose interruptions or dose modifications [76, 77]. Additional cumulative experience will be required to determine whether imatinib monotherapy post transplant will improve RFS or conversely, lead to development of resistance.

Treatment of Elderly Patients with Ph-Positive ALL

The prognosis of ALL in elderly patients has traditionally been poor, irrespective of the presence or absence of the Ph chromosome [2]. Overall CR rates with frontline ALL chemotherapy regimens yield CR rates of 46–79%, with 3-year OS rates less than 20% [2]. Intolerance of chemotherapy, inability to undergo allogeneic SCT owing to comorbidities, and heretofore still unrecognized differences in the biology of the disease account for the inferior outcomes in the elderly subgroup compared with their younger counterparts. An optimal treatment approach to the elderly patient with Ph-positive ALL is paramount, particularly since the incidence of the Ph chromosome increases with advancing age. Several approaches using imatinib-based therapy for elderly patients with de novo Ph-positive ALL have been explored (Table 15.2).

In the Gruppo Italiano Malattie EMatologiche dell'Adulto Vignetti (GIMEMA) study for patients aged 60 years or older with de novo Ph-positive ALL, the efficacy of induction therapy with high-dose imatinib (800 mg) and intermediate dose oral prednisone (40 mg/m^2 daily days 1–45) was evaluated [68]. Nearly all patients achieved CR; however, only one molecular CR was observed. Therapy with single agent imatinib was continued indefinitely until disease recurrence, with a median CR duration and OS of 8 and 12 months, respectively. Fourteen patients (48%) relapsed within a median of 14 months (range, 3–28 months). Thirteen patients remained in continuous CR after a median of 10 months (range, 1–32 months) whereas two others died in CR.

In the study Group for Research on Adult Acute Lymphocytic Leukemia (GRAALL) AFR09, 30 patients aged 55 years and older were treated with induction chemotherapy after a prephase of corticosteroids, followed by intermediate dose (600 mg) imatinib alternating with consolidation chemotherapy [69]. Improvements in the 1-year DFS and OS rates were observed compared with historical controls (58% versus 11%, $p = 0.0003$ and 66% versus 43%, $p = 0.005$, respectively); however, the relapse rate approached 60%. Notably, there was relatively minimal use of imatinib in the consolidation and maintenance phases (3 blocks of 60 days over a 730 day period) compared with other imatinib-based regimens. No data was provided regarding the incidence of ABL KD mutations at the time of disease recurrence.

Ottmann and colleagues [67] conducted a randomized study of frontline induction therapy with single agent intermediate dose imatinib versus standard chemotherapy for patients with de novo Ph-positive ALL older than 55 years of age (median age 68 years), followed by consolidation with concurrent imatinib and chemotherapy in both arms. The CR rate with imatinib was superior to chemotherapy (96% versus 50%, respectively) owing to induction mortality and disease resistance in the latter arm. Patients refractory to the induction chemotherapy were often successfully salvaged with imatinib plus chemotherapy. However, there were no significant differences in long-term outcome between the two frontline approaches; overall 2-year OS rate was 42% (Table 15.2). Molecular CR rates were similar for the two arms, but occurred earlier in the imatinib induction arm. Achievement of a molecular CR with either approach was associated with a longer median DFS (18.3 versus 7.2 months, $p = .002$). Disease recurrence appeared to be associated with a high rate of ABL KD mutations [78].

The optimal therapy for elderly patients with de novo Ph-positive ALL has yet to be defined, but may be further delineated with the advent of the novel TKIs developed to counter mechanisms of resistance to imatinib.

Mechanisms of Resistance to Tyrosine Kinase Inhibitors

In the GRAAPH 2003 study, prephase corticosteroid insensitivity appeared to predict a higher probability of disease recurrence despite incorporating imatinib earlier into the chemotherapy regimen (the induction phase rather than delaying until the consolidation phase) [65]. Relapse rates after imatinib-based frontline chemotherapy with or without allogeneic SCT ranged from 19% to 32% in the studies confined to younger patients (Table 15.2) [60, 61, 63]. Relapse rates after imatinib-based regimens tailored for the elderly group appear higher, ranging from 41% to 60%, likely related to inherent differences in the biological features of Ph-positive ALL with older age. Dose attenuation of the chemotherapy and/or higher frequency of ABL KD mutations partly account for age-related differences in outcomes [67, 69, 79].

ABL Kinase Domain Mutations

Imatinib continues to have a favorable toxicity profile with accumulating clinical experience [54]. However, resistance to imatinib has now emerged as a therapeutic challenge (Table 15.3). Several resistance mechanisms have been identified, including acquisition of point mutations in the ABL KD (Fig. 15.2). ABL KD mutations that directly impede contact between imatinib and BCR-ABL, such as the gatekeeper mutations T315I or F317L, appear to be the most influential [93]. Other KD mutations alter the spatial conformation of the BCR-ABL protein by affecting one of the two flexible loops: (1) the P-loop containing the ATP binding pocket, or (2) the activating loop [80, 94, 95]. To date, more than 50 ABL KD mutations have been identified. Although the prognostic significance of several of these mutations remains unclear, the T315I KD mutation has been associated with a particularly adverse outcome. It has been identified in up to 20% of imatinib-resistant Ph-positive ALL cases and also confers resistance to the second-generation TKIs nilotinib and dasatinib [78].

Data on the frequency of ABL KD mutations in Ph-positive ALL have been relatively sparse until recently. In the elderly GMALL study for Ph-positive ALL, the incidence of ABL KD mutations (by direct cDNA sequencing) at the time of disease recurrence was 84% [67]. In cases

Table 15.3 Mechanisms of resistance to imatinib

BCR-ABL dependent
  Amplification of BCR-ABL [80]
  ABL kinase domain mutations
BCR-ABL independent
  Clonal evolution [81]
  Expression Ikaros (*IKZF1*) isoform 6 [82]
  Activation of alternative signaling pathways (e.g., Src) [83]
Cellular uptake and efflux
  Increased binding to α1-acid glycoprotein-1 [84]
  Increased MDR1 gene expression and/or permeability glycoprotein (PgP) [85, 86]
  Decreased organic cation transporter-1 (OCT-1) mediated influx [87, 88]
Stromal dysregulation
  Downregulation chemokine receptor 4 (CXCR4) [89]
Miscellaneous
  Stem cell quiescence [90]
  Noncompliance [91]

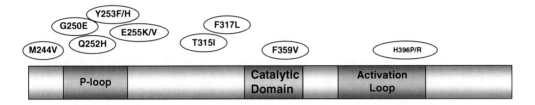

		Imatinib		Dasatinib		Nilotinib	
		Cellular IC50 (nmol/L)	Fold Change	Cellular IC50 (nmol/L)	Fold Change	Cellular IC50 (nmol/L)	Fold Change
	Wild type	260–500	1	0.8	1	13–25	1
	M244V	2000	4–8	1.3	2	38	1.5–3
P-loop	G250E	1350–3900	3–15	1.8	2	48–219	4–16
	Q252H	1200–2900	2.5–11	3.4	4	16–70	1–5
	Y253F	3475	7–13	1.4	2	125	10
	Y253H	> 10,000	> 20	1.3	2	450–750	35–60
	E255K/V	4400–8400	9–32	5.6–11	7–14	200–680	8–52
	T315I	> 10,000	> 20	> 200	> 250	> 2000	> 154
	F317L	810–1500	1.6–6	7.4	9	50–80	2–6
Catalytic domain	F359V	1200–1325	2.5–5	2.2	3	175	7–13
Activation loop	H396P/R	850–4200	1.7–16	0.6–1.3	0.8–3	41	1.6–3

Fig. 15.2 Over 50 ABL kinase domain mutations have been identified with differential potency of the tyrosine kinase inhibitors imatinib, dasatinib and nilotinib [65, 66]. Selected mutations with clinical relevance are depicted. *IC* inhibitory concentration. This figure was originally published in *Blood*. D.A. Thomas [92]. © The American Society of Hematology

harboring ABL KD mutations, P-loop mutations predominated at a frequency of 57%, followed by the T315I mutation at 19% [78]. The mutated clone comprised over 50% of the ABL clones in all cases of recurrence. Pfeifer et al. [78] also demonstrated that these ABL KD mutations could by detected in nearly 40% of de novo imatinib-naïve Ph-positive ALL cases with more sensitive techniques such as high-performance liquid chromatography. The distribution of mutations was similar to the relapsed experience, with P-loop mutations in 80% and the T315I mutation in 17%. However, the mutated ABL clone always comprised less than 2% of the de novo sample, in contrast to predominance of the mutated clone upon disease recurrence, and was below the level of detection when assayed by direct cDNA sequencing.

The presence of ABL KD mutations prior to imatinib-based therapy did not correlate with established prognostic factors. There was no difference in the probability of achieving CR or molecular CR based on the presence or absence of ABL KD mutations at diagnosis. There was no difference in CR or molecular CR rates for those harboring the T315I mutation at diagnosis, but a more rapid disease recurrence was noted in these cases. Nearly all the cases of de novo Ph-positive ALL with detectable ABL KD mutations at diagnosis subsequently relapsed, compared with 50% of those without mutations. In nearly all cases where an ABL KD mutation was present pretreatment, the same mutation was noted at the time of disease recurrence. Conversely, approximately 67% of patients without an ABL KD mutation prior to imatinib subsequently exhibited a dominant mutant clone at the time of disease recurrence. Whether imatinib resistance acquired via ABL KD mutations is predominantly a result of outgrowth of preexisting mutant KD clones present prior to therapy (and not eradicated by chemotherapy) or selection pressure related to continuous exposure to TKI remains to be discerned.

The discovery of novel, acquired ABL KD mutations has also been reported in Ph-positive ALL after sequential therapy with imatinib followed by the second-generation TKI dasatinib. Soverini et al. [96] reported the development of T315A and F317I KD mutations (as opposed to T315I or F317L), which are inherently resistant to dasatinib. These ABL KD mutations could be suppressed by either imatinib or nilotinib owing to the lower IC_{50} with these compounds, although retreatment with imatinib after a prior failure would likely be ineffective owing to the potential role of other coexisting mechanisms of resistance. Resistance screening with nilotinib, the other second generation TKI, yielded only a limited spectrum of point mutations [97]. This suggested the potential for a lower rate of ABL KD mutations after nilotinib therapy; however, additional analyses of ongoing clinical trials are needed to support this contention.

Other Mechanisms of Resistance to Imatinib

IKZF1 (Ikaros) functions as a critical regulator of normal lymphocyte development and is involved in the rapid development of leukemia in mice expressing non-DNA binding isoforms [98]. More recently, *IKZF1* inactivating mutations (complete or partial deletions which result in dominant negative isoforms) have been identified in Ph-positive ALL via single nucleotide polymorphism (SNP) array analysis [82]. In particular, the Ik6 isoform, which lacks all 4 N-terminal zinc fingers responsible for DNA binding, was identified in approximately 85% of Ph-positive ALL cases resistant to imatinib or dasatinib. *IKZF1* inactivating mutations have also been associated with a poor prognosis in Ph-negative pediatric ALL [99]. Although these cases do not harbor the *BCR-ABL* fusion gene, they have gene expression signatures similar to Ph-positive ALL [100].

Other mechanisms of resistance to imatinib and other TKIs include increased drug efflux [101], amplification of the *BCR-ABL* gene [80], and signaling independence of *BCR-ABL* after secondary transforming events (e.g., Src kinase pathway [83]). Imatinib is a substrate of the drug efflux permeability glycoprotein (PgP). Increased expression of PgP can decrease intracellular concentrations of imatinib [85, 86]. In addition, imatinib uptake is dependent on the organic cation transporter-1 (OCT-1) [101]. Low OCT-1 activity has been observed in Ph-positive CML patients with suboptimal response to imatinib; its relevance in Ph-positive ALL is under investigation [87]. Constitutive activation of downstream signaling molecules that result in activation of BCR-ABL independent pathways include the Src family kinases Lyn, Hck, and Fgr [102]. Imatinib-resistant CML cell lines that overexpress Lyn and Hck undergo apoptosis when exposed to dual Src and BCR-ABL TKIs [103]. Theoretically, dose escalation of imatinib or use of more potent ABL inhibitors could circumvent the first two events; whereas use of novel Src inhibitors or multitargeted kinase inhibitors would be required to restore sensitivity in the latter case.

Other potential applications of MRD may include the ability to guide the level of immunosuppression and the dose and frequency of donor lymphocyte infusions applied following allogeneic transplantation. MRD also has a potentially valuable role to play in the evaluation of novel anti-leukemic therapies and in supporting the design of early phase clinical trials.

Emerging Indicators for Response Assessment

Pharmacological

An interesting association between the efficacy of serum asparagine depletion and clinical outcome was recently reported. Rapid depletion of asparagine by the therapeutic enzyme asparaginase results in selective killing of lymphoblasts and is now established as a key component of ALL therapy (refer to the Chap. 10). Wetzler et al. suggested that those patients who failed to achieve depletion of serum asparagine during induction or early intensification experienced a shorter disease-free survival (DFS) [50]. This observation requires validation in larger prospective studies, but may have important utility as a surrogate marker of response. Importantly, it also represents a good example of how response assessment may allow clinicians to implement individualized changes to dose and schedule of specific components of therapy.

Epigenetics

Much research interest is currently focused on the epigenetic control of gene expression in leukemic blasts, such as aberrant DNA methylation patterns. In terms of response assessment, recently published data suggests an association between residual methylation of specific genes at the time of morphological remission, with disease-free and overall survival [51]. Although this study did not examine whether this association was independent of MRD status in those patients with residual p73 methylation, this is nonetheless interesting data that deserves further study and in principle could help further refine post-remission risk stratification and impact upon therapeutic decisions.

Conclusions

The outcome following therapy of ALL in adults remains unsatisfactory. The broad application of further intensification of therapy however has limitations, highlighting an urgent need for individualized, dynamic risk-adapted therapy. The prognostic importance of response assessment in this disease has been recognized for over 3 decades but recent advances in the analysis of minimal residual disease are potentially of great significance. Clinical and laboratory data derived largely from national and international collaborative clinical trials, in concert with rapid advances and improved reliability of molecular biology methodology have not only allowed its powerful prognostic significance to be realized but, tantalizingly, may soon begin to impact directly on individual therapeutic choices. Employing flow cytometry to detect a leukemia-associated phenotype or PCR to detect patient-specific rearrangements of antigen-receptor genes are undoubtedly reliable and sensitive approaches, although these assays can be quite complex and will represent a challenge to standardize and implement with sufficient accuracy to allow definition as a standard of care.

Although an extremely promising strategy, at the present time it remains unproven that the early detection of MRD will translate into an effective opportunity to alter the disease course in such a way as to impact upon the survival of adults with acute lymphoblastic leukemia. Nonetheless, these improvements are anticipated and should be clarified in the coming years as the ongoing prospective studies begin to report. It is to be hoped that this significant progress made in the assessment of response to therapy will be realized to allow more adults with ALL to be cured of their disease with a minimum of treatment-related complications.

References

1. Durrant, I. J., Prentice, H. G., & Richards, S. M. (1997). Intensification of treatment for adults with acute lymphoblastic leukemia: Results of U.K. Medical Research Council randomized trial UKALL XA. Medical Research Council Working Party on Leukemia in Adults. *British Journal of Haematology, 99*(1), 84–92.
2. Fielding, A. K., Richards, S. M., Chopra, R., et al. (2007). Outcome of 609 adults after relapse of acute lymphoblastic leukemia (ALL); an MRC UKALL12/ECOG 2993 study. *Blood, 109*(3), 944–950.
3. Rowe, J. M. (2009). Optimal management of adults with ALL. *British Journal of Haematology, 144*(4), 468–483.
4. Tavernier, E., Boiron, J. M., Huguet, F., et al. (2007). Outcome of treatment after first relapse in adults with acute lymphoblastic leukemia initially treated by the LALA-94 trial. *Leukemia, 21*(9), 1907–1914.
5. Bruggemann, M., Raff, T., Flohr, T., et al. (2006). Clinical significance of minimal residual disease quantification in adult patients with standard-risk acute lymphoblastic leukemia. *Blood, 107*(3), 1116–1123.
6. Hoelzer, D., Thiel, E., Loffler, H., et al. (1988). Prognostic factors in a multicenter study for treatment of acute lymphoblastic leukemia in adults. *Blood, 71*(1), 123–131.
7. Moorman, A. V., Harrison, C. J., Buck, G. A., et al. (2007). Karyotype is an independent prognostic factor in adult acute lymphoblastic leukemia (ALL): Analysis of cytogenetic data from patients treated on the Medical Research Council (MRC) UKALLXII/Eastern Cooperative Oncology Group (ECOG) 2993 trial. *Blood, 109*(8), 3189–3197.
8. Nachman, J. B., Sather, H. N., Sensel, M. G., et al. (1998). Augmented post-induction therapy for children with high-risk acute lymphoblastic leukemia and a slow response to initial therapy. *The New England Journal of Medicine, 338*(23), 1663–1671.
9. Bassan, R., Spinelli, O., Oldani, E., et al. (2009). Improved risk classification for risk-specific therapy based on the molecular study of MRD in adult ALL. *Blood, 113*(18), 4153–4162.
10. Borowitz, M. J., Devidas, M., Hunger, S. P., et al. (2008). Clinical significance of minimal residual disease in childhood acute lymphoblastic leukemia and its relationship to other prognostic factors: A Children's Oncology Group study. *Blood, 111*(12), 5477–5485.
11. Coustan-Smith, E., Sancho, J., Behm, F. G., et al. (2002). Prognostic importance of measuring early clearance of leukemic cells by flow cytometry in childhood acute lymphoblastic leukemia. *Blood, 100*(1), 52–58.
12. Flohr, T., Schrauder, A., Cazzaniga, G., et al. (2008). Minimal residual disease-directed risk stratification using real-time quantitative PCR analysis of immunoglobulin and T-cell receptor gene rearrangements in the international multicenter trial AIEOP-BFM ALL 2000 for childhood acute lymphoblastic leukemia. *Leukemia, 22*(4), 771–782.
13. Foroni, L., Coyle, L. A., Papaioannou, M., et al. (1997). Molecular detection of minimal residual disease in adult and childhood acute lymphoblastic leukemia reveals differences in treatment response. *Leukemia, 11*(10), 1732–1741.
14. Mortuza, F. Y., Papaioannou, M., Moreira, I. M., et al. (2002). Minimal residual disease tests provide an independent predictor of clinical outcome in adult acute lymphoblastic leukemia. *Journal of Clinical Oncology, 20*(4), 1094–1104.
15. Vidriales, M. B., Perez, J. J., Lopez-Berges, M. C., et al. (2003). Minimal residual disease in adolescent (older than 14 years) and adult acute lymphoblastic leukemias: Early immunophenotypic evaluation has high clinical value. *Blood, 101*(12), 4695–4700.
16. Zhou, J., Goldwasser, M. A., Li, A., et al. (2007). Quantitative analysis of minimal residual disease predicts relapse in children with B-lineage acute lymphoblastic leukemia in DFCI ALL Consortium Protocol 95-01. *Blood, 110*(5), 1607–1611.
17. Raff, T., Gokbuget, N., Luschen, S., et al. (2007). Molecular relapse in adult standard-risk ALL patients detected by prospective MRD monitoring during and after maintenance treatment: Data from the GMALL 06/99 and 07/03 trials. *Blood, 109*(3), 910–915.
18. Sallan, S. E., Cammita, B. M., Cassady, J. R., Nathan, D. G., & Frei, E., 3rd. (1978). Intermittent combination chemotherapy with adriamycin for childhood acute lymphoblastic leukemia: Clinical results. *Blood, 51*(3), 425–433.

19. Gaynon, P. S., Desai, A. A., Bostrom, B. C., et al. (1997). Early response to therapy and outcome in childhood acute lymphoblastic leukemia: A review. *Cancer, 80*(9), 1717–1726.
20. Steinherz, P. G., Gaynon, P. S., Breneman, J. C., et al. (1996). Cytoreduction and prognosis in acute lymphoblastic leukemia–the importance of early marrow response: Report from the Childrens Cancer Group. *Journal of Clinical Oncology, 14*(2), 389–398.
21. Gaynor, J., Chapman, D., Little, C., et al. (1988). A cause-specific hazard rate analysis of prognostic factors among 199 adults with acute lymphoblastic leukemia: The Memorial Hospital experience since 1969. *Journal of Clinical Oncology, 6*(6), 1014–1030.
22. Hoelzer, D., Thiel, E., Loffler, H., et al. (1984). Intensified therapy in acute lymphoblastic and acute undifferentiated leukemia in adults. *Blood, 64*(1), 38–47.
23. Linker, C. A., Levitt, L. J., O'Donnell, M., Forman, S. J., & Ries, C. A. (1991). Treatment of adult acute lymphoblastic leukemia with intensive cyclical chemotherapy: A follow-up report. *Blood, 78*(11), 2814–2822.
24. Larson, R. A., Dodge, R. K., Burns, C. P., et al. (1995). A five-drug remission induction regimen with intensive consolidation for adults with acute lymphoblastic leukemia: Cancer and leukemia group B study 8811. *Blood, 85*(8), 2025–2037.
25. Donadieu, J., & Hill, C. (2001). Early response to chemotherapy as a prognostic factor in childhood acute lymphoblastic leukemia: A methodological review. *British Journal of Haematology, 115*(1), 34–45.
26. Lilleyman, J. S. (1998). Clinical importance of speed of response to therapy in childhood lymphoblastic leukemia. *Leukaemia & Lymphoma, 31*(5–6), 501–506.
27. Sebban, C., Browman, G. P., Lepage, E., & Fiere, D. (1995). Prognostic value of early response to chemotherapy assessed by the day 15 bone marrow aspiration in adult acute lymphoblastic leukemia: A prospective analysis of 437 cases and its application for designing induction chemotherapy trials. *Leukemia Research, 19*(11), 861–868.
28. Kaspers, G. J., Pieters, R., Van Zantwijk, C. H., Van Wering, E. R., Van Der Does-Van Den Berg, A., & Veerman, A. J. (1998). Prednisolone resistance in childhood acute lymphoblastic leukemia: Vitro-vivo correlations and cross-resistance to other drugs. *Blood, 92*(1), 259–266.
29. Holleman, A., den Boer, M. L., de Menezes, R. X., et al. (2006). The expression of 70 apoptosis genes in relation to lineage, genetic subtype, cellular drug resistance, and outcome in childhood acute lymphoblastic leukemia. *Blood, 107*(2), 769–776.
30. Annino, L., Vegna, M. L., Camera, A., et al. (2002). Treatment of adult acute lymphoblastic leukemia (ALL): Long-term follow-up of the GIMEMA ALL 0288 randomized study. *Blood, 99*(3), 863–871.
31. Sorich, M. J., Pottier, N., Pei, D., et al. (2008). In vivo response to methotrexate forecasts outcome of acute lymphoblastic leukemia and has a distinct gene expression profile. *PLoS Medicine, 5*(4), e83.
32. Campana, D. (2008). Molecular determinants of treatment response in acute lymphoblastic leukemia. *Hematology (American Society of Hematology Education Program), 2008*, 366–373.
33. Lazarus, H. M., Richards, S. M., Chopra, R., et al. (2006). Central nervous system involvement in adult acute lymphoblastic leukemia at diagnosis: Results from the international ALL trial MRC UKALL XII/ECOG E2993. *Blood, 108*(2), 465–472.
34. Bromberg, J. E., Breems, D. A., Kraan, J., et al. (2007). CSF flow cytometry greatly improves diagnostic accuracy in CNS hematologic malignancies. *Neurology, 68*(20), 1674–1679.
35. Hegde, U., Filie, A., Little, R. F., et al. (2005). High incidence of occult leptomeningeal disease detected by flow cytometry in newly diagnosed aggressive B-cell lymphomas at risk for central nervous system involvement: The role of flow cytometry versus cytology. *Blood, 105*(2), 496–502.
36. Schinstine, M., Filie, A. C., Wilson, W., Stetler-Stevenson, M., & Abati, A. (2006). Detection of malignant hematopoietic cells in cerebral spinal fluid previously diagnosed as atypical or suspicious. *Cancer, 108*(3), 157–162.
37. Finn, W. G., Peterson, L. C., James, C., & Goolsby, C. L. (1998). Enhanced detection of malignant lymphoma in cerebrospinal fluid by multiparameter flow cytometry. *American Journal of Clinical Pathology, 110*(3), 341–346.
38. French, C. A., Dorfman, D. M., Shaheen, G., & Cibas, E. S. (2000). Diagnosing lymphoproliferative disorders involving the cerebrospinal fluid: Increased sensitivity using flow cytometric analysis. *Diagnostic Cytopathology, 23*(6), 369–374.
39. Pine, S. R., Yin, C., Matloub, Y. H., et al. (2005). Detection of central nervous system leukemia in children with acute lymphoblastic leukemia by real-time polymerase chain reaction. *The Journal of Molecular Diagnostics, 7*(1), 127–132.
40. Pui, C. H., & Howard, S. C. (2008). Current management and challenges of malignant disease in the CNS in paediatric leukemia. *The Lancet Oncology, 9*(3), 257–268.
41. Burger, B., Zimmermann, M., Mann, G., et al. (2003). Diagnostic cerebrospinal fluid examination in children with acute lymphoblastic leukemia: Significance of low leukocyte counts with blasts or traumatic lumbar puncture. *Journal of Clinical Oncology, 21*(2), 184–188.

42. Gajjar, A., Harrison, P. L., Sandlund, J. T., et al. (2000). Traumatic lumbar puncture at diagnosis adversely affects outcome in childhood acute lymphoblastic leukemia. *Blood, 96*(10), 3381–3384.
43. te Loo, D.M., Kamps, W.A., van der Does-van den Berg, A., van Wering, E.R., de Graaf, S.S. (2006). Prognostic significance of blasts in the cerebrospinal fluid without pleiocytosis or a traumatic lumbar puncture in children with acute lymphoblastic leukemia: Experience of the Dutch Childhood Oncology Group. *Journal of Clinical Oncology, 24*(15), 2332–2336
44. Pui, C. H., Sandlund, J. T., Pei, D., et al. (2004). Improved outcome for children with acute lymphoblastic leukemia: Results of Total Therapy Study XIIIB at St Jude Children's Research Hospital. *Blood, 104*(9), 2690–2696.
45. Pui, C. H. (2006). Central nervous system disease in acute lymphoblastic leukemia: Prophylaxis and treatment. *Hematology American Society of Hematology Education Program, 2006*(1), 142–146.
46. Campana, D., & Pui, C. H. (1995). Detection of minimal residual disease in acute leukemia: Methodologic advances and clinical significance. *Blood, 85*(6), 1416–1434.
47. Coustan-Smith, E., Ribeiro, R. C., Stow, P., et al. (2006). A simplified flow cytometric assay identifies children with acute lymphoblastic leukemia who have a superior clinical outcome. *Blood, 108*(1), 97–102.
48. Seibel, N. L., Steinherz, P. G., Sather, H. N., et al. (2008). Early postinduction intensification therapy improves survival for children and adolescents with high-risk acute lymphoblastic leukemia: A report from the Children's Oncology Group. *Blood, 111*(5), 2548–2555.
49. Lo Coco, F., Diverio, D., Avvisati, G., et al. (1999). Therapy of molecular relapse in acute promyelocytic leukemia. *Blood, 94*(7), 2225–2229.
50. Wetzler, M., Sanford, B. L., Kurtzberg, J., et al. (2007). Effective asparagine depletion with pegylated asparaginase results in improved outcomes in adult acute lymphoblastic leukemia: Cancer and Leukemia Group B Study 9511. *Blood, 109*(10), 4164–4167.
51. Yang, H., Kadia, T., Xiao, L., et al. (2009). Residual DNA methylation at remission is prognostic in adult Philadelphia chromosome-negative acute lymphocytic leukemia. *Blood, 113*(9), 1892–1898.

88. Howard, S. C., & Pui, C. H. (2002). Endocrine complications in pediatric patients with acute lymphoblastic leukemia. *Blood Reviews, 16,* 225–243.
89. Derijk, R. H., & de Kloet, E. R. (2008). Corticosteroid receptor polymorphisms: determinants of vulnerability and resilience. *European Journal of Pharmacology, 583,* 303–311.
90. Derijk, R. H., Schaaf, M., & de Kloet, E. R. (2002). Glucocorticoid receptor variants: clinical implications. *The Journal of Steroid Biochemistry and Molecular Biology, 81,* 103–122.
91. Fleury, I., Primeau, M., Doreau, A., et al. (2004). Polymorphisms in genes involved in the corticosteroid response and the outcome of childhood acute lymphoblastic leukemia. *American Journal of Pharmacogenomics, 4,* 331–341.
92. Tissing, W. J., Meijerink, J. P., den Boer, M. L., et al. (2005). Genetic variations in the glucocorticoid receptor gene are not related to glucocorticoid resistance in childhood acute lymphoblastic leukemia. *Clinical Cancer Research, 11,* 6050–6056.
93. Fleury, I., Beaulieu, P., Primeau, M., Labuda, D., Sinnett, D., & Krajinovic, M. (2003). Characterization of the BclI polymorphism in the glucocorticoid receptor gene. *Clinical Chemistry, 49,* 1528–1531.
94. Peeters, G. M., van Schoor, N. M., van Rossum, E. F., Visser, M., & Lips, P. (2008). The relationship between cortisol, muscle mass and muscle strength in older persons and the role of genetic variations in the glucocorticoid receptor. *Clinical Endocrinology (Oxford), 69,* 673–682.
95. Aguilera, G., Nikodemova, M., Wynn, P. C., & Catt, K. J. (2004). Corticotropin releasing hormone receptors: two decades later. *Peptides, 25,* 319–329.
96. Tantisira, K. G., Lake, S., Silverman, E. S., et al. (2004). Corticosteroid pharmacogenetics: association of sequence variants in CRHR1 with improved lung function in asthmatics treated with inhaled corticosteroids. *Human Molecular Genetics, 13,* 1353–1359.
97. Kamdem, L. K., Hamilton, L., Cheng, C., et al. (2008). Genetic predictors of glucocorticoid-induced hypertension in children with acute lymphoblastic leukemia. *Pharmacogenetics and Genomics, 18,* 507–514.
98. Jones, T. S., Kaste, S. C., Liu, W., et al. (2008). CRHR1 polymorphisms predict bone density in survivors of acute lymphoblastic leukemia. *Journal of Clinical Oncology, 26,* 3031–3037.
99. Franchimont, D., Martens, H., Hagelstein, M. T., et al. (1999). Tumor necrosis factor alpha decreases, and interleukin-10 increases, the sensitivity of human monocytes to dexamethasone: potential regulation of the glucocorticoid receptor. *The Journal of Clinical Endocrinology and Metabolism, 84,* 2834–2839.
100. Lauten, M., Matthias, T., Stanulla, M., Beger, C., Welte, K., & Schrappe, M. (2002). Association of initial response to prednisone treatment in childhood acute lymphoblastic leukaemia and polymorphisms within the tumour necrosis factor and the interleukin-10 genes. *Leukemia, 16,* 1437–1442.
101. Lo, H. W., & Ali-Osman, F. (2007). Genetic polymorphism and function of glutathione S-transferases in tumor drug resistance. *Current Opinion in Pharmacology, 7,* 367–374.
102. Anderer, G., Schrappe, M., Brechlin, A. M., et al. (2000). Polymorphisms within glutathione S-transferase genes and initial response to glucocorticoids in childhood acute lymphoblastic leukaemia. *Pharmacogenetics, 10,* 715–726.
103. Stanulla, M., Schrappe, M., Brechlin, A. M., Zimmermann, M., & Welte, K. (2000). Polymorphisms within glutathione S-transferase genes (GSTM1, GSTT1, GSTP1) and risk of relapse in childhood B-cell precursor acute lymphoblastic leukemia: a case-control study. *Blood, 95,* 1222–1228.
104. Meissner, B., Stanulla, M., Ludwig, W. D., et al. (2004). The GSTT1 deletion polymorphism is associated with initial response to glucocorticoids in childhood acute lymphoblastic leukemia. *Leukemia, 18,* 1920–1923.
105. Kishi, S., Yang, W., Boureau, B., et al. (2004). Effects of prednisone and genetic polymorphisms on etoposide disposition in children with acute lymphoblastic leukemia. *Blood, 103,* 67–72.
106. Rollinson, S., Roddam, P., Kane, E., et al. (2000). Polymorphic variation within the glutathione S-transferase genes and risk of adult acute leukaemia. *Carcinogenesis, 21,* 43–47.
107. Krajinovic, M., Labuda, D., Mathonnet, G., et al. (2002). Polymorphisms in genes encoding drugs and xenobiotic metabolizing enzymes, DNA repair enzymes, and response to treatment of childhood acute lymphoblastic leukemia. *Clinical Cancer Research, 8,* 802–810.
108. Celander, M., Weisbrod, R., & Stegeman, J. J. (1997). Glucocorticoid potentiation of cytochrome P4501A1 induction by 2, 3, 7, 8-tetrachlorodibenzo-p-dioxin in porcine and human endothelial cells in culture. *Biochemical and Biophysical Research Communications, 232,* 749–753.
109. Monostory, K., Kohalmy, K., Prough, R. A., Kobori, L., & Vereczkey, L. (2005). The effect of synthetic glucocorticoid, dexamethasone on CYP1A1 inducibility in adult rat and human hepatocytes. *FEBS Letters, 579,* 229–235.
110. Yiannakouris, N., Yannakoulia, M., Melistas, L., Chan, J. L., Klimis-Zacas, D., & Mantzoros, C. S. (2001). The Q223R polymorphism of the leptin receptor gene is significantly associated with obesity and predicts a small percentage of body weight and body composition variability. *The Journal of Clinical Endocrinology and Metabolism, 86,* 4434–4439.
111. Nishiyama, K., Tanaka, Y., Nakajima, K., et al. (2005). Polymorphism of the solute carrier family 12 (sodium/chloride transporters) member 3, SLC12A3, gene at exon 23 (+78G/A: Arg913Gln) is associated with elevation

of urinary albumin excretion in Japanese patients with type 2 diabetes: a 10-year longitudinal study. *Diabetologia, 48,* 1335–1338.

112. Cavalli, S. A., Hirata, M. H., Salazar, L. A., et al. (2000). Apolipoprotein B gene polymorphisms: prevalence and impact on serum lipid concentrations in hypercholesterolemic individuals from Brazil. Clinica chimica acta. *International Journal of Clinical Chemistry, 302,* 189–203.

113. Van Veldhuizen, P. J., Neff, J., Murphey, M. D., Bodensteiner, D., & Skikne, B. S. (1993). Decreased fibrinolytic potential in patients with idiopathic avascular necrosis and transient osteoporosis of the hip. *American Journal of Hematology, 44,* 243–248.

114. Halleux, C. M., Declerck, P. J., Tran, S. L., Detry, R., & Brichard, S. M. (1999). Hormonal control of plasminogen activator inhibitor-1 gene expression and production in human adipose tissue: stimulation by glucocorticoids and inhibition by catecholamines. *The Journal of Clinical Endocrinology and Metabolism, 84,* 4097–4105.

115. French, D., Hamilton, L. H., Mattano, L. A., Jr., et al. (2008). A PAI-1 (SERPINE1) polymorphism predicts osteonecrosis in children with acute lymphoblastic leukemia: a report from the Children's Oncology Group. *Blood, 111,* 4496–4499.

116. Kathiresan, S., Gabriel, S. B., Yang, Q., et al. (2005). Comprehensive survey of common genetic variation at the plasminogen activator inhibitor-1 locus and relations to circulating plasminogen activator inhibitor-1 levels. *Circulation, 112,* 1728–1735.

117. Ferrari, P., Schroeder, V., Anderson, S., et al. (2002). Association of plasminogen activator inhibitor-1 genotype with avascular osteonecrosis in steroid-treated renal allograft recipients. *Transplantation, 74,* 1147–1152.

118. Bosma, P. J., Chowdhury, J. R., Bakker, C., et al. (1995). The genetic basis of the reduced expression of bilirubin UDP-glucuronosyltransferase 1 in Gilbert's syndrome. *The New England Journal of Medicine, 333,* 1171–1175.

119. Kantarjian, H., Giles, F., Wunderle, L., et al. (2006). Nilotinib in imatinib-resistant CML and Philadelphia chromosome-positive ALL. *The New England Journal of Medicine, 354,* 2542–2551.

120. Singer, J. B., Shou, Y., Giles, F., et al. (2007). UGT1A1 promoter polymorphism increases risk of nilotinib-induced hyperbilirubinemia. *Leukemia, 21,* 2311–2315.

121. Mayor, N. P., Shaw, B. E., Hughes, D. A., et al. (2007). Single nucleotide polymorphisms in the NOD2/CARD15 gene are associated with an increased risk of relapse and death for patients with acute leukemia after hematopoietic stem-cell transplantation with unrelated donors. *Journal of Clinical Oncology, 25,* 4262–4269.

122. Ogura, Y., Inohara, N., Benito, A., Chen, F. F., Yamaoka, S., & Nunez, G. (2001). Nod2, a Nod1/Apaf-1 family member that is restricted to monocytes and activates NF-kappaB. *The Journal of Biological Chemistry, 276,* 4812–4818.

123. Hampe, J., Grebe, J., Nikolaus, S., et al. (2002). Association of NOD2 (CARD 15) genotype with clinical course of Crohn's disease: a cohort study. *Lancet, 359,* 1661–1665.

124. Hugot, J. P., Chamaillard, M., Zouali, H., et al. (2001). Association of NOD2 leucine-rich repeat variants with susceptibility to Crohn's disease. *Nature, 411,* 599–603.

125. Mayor, N. P., Shaw, B. E., Madrigal, J. A., & Marsh, S. G. (2008). No impact of NOD2/CARD15 on outcome after SCT: a reply. *Bone Marrow Transplantation, 42,* 837–838.

126. Elmaagacli, A. H., Koldehoff, M., Hindahl, H., et al. (2006). Mutations in innate immune system NOD2/CARD 15 and TLR-4 (Thr399Ile) genes influence the risk for severe acute graft-versus-host disease in patients who underwent an allogeneic transplantation. *Transplantation, 81,* 247–254.

127. Holler, E., Rogler, G., Herfarth, H., et al. (2004). Both donor and recipient NOD2/CARD15 mutations associate with transplant-related mortality and GvHD following allogeneic stem cell transplantation. *Blood, 104,* 889–894.

128. Granell, M., Urbano-Ispizua, A., Arostegui, J. I., et al. (2006). Effect of NOD2/CARD15 variants in T-cell depleted allogeneic stem cell transplantation. *Haematologica, 91,* 1372–1376.

129. Holler, E., Rogler, G., Brenmoehl, J., et al. (2006). Prognostic significance of NOD2/CARD15 variants in HLA-identical sibling hematopoietic stem cell transplantation: effect on long-term outcome is confirmed in 2 independent cohorts and may be modulated by the type of gastrointestinal decontamination. *Blood, 107,* 4189–4193.

130. Croucher, P. J., Mascheretti, S., Hampe, J., et al. (2003). Haplotype structure and association to Crohn's disease of CARD15 mutations in two ethnically divergent populations. *European Journal of Human Genetics, 11,* 6–16.

131. Ansari, M., & Krajinovic, M. (2007). Pharmacogenomics in cancer treatment defining genetic bases for inter-individual differences in responses to chemotherapy. *Current Opinion in Pediatrics, 19,* 15–22.

132. Ansari, M., & Krajinovic, M. (2007). Pharmacogenomics of acute leukemia. *Pharmacogenomics, 8,* 817–834.

Chapter 21
Late Consequences of Therapy of Acute Lymphoblastic Leukemia

Mark R. Litzow

Introduction

In 1948, Farber and colleagues published the first report of temporary remissions of children with acute lymphoblastic leukemia (ALL) who were treated with the folic acid antagonist, aminopterin [1]. The use of antimetabolites combined with corticosteroids began to result in long-term remissions of children with ALL and subsequent long-term cures [2]. The tremendous success in the treatment of ALL through the introduction of new antileukemic agents and optimal use of these drugs has led to increases in the probability of overall survival from 20% in the early 1960s to approximately 80% in the 1990s. More recent studies suggest that a cure rate approaching 90% is attainable (Fig. 21.1) [3].

The radiation and drug combinations used in the treatment of ALL are not without toxicity at both the cellular and organ levels. The range of toxicities of the specific agents is beyond the scope of this review but has been well-outlined elsewhere [4]. These toxicities combined with the cure and long-term survival of most pediatric patients with ALL has resulted in the development of multiple long-term sequelae (Table 21.1). This review will outline these sequelae by organ system and by their impact on quality of life, psychosocial functioning, and development of second malignancies. A conceptual model of how these different factors interact in cancer survivors is shown in Fig. 21.2.

Cohort Studies

Studies of large numbers of children from single centers or from population-based reviews have confirmed the improvements in survival over time and have also documented the physical and psychosocial impact of these treatments [6, 7]. Long-term follow-up of a cohort of 856 patients treated at St. Jude's Hospital between 1962 and 1992 was conducted. Half of the patients relapsed, eight died in remission, and 44 patients developed a second malignancy. Of these 44 second malignancies, 41 of them were related to radiation therapy (RT). The risk of a second malignancy in those who received RT was significantly higher than in those who did not ($p = 0.04$). Many of these second malignancies were benign or low grade. For the irradiated group, the death rate was slightly higher than the expected rate for the general U. S. population (standardized mortality ratio 1.90, 95% confidence intervals (CI) 1.12–3.00). For patients who did not receive RT, their survival did not differ from the population norm. Rates of marriage, employment, and health insurance coverage were also

M.R. Litzow (✉)
Hematology Mayo Clinic, Rochester, MN, USA
e-mail: litzow.mark@mayo.edu

A.S. Advani and H.M. Lazarus (eds.), *Adult Acute Lymphocytic Leukemia*, Contemporary Hematology,
DOI 10.1007/978-1-60761-707-5_21, © Springer Science+Business Media, LLC 2011

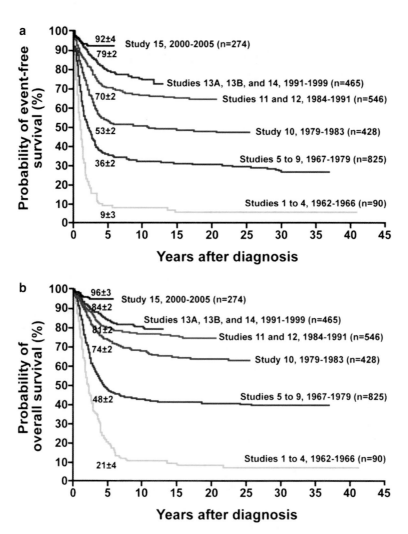

Fig. 21.1 Kaplan–Meier analyses of event-free survival (Panel **a**) and overall survival (Panel **b**) in 2,628 children with newly diagnosed ALL. The patients participated in 15 consecutive studies conducted at St. Jude Children's Research Hospital from 1962 to 2005. The five-year event-free and overall survival estimates ({±}SE) are shown, except for Study 15, for which preliminary results at four years are provided. The results demonstrate steady improvement in clinical outcome over the past four decades. The difference in event-free and overall survival rates has narrowed in the recent periods, suggesting that relapses or second cancers that occur after contemporary therapy are more refractory to treatment (From [3])

similar to national averages for patients who did not receive RT. However, in the irradiated group, unemployment rates were higher and marriage rates in women were lower despite similar health insurance rates [7].

Some of the most comprehensive outcome data on long-term survivors of childhood ALL comes from the Childhood Cancer Survivor Study (CCSS). This epidemiological study assessed patients who have had all types of childhood cancer [8]. A recent report from the CCSS documented the long-term follow-up and sequelae of treatment after 25 years among survivors of childhood ALL [9]. Of 5,760 patients who had survived their ALL for an initial 5 years, the cumulative mortality at 25 years was 13%. Survival at 25 years was 96% in those treated without RT and 87% in those who received RT. Recurrent ALL afflicted 483 patients and second neoplasms occurred in 89 patients. Among 185 survivors who reported second neoplasms, a total of 199 non-melanomatous skin cancer

Functional *NOTCH1* is a trans-membrane receptor complex consisting of extracellular (NEC) and trans-membrane (NTM) subunits non-covalently bound through heterodimerization domain (HD). After ligand binding, a cascade of proteolytic cleavages (final cleavage is catalyzed by γ-secretase complex) liberates intracellular *NOTCH1* (ICN). ICN translocates into the nucleus where it becomes part of a large transcription activator complex [31].

Several important studies strongly implicate constitutive *NOTCH1* upregulation in murine T-ALL models. Mice transplanted with bone marrow expressing directly or indirectly activated *NOTCH1* develop T-cell neoplasms [32, 33]. In *TAL1* model of murine T-ALL, 74% of tumors harbored activating *NOTCH1* mutations. Cell lines from these tumors undergo G0/G1 arrest and apoptosis when treated with a γ-secretase inhibitor, indicating crucial leukemogenic role for *NOTCH1* [23]. In a different study, *NOTCH1* activating mutations in either *PEST* or *HD* domains were found in 13 out of 19 murine T-ALL cell lines and in 29 of 49 primary tumors derived from mice spontaneously developing T-ALL (*SCL/LMO1*, *OLIG2/LMO1*, *OLIG2*, *LMO1*, *NUP98/HOXD13, and p27$^{-/-}$/SMAD3$^{+/-}$* strains) [22].

Recent studies in human T-ALL confirm an important role for *NOTCH1* in leukemogenesis. *NOTCH1* activating mutations have been found in the *HD* domain and the *PEST* domain in 56% of T-ALL from all of the molecular subtypes [7]. Mutations in the *HD* domain, found in 44% of T-ALL, confer ligand independent *ICN* production; mutations in the *PEST* domain, observed in 30% of T-ALL, extend the half-life of the *ICN* transcription complex. Combined mutations of the *HD* and *PEST* domains, found in 17% of cases, have a synergistic effect on *NOTCH1* activation. The finding of *NOTCH1* mutations in all molecular subtypes of T-ALL suggest that they occur in immature progenitors and might be a prenatal event. To support this hypothesis, one report identified *NOTCH1* mutation in neonatal blood sample prior to T-ALL development; the sample was negative for *SIL-TAL1* fusion [24]. Both genetic events were present in diagnostic samples after the patient was diagnosed with T-ALL. The authors hypothesized that *NOTCH1* is an early (possibly prenatal) or initiating event that was complemented by later (postnatal) *SIL-TAL1* fusion to complete leukemogenesis. Furthermore, in a recent study, blockade of *NOTCH1* signaling at two dependent steps suppressed the growth and survival of *NOTCH1*-transformed T-ALL cells [25]. Firstly, inhibitors of presenilin, required for proteolysis of membrane-bound *NOTCH1* and liberation of *ICN*, induced growth suppression and apoptosis of the murine T-ALL cell line. Secondly, 62-aminoacid *MAML1* (Mastermind-like-1 factor – *NOTCH* coactivator)-derived peptide, which forms transcriptionally inert complex with *ICN*, specifically inhibited growth of both murine and human NOTCH1-transformed T-ALL lines.

The intrinsic mechanisms of *NOTCH1*-induced leukemogenesis are still unknown and might result from the deregulation of cell cycle control and other normal functions [34] and self-renewal capacity of early lymphoid progenitors and/or stem cells [35]. The m-TOR pathway was recently identified as one of the possible *NOTCH1*-downstream events. Using 13 T-ALL cell lines and DNA-microarray screen, it has been determined that GSI (γ-secretase inhibitor)-induced hypophosphorylation of multiple signaling proteins in mTOR pathway, was rescued by expression of the *ICN* and mimicked by *MAML1* confirming *NOTCH1* specificity. The effect of GSI was also rescued by expression of *c-Myc*, a direct transcriptional target of *NOTCH1*, implicating *c-Myc* as an intermediary between *NOTCH1* and mTOR [36]. Rap1 signaling has been suggested by another study to be a possible upstream event in *NOTCH1* transformation. Transplantation of hematopoetic progenitors expressing Rap1 guanine nucleoside exchange factor into normal recipients resulted in markedly enhanced expression of *NOTCH1* as well as target downstream genes, including c-Myc and eventually led to *NOTCH1*-dependent T-ALL [33].

Other Signaling pathways. Multiple other molecular pathways were identified or suspected in either animal or human studies to play a role in T-ALL leukemogenesis. A comprehensive review of recently published studies can be found elsewhere [8]. From a translational research standpoint, two of these pathways deserve mentioning here because of possible therapeutic intervention with novel targeted agents.

ABL1 is a well-known ubiquitously expressed cytoplasmic tyrosine kinase, encoded by a gene mapping on 9q34. The t(9;22)(q34;q11) encoding the *BCR-ABL1* fusion protein kinase [37], is characteristic of chronic myeloid leukemia and is also expressed in 25% of precursor B-cell ALL and only rarely (1%) in T-ALL [38, 39]. Specific for T-ALL, *NUP214-ABL1* was identified in up to 6% of T-ALL patients [18, 19]. This fusion gene is found on amplified episomes, which are not detected cytogenetically [40]. Molecular detection by FISH or RT-PCR is usually required to diagnose these cases. Other partners that encode fusion genes with *ABL1* were described in T-ALL but are exceptionally rare [41, 42]. All these gene fusions result in constitutive activation of *ABL1*-mediated kinase activity leading to the upregulation of survival and proliferation pathways. In addition, it has recently been shown that *ABL1* plays a role in TCR signaling [43]. Of special interest, imatinib, a specific inhibitor of *ABL1*, appears to be effective in controlling the activity of the kinase regardless of the fusion partner in vitro, which creates a therapeutic promise for these specific T-ALL cases.

The *RAS* proteins play a critical role in transmitting survival signals. *RAS* mutations were found in multiple cancers including leukemias [44]. Activating mutations in *N-RAS* have been detected in up to 10% of pediatric T-ALL in a Japanese study of 125 patients [45]. Other reports suggested that *RAS* is highly activated in 50% of pediatric T-ALL implicating a major role in disease pathogenesis [46]. These findings support therapeutic trials of farnesytransferase inhibitors in this patient population [47].

Finally, upregulation of signaling pathways involving *JAK2* and *FLT3* activation via gene-fusion or gene-duplication, respectively, were found in a small number of T-ALL cases [48–50]. Specific inhibitors of these kinases are being developed and might find use in the near future for targeted therapies in specific patient subgroups.

Factors Predicting Clinical Outcomes in T-ALL

In the recent decade, improved clinical protocols have overcome multiple adverse prognostic indicators in both B-cell and T-cell ALL. The strategies contributing to this progress include intensification of treatments, aggressive central nervous system (CNS) prophylaxis, upfront risk stratification and more appropriate use of allogeneic hematopoietic cell transplantation, more aggressive use of L-asparaginase products and others. While in the past considered to be a high-risk phenotype, as a group, T-ALL has outcomes comparable to or superior to B-ALL when current treatment protocols are applied [51–53]. Outcomes in pediatric T-ALL continue to be highly superior to outcomes in adult T-ALL. Five-year event-free survivals (EFS) as high as ≥80% have been reported in children treated on several cooperative group protocols [54–56]. Several groups of disease- and host-related factors have emerged as strong predictors of treatment outcome in T-ALL.

Genetic aberrations affecting outcomes. Several recently described chromosomal abnormalities and genetically silent deregulations of signaling pathways were found to correlate with treatment outcomes in T-ALL (Table 12.3). Translocation [11, 19] (q23;p13.3) encoding the fusion product of *MLL* (mixed lineage leukemia) gene and *ENL* (eleven nineteen leukemia) gene is frequently found in young adolescents and carries a better prognosis [16]. This is in sharp contrast with the majority of other translocations involving *MLL* that confer an especially poor outcome. This includes *AF10, AF6, AF4,* and *AFX1* gene partners [61–63].

The class II orphan homeobox *HOX11* (*TLX1*) over-expression resulting from t(10;14)(q24;q11) and t(7;10)(q34;q24) translocations that puts *HOX11* gene under a strong *TCRA* and *TCRB* promoters, respectively [65], was reported to portend a favorable outcome in the recent study of two cooperative group trials in T-ALL patients [13]. While the complete remission rate did not differ in

Table 12.3 Prognostic significance of selected chromosomal aberration in T-cell acute lymphoblastic leukemia

Genetic aberration	Frequency in T-ALL (%)	Effect on prognosis
t(5;14)(q35;q32) *HOX11L2*	18–23	Poor [57]
		Neutral [58]
t(10;14)(q24;q11) *HOX11(TLX1)* t(7;10)(q34;q24)	31	Favorable [13]
del(6q) Unknown	20–31	Poor [59, 60]
TAL1/LYL1	45	Poor [5]
t(11;19)(q23;p13) *MLL/ENL*	8 (all *MLL*)	Favorable [16]
Other 11q23/*MLL*		Poor [61]
t(4;11)(q21;q23) *MLL/AF4*		Poor [62, 63]
t(10;11)(p13;q14) *CALM-AF10*	10	Favorable [14]
del(9q) p16	65	Poor [64]

HOX11+ and *HOX11−* T-ALL patients, the leukemia-specific survival was significantly better in patients with *HOX11* over-expression.

Cryptic deletion of the *INK4/ARF* locus on 9q21 is the most frequent anomaly in T-ALL [20, 66]. These deletions target the *CDKN2A(p16/p14)* and in part *CDKN2B(p15)* genes. Homozygous and heterozygous deletions are detected by FISH in 65% and 15% of T-ALLs, respectively. It has been reported that T-ALL patients harboring homozygous del(9q21) have a significantly worse 5-year EFS then patients with germline p16 [64].

Pharmacodynamic factors affecting outcome. Host factors can significantly influence treatment efficacy and outcomes [67, 68]. Examples include genetic polymorphism of drug-metabolizing enzymes, specifically the hepatic P450 system, drug transporters, receptors, and targets. Concomitant medications can severely impact clearance or metabolism of the anti-leukemic agents. Anticonvulsant drugs (phenytoin, phenobarbital, etc.) can significantly increase cytochrome P450 activity in the liver, thereby enhancing clearance and reducing efficacy of chemotherapeutic agents and adversely affecting outcome [69].

A recent study of folate pathway gene expression in ALL patients found much lower levels of folylpolyglutamate synthetase (FPGS), a critical enzyme that determines cytosolic glutamation of methotrexate (MTX → MTXPG), and MTX anti-tumor activity, in T-ALL compared to all other ALL subtypes [70]. Suboptimal accumulation of MTXPG in T-ALL blasts might be responsible for reduced anti-leukemic activity of MTX. Consistent with these findings, recent clinical trials suggested improved outcomes in T-ALL patients with the use of very high doses of MTX [71, 72].

Global gene expression patterns affecting outcomes. DNA-array technology has emerged as a new dimension in studying genetic deregulations in T-ALL and other leukemias [5]. It allows large-scale screening of expression profiles in leukemic blasts, determination of pathogenetic mechanisms and identification of molecular predictors of outcomes after modern therapies.

Analysis of gene expression patterns in T-ALL blasts and statistical correlation with clinical outcomes identified a molecular predictive model based on the expression of three genes, *TTK, CD2, and AHNAK* in a recent study [73]. These genes were selected from a set of 19 genes that were differentially expressed in patients with sustained CR for more then 2 years and those who relapsed within this period of time. *AHNAK* had increased expression in blasts from patients who subsequently experienced a relapse, whereas high expression of *CD2* and *TTK* were found in patients who remained in remission. This three-gene model correctly classifies 71% of outcomes in this study of 33 patients with T-ALL. In addition, interleukin 8 (*IL-8*) was highly expressed in refractory T-ALL cells from patients who failed induction therapy. Expression of *CD2*, but not *TTK* or *AHNAK*, was similarly found to predict poor outcomes in pediatric T-ALL [74, 75].

Treatment Outcomes in T-ALL

Improved treatments in the last decade have abolished the adverse prognostic influence of multiple disease factors including T-cell phenotype. Complete response rates as high as 85–90% and 5-year leukemia-free survival rates of 45–50% can be obtained with modern therapies in adults with T-ALL. Children with T-ALL fair even better after contemporary pediatric treatment protocols with a 3-year event-free survival rate reaching 85%. While prospective clinical trials focusing on T-ALL are lacking due to a low incidence of this leukemia, multiple pediatric and adult study groups have reported outcomes in T-ALL patients enrolled into prospective ALL protocols. Selected clinical trials are presented in Table 12.4.

Several conclusions can be made from these studies. Firstly, pediatric T-ALL patients have significantly better survival rates than adults (Table 12.5). Factors influencing this difference are likely to be the same as for B-ALL and include, but are not limited to, higher intensity of pediatric protocols; more rigorous adherence to treatment doses and schedules in children compared to adult patients due to higher tolerance of treatment toxicities by pediatric oncologists, "treatment culture" and lack of autonomy of children; presence of comorbidities in older adults precluding the use of

Table 12.4 Clinical outcomes in selected pediatric and adult ALL trials according to disease phenotype

Study Group	B-lineage	T-lineage	P value
Childhood ALL (EFS%)			
ALL-BFM 86 (6-year)	77	73 [76]	0.096
ALL-BFM 90 (6-year)	82	61 [72]	NR
AIEOP-ALL 82 (8-year)	63	55 [54]	NR
AIEOP-ALL 87 (8-year)	68	78[54]	NR
AIEOP-ALL 88 (8-year)	73	83 [54]	NR
AIEOP-ALL 91 (8-year)	78	65 [54]	NR
CCG 1989-95 (8-year)	78	79 [77]	NR
DCLSG ALL-8 (5-year)	73	83 [55]	0.31
CLCG-EORTC (8-year)	69	62 [78]	NR
NOPHO (5-year)	85	75 [79]	<0.01
DFCI-91-01 (5-year)	84	79 [56]	0.34
SJCRH XIIIB (5-year)	83	72 [52]	0.17
UKALL XI (10-year)	65	52 [80]	0.04
Adult ALL (OS%)			
MDACC (5-year)	45	48 [81]	0.18
LALA 94 (5-year)	34	32 [82]	NR
GIMEMA (8-year)	30	27 [83]	NR
JALSG-ALL93 (6-year)	36	42 [84]	0.85
UCSF (5-year)	66	48 [85]	NR
EHH (8-year)	17	36 S	0.05

EFS Event-free survival, *OS* overall survival, *BFM* Berlin–Frankfurt–Munster study group; *AIEOP* Italian Association of Pediatric Hematology Oncology, *CCG* Children Cancer Group, *DCLSG* Dutch Childhood Leukemia Study Group, *CLCG-EORTC* Children Leukemia Cooperative Group – European Organization for Research and treatment of Cancer, *NOPHO* Nordisk Forening for Pediatrisk Hematologi og Oncologi, *DFCI* Dana Farber Cancer Institute, *SJCRH* St. Jude Cancer Research Hospital, *UKALL* United Kingdom ALL Study Group, *MDACC* MD Anderson Cancer Center, *LALA* Leucemie Aigue Lymphoblastique de l'Adulte, *GIMEMA* Gruppo Italiano Malattie Ematologiche dell'Adulto, *JALSG* Japan Adult Leukemia Study Group, *UCSF* University of California at San Francisco, *EHH* Edouard Herriot Hospital, *NR* not reported

Table 12.5 T-ALL: clinical observations

- Pediatric T-ALL patients have better survival than adult T-ALL patients.
- Survivals of both pediatric and adult T-ALL patients are higher in modern clinical trials than in historical data.
- Survival of T-ALL patients appears equal or superior to B-ALL patients when treated with modern regimens.
- T-ALL represents a group of T-cell neoplasms with diverse biology, clinical behavior, prognosis, and outcomes. This diversity is likely related to molecular genetics and pathogenesis.

intensive regimens required for cure; higher proportions of children being treated on clinical protocols at the academic centers versus by community adult oncologists [86]; and higher rates of adverse prognostic features in adult T-ALL, most notably cytogenetic aberrations compared to childhood T-ALL. Secondly, more recent trials report better survival in both pediatric and adult T-ALL when compared to trials 2–3 decades ago. This is most pronounced in patients treated within the same cooperative groups and single institutions over the span of several decades when outcomes are compared between different time periods [54, 79, 87]. Analyses of changes in clinical protocols might suggest what specific interventions led to improvement in outcomes (discussed below). Thirdly, in contradiction to earlier reports assigning a poor prognosis to ALL patients with T-cell phenotype, survival of both pediatric and adult T-ALL patients appears to be more favorable than patients with B-cell ALL, with the exception of a small proportion of T-ALL patients harboring adverse chromosomal aberrations discussed above [71]. Fourthly, it is becoming increasingly clear that T-ALL represents a group of aggressive lymphoid neoplasms with a diverse biology, response to treatments and prognosis and should not be viewed as a single clinico-pathologic entity [8]. Future clinical studies should attempt to incorporate risk stratification algorithms based on current knowledge of molecular pathogenesis, cytogenetic profile of the leukemic blasts and clinical predictors of outcome, although with the relative rarity of these subpopulations, this presents a significant challenge.

Several changes in the treatment protocols appear to have a favorable impact on the outcomes, including long-term survival, in patients with T-ALL.

High-dose methotrexate. The use of very-high-dose methotrexate (≥ 4 g/m^2) in the consolidation protocols may have improved CR rates and survival in adult and pediatric T-ALL patients. Pediatric Oncology Group (POG) 9404 study for T-ALL and advanced stage T-LBL evaluated the efficacy of high-dose methotrexate (5 g/m^2, given every 3 weeks for 4 doses) added to the backbone of DFCI-87-01 treatment protocol. The data showed that high-dose methotrexate significantly improved outcome for both T-ALL and T-LBL. The 3-year event-free survival (EFS) was encouraging at 85% and 87%, respectively [71]. Of particular interest was the observation that the impact of high-dose methotrexate was particularly striking in patients with leukocyte count $\geq 50 \times 10^9$/L, generally considered a high-risk feature. ALL-BFM study group reported similar improvement in survival outcomes in pediatric T-ALL patients after high-dose methotrexate was introduced into treatment protocols, yielding promising 6-year EFS of 83% [76]. These results are consistent with a lower accumulation of methotrexate polyglutamates (i.e., active metabolite) in T-ALL blasts compared to B-cell precursor ALL, requiring higher doses and hence, serum concentrations for adequate therapeutic effect [70]. The role of high-dose methotrexate in adult T-ALL is less clear from current evidence and should be addressed in future studies.

High-dose l-asparaginase. Studies in both adult and pediatric ALL suggested that protracted use of high-dose l-asparaginase might be beneficial for T-ALL patients. One of the first pieces of evidence came from the Pediatric Oncology Group (POG) study of 552 children with T-ALL and T-LBL [88]. All patients received aggressive remission induction and then were randomized to receive or not receive high-dose, intensive l-asparaginase consolidation given weekly for 20 weeks. The high-dose asparaginase regimen was significantly superior to the control regimen in both T-ALL and T-LBL. Four-year continuous remission rates (CRR) for the asparaginase group and control group were 68% and 55% ($P = 0.002$), respectively in T-ALL patients. Corresponding CRR for T-LBL patients were 78% and 64%, respectively ($P=0.048$). This largest trial to date in T-ALL patients demonstrated significant improvement in outcomes for these patients with addition of high-dose L-asparaginase to aggressive chemotherapy regimens. Echoing this finding in pediatric population, in a recent report by the CALGB study group, T-ALL patients treated on Protocol 9511 were evaluated for the level of asparagine depletion and its correlation with treatment outcome. Investigators found that effective and meaningful asparagine depletion can be achieved with intensified dosing of PEG-asparaginase, and secondly, that the successful depletion was achieved much more commonly in T-ALL than in B-ALL adult patients (92% vs 68%) [89]. The study also demonstrated that survival rates for the entire study population strongly correlated with effective asparagine depletion. Additional evidence of significant improvement in outcome after intensification of L-asparaginase dosing was also provided in successive pediatric trials reported by the Dana Farber Cancer Institute (DFCI) Consortium and Italian Association of Pediatric Hematology and Oncology (AIEOP). Five-year EFS (DFCI) and 8-year EFS (AIEOP) for T-ALL in the recent Protocols DFCI 91-01 and AIEOP 87 were 79% [56] and 78% [54], respectively. These results compared favorably to previous protocols with less intense L-asparaginase regimens and similar chemotherapy backbones. The importance of understanding the pharmacokinetics and pharmacodynamics of various L-asparaginase preparations was underscored by the reports from the Dutch DCLSG consortium and the Italian AIEOP consortium that observed no benefit from high-dose Erwinia L-asparaginase use in pediatric protocols ALL-8 and BFM, respectively, in contrast to other studies where the use of high-dose *E. coli* or PEG-asparaginase provided meaningful improvement in outcomes [55, 90]. Similarly, the DFCI consortium reported inferior outcomes with Erwinia asparaginase compared to the *E. coli* product [91]. To improve pharmacokinetic properties and possibly modify toxicity profile of L-asparaginase products, native *E. coli* ASNase was covalently bound with 5,000 Da of monomethoxypolyethylene glycol. PEG-ASNase (PEG-asparaginase) retains enzymatic activity but has reduced immunogenicity and a fivefold greater half life than the native product. In a recent pharmacokinetic study in pediatric ALL patients, the use of PEG-asparaginase resulted in a high-level serum enzyme activity and asparagine depletion in serum and CSF [92]. Furthermore, a randomized comparison of native *E. coli* ASNase and PEG-asparaginase in children with previously untreated ALL showed that PEG-asparaginase was associated with an improved prolonged serum ASNase activity, lower incidence of high titer antibodies to ASNase, and a more rapid clearance of lymphoblasts in the bone marrow [93]. When used in children with relapsed and refractory ALL, dose-dense weekly PEG-asparaginase circumvented rapid systemic clearance seen in some of these patients and resulted in a higher remission induction rate than the biweekly schedule (97% with weekly schedule vs .82% with biweekly) [94]. These studies provide initial evidence of superiority of PEG-asparaginase over native enzyme and provide a rationale for incorporation of polyethylene-glycol-conjugated ASNase into future clinical protocols.

Cranial radiotherapy. The realization of the high-risk of CNS relapse in T-ALL patients with high WBC at diagnosis (>100,000/ul) and benefit of cranial irradiation for this group has been gleaned from comparison of the ALL-BFM 90 and AIEOP-ALL 91 studies [72, 95]. Lack of prophylactic cranial radiotherapy was associated with a higher risk of systemic relapses in the latter study. In addition, the ALL-BFM 90 trial provided evidence that 12 Gy cranial irradiation is as effective as 18 Gy, with a potential reduction for neurotoxicity. However, patients with WBC at diagnosis <100,000/ul might fare better with intrathecal therapy combined with four cycles high-dose systemic methotrexate due to a reduced rate of neurotoxicity and long-term, cognitive deficits from this approach compared to cranial irradiation (UKALL XI) [80].

Allogeneic hematopoietic cell transplantation for high-risk patients. A major improvement in long-term survival in both adult and pediatric ALL including T-ALL has been obtained by stratifying patients to consolidative allogeneic hematopoietic cell transplantation (HCT) based on the high-risk features at diagnosis and/or during treatment. High-risk clinical features shared with B-ALL include age older than 35 years, failure to achieve CR after 1 cycle of induction and presence of minimal residual disease after completion of therapy. Specific T-ALL associated high risk features suggested from numerous trials include peripheral blood leukocytosis >100,000/ul, pro-T-ALL (TI) immunophenotype, t(4; 11), t(1; 19,) and t(10; 11). The GOELAMS group reported meaningful improvement in the achievement of CR and survival in high-risk T-ALL patients treated with allogeneic HCT compared to delayed autologous HCT with encouraging median PFS and OS reaching 57.6 and 60.9 months, respectively [96]. French investigators from Edouard Herriot Hospital (Lyon, France) reported their experience in 378 ALL patients diagnosed with ALL between 1978 and 1999. In this study, the most significant improvement in survival was observed in T-ALL patients receiving allogeneic HCT. The 3-year OS after HCT in first CR was 74% in T-cell lineage, while it was less then 50% in B-cell lineage ALL [87].

Novel and Investigational Therapies

The understanding of intrinsic mechanisms in leukemogenesis and advances in biopharmaceutical technologies opened a new era in the development of novel chemotherapeutic and targeted/biologic agents for both B-cell and T-cell ALL. Many of these agents are in various stages of clinical development or have entered human trials.

Several novel nucleoside analogues, including clofarabine, forodesine, and nelarabine, have shown promise in both pediatric and adult T-ALL. Both, forodesine and nelarabine target human/mammalian purine nucleoside phosphorylase (PNP) via direct inhibition and by serving as a resistant substrate, respectively. The major role for mammalian PNP is to catalyze the cleavage of several substrates, including guanosine and deoxyguanosine (dGuo) to their corresponding base and sugar 1-phosphate by phosphorolysis [97]. The impetus for a PNP inhibitor search emerged from the observation that patients with rare hereditary PNP deficiency develop immunodeficiency syndrome with profound T-cell depletion and only minor changes in the humoral system [98]. Forodesine, a potent PNP-inhibitor, was designed based on the transition-state structure stabilized by the enzyme. Preclinical studies demonstrated that the cytotoxic activity of forodesine in the presence of dGuo was selective to T-lymphocytes [99]. High deoxynucleoside kinase and low nucleotidase levels make T-cells more sensitive to forodesine-induced inhibition/apoptosis. A Phase I clinical trial of forodesine in advanced T-cell malignancies demonstrated significant antitumor activity that correlated with an increased plasma forodesine and dGuo, and an accumulation of intracellular dGuo-triphosphate [100]. Nelarabine (506U78), the 6-methoxy derivative of araG, which is rapidly deaminated by adenosine deaminase in vivo to araG, its active form [101], is a PNP-resistant substrate that induces competitive inhibition of the enzyme. It demonstrated significant cytotoxicity against T-lymphoid lineage [102, 103]. In the initial trial of nelarabine in multiple hematologic malignancies, it was determined that the highest activity was in patients with precursor T-cell neoplasms (T-ALL and T-LBL) [104]. Subsequently, a CALGB/SWOG intergroup study (C19801) reported results of nelarabine in adult patients with relapsed and refractory T-ALL/T-LBL [105]. Twenty-six patients were treated and the response rate (CR/PR) was 41% with 31% of the patients achieving CR. Even higher activity was documented in a phase II pediatric trial in which 34 T-ALL/LBL patients in first relapse (stratum 1) and 36 patients in second relapse (stratum 2) were treated and the rates of overall (complete) responses were 55% (48%) for stratum 1 and 27% (23%) for stratum 2 [106]. These results are very encouraging for this very difficult group of patients and led to approval of nelarabine by the FDA for treatment of relapsed/refractory T-cell ALL/LBL [107].

Clofarabine, a novel nucleoside analogue, has been shown to have several mechanisms of anti-leukemic action: (1) it is incorporated into the DNA and inhibits DNA elongation and DNA repair; (2) it is a potent inhibitor of ribonucleotide reductase, depleting primarily dCTP and dATP pools; and (3) it may directly induce apoptosis by altering mitochondrial membrane and subsequently enabling

Table 12.6 Novel agents in trials for treatment of T-cell acute lymphoblastic leukemia

Agent	Mechanism of action	Subtype of leukemia targeted
MK0752	γ-secretase inhibition (interference with NOTCH signaling)	T-cell
PKC412	FMS-like tyrosine kinase3 inhibition	*MLL*-rearranged
MLN518		
CEP701		
Tipifarnib	Farnesyltransferase inhibition	T- and B-cell
Decitabine	DNA demethylation	T- and B-cell
5-Azacitidine		
Vorinostat	Histone deacetylase inhibition	T- and B-cell
MS-275		
Bortezomib PS-341	Ubiquitin proteosome inhibition	T- and B-cell
Clofarabine	Deoxyadenosine analogue	T- and B-cell
Forodesine	Purine nucleoside phosphorilase inhibition	T-cell
Alemtuzumab	Anti-CD52 humanized MAB	CD52+

release of cytochrome C [108]. Due to its high efficacy observed in phase II clinical trials, clofarabine was granted FDA approval for treatment of relapsed or refractory childhood B-ALL [109, 110]. Recent anecdotal evidence suggests that clofarabine might have substantial activity in T-ALL [111].

Among targeted agents in development, UCN-01, a cell cycle checkpoint inhibitor, presents interesting activity in T-ALL. UCN-01 (7-hydroxy-staurosporine) inhibits cyclin-dependent kinase activity, important in transition checkpoint regulation, and demonstrates anti-proliferative activity in multiple human tumor cell lines. Pediatric T-ALL cells lacking p16 expression, a cyclin-dependent kinase inhibitor, have been found to be differentially sensitive to UCN-01, suggesting that p16 protein expression status may influence the cytotoxicity of UCN-01 in T-ALL blasts and that this agent may be active in p16-negative T-ALL [112].

Several other targeted agents are undergoing clinical development and might find use in T-ALL in the future. Table 12.6 lists selected antileukemic agents being tested in clinical trials.

T-ALL: Future Directions

Recent scientific discoveries and numerous clinical trials have made a significant impact on outcomes in adult and pediatric patients with T-ALL. Higher rates of CR, incorporation of intensified consolidation protocols, use of aggressive CNS prophylaxis and up-front stratification of patients with high risk disease to consolidative allogeneic HCT have all contributed to this success. Introduction of novel agents, such as nelarabine, and progress in reduced-intensity conditioning transplants have brought further gains to these patients. However, despite the excitement of this progress, significant proportion of pediatric patients and majority of adults with T-ALL will experience failures of initial therapies and leukemia relapse after achievement of CR and will subsequently succumb to their disease. This identifies an acute need for further research in disease biology and clinical arena. Several directions should be pursued.

Advances in molecular biology identified specific pathways in leukemogenesis that are attractive targets for small molecule inhibitors. Use of these agents in combination with established chemotherapy might restore sensitivity of resistant leukemic blasts without adding significant toxicities, improve CR rates and ultimately affect outcomes of treatment. Among targeted agents, monoclonal antibodies are certainly underutilized in ALL protocols and should be incorporated into future clinical trials. The combination of rituximab with chemotherapy for CD20-positive B-cell ALL was the first step in this direction and showed promising preliminary results [113]. Other attractive targets for B-cell ALL are CD22 and CD19. Several anti-CD19 antibody agents were tested in phase I clinical trials but results are not conclusive [114]. Far less experience with monoclonal antibody therapy is available for T-ALL, but studies are underway with anti-CD25 and anti-CD52 antibodies in adult T-ALL/LBL. It is likely that the greatest benefit of using monoclonal antibodies will be in combination with chemotherapy. The hope is that this will improve the rate of CR, quality of CR, and lead to eradication of minimal residual disease.

Current maintenance protocols generally utilize low-dose chemotherapy, most commonly, combinations of oral methotrexate, 6-mercaptopurine and corticosteroids with infusional vincristine. While a positive impact has been reported in nonrandomized trials, the magnitude of this benefit is modest. Novel agents with a potential effect on leukemic "stem cells" might produce meaningful improvement in the cure rate and incidence of relapse after attainment of CR. Epigenetic agents including histone deacetylase inhibitiors and hypomethylating are agent, attractive candidates with toxicity profiles acceptable for long-term use.

Further improvements in molecular risk stratification will help to better identify patients with poor-risk cytogenetic and cryptic aberrations who are candidates for allogeneic HCT in first remission. The majority of recently identified genetic events with either poor or favorable prognosis are not detected by conventional clinical methods. Many pathways that are linked to poor prognosis are not associated with specific mutations but could be identified via gene expression profiles. Incorporation of known aberrations into an "ALL-chip" based on DNA-array technology would be a significant advance in prognostic models.

Modifying existing agents to produce higher efficacy and lower toxicity is another direction to improve outcomes. A recently developed recombinant form of asparaginase may be less immunogenic than other products. The use of liposomal daunorubicin and vincristine might decrease cardiotoxicity and neurotoxicity, respectively, while improving efficacy due to increased *area under the curve* (AUC). Liposomal cytarabine is being tested and showed promising results as an intrathecal agent with increased half-life and better control of central nervous system disease [115].

T-cell ALL is a rare neoplasm and recent advances suggest heterogeneity of pathogenesis and clinical behavior. Multi-institutional collaboration is necessary to answer existing questions and perform prospective clinical studies focusing specifically on this group of patients. Such studies with the innovations discussed above may further improve the cure rates in T-ALL in both pediatric and adult patients.

References

1. Bene, M. C., Castoldi, G., Knapp, W., Ludwig, W. D., Matutes, E., Orfao, A., et al. (1995). Proposals for the immunological classification of acute leukemias. European group for the immunological characterization of leukemias (EGIL). *Leukemia, 9*(10), 1783–1786.
2. Asnafi, V., Beldjord, K., Boulanger, E., Comba, B., Le Tutour, P., Estienne, M. H., et al. (2003). Analysis of TCR, pT alpha, and RAG-1 in T-acute lymphoblastic leukemias improves understanding of early human T-lymphoid lineage commitment. *Blood, 101*(7), 2693–2703.
3. Harrison, C. J., & Foroni, L. (2002). Cytogenetics and molecular genetics of acute lymphoblastic leukemia. *Reviews in Clinical and Experimental Hematology, 6*(2), 91–113. discussion 200-2.
4. Ferrando, A. A., Armstrong, S. A., Neuberg, D. S., Sallan, S. E., Silverman, L. B., Korsmeyer, S. J., et al. (2003). Gene expression signatures in MLL-rearranged T-lineage and B-precursor acute leukemias: Dominance of HOX dysregulation. *Blood, 102*(1), 262–268.
5. Ferrando, A. A., Neuberg, D. S., Staunton, J., Loh, M. L., Huard, C., Raimondi, S. C., et al. (2002). Gene expression signatures define novel oncogenic pathways in T cell acute lymphoblastic leukemia. *Cancer Cell, 1*(1), 75–87.
6. Soulier, J., Clappier, E., Cayuela, J. M., Regnault, A., Garcia-Peydro, M., Dombret, H., et al. (2005). HOXA genes are included in genetic and biologic networks defining human acute T-cell leukemia (T-ALL). *Blood, 106*(1), 274–286.

7. Weng, A. P., Ferrando, A. A., Lee, W., Morris, J. P., 4th, Silverman, L. B., Sanchez-Irizarry, C., et al. (2004). Activating mutations of NOTCH1 in human T cell acute lymphoblastic leukemia. *Science, 306*(5694), 269–271.

8. Graux, C., Cools, J., Michaux, L., Vandenberghe, P., & Hagemeijer, A. (2006). Cytogenetics and molecular genetics of T-cell acute lymphoblastic leukemia: From thymocyte to lymphoblast. *Leukemia, 20*(9), 1496–1510.

9. Cauwelier, B., Dastugue, N., Cools, J., Poppe, B., Herens, C., De Paepe, A., et al. (2006). Molecular cytogenetic study of 126 unselected T-ALL cases reveals high incidence of TCRbeta locus rearrangements and putative new T-cell oncogenes. *Leukemia, 20*(7), 1238–1244.

10. Bernard, O. A., Busson-LeConiat, M., Ballerini, P., Mauchauffe, M., Della Valle, V., Monni, R., et al. (2001). A new recurrent and specific cryptic translocation, t(5;14)(q35;q32), is associated with expression of the Hox11L2 gene in T acute lymphoblastic leukemia. *Leukemia, 15*(10), 1495–1504.

11. Iolascon, A., Faienza, M. F., Coppola, B., Moretti, A., Basso, G., Amaru, R., et al. (1997). Frequent clonal loss of heterozygosity (LOH) in the chromosomal region 1p32 occurs in childhood T cell acute lymphoblastic leukemia (T-ALL) carrying rearrangements of the TAL1 gene. *Leukemia, 11*(3), 359–363.

12. Bergeron, J., Clappier, E., Radford, I., Buzyn, A., Millien, C., Soler, G., et al. (2007). Prognostic and oncogenic relevance of TLX1/HOX11 expression level in T-ALLs. *Blood, 110*(7), 2324–2330.

13. Ferrando, A. A., Neuberg, D. S., Dodge, R. K., Paietta, E., Larson, R. A., Wiernik, P. H., et al. (2004). Prognostic importance of TLX1 (HOX11) oncogene expression in adults with T-cell acute lymphoblastic leukaemia. *Lancet, 363*(9408), 535–536.

14. Asnafi, V., Radford-Weiss, I., Dastugue, N., Bayle, C., Leboeuf, D., Charrin, C., et al. (2003). CALM-AF10 is a common fusion transcript in T-ALL and is specific to the TCRgammadelta lineage. *Blood, 102*(3), 1000–1006.

15. Hayette, S., Tigaud, I., Maguer-Satta, V., Bartholin, L., Thomas, X., Charrin, C., et al. (2002). Recurrent involvement of the MLL gene in adult T-lineage acute lymphoblastic leukemia. *Blood, 99*(12), 4647–4649.

16. Rubnitz, J. E., Camitta, B. M., Mahmoud, H., Raimondi, S. C., Carroll, A. J., Borowitz, M. J., et al. (1999). Childhood acute lymphoblastic leukemia with the MLL-ENL fusion and t(11;19)(q23;p13.3) translocation. *Journal of Clinical Oncology, 17*(1), 191–196.

17. Tsutsumi, S., Taketani, T., Nishimura, K., Ge, X., Taki, T., Sugita, K., et al. (2003). Two distinct gene expression signatures in pediatric acute lymphoblastic leukemia with MLL rearrangements. *Cancer Research, 63*(16), 4882–4887.

18. Graux, C., Cools, J., Melotte, C., Quentmeier, H., Ferrando, A., Levine, R., et al. (2004). Fusion of NUP214 to ABL1 on amplified episomes in T-cell acute lymphoblastic leukemia. *Nature Genetics, 36*(10), 1084–1089.

19. Graux, C., Stevens-Kroef, M., Lafage, M., Dastugue, N., Harrison, C. J., Mugneret, F., et al. (2009). Heterogeneous patterns of amplification of the NUP214-ABL1 fusion gene in T-cell acute lymphoblastic leukemia. *Leukemia, 23*, 125–133.

20. Hebert, J., Cayuela, J. M., Berkeley, J., & Sigaux, F. (1994). Candidate tumor-suppressor genes MTS1 (p16INK4A) and MTS2 (p15INK4B) display frequent homozygous deletions in primary cells from T- but not from B-cell lineage acute lymphoblastic leukemias. *Blood, 84*(12), 4038–4044.

21. Sinclair, P. B., Sorour, A., Martineau, M., Harrison, C. J., Mitchell, W. A., O'Neill, E., et al. (2004). A fluorescence in situ hybridization map of 6q deletions in acute lymphocytic leukemia: Identification and analysis of a candidate tumor suppressor gene. *Cancer Research, 64*(12), 4089–4098.

22. Lin, Y. W., Nichols, R. A., Letterio, J. J., & Aplan, P. D. (2006). Notch1 mutations are important for leukemic transformation in murine models of precursor-T leukemia/lymphoma. *Blood, 107*(6), 2540–2543.

23. O'Neil, J., Calvo, J., McKenna, K., Krishnamoorthy, V., Aster, J. C., Bassing, C. H., et al. (2006). Activating Notch1 mutations in mouse models of T-ALL. *Blood, 107*(2), 781–785.

24. Eguchi-Ishimae, M., Eguchi, M., Kempski, H., & Greaves, M. (2008). NOTCH1 mutation can be an early, prenatal genetic event in T-ALL. *Blood, 111*(1), 376–378.

25. Weng, A. P., Nam, Y., Wolfe, M. S., Pear, W. S., Griffin, J. D., Blacklow, S. C., et al. (2003). Growth suppression of pre-T acute lymphoblastic leukemia cells by inhibition of notch signaling. *Molecular and Cellular Biology, 23*(2), 655–664.

26. Garcia-Peydro, M., de Yebenes, V. G., & Toribio, M. L. (2003). Sustained Notch1 signaling instructs the earliest human intrathymic precursors to adopt a gammadelta T-cell fate in fetal thymus organ culture. *Blood, 102*(7), 2444–2451.

27. Radtke, F., Wilson, A., Stark, G., Bauer, M., van Meerwijk, J., MacDonald, H. R., et al. (1999). Deficient T cell fate specification in mice with an induced inactivation of Notch1. *Immunity, 10*(5), 547–558.

28. Ciofani, M., Schmitt, T. M., Ciofani, A., Michie, A. M., Cuburu, N., Aublin, A., et al. (2004). Obligatory role for cooperative signaling by pre-TCR and notch during thymocyte differentiation. *Journal of Immunology, 172*(9), 5230–5239.

29. Wolfer, A., Wilson, A., Nemir, M., MacDonald, H. R., & Radtke, F. (2002). Inactivation of Notch1 impairs VDJbeta rearrangement and allows pre-TCR-independent survival of early alpha beta lineage thymocytes. *Immunity, 16*(6), 869–879.

30. Nie, L., Xu, M., Vladimirova, A., & Sun, X. H. (2003). Notch-induced E2A ubiquitination and degradation are controlled by MAP kinase activities. *The EMBO Journal, 22*(21), 5780–5792.
31. Schweisguth, F. (2004). Regulation of notch signaling activity. *Current Biology, 14*(3), R129–R138.
32. Pear, W. S., Aster, J. C., Scott, M. L., Hasserjian, R. P., Soffer, B., Sklar, J., et al. (1996). Exclusive development of T cell neoplasms in mice transplanted with bone marrow expressing activated notch alleles. *The Journal of Experimental Medicine, 183*(5), 2283–2291.
33. Wang, S. F., Aoki, M., Nakashima, Y., Shinozuka, Y., Tanaka, H., Taniwaki, M., et al. (2008). Development of notch-dependent T-cell leukemia by deregulated Rap1 signaling. *Blood, 111*(5), 2878–2886.
34. Aster, J. C. (2005). Deregulated NOTCH signaling in acute T-cell lymphoblastic leukemia/lymphoma: New insights, questions, and opportunities. *International Journal of Hematology, 82*(4), 295–301.
35. Duncan, A. W., Rattis, F. M., DiMascio, L. N., Congdon, K. L., Pazianos, G., Zhao, C., et al. (2005). Integration of notch and Wnt signaling in hematopoietic stem cell maintenance. *Nature Immunology, 6*(3), 314–322.
36. Chan, S. M., Weng, A. P., Tibshirani, R., Aster, J. C., & Utz, P. J. (2007). Notch signals positively regulate activity of the mTOR pathway in T-cell acute lymphoblastic leukemia. *Blood, 110*(1), 278–286.
37. Wong, S., & Witte, O. N. (2004). The BCR-ABL story: Bench to bedside and back. *Annual Review of Immunology, 22*, 247–306.
38. Pui, C. H., Relling, M. V., & Downing, J. R. (2004). Acute lymphoblastic leukemia. *The New England Journal of Medicine, 350*(15), 1535–1548.
39. Quentmeier, H., Cools, J., Macleod, R. A., Marynen, P., Uphoff, C. C., & Drexler, H. G. (2005). e6-a2 BCR-ABL1 fusion in T-cell acute lymphoblastic leukemia. *Leukemia, 19*(2), 295–296.
40. Ballerini, P., Busson, M., Fasola, S., van den Akker, J., Lapillonne, H., Romana, S. P., et al. (2005). NUP214-ABL1 amplification in t(5;14)/HOX11L2-positive ALL present with several forms and may have a prognostic significance. *Leukemia, 19*(3), 468–470.
41. De Keersmaecker, K., Graux, C., Odero, M. D., Mentens, N., Somers, R., Maertens, J., et al. (2005). Fusion of EML1 to ABL1 in T-cell acute lymphoblastic leukemia with cryptic t(9;14)(q34;q32). *Blood, 105*(12), 4849–4852.
42. De Keersmaecker, K., Lahortiga, I., Graux, C., Marynen, P., Maertens, J., Cools, J., et al. (2006). Transition from EML1-ABL1 to NUP214-ABL1 positivity in a patient with acute T-lymphoblastic leukemia. *Leukemia, 20*(12), 2202–2204.
43. Zipfel, P. A., Zhang, W., Quiroz, M., & Pendergast, A. M. (2004). Requirement for Abl kinases in T cell receptor signaling. *Current Biology, 14*(14), 1222–1231.
44. Neubauer, A., Dodge, R. K., George, S. L., Davey, F. R., Silver, R. T., Schiffer, C. A., et al. (1994). Prognostic importance of mutations in the ras proto-oncogenes in de novo acute myeloid leukemia. *Blood, 83*(6), 1603–1611.
45. Yokota, S., Nakao, M., Horiike, S., Seriu, T., Iwai, T., Kaneko, H., et al. (1998). Mutational analysis of the N-ras gene in acute lymphoblastic leukemia: A study of 125 Japanese pediatric cases. *International Journal of Hematology, 67*(4), 379–387.
46. von Lintig, F. C., Huvar, I., Law, P., Diccianni, M. B., Yu, A. L., & Boss, G. R. (2000). Ras activation in normal white blood cells and childhood acute lymphoblastic leukemia. *Clinical Cancer Research, 6*(5), 1804–1810.
47. Goemans, B. F., Zwaan, C. M., Harlow, A., Loonen, A. H., Gibson, B. E., Hahlen, K., et al. (2005). In vitro profiling of the sensitivity of pediatric leukemia cells to tipifarnib: Identification of T-cell ALL and FAB M5 AML as the most sensitive subsets. *Blood, 106*(10), 3532–3537.
48. Paietta, E., Ferrando, A. A., Neuberg, D., Bennett, J. M., Racevskis, J., Lazarus, H., et al. (2004). Activating FLT3 mutations in CD117/KIT(+) T-cell acute lymphoblastic leukemias. *Blood, 104*(2), 558–560.
49. Peeters, P., Raynaud, S. D., Cools, J., Wlodarska, I., Grosgeorge, J., Philip, P., et al. (1997). Fusion of TEL, the ETS-variant gene 6 (ETV6), to the receptor-associated kinase JAK2 as a result of t(9;12) in a lymphoid and t(9;15;12) in a myeloid leukemia. *Blood, 90*(7), 2535–2540.
50. Van Vlierberghe, P., Meijerink, J. P., Stam, R. W., van der Smissen, W., van Wering, E. R., Beverloo, H. B., et al. (2005). Activating FLT3 mutations in CD4+/CD8- pediatric T-cell acute lymphoblastic leukemias. *Blood, 106*(13), 4414–4415.
51. Pui, C. H., & Evans, W. E. (2006). Treatment of acute lymphoblastic leukemia. *The New England Journal of Medicine, 354*(2), 166–178.
52. Pui, C. H., Sandlund, J. T., Pei, D., Campana, D., Rivera, G. K., Ribeiro, R. C., et al. (2004). Improved outcome for children with acute lymphoblastic leukemia: Results of total therapy study XIIIB at St Jude Children's Research hospital. *Blood, 104*(9), 2690–2696.
53. Rowe, J. M., Buck, G., Burnett, A. K., Chopra, R., Wiernik, P. H., Richards, S. M., et al. (2005). Induction therapy for adults with acute lymphoblastic leukemia: Results of more than 1500 patients from the international ALL trial: MRC UKALL XII/ECOG E2993. *Blood, 106*(12), 3760–3767.
54. Conter, V., Arico, M., Valsecchi, M. G., Basso, G., Biondi, A., Madon, E., et al. (2000). Long-term results of the Italian association of pediatric hematology and oncology (AIEOP) acute lymphoblastic leukemia studies, 1982–1995. *Leukemia, 14*(12), 2196–2204.

55. Kamps, W. A., Bokkerink, J. P., Hakvoort-Cammel, F. G., Veerman, A. J., Weening, R. S., van Wering, E. R., et al. (2002). BFM-oriented treatment for children with acute lymphoblastic leukemia without cranial irradiation and treatment reduction for standard risk patients: Results of DCLSG protocol ALL-8 (1991–1996). *Leukemia, 16*(6), 1099–1111.

56. Silverman, L. B., Gelber, R. D., Dalton, V. K., Asselin, B. L., Barr, R. D., Clavell, L. A., et al. (2001). Improved outcome for children with acute lymphoblastic leukemia: Results of Dana-Farber consortium protocol 91-01. *Blood, 97*(5), 1211–1218.

57. Ballerini, P., Blaise, A., Busson-Le Coniat, M., Su, X. Y., Zucman-Rossi, J., Adam, M., et al. (2002). HOX11L2 expression defines a clinical subtype of pediatric T-ALL associated with poor prognosis. *Blood, 100*(3), 991–997.

58. Cave, H., Suciu, S., Preudhomme, C., Poppe, B., Robert, A., Uyttebroeck, A., et al. (2004). Clinical significance of HOX11L2 expression linked to t(5;14)(q35;q32), of HOX11 expression, and of SIL-TAL fusion in childhood T-cell malignancies: Results of EORTC studies 58881 and 58951. *Blood, 103*(2), 442–450.

59. Burkhardt, B., Bruch, J., Zimmermann, M., Strauch, K., Parwaresch, R., Ludwig, W. D., et al. (2006). Loss of heterozygosity on chromosome 6q14-q24 is associated with poor outcome in children and adolescents with T-cell lymphoblastic lymphoma. *Leukemia, 20*(8), 1422–1429.

60. Burkhardt, B., Moericke, A., Klapper, W., Greene, F., Salzburg, J., Damm-Welk, C., et al. (2008). Pediatric precursor T lymphoblastic leukemia and lymphoblastic lymphoma: Differences in the common regions with loss of heterozygosity at chromosome 6q and their prognostic impact. *Leukaemia & Lymphoma, 49*(3), 451–461.

61. Pui, C. H., Gaynon, P. S., Boyett, J. M., Chessells, J. M., Baruchel, A., Kamps, W., et al. (2002). Outcome of treatment in childhood acute lymphoblastic leukaemia with rearrangements of the 11q23 chromosomal region. *Lancet, 359*(9321), 1909–1915.

62. Armstrong, S. A., & Look, A. T. (2005). Molecular genetics of acute lymphoblastic leukemia. *Journal of Clinical Oncology, 23*(26), 6306–6315.

63. Mancini, M., Scappaticci, D., Cimino, G., Nanni, M., Derme, V., Elia, L., et al. (2005). A comprehensive genetic classification of adult acute lymphoblastic leukemia (ALL): Analysis of the GIMEMA 0496 protocol. *Blood, 105*(9), 3434–3441.

64. Ramakers-van Woerden, N. L., Pieters, R., Slater, R. M., Loonen, A. H., Beverloo, H. B., van Drunen, E., et al. (2001). In vitro drug resistance and prognostic impact of p16INK4A/P15INK4B deletions in childhood T-cell acute lymphoblastic leukaemia. *British Journal of Haematology, 112*(3), 680–690.

65. Hatano, M., Roberts, C. W., Minden, M., Crist, W. M., & Korsmeyer, S. J. (1991). Deregulation of a homeobox gene, HOX11, by the t(10;14) in T cell leukemia. *Science, 253*(5015), 79–82.

66. Cayuela, J. M., Madani, A., Sanhes, L., Stern, M. H., & Sigaux, F. (1996). Multiple tumor-suppressor gene 1 inactivation is the most frequent genetic alteration in T-cell acute lymphoblastic leukemia. *Blood, 87*(6), 2180–2186.

67. Evans, W. E., & McLeod, H. L. (2003). Pharmacogenomics–drug disposition, drug targets, and side effects. *The New England Journal of Medicine, 348*(6), 538–549.

68. Evans, W. E., & Relling, M. V. (2004). Moving towards individualized medicine with pharmacogenomics. *Nature, 429*(6990), 464–468.

69. Relling, M. V., Pui, C. H., Sandlund, J. T., Rivera, G. K., Hancock, M. L., Boyett, J. M., et al. (2000). Adverse effect of anticonvulsants on efficacy of chemotherapy for acute lymphoblastic leukaemia. *Lancet, 356*(9226), 285–290.

70. Kager, L., Cheok, M., Yang, W., Zaza, G., Cheng, Q., Panetta, J. C., et al. (2005). Folate pathway gene expression differs in subtypes of acute lymphoblastic leukemia and influences methotrexate pharmacodynamics. *Journal of Clinical Investigation, 115*(1), 110–117.

71. Pui, C. H., Sallan, S., Relling, M. V., Masera, G., & Evans, W. E. (2001). International childhood acute lymphoblastic leukemia workshop: Sausalito, CA, 30 November–1 December 2000. *Leukemia, 15*(5), 707–715.

72. Schrappe, M., Reiter, A., Ludwig, W. D., Harbott, J., Zimmermann, M., Hiddemann, W., et al. (2000). Improved outcome in childhood acute lymphoblastic leukemia despite reduced use of anthracyclines and cranial radiotherapy: Results of trial ALL-BFM 90. German-Austrian-Swiss ALL-BFM study group. *Blood, 95*(11), 3310–3322.

73. Chiaretti, S., Li, X., Gentleman, R., Vitale, A., Vignetti, M., Mandelli, F., et al. (2004). Gene expression profile of adult T-cell acute lymphocytic leukemia identifies distinct subsets of patients with different response to therapy and survival. *Blood, 103*(7), 2771–2778.

74. Uckun, F. M., Steinherz, P. G., Sather, H., Trigg, M., Arthur, D., Tubergen, D., et al. (1996). CD2 antigen expression on leukemic cells as a predictor of event-free survival after chemotherapy for T-lineage acute lymphoblastic leukemia: A children's cancer group study. *Blood, 88*(11), 4288–4295.

75. Yeoh, E. J., Ross, M. E., Shurtleff, S. A., Williams, W. K., Patel, D., Mahfouz, R., et al. (2002). Classification, subtype discovery, and prediction of outcome in pediatric acute lymphoblastic leukemia by gene expression profiling. *Cancer Cell, 1*(2), 133–143.

76. Reiter, A., Schrappe, M., Ludwig, W. D., Hiddemann, W., Sauter, S., Henze, G., et al. (1994). Chemotherapy in 998 unselected childhood acute lymphoblastic leukemia patients. Results and conclusions of the multicenter trial ALL-BFM 86. *Blood, 84*(9), 3122–3133.

77. Gaynon, P. S., Trigg, M. E., Heerema, N. A., Sensel, M. G., Sather, H. N., Hammond, G. D., et al. (2000). Children's cancer group trials in childhood acute lymphoblastic leukemia: 1983–1995. *Leukemia, 14*(12), 2223–2233.

78. Vilmer, E., Suciu, S., Ferster, A., Bertrand, Y., Cave, H., Thyss, A., et al. (2000). Long-term results of three randomized trials (58831, 58832, 58881) in childhood acute lymphoblastic leukemia: A CLCG-EORTC report. Children leukemia cooperative group. *Leukemia, 14*(12), 2257–2266.

79. Gustafsson, G., Schmiegelow, K., Forestier, E., Clausen, N., Glomstein, A., Jonmundsson, G., et al. (2000). Improving outcome through two decades in childhood ALL in the nordic countries: The impact of high-dose methotrexate in the reduction of CNS irradiation. Nordic society of pediatric haematology and oncology (NOPHO). *Leukemia, 14*(12), 2267–2275.

80. Hill, F. G., Richards, S., Gibson, B., Hann, I., Lilleyman, J., Kinsey, S., et al. (2004). Successful treatment without cranial radiotherapy of children receiving intensified chemotherapy for acute lymphoblastic leukaemia: Results of the risk-stratified randomized central nervous system treatment trial MRC UKALL XI (ISRC TN 16757172). *British Journal Haematology, 124*(1), 33–46.

81. Kantarjian, H., Thomas, D., O'Brien, S., Cortes, J., Giles, F., Jeha, S., et al. (2004). Long-term follow-up results of hyperfractionated cyclophosphamide, vincristine, doxorubicin, and dexamethasone (hyper-CVAD), a dose-intensive regimen, in adult acute lymphocytic leukemia. *Cancer, 101*(12), 2788–2801.

82. Thomas, X., Boiron, J. M., Huguet, F., Dombret, H., Bradstock, K., Vey, N., et al. (2004). Outcome of treatment in adults with acute lymphoblastic leukemia: Analysis of the LALA-94 trial. *Journal of Clinical Oncology, 22*(20), 4075–4086.

83. Annino, L., Vegna, M. L., Camera, A., Specchia, G., Visani, G., Fioritoni, G., et al. (2002). Treatment of adult acute lymphoblastic leukemia (ALL): Long-term follow-up of the GIMEMA ALL 0288 randomized study. *Blood, 99*(3), 863–871.

84. Takeuchi, J., Kyo, T., Naito, K., Sao, H., Takahashi, M., Miyawaki, S., et al. (2002). Induction therapy by frequent administration of doxorubicin with four other drugs, followed by intensive consolidation and maintenance therapy for adult acute lymphoblastic leukemia: The JALSG-ALL93 study. *Leukemia, 16*(7), 1259–1266.

85. Linker, C., Damon, L., Ries, C., & Navarro, W. (2002). Intensified and shortened cyclical chemotherapy for adult acute lymphoblastic leukemia. *Journal of Clinical Oncology, 20*(10), 2464–2471.

86. Schiffer, C. A. (2003). Differences in outcome in adolescents with acute lymphoblastic leukemia: A consequence of better regimens? Better doctors? Both? *Journal of Clinical Oncology, 21*(5), 760–761.

87. Thomas, X., Danaila, C., Le, Q. H., Sebban, C., Troncy, J., Charrin, C., et al. (2001). Long-term follow-up of patients with newly diagnosed adult acute lymphoblastic leukemia: A single institution experience of 378 consecutive patients over a 21-year period. *Leukemia, 15*(12), 1811–1822.

88. Amylon, M. D., Shuster, J., Pullen, J., Berard, C., Link, M. P., Wharam, M., et al. (1999). Intensive high-dose asparaginase consolidation improves survival for pediatric patients with T cell acute lymphoblastic leukemia and advanced stage lymphoblastic lymphoma: A pediatric oncology group study. *Leukemia, 13*(3), 335–342.

89. Wetzler, M., Sanford, B. L., Kurtzberg, J., DeOliveira, D., Frankel, S. R., Powell, B. L., et al. (2007). Effective asparagine depletion with pegylated asparaginase results in improved outcomes in adult acute lymphoblastic leukemia: Cancer and leukemia group B study 9511. *Blood, 109*(10), 4164–4167.

90. Rizzari, C., Valsecchi, M. G., Arico, M., Conter, V., Testi, A., Barisone, E., et al. (2001). Effect of protracted high-dose L-asparaginase given as a second exposure in a Berlin-Frankfurt-Munster-based treatment: Results of the randomized 9102 intermediate-risk childhood acute lymphoblastic leukemia study – A report from the Associazione Italiana Ematologia Oncologia Pediatric. *Journal of Clinical Oncology, 19*(5), 1297–1303.

91. Moghrabi, A., Levy, D. E., Asselin, B., Barr, R., Clavell, L., Hurwitz, C., et al. (2007). Results of the dana-farber cancer institute ALL consortium protocol 95-01 for children with acute lymphoblastic leukemia. *Blood, 109*(3), 896–904.

92. Hawkins, D. S., Park, J. R., Thomson, B. G., Felgenhauer, J. L., Holcenberg, J. S., Panosyan, E. H., et al. (2004). Asparaginase pharmacokinetics after intensive polyethylene glycol-conjugated L-asparaginase therapy for children with relapsed acute lymphoblastic leukemia. *Clinical Cancer Research, 10*(16), 5335–5341.

93. Avramis, V. I., Sencer, S., Periclou, A. P., Sather, H., Bostrom, B. C., Cohen, L. J., et al. (2002). A randomized comparison of native *Escherichia coli* asparaginase and polyethylene glycol conjugated asparaginase for treatment of children with newly diagnosed standard-risk acute lymphoblastic leukemia: A children's cancer group study. *Blood, 99*(6), 1986–1994.

94. Abshire, T. C., Pollock, B. H., Billett, A. L., Bradley, P., & Buchanan, G. R. (2000). Weekly polyethylene glycol conjugated L-asparaginase compared with biweekly dosing produces superior induction remission rates in childhood relapsed acute lymphoblastic leukemia: A pediatric oncology group study. *Blood, 96*(5), 1709–1715.

95. Conter, V., Schrappe, M., Arico, M., Reiter, A., Rizzari, C., Dordelmann, M., et al. (1997). Role of cranial radiotherapy for childhood T-cell acute lymphoblastic leukemia with high WBC count and good response to prednisone. Associazione Italiana Ematologia Oncologia Pediatrica and the Berlin-Frankfurt-Munster groups. *Journal of Clinical Oncology, 15*(8), 2786–2791.

96. Hunault, M., Harousseau, J. L., Delain, M., Truchan-Graczyk, M., Cahn, J. Y., Witz, F., et al. (2004). Better outcome of adult acute lymphoblastic leukemia after early genoidentical allogeneic bone marrow transplantation (BMT) than after late high-dose therapy and autologous BMT: A GOELAMS trial. *Blood, 104*(10), 3028–3037.

97. Parks, R. E., Jr., & Agarwal, R. P. (1972). In P. D. Boyer (Ed.), *The Enzymes* (pp. 483–514). New York: Academic.

98. Giblett, E. R., Anderson, J. E., Cohen, F., Pollara, B., & Meuwissen, H. J. (1972). Adenosine-deaminase deficiency in two patients with severely impaired cellular immunity. *Lancet, 2*(7786), 1067–1069.

99. Kicska, G. A., Long, L., Horig, H., Fairchild, C., Tyler, P. C., Furneaux, R. H., et al. (2001). Immucillin H, a powerful transition-state analog inhibitor of purine nucleoside phosphorylase, selectively inhibits human T lymphocytes. *Proceedings of the National Academy of Sciences of the United States of America, 98*(8), 4593–4598.

100. Gandhi, V., Kilpatrick, J. M., Plunkett, W., Ayres, M., Harman, L., Du, M., et al. (2005). A proof-of-principle pharmacokinetic, pharmacodynamic, and clinical study with purine nucleoside phosphorylase inhibitor immucillin-H (BCX-1777, forodesine). *Blood, 106*(13), 4253–4260.

101. Lambe, C. U., Averett, D. R., Paff, M. T., Reardon, J. E., Wilson, J. G., & Krenitsky, T. A. (1995). 2-amino-6-methoxypurine arabinoside: An agent for T-cell malignancies. *Cancer Research, 55*(15), 3352–3356.

102. Cohen, A., Lee, J. W., & Gelfand, E. W. (1983). Selective toxicity of deoxyguanosine and arabinosyl guanine for T-leukemic cells. *Blood, 61*(4), 660–666.

103. Hebert, M. E., Greenberg, M. L., Chaffee, S., Gravatt, L., Hershfield, M. S., Elion, G. B., et al. (1991). Pharmacologic purging of malignant T cells from human bone marrow using 9-beta-D-arabinofuranosylguanine. *Transplantation, 52*(4), 634–640.

104. Kurtzberg, J., Ernst, T. J., Keating, M. J., Gandhi, V., Hodge, J. P., Kisor, D. F., et al. (2005). Phase I study of 506U78 administered on a consecutive 5-day schedule in children and adults with refractory hematologic malignancies. *Journal of Clinical Oncology, 23*(15), 3396–3403.

105. DeAngelo, D. J., Yu, D., Johnson, J. L., Coutre, S. E., Stone, R. M., Stopeck, A. T., et al. (2007). Nelarabine induces complete remissions in adults with relapsed or refractory T-lineage acute lymphoblastic leukemia or lymphoblastic lymphoma: Cancer and leukemia group B study 19801. *Blood, 109*(12), 5136–5142.

106. Berg, S. L., Blaney, S. M., Devidas, M., Lampkin, T. A., Murgo, A., Bernstein, M., et al. (2005). Phase II study of nelarabine (compound 506U78) in children and young adults with refractory T-cell malignancies: A report from the children's oncology group. *Journal of Clinical Oncology, 23*(15), 3376–3382.

107. Cohen, M. H., Johnson, J. R., Massie, T., Sridhara, R., McGuinn, W. D., Jr., Abraham, S., et al. (2006). Approval summary: Nelarabine for the treatment of T-cell lymphoblastic leukemia/lymphoma. *Clinical Cancer Research, 12*(18), 5329–5335.

108. Bonate, P. L., Arthaud, L., Cantrell, W. R., Jr., Stephenson, K., Secrist, J. A., 3rd, & Weitman, S. (2006). Discovery and development of clofarabine: A nucleoside analogue for treating cancer. *Nature Reviews. Drug Discovery, 5*(10), 855–863.

109. Jeha, S., Gandhi, V., Chan, K. W., McDonald, L., Ramirez, I., Madden, R., et al. (2004). Clofarabine, a novel nucleoside analog, is active in pediatric patients with advanced leukemia. *Blood, 103*(3), 784–789.

110. Jeha, S., Gaynon, P. S., Razzouk, B. I., Franklin, J., Kadota, R., Shen, V., et al. (2006). Phase II study of clofarabine in pediatric patients with refractory or relapsed acute lymphoblastic leukemia. *Journal of Clinical Oncology, 24*(12), 1917–1923.

111. Choi, J., & Foss, F. (2006). Efficacy of low dose clofarabine in refractory precursor T- acute lymphoblastic leukemia. *The Yale Journal of Biology and Medicine, 79*(3–4), 169–172.

112. Omura-Minamisawa, M., Diccianni, M. B., Batova, A., Chang, R. C., Bridgeman, L. J., Yu, J., et al. (2000). In vitro sensitivity of T-cell lymphoblastic leukemia to UCN-01 (7-hydroxystaurosporine) is dependent on p16 protein status: A pediatric oncology group study. *Cancer Research, 60*(23), 6573–6576.

113. Thomas, D. A., Faderl, S., O'Brien, S., Bueso-Ramos, C., Cortes, J., Garcia-Manero, G., et al. (2006). Chemoimmunotherapy with hyper-CVAD plus Rituximab for the treatment of adult Burkitt and Burkitt-type lymphoma or acute lymphoblastic leukemia. *Cancer, 106*(7), 1569–1580.

114. Gokbuget, N., & Hoelzer, D. (2004). Treatment with monoclonal antibodies in acute lymphoblastic leukemia: Current knowledge and future prospects. *Annals of Hematology, 83*(4), 201–205.

115. Phuphanich, S., Maria, B., Braeckman, R., & Chamberlain, M. (2007). A pharmacokinetic study of intra-CSF administered encapsulated cytarabine (DepoCyt) for the treatment of neoplastic meningitis in patients with leukemia, lymphoma, or solid tumors as part of a phase III study. *Journal of Neurooncology, 81*(2), 201–208.

Chapter 13
Burkitt Lymphoma and Leukemia

Kevin A. David, Mark Roberts, LoAnn C. Peterson,
and Andrew M. Evens

Introduction

Burkitt lymphoma and Burkitt leukemia are highly aggressive B-cell malignancies characterized genetically by constitutive activation of the *c-myc* oncogene and clinically by a rapid growth phase often with extranodal presentation including frequent central nervous system (CNS) involvement. The aggressiveness of this malignancy, with a tumor doubling time of 24–48 h, necessitates prompt initiation of therapy. The British surgeon Denis Burkitt first described this disease entity in 1958 after observing a clustering of cases of children with jaw tumors spanning central East Africa [1]. He found that while surgical resection was not particularly effective against the disease, chemotherapy could treat, and in some cases, cure these neoplasms. Survival rates improved significantly first in children through the use of shorter duration, dose-intensive systemic chemotherapy protocols with early prophylaxis/treatment of the CNS. Similar therapeutic regimens have been adapted in adults using intensive multi-agent chemotherapy plans, which have resulted in similarly improved long-term survival rates.

The World Health Organization (WHO) Classification of Tumours of Hematopoietic and Lymphoid Tissues (2008) considers Burkitt lymphoma and Burkitt leukemia as different clinical manifestations of the same genetic disease [2]. This malignancy was originally termed "undifferentiated non-Burkitt's lymphoma" in the Rappaport classification [3, 4]. Under the French-American-British (FAB) Cooperative Group classification, Burkitt lymphoma with greater than 25% bone marrow involvement was referred to as L3 acute lymphoblastic leukemia (ALL) [5]. Three clinical/pathologic variants of Burkitt lymphoma have been described: the *endemic* form, commonly observed in equatorial Africa; the *sporadic* form, occurring in other geographic areas, and the *immunodeficiency* subtype, associated with human immunodeficiency virus (HIV) infection. Recent advances in the development of intensive chemotherapy regimens, as well as the incorporation of monoclonal antibodies and stem cell transplantation into treatment approaches, continue to foster improvements in patient outcomes.

Epidemiology

Burkitt lymphoma accounts for approximately 1% of all non-Hodgkin lymphomas (NHLs) [6]. An analysis of 114,548 newly diagnosed lymphoid neoplasms in 12 Surveillance, Epidemiology, and End Results (SEER) Registries (estimated to account for 14% of the US population) between 1992

A.M. Evens (✉)
Department of Medicine, Division of Hematology/Oncology, Northwestern University Feinberg School
of Medicine, Robert H. Lurie Comprehensive Cancer Center, Chicago, IL, USA
e-mail: a-evens@northwestern.edu

A.S. Advani and H.M. Lazarus (eds.), *Adult Acute Lymphocytic Leukemia*, Contemporary Hematology,
DOI 10.1007/978-1-60761-707-5_13, © Springer Science+Business Media, LLC 2011

and 2001 found approximately 1,100 new cases of Burkitt lymphoma and leukemia with an incidence rate of 0.30/100,000 person-years [7]. A male predominance was seen among cases in the analysis, with male:female incidence rate ratios of 3.3, 3.8, and 2.2 among whites, blacks, and Asians, respectively.

Endemic disease most commonly occurs in children of equatorial Africa. The incidence is particularly high in Eastern Africa, where, for example, the age-standardized incidence rate in Kyadondo County, Uganda was 4.73 per 100,000 for boys aged 0–14 and 2.98 per 100,000 for girls in the 1990s [8].

The overall risk of Burkitt lymphoma is increased approximately 200-fold in patients with HIV and acquired immune deficiency syndrome (AIDS) compared to people without AIDS [9, 10]. Burkitt lymphoma and leukemia constitute approximately 7–20% of HIV-related lymphoma [9, 11]. While the use of highly active antiretroviral therapy (HAART) has reduced the incidence of AIDS-related NHLs, in general, it has not impacted the incidence of Burkitt lymphoma and leukemia, likely due to the lack of correlation of CD4 cell count with disease development. An analysis by Biggar et al. of 325,516 adults with AIDS calculated the relative risk of Burkitt lymphoma and leukemia diagnosis in 1996–2002 (post-HAART era) compared to 1990–1995 (pre-HAART era) as 0.92 (95% CI 0.64–1.33). While declines in CD4 cell count yielded an increased risk of non-Burkitt NHL development during the post-HAART era, the same correlation was not seen in Burkitt lymphoma and leukemia, as the hazard ratio for their development per 50 CD4 cell count/μL decline was found to be 0.93 (95% CI 0.83–1.04 in 1990–1995 and 95% CI 0.81–1.06 in 1996–2002) [11].

Pathogenesis

Role of c-myc

The helix-loop-helix leucine zipper transcription factor *c-myc* regulates proteins involved in a variety of cell processes, including cellular differentiation, growth, adhesion, apoptosis, angiogenesis, and cell cycle regulation. The exact array of genes under the influence of *c-myc* is still being elucidated; however, it is clear that lymphomagenesis is related to *c-myc* dysregulation. In experimental models, dysregulation of *c-myc* results in a slowing of cellular differentiation, impaired exit from the cell cycle, and increased angiogenesis [12]. Cell cycle progression genes under *c-myc* control include *cyclin D1*, *cyclin D2*, and *p21*; apoptosis-related genes include *Bax*, *Fas/Fas ligand*, and *p53*; while cell adhesion–related processes include LFA-1 and collagen production [13, 14]. Point mutations, translocations, gene amplification, and enhanced translation all likely contribute to oncogenic aberrancies in *c-myc* activity [15]. Three *c-myc* translocations have been directly implicated in the pathogenesis of Burkitt lymphoma and leukemia cases: 80% of cases exhibit the t(8;14) translocation, characterized by the juxtaposition of the *c-myc* gene on chromosome 8 with immunoglobulin heavy chain (IgH) enhancers on chromosome 14 leading to increased *c-myc* RNA expression and protein upregulation. The remaining 20% of cases involve translocations between either chromosomes 2 and 8 leading to t(2;8)(p12;q24), resulting in *c-myc* upregulation by k-light chain enhancer elements, or chromosomes 8 and 22 leading to t(8;22)(q24;q11), resulting in gene upregulation by λ-light chain enhancers [14, 16, 17].

Each of the three clinical variants of Burkitt lymphoma and leukemia is characterized by differences in the translocational breakpoints of chromosome 8. Endemic disease typically harbors a chromosome 8 breakpoint lying approximately 100 kb upstream of *c-myc* exon 1, while chromosome 14 breakpoints occur in the joining segments of the *IgH* gene, placing the *c-myc* promoter under the control of the *IgH* Eμ enhancer [14, 16, 18–20]. Sporadic and HIV-associated variants are characterized

BCR/ABL*pos* ALL

In 1997, a preliminary analysis in 144 patients enrolled in ECOG's phase III adult ALL trial, E2993, suggested an association between BCR/ABL positivity and expression of CD25, the α-chain of the interleukin-2 receptor [19]. In that study, data were simply expressed as the percentage of blasts, which stained for CD25 with fluorescence intensity greater than 98% of the negative isotype control, without defining a positive threshold. In BCR/ABL[neg] blast cell populations, a median of 3% of blasts expressed CD25 (range 1–11%), compared with a median of 23% of CD25[pos] lymphoblasts (range 5–68%) in BCR/ABL[pos] cases (*p*=0.00006). Despite this strong association, subsequent claims regarding a unique immunophenotype displayed by BCR/ABL[pos] B-lineage ALL emphasized solely a pattern of constant CD10, CD34, CD33, and CD13, but low CD38 expression [52, 57, 58]. This may have been attributable to the more accepted, though questionable routine to define antigen positivity with >20% of blasts staining for a given antibody. The recent final analysis of E2993 firmly established the role of CD25 as a surrogate antigen for BCR/ABL positivity by classification tree analysis [20]. Most importantly, it showed that expression of CD25 on as few as ≥5% of BCR/ABL lymphoblasts significantly decreased overall survival when compared to CD25[neg] BCR/ABL[pos] lymphoblasts, which comprised a small subset of E2993 patients. In fact, CD25[neg] BCR/ABL[pos] patients had an overall survival comparable to that of BCR/ABL[neg] B-lineage ALL. This striking observation could not be explained by an effect of interleukin-2, since CD25[pos] lymphoblasts expressed the γ- but not the β-chain of the interleukin-2 receptor, in addition to CD25, the receptor's α-chain [20]. The fact that CD25 expression correlated with increased expression of stem cell markers, such as CD133, CD105, CD109, CD135, and CD123, in BCR/ABL[pos] lymphoblasts suggests that CD25[pos] BCR/ABL[pos] lymphoblasts are arrested at an immature, potentially stem cell level of B-cell differentiation.

As exemplified with data from E2993 in Table 23.2 [20], the dual expression of CD33 and CD13 in BCR/ABL[pos] lymphoblasts is independent of the stage of B-cell maturation, opposite to what is seen in BCR/ABL[neg] B-lineage ALL (compare to Table 23.1).

CD117*pos* ALL with or Without FLT3 Gene Mutations

CD117, the stem cell factor receptor, is much more frequently expressed by leukemic myeloblasts than lymphoblasts. Although CD117[pos] ALL belongs more often to the T-cell lineage, a few cases with B-cell immunophenotype have been reported [3, 59, 60]. In normal lymphopoiesis, a fraction of CD3/CD4/CD8-triple negative, CD34[pos] thymocytes, which have not yet rearranged their T-cell receptor genes, express high levels of CD117 [59]. In these thymocytes, expression of CD117 coincides with that of CD135, the FLT3 receptor tyrosine kinase encoded by the FLT3 gene [61, 62].

Table 23.2 Antigen expression in BCR/ABL[pos] B-lineage ALL patients from ECOG protocol E2993 (*N*=160)

B-ALL maturation stage	*N*	Percentage of patients with antigen expression on ≥30% of leukemic lymphoblasts			
		CD33	CD13	CD65(s)	CD15
Pro-B/Pre-Pre-B	6	40	60	20	25
Early Pre-B	141	67	79	2	4
Pre-B; transitional Pre-B	13	53	75	0	9

Pro/Pre-Pre B ALL, CD10[neg]; Early Pre-B ALL, CD10[pos]; Pre-B ALL, intracytoplasmic μ[pos]; Transitional Pre-B ALL, both intracytoplasmic and surface μ[pos]

Treatment of these T-cell progenitors with stem cell factor and FLT3 ligand propagates their differentiation along the myeloid lineage, while stem cell factor together with interleukin-7 induces their differentiation into mature T-lymphocytes [62].

Activating mutations of the FLT3 gene (internal tandem duplications, ITD, or point mutations) are the most common known genetic abnormalities in AML, but they rarely occur in ALL [61]. ECOG reported that CD117^{pos} T-lineage lymphoblasts, which may present with MPO antibody reactivity in a fraction of the T-lymphoblasts, contained FLT3-gene mutations (predominantly FLT3-ITD), provided that the blasts presented with the following unique immunophenotype: surface CD3^{neg}CD5^{neg}CD4^{neg}CD8^{neg}, positive for CD34, CD2, CD7, TdT, CD62L, CD13, CD135, and positive for T-cell lineage-specific intracytoplasmic CD3 [14]. In further support of a T-lineage affiliation, these FLT3-mutated lymphoblasts overexpressed LYL1 and LMO2 oncogenes [14], transcription factors, which have been associated with an early CD34^{pos} thymocyte phenotype in pediatric T-ALL [63]. The flow cytometric presentation of a typical case of CD117^{pos} FLT3-gene mutated T-ALL is demonstrated in Fig. 23.1.

Van Vlierberghe et al. [64] subsequently stated that in pediatric T-ALL CD117 mRNA (not protein) expression was not invariably associated with FLT3-gene mutations. Their finding that most pediatric cases expressed CD117 mRNA is intriguing but suggests that, similar to what is reported for MPO transcripts [54], CD117 mRNA might undergo posttranscriptional downregulation in ALL. After their publication in *Blood* [14], Paietta et al. realized that any deviation from the unique immune profile described above decreased the likelihood of finding FLT3-gene mutations in CD117^{pos} T-lymphoblasts (unpublished). CD117^{pos} T-ALL lacking FLT3-gene mutations expressed CD5, frequently expressed CD33 instead of CD13, and commonly lacked CD34 and CD62L. A close association between CD117 and CD13 expression in surface CD3^{neg} T-ALL has been previously reported [65]. In summary, these findings restrict FLT3-gene mutations in T-ALL to the most immature T-lymphoid maturation stage, triple surface CD4/CD8/CD3^{neg}, positive for the stem cell marker, CD34, and the cell adhesion selectin, CD62L, with overexpression of the LYL1 oncogene [63, 66].

While all of the FLT3-gene mutated cases with T-lineage phenotype on E2993 expressed the published unique CD117^{pos} antigen profile (5% of T-ALL) [14], the investigators found three patients with FLT3-ITD^{pos} B-lineage ALL (0.6% of B-Lineage ALL) (Paietta et al., unpublished). These B-lymphoblasts lacked CD117 and expressed CD19, CD10, and CD33; one of these cases contained BCR/ABL transcripts. In pediatric T-ALL, the LYL1-overexpressing, most immature cases (analogous to FLT3-gene mutated CD117^{pos} T-ALL) demonstrate relative resistance to standard chemotherapy [63]. Despite the low frequency of FLT3-gene mutations in adult ALL, the availability of a variety of FLT3-kinase inhibitors suggests a potential targeted approach in the treatment of this small ALL patient cohort.

Fig. 23.1 Illustrates the flow cytometric presentation of a case of CD117^{pos} FLT3-ITD^{pos} T-ALL with the unique immunophenotype described in the text. (**a**) Demonstrates the scattergram of isolated bone marrow mononuclear cells (MNC) according to cell size (FSC) and granularity (SSC). MNCs consisted of a residual normal myeloid component (MY), monocytes (MO), and a dominant fraction with low granularity but variable size (LY, lymphocytes, and BL, blasts). (**b**) Demonstrates staining of the lymphoblasts with CD34, the antibody that was used to gate the blasts in all other antibody combinations. Noteworthy, CD34 intensity ranged widely. However, as seen in contour plot 1c, all of the CD34-gated blasts expressed CD117 confirming that they all were part of the leukemia population. (**c**) Shows that CD34^{pos} blasts expressed CD117 but lack predominantly surface CD3. Although in this contour plot, CD3 is conjugated with fluorescein-isothiocyanate, which usually yields weak CD3 staining, this weak surface CD3 expression was reproduced with other fluorochromes. (**d**) Shows co-expression of CD7 and CD13 by the blast cells. The *arrow* points at a tiny subpopulation of CD7^{pos}CD13^{neg} cells, which could represent normal T-lymphocytes (<0.5% of MNC). Contour plot (**e**) shows that CD34^{pos}CD117^{pos} lymphoblasts expressed intracytoplasmic CD3, a specific marker for the T-cell lineage. Contour plot (**f**) demonstrates the strong expression of surface CD2 in the absence of CD5

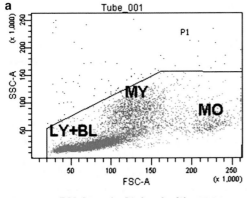

BM Sample Stained with CD34

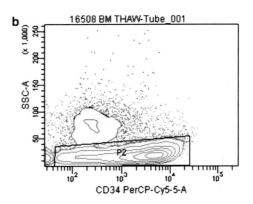

Staining of lymphoblasts with CD34

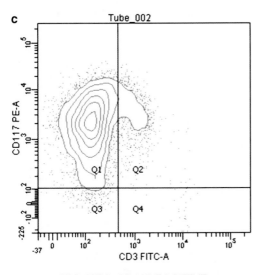

CD3 NEG CD117 POSITIVE

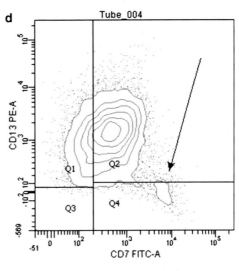

CD7 AND CD13 DOUBLE POSITIVE

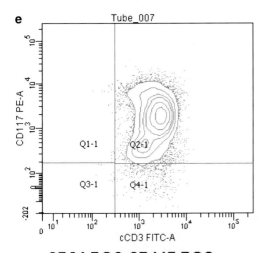

CD34 POS CD117 POS
Lymphoblasts express
intracytoplasmic CD3

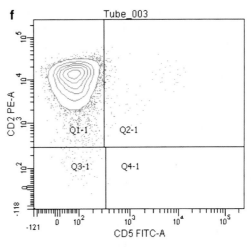

CD2 POS
CD5 NEG

NOTCH1-Mutated T-ALL with Myeloid Features

Aberrant, ligand-independent activation of NOTCH1-receptor signaling is a hallmark finding in T-ALL [67]. Activating NOTCH1 gene mutations are found in >50% of pediatric T-ALLs [68] and carry a favorable diagnosis [69, 70]. While a comparably high frequency of NOTCH1 mutations has been found in adult T-ALL cases [71], prognostic implications remain controversial.

Despite the high incidence of NOTCH1 gene mutations in T-ALL, information regarding an immunophenotypic correlate is remarkably scarce. A predominance of the common cortical T-cell maturation stage among NOTCH1-mutated patients has been observed in children [69]. Cortical thymocyte T-ALL represents an intermediate stage of differentiation, characterized by expression of CD1, double positivity for CD4/CD8, and occasional appearance of CD10 [3]. In children as well as adult T-ALL, the CD1^{pos} cortical thymocyte immunophenotype has been associated with favorable outcome when compared with other immunophenotypic profiles [7, 72, 73]. In pediatric T-ALL, this cortical thymocyte stage is furthermore characterized by constitutive HOX11 oncogene expression [63], which carries favorable prognosis both in pediatric [63, 74, 75] and adult disease [10, 76]. This raises the question whether the superior outcome in early cortical thymocyte T-ALL in children is related to NOTCH1-mutation or HOX11 expression.

Contrary to what is seen in pediatric NOTCH1-mutated T-ALL [69], the recent analysis of phenotypic characteristics of NOTCH1-mutated patients in adult ALL trial, E2993, surprisingly showed that only one-third of patients demonstrated the typical cortical thymocyte phenotype with surface CD3^{neg}, CD1^{pos}, and double CD4/CD8^{pos} antigen profile [77]. As a side note, since there is no standardized nomenclature for thymocyte differentiation stages in T-ALL, this chapter will simply refer to cortical thymocyte T-ALL in the presence of CD1 and simultaneous expression of CD4/CD8. Wouters et al. [78] described a novel "AML" subtype characterized by mutations in NOTCH1 and silenced CEBPA gene. Careful evaluation of their data, however, points strongly at an affiliation of these cases with the T-lymphoid rather than myeloid lineage. By flow cytometry, their NOTCH1-mutated cases expressed CD7, CD34, TdT, CD33, and CD13; remarkably though there were high levels of mRNA for CD3, weak expression of surface CD3 in one of the six specimens, rearrangements of T-cell receptor genes, and expression of the T-cell-specific Src-family kinase LCK. Unfortunately, these investigators had made the diagnosis of "AML" based on FAB criteria and had tested neither cCD3 nor MPO flow cytometrically. Although not proven by gene expression profiling, these cases [78] illustrate close similarity to CD1^{neg} NOTCH1-mutated T-ALLs from E2993, which demonstrated dual expression of CD33 and CD13 in 7/12 cases, and CD13 alone in the remaining five [77]. In all NOTCH1-mutated T-ALL patients from E2993, T-lineage affiliation was unequivocally confirmed by staining for cCD3 and absence of MPO reactivity. Thus, there is a possibility that a difference in T-cell differentiation levels associated with NOTCH1 mutation could account for distinct prognostic implications in children versus adults.

T-ALL with HOX11/TLX1 Overexpression

The regulation and subsequent expression of homeobox containing HOX genes is tightly linked to the development of acute leukemias [79, 80]. Both in pediatric and adult T-ALL, deregulation of the HOX11/TLX1 gene, which is situated at chromosome 10q24, is found much more frequently (about 20% of adults and 5% of children) [76] than 10q24 translocations which yield HOX11/TLX1 gene activation (8–10% in adults and <1% in children) [74, 76]. Because standard karyotyping may not reveal the (10,14)(q24;q11) or (7,10)(q35;q24) translocations, the definition of an immunophenotypic surrogate is of great interest, given that HOX11/TLX1 overexpression is associated with favorable outcome both in pediatric [63, 74, 75] and adult T-ALL [10, 76]. It appears

Chapter 2
Acute Lymphocytic Leukemia – Clinical Features and Making the Diagnosis

Olga Frankfurt, LoAnn Petersen, and Martin S. Tallman

Presentation: Signs, Symptoms and Laboratory Features

The clinical presentation of acute lymphocytic leukemia (ALL) may range from insidious nonspecific symptoms to severe acute life-threatening manifestations, reflecting the extent of bone marrow involvement and degree of extramedullary spread (Table 2.1). In younger patients anemia-induced fatigue may be the only presenting feature. Dyspnea, angina, dizziness, and lethargy may reflect the degree of anemia in older patients presenting with ALL. Approximately half of all patients may present with fever attributable to the pyrogenic cytokines, such as IL-1, IL-6, TNF, released from the leukemic cells, infection, or both. Arthralgia and bone pain due to the bone marrow expansion by the leukemic cells and occasionally necrosis can be observed, although less commonly in adults compared to children. Pallor, petechiae, and ecchymosis in the skin and mucous membranes due to thrombocytopenia, DIC, or a combination of the above may be observed. ALL may present with either leukopenia (~20%) or moderate ($50\%-5-25 \times 10^9$/L) and severe leukocytosis ($10\%->100 \times 10^9$/L). Neutropenia is common. The majority of patients present with platelet counts less than 100×10^9/L (75%), while 15% have platelet counts of less than 10×10^9/L.

Superior Vena Cava Syndrome/Mediastinal Mass

Patients with ALL (particularly T-ALL), may present with symptoms of cough, dyspnea, stridor, or dysphagia from tracheal and esophageal compression by a mediastinal mass (15% of patients) (Fig. 2.1). Compression of the great vessels by a bulky mediastinal mass also may lead to the life-threatening superior vena cava syndrome. In addition to the above mentioned symptoms, patient may develop cyanosis, facial edema, increased intracranial pressure, and syncope.

Neurological Complications

At the time of the diagnosis, 5–10% of adult patients with ALL have evidence of leukemic involvement of the central nervous system (CNS) [1–6]. Patients with T-cell phenotype, leukocytosis (WBC $>100 \times 10^9$/L), and the presence of mediastinal mass are at a higher risk of CNS leukemia.

O. Frankfurt (✉)
Department of Medicine, Division of Hematology and Oncology, Robert H. Lurie Comprehensive Cancer Center, Feinberg School of Medicine, Northwestern University, Chicago, IL USA
e-mail: o-frankfurt@northwestern.edu

A.S. Advani and H.M. Lazarus (eds.), *Adult Acute Lymphocytic Leukemia*, Contemporary Hematology, DOI 10.1007/978-1-60761-707-5_2, © Springer Science+Business Media, LLC 2011

Table 2.1 Clinical features of adult acute lymphocytic leukemias

Clinical and laboratory findings	Signs and symptoms
Anemia	Pallor, fatigue, exertional dyspnea, CHF
Neutropenia	Fever (~50%), infection (<30%)
Thrombocytopenia	Petechiae, ecchymosis, retinal hemorrhages
Leukocytosis (10% of patients with WBC>100,000)	Hepatomegaly, splenomegaly (~50%), lymphadenopathy
	Bone pain and joint pain (5–20%)
	Leukemia cutis
Leukostasis	Dyspnea, hypoxia, mental status changes
Mediastinal Mass (80% of patients with T-cell ALL)	Cough, dyspnea, chest pain
CNS involvement (<10%)	Headache, diplopia, cranial neuropathies, particularly cranial nerves VI, VIII, papilledema, nausea, vomiting
Testicular involvement (<1%)	Painless testicular/scrotal enlargement
Elevated prothrombin time (PT), partial thromboplastin time (PTT), low fibrinogen	Intracranial bleeding, DIC
Acute renal failure (uncommon), acidosis, hypekalemia, hyperphosphatemia, hypocalcemia, elevated serum LDH and, uric acid level	Tumor lysis syndrome

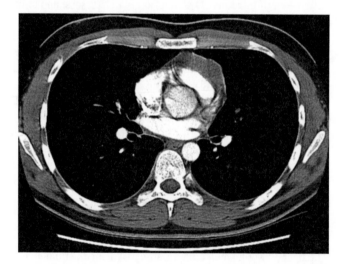

Fig. 2.1 60×20 mm anterior mediastinal mass in the thymic bed of a 22-year-old patient presenting with T-ALL

CNS involvement may manifest as generalized headache and papilledema from elevated intracranial pressure; visual impairment due to the unilateral and bilateral optic nerve infiltration; as well as direct ocular involvement via infiltration of the orbit, retina, iris, cornea, conjunctiva; trigeminal neuralgia secondary to seventh cranial nerve infiltration and leukemic meningitis; transverse myelopathy; and epidural spinal cord compression [7–9]. In a study of 36 patients with CNS leukemia (46 episodes of CNS involvement) 21.7% of the episodes involved the cranial nerves, most commonly the bulbar motor, facial, and optic nerves [10].

Testicular Involvement

In adults, testicular involvement with ALL is uncommon at the time of diagnosis (<1%) (Fig. 2.2). However, it is frequently observed at the time of disease recurrence, typically heralding systemic

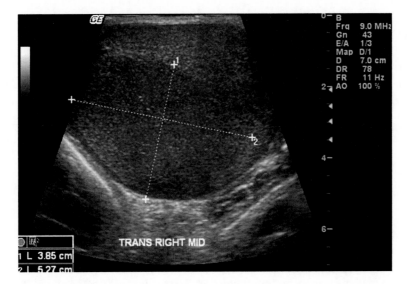

Fig. 2.2 Testicular involvement with T-ALL. 3.85 cm × 5.27 cm hypoechoic lesion involving the right testicle in a 23-year-old male with T-ALL

relapse within months. It may present with painless lesions, often involving the endothelial side of the interstitium of one or both testis, as well as increased testicular size and firmness [11]. Hydrocele resulting from lymphatic obstruction may also present with painless scrotal enlargement and is readily identified by ultrasonography.

Other Organ Involvement

Leukemic cells may infiltrate virtually any organ system. Lymphadenopathy and hepatosplenomegaly are frequently observed, more commonly in T-cell disease. Patients presenting with diffuse abdominal pain require immediate evaluation by the surgeon, due to a high mortality rate (100%) from bowel perforation attributable to leukemic infiltrates [12]. Cases of splenic rupture from leukemic infiltrates, priapism due to leukostasis in the corpora cavernosa and dorsal vein, and sacral involvement in ALL have been described [13, 14]. Asymmetric arthritis involving larger joints attributed to the direct leukemic infiltration of the synovial membrane and fluid, hemorrhage in the synovial space, and secondary metabolic and immunologic disturbances may rarely herald the onset of ALL in adults [15–18]. Other uncommon presenting features include direct skin infiltration (leukemia cutis), enlarged salivary glands, and epidural spinal cord compression [19].

Hyperleukocytosis and Leukostasis

Although hyperleukocytosis is a common presenting feature (10–30%) in patients with ALL, particularly with T-cell phenotype, 11q23, and t(9;22) chromosomal rearrangements, symptomatic leukostasis is exceedingly rare [20, 21]. While WBC count is a major factor contributing to microvessel occlusion seen with leukostasis, other features, such as activation of adhesion cell surface markers and mechanical properties of the leukemic blasts, are likely to be important. For example, the stiffness of myeloid blasts, as measured by atomic force microscopy, is 18 times that of lymphoid blasts [22]. This difference in deformability of the cells may at least partially explain the increased frequency of leukostasis in acute myeloid leukemia (AML) compared to than in ALL. Presence of symptoms suggestive of leukostasis, such as headache, blurred vision, dyspnea, hypoxia, constitute a medical emergency and efforts should be made to lower the WBC rapidly. The role of leukapheresis to reduce tumor burden in patients with ALL and leukocytosis remains controversial. Historically, leukapheresis has been used in ALL patients presenting with neurological and pulmonary symptoms of leukostasis or a blast count exceeding $100\text{--}200 \times 10^9/L$ [23].

DIC

Disseminated intravascular coagulation (DIC) is a known complication of adult ALL and has been reported in 10–16% of patients at presentation [24]. Hypofibrinogenemia (<100 mg/dL) was detected in 41% of patients with ALL at the time of diagnosis and after initiation of therapy [25]. Hemorrhagic symptoms usually are mild; however, serious hemorrhage occurs in 20% of patients with laboratory evidence of DIC [24]. Patients who develop DIC tend to have higher WBC ($77.9 \times 10^9/L$ vs. $9.4 \times 10^9/L$) counts and a higher frequency of palpable spleens than patients who do not develop DIC. However, no statistically significant relationship has been established between DIC and age, FAB subtype, immunophenotype, karyotype, LDH, and percentage of blasts in the bone marrow. An etiologic link between CD34 expression and DIC has been suggested [26].

Metabolic Complications

Severe metabolic abnormalities may accompany the initial diagnosis of ALL [27].

Patients with high leukemic burden are at risk of developing acute tumor lysis syndrome (ATLS), manifested by hyperuricemia, hyperkalemia, hyperphosphatemia, and secondary hypocalcemia. Such electrolyte abnormalities may lead to the development of oliguric renal failure due to the tubular precipitation of urate and calcium phosphate crystals, fatal cardiac arrhythmias, hypocalcemic tetany, and seizures.

Hyperkalemia, defined by a serum potassium concentration of >6 mmol/L, caused by massive cellular degradation, may precipitate significant neuromuscular (muscle weakness, cramps, paresthesias) and potentially life threatening cardiac (asystole, ventricular tachycardia, and ventricular fibrillation) abnormalities [28].

Hypocalcemia, one of the most dangerous sequelae of ATLS, may result in potentially lethal cardiac (ventricular arrhythmias, heart block) and neurological (hallucination, seizures, coma) manifestations [28].

Severe *hypercalcemia* is a rare, yet serious manifestation of ALL, reported in <5% patients at diagnosis [29]. Patients may experience severe malaise, diffuse abdominal pain, emesis, and changes in mental status. Both humoral and local mechanisms have been implicated in the pathogenesis of hypercalcemia in ALL [30]. Paraneoplastic production of parathyroid hormone-related protein (PTHrP) is thought to be responsible for hypercalcemia via a humoral effect, while osteolytic skeletal metastasis and cytokines, such as TNF-α, IL-6, and IL-2 may be responsible for local osteolytic hypercalcemia [31, 32]. Occasionally, a combination of high calcium and phosphorus concentration leads to the calcinosis cutis syndrome – an aberrant deposition of calcium salts in the skin [33].

Lactic Acidosis

Primary leukemia-induced lactic acidosis (LA) is a rare yet potentially fatal event, characterized by low arterial pH due to the accumulation of blood lactate. It has been suggested that LA occurring in the setting of hematological malignancy is associated with an extremely poor prognosis [34]. Lactate, the end product of anaerobic glycolysis, is metabolized to glucose by the liver and kidneys. Because leukemic cells have a high rate of glycolysis even in the presence of oxygen and produce a large quantity of lactate, LA may result from an imbalance between lactate production and hepatic lactate utilization [34]. Several factors may contribute to the high rate of glycolysis. Overexpression or aberrant expression of glycolytic enzymes, such as hexokinase, the first rate-limiting enzyme in the glycolytic pathway [35] allows leukemic blasts to proliferate rapidly and survive for prolonged periods [36]. Although insulin normally regulates the expression of this enzyme, insulin-like growth factors (IGFs) that are overexpressed by malignant leukemic cells, can mimic insulin activity [37–39]. LA is frequently associated with ATLS and its extent is correlated with the severity of ATLS. Typically, the patient with lactic acidosis presents with weakness, tachycardia, nausea, mental status changes, hyperventilation, and hypotension, which may progress to frank shock as acidosis worsens. Laboratory studies show a decreased blood pH (<7.37), a widened anion gap (>18), and a low serum bicarbonate.

Making the Diagnosis

The diagnosis of ALL is typically established by the examination of peripheral smear and bone marrow (BM) aspirate and core biopsy (Figs. 2.3 and 2.4). It is based on cell morphology, cytochemistry, as well as immunophenotypic, cytogenetic, and molecular features. Biologically, ALL and lymphoblastic lymphoma (LBL) are considered to be the same disorder and when it involves both the nodal structures and peripheral blood/BM, the distinction is arbitrary. By convention, the diagnosis of LBL is used when the process is confined to nodal structures with no or minimal involvement of peripheral blood and the bone marrow. In many clinical protocols, marrow involvement with >25% lymphoblasts is used to differentiate ALL from LBL.

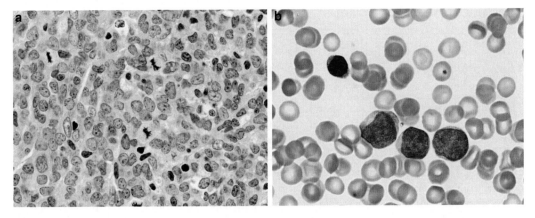

Fig. 2.3 Peripheral smear and a core biopsy from a patient with Ph+ B-ALL. (**a**) Core biopsy from a patient with Ph+ B-ALL, demonstrating numerous lymphoblasts with a high mitotic rate. (**b**) Peripheral smear from a patient with Ph+ B-ALL, demonstrating 3 larger blasts next to a normal mature lymphocyte

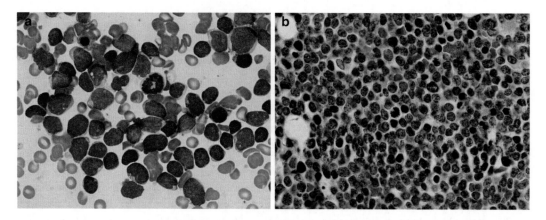

Fig. 2.4 Bone marrow aspirate and core biopsy from a patient with T-ALL. (**a**) Bone marrow core biopsy from a patient with T-ALL, demonstrating extensive involvement with leukemic blasts and a high mitotic rate. (**b**) Bone marrow aspirate from a patient with T-ALL, demonstrating a large number of blasts

To evaluate for the presence of CNS involvement, a lumbar puncture (LP) is typically performed on patients with ALL. The presence of at least 5 leukocytes per µL of CSF (with leukemic blasts apparent in the sample) or the presence of cranial nerve palsies defines CNS leukemia. There is an ongoing debate regarding the clinical significance of leukemic blasts present in the CSF sample at a level <5 WBC/µL (CNS2 status). In several, but not all trials, CNS2 status was linked to an increased risk of CNS and systemic relapse, likely due to the difference in the efficacy of systemic and CNS-directed therapy between the studies [40, 41] The timing of performing diagnostic LP is not universally agreed upon. Historically, LP was often postponed until blasts were cleared from the peripheral blood, to avoid "seeding" of the CSF and obtaining false positive results due to contamination of the sample with blood as a result of traumatic puncture. Recently, there has been a tendency to follow pediatric protocols for young adults where LP is performed on day one of starting chemotherapy. Regardless of the timing, traumatic lumbar puncture *should be avoided*. The previously shown increased risk of CNS relapse and poor event-free survival associated with traumatic lumbar puncture may be overcome by more intensive therapy [42, 43]. However, in the setting of traumatic lumbar puncture, the *efficacy* of intrathecal chemotherapy might be compromised as the result of the collapse of the thecal sac due to the hematoma or CNS fluid collection [42].

It has been our practice to provide intensive systemic and intrathecal therapy to patients identified as having CNS2 status or traumatic LP with the presence of blasts, to reduce the risk of relapse.

Morphologic Assessment

The evaluation of ALL begins with morphologic analysis of the peripheral blood and bone marrow aspirate smears. The FAB classification describing three morphologic subtypes (L1, L2, and L3) is primarily of *historic* significance, but highlights well the range of morphological appearance of the leukemic blasts in terms of cell size, amount of cytoplasm, prominence of nucleoli, and degree of cytoplasmic basophilia. The appearance of the leukemic blasts vary from small cells with coarsely reticular nuclear chromatin pattern, scant cytoplasm, and indistinct nucleoli to larger cells with finely dispersed nuclear chromatin, moderately abundant cytoplasm, and prominent nucleoli. Vacuoles might be present, but only rarely are they as prominent as in Burkitt lymphoma. Cytoplasmic granules are found in a small number of cases. Auer rods are absent. Morphologically, acute B-cell leukemia is indistinguishable from T-cell ALL.

The bone marrow biopsy sections involved with ALL are typically markedly hypercellular, but may be normocellular or hypocellular in rare cases. The bone marrow is replaced by a uniform, diffuse proliferation of lymphoblasts; normal hematopoietic cells are markedly reduced. In most cases the lymphoblasts are monotonous in appearance with finely dispersed chromatin patterns, scant cytoplasm, round to oval, indented or convoluted nuclei and variably conspicuous nucleoli. Mitotic activity is variable but is usually brisk and mitotic figures are almost always easy to identify. Reticulin fibrosis is present in a minority of cases.

Cytochemical Assessment

There is no cytochemical stain that is pathognomonic for the ALL. Lymphoblasts are always negative for myeloperoxidase. They are typically negative for Sudan black-B but rare cases might be positive. PAS (periodic acid-Shiff) is often positive in the form of coarse granules or clumps in the cytoplasm. Nonspecific esterase may be positive in a minority of cases, usually in a focal or punctuate pattern of reactivity in a proportion of the blasts. Acid phosphatase is typically negative but may be present in the form of weak scattered granular positivity.

Immunophenotypic Assessment

In adult ALL, approximately 75% of cases are of B- and 25% of T-lineage. However, lineage assignment of ALL cannot be established by the morphologic evaluation alone. Immunophenotyping is essential in the work-up of patients with ALL. Immunophenotyping by flow cytometry became a preferred method of lineage assessment due to its ease of application in clinical settings and to its ability to analyze multiple antigens simultaneously on each cell. Immunohistochemical stains on bone marrow biopsy sections can be performed as an alternative since a wide variety of antibodies to both lymphoid- and myeloid-associated antigens reactive in paraffin-embedded sections are now available. Most leukocyte antigens lack specificity; hence, a *panel* of antibodies is required to establish the diagnosis and to distinguish among the different immunologic subtypes of leukemic cells.

The lymphoblasts in B-ALL are almost always positive for the B-cell markers: CD19, cytoplasmic CD79a, and cytoplasmic CD22. None of these markers by itself are specific for B-lineage leukemia, but their expression on the lymphoblasts in combination strongly supports the diagnosis. CD20 is specific for B-lineage, but is often dimly expressed or negative in B-ALL. CD79a and PAX5 are the most frequently utilized antibodies to document B-cell differentiation in *tissue sections*; however, they are not specific. CD79a reacts with some cases of T-ALL and both CD79a and PAX5 can react with cases of AML. HLA-DR is present on the lymphoblasts of most cases of B-ALL. Most cases lack surface immunoglobulins, but their presence, often in low density, does not preclude the diagnosis of B-ALL. TdT (terminal deoxynucleotidyl transferase) is expressed in most cases of B-ALL, while CD34 expression is identified in approximately 75% of cases. CD10 is present on the lymphoblasts in about 25% cases of *adult* B-ALL.

Based on various combinations of antigen expression, B-ALL can be further divided into immunophenotypic subtypes, which *roughly* parallel the stages of normal B-lymphocytes maturation (Table 2.2). However, in virtually all cases the lymphoblasts exhibit incomplete maturation and immunophenotypic asynchrony and aberrancy that deviates from the spectrum of antigen expression typical of normal B lymphocytes stages of maturation. The clinical and prognostic significance of these subtypes have been overcome by the cytogenetic characteristics and modern therapeutic approach.

Table 2.2 Immunophenotypes of ALL (From [44])

Subtype	Characteristic markers	Frequency in adult ALL
Precursor B-cell	CD19$^+$ CD22$^+$, CD79a$^+$, cIg$^{+/-}$, PAX5, sIgμ$^-$, HLA-DR$^+$ CD20, CD34 – variable expression CD45 – may be absent	~70–75%
Early precursor (pre-pre or pro-)-B cell	CD19$^+$, cCD79a$^+$, cCD22$^+$, TdT$^+$, CD10$^-$	~10%
Common (early pre)-B cell	CD10$^+$	~50–65%
Pre-B cell	CD10$^{+/-}$, c-μ$^+$	~10%
Precursor T-cell	TdT$^+$, CD7$^+$, cCD3$^+$ (lineage specific); HLA-DR$^{+/-}$, CD1a$^{+/-}$, CD2$^{+/-}$, CD4$^{+/-}$, CD5$^{+/-}$, CD7$^{+/-}$, CD8$^{+/-}$	~20–25%
Pro-T	cCD3$^+$, CD7$^+$, CD2$^-$, CD1a$^-$, CD34$^{+/-}$CD4$^-$, CD8$^-$	
Pre-T	cCD3$^+$, CD7$^+$, CD2$^+$, CD1a$^-$, CD34$^{+/-}$CD4$^-$, CD8$^-$	
Cortical T	cCD3$^+$, CD7$^+$, CD2$^+$, CD1a$^+$, CD34$^-$CD4$^+$, CD8$^+$	
Medullary T	cCD3$^+$, CD7$^+$, CD2$^+$, CD1a$^-$, CD34$^-$sCD3$^+$; either CD4$^+$ or CD8$^+$	

cCD3 – cytoplasmic CD3; c-μ$^+$ – cytoplasmic chains; cIg – cytoplasmic immunoglobulin; sIg – surface immunoglobulin; TdT – terminal deoxynucleotidyl transferase

In T-ALL, the lymphoblasts express the T-cell associated antigens – CD7, CD5 and CD2 – in over 90% of cases. Cell surface expression of CD3 is often lacking in T-ALL, but cytoplasmic CD3 is present in virtually *all cases* and is considered the most specific marker for T-lineage. CD1a positivity and co-expression of CD4 and CD8 are found in approximately 1/3 of cases. TdT is positive in most cases and CD34 expression is variable. CD10 may be positive. Based on the type and pattern of antigen expression T-ALL may be stratified into categories corresponding to various stages of intrathymic differentiation (Table 2.2).

Up to 50% of patients with B- or T-ALL may co-express both lymphoid and myeloid markers [45]. The most frequently co-expressed myeloid markers are CD13 and CD33. Their presence does not exclude ALL nor indicate a mixed phenotype. The lymphoblasts in ALL are negative for myeloperoxidase, a more specific marker for myeloid lineage than CD13 and CD33. Over the years, there has been a debate whether the presence of myeloid antigens confers a worse survival [45]. It appears that with modern therapeutic approaches, the presence of myeloid antigens has no prognostic significance [46].

Genetic Analysis

Recurrent genetic alterations occur in 66–85% of patients with ALL and can be detected by the traditional cytogenetic analysis, fluorescent in situ hybridization (FISH), and reverse transcriptase polymerase chain reaction (RT-PCR) [47–50]. These diagnostic tools allow for the precise determination of specific ALL genotype that provide important prognostic and therapeutic information (Table 2.3). In fact, cytogenetics is the single-most important prognostic factor of overall survival (OS) and relapse-free survival (RFS) in patients with ALL [48] (Fig. 2.5). The results of the recently published UKALLXII/ECOG2993 trial highlighted the prognostic significance and further defined cytogenetic abnormalities for adult patients with ALL [49]. Patients with Philadelphia positive (Ph+) chromosome, t(4;11), t(8;14), complex karyotype (defined by at least five chromosomal abnormalities), or low hypodiploidy/near triploidy had significantly inferior rates of event-free survival (EFS) and OS compared to patients with high hyperdiploidy or del(9p). Among the Ph$^-$ ALL patients, t(8;14), complex karyotype, and low hypodiploidy/near triploidy were significant

The Société Française d'Oncologie Pediatrique also achieved impressive cure rates with the Lymphomes Malins B (LMB) protocols that incorporated a cytoreductive phase of cyclophosphamide, vincristine, and prednisone with the goal of diminishing the tumor burden while minimizing tumor lysis and myelosuppression, followed by induction consisting of vincristine, cyclophosphamide, doxorubicin, high-dose methotrexate, and prednisone. Consolidation in the LMB 84 trial consisted of cytarabine and methotrexate, while this phase of therapy incorporated etoposide and cytarabine in the LMB 86 trial [90]. The two most recently reported LMB protocols have been LMB 89 and LMB 96. The aims of LMB 89 were to confirm the results of the earlier LMB protocols and to adapt treatment strategies to tumor burden and to the initial response to chemotherapy [91]. A total of 561 eligible patients younger then 18 years with Burkitt lymphoma, DLBCL, or L3 ALL were enrolled and classified into one of three treatment groups based on the Murphy staging system – group A consisting of those with completely resected stage I or abdominal stage II disease; group B consisting of those with unresected stage I, non-abdominal stage II, any stage III or IV disease or L3 ALL without CNS involvement and fewer than 70% bone marrow blasts; and group C consisting of those patients with CNS involvement or L3 ALL with at least 70% bone marrow blasts. Burkitt lymphoma was confirmed by central pathologic review in 420 patients. Fifty-two patients were assigned to group A, the lowest risk group, and received two courses of induction therapy with cyclophosphamide, vincristine, prednisone, and adriamycin (COPAD). A total of 386 patients were treated in group B, the intermediate risk group; they received one course of prephase chemotherapy consisting of cyclophosphamide, vincristine, prednisone (COP) and intrathecal methotrexate followed by two courses of induction chemotherapy that consisted of cyclophosphamide, vincristine, prednisone, adriamycin, and methotrexate – similar to the COPAD induction of group A with the addition of systemic and intrathecal methotrexate. Group B patients then went on to receive two courses of consolidation high-dose methotrexate and cytarabine with intrathecal methotrexate and cytarabine. Finally, they received one course of maintenance chemotherapy comprising cyclophosphamide, adriamycin, high-dose methotrexate, intrathecal methotrexate, prednisone, and vincristine. The 123 patients in group C received one cycle of COP prephase therapy, two cycles of COPADM induction therapy modified to include intrathecal cytarabine and an escalated dose of high-dose methotrexate, and two cycles of consolidation containing infusional and high-dose cytarabine and VP-16, followed by four cycles of maintenance chemotherapy and CNS irradiation for those with CNS involvement. A CR was obtained in 97% of patients. With a median follow-up of 64 months, median 5-year OS and EFS were 92.5% and 91%, respectively, for the entire study population. Those same rates, respectively, were 100% and 98% in group A; 94% and 92% for group B; and 85% and 84% for group C. The main toxicities of therapy were febrile neutropenia (75% of patients), mucositis, and myelosuppression requiring transfusions. The study confirmed that children with a lower disease burden could be effectively treated with less intensive therapy and concluded that pediatric DLBCL could be treated like Burkitt lymphoma.

Given these results, the same group developed the FAB/LMB96 protocol to evaluate the feasibility of reducing the treatment intensity for patients with intermediate-risk (group B, as above) disease, with a regimen modified from the LMB89 protocol [92]. A total of 637 patients were analyzed in this study, in which those patients with early responsive disease (>20% tumor response at day 7) were randomized among four arms in a factorial design, with two arms containing a 50% reduction in the cyclophosphamide dose in the second induction course (COPADM) and two arms omitting the maintenance chemotherapy course. Neither the reduction of the cyclophosphamide dose nor the omission of the maintenance chemotherapy phase impacted OS or EFS.

Cairo et al. on behalf of the FAB/LMB96 International Study Committee, investigated the feasibility of shortening treatment for children with high-risk disease (group C as described in the LMB89 protocol, above) [93]. The trial enrolled 235 eligible patients and 199 patients with a >20% response to COP prephase therapy who were randomized to either standard FAB/LMB96 protocol therapy or to reduced intensity/duration therapy, in which the consolidation high-dose cytarabine and etoposide doses of the consolidation phase were reduced. Additionally, patients in the experimental reduced intensity/duration arm received only one cycle of maintenance therapy compared to the standard four cycles. Randomization was halted in the middle of the trial after an interim analysis suggested a benefit to the standard-therapy arm.

Adult Trials

Building upon the backbone of promising therapeutic regimens in pediatric populations, studies of adult patients published in the 1990s utilized similar regimens incorporating shorter-duration, high-intensity strategies with non-cross-resistant agents, with minimal treatment breaks, and thorough CNS prophylaxis (Tables 13.4 and 13.5). Among the earliest studies showing successful results with this strategy were reports from Stanford University and Vanderbilt University. The Stanford group treated 18 adult patients with high-dose cyclophosphamide, doxorubicin, vincristine, prednisone, high-dose methotrexate, and intrathecal methotrexate [104]. Chemotherapy was administered every 21 days for six to ten cycles. Patients with abdominal masses greater than 10 cm in size received radiation. The study had a median follow-up of 1.2 years with actuarial survival of 6% and relapse-free survival of 71%. The Vanderbilt group treated 20 patients with an intensive inpatient regimen containing cyclophosphamide, etoposide, vincristine, bleomycin, methotrexate, and prednisone [105]. In patients without CNS disease, intrathecal chemotherapy was administered at the individual investigator's discretion. CR was achieved in 85% of patients; 65% of patients remained disease-free at a median follow-up of 29 months.

Soussain et al. performed a retrospective analysis of adults with L3 ALL or SNCCL treated with the LMB protocols. Eighty-nine percent of patients achieved a CR. The 3-year OS rate was 74%. Among patients with Murphy stage I and II disease, the 3-year OS rate was 100%; among patients with stage III disease 80%; and among those with stage IV disease and L3 ALL 57% [90]. A multicenter prospective trial of the LMB95 protocol enrolled 72 adult patients, stratifying them into three groups based on the risk factors of modified St. Jude stage, resection status, CNS involvement, and bone marrow involvement [95]. Treatment was based on the pediatric LMB protocols, albeit with some dose modifications. Seventy-two percent of patients achieved a CR. The remaining 28% of patients failed to respond to treatment and died – three due to treatment toxicity and 16 due to their disease. With a median follow-up of 32 months, 2-year EFS and OS rates were 65% and 70%, respectively.

Based on the experience of the BFM pediatric trials, the German Multicenter Study Group for Treatment of Adult ALL (GMALL) utilized three protocols for adults with L3 ALL – the conventional ALL protocol 01/81, and modified pediatric regimens B-NHL83 and B-NHL86 [94]. ALL 01/81, which included nine patients in the GMALL report comprised an 8-week induction consisting of vincristine, prednisone, daunorubicin, L-asparaginase, cyclophosphamide, cytarabine, 6-mercaptopurine (6-MP), intrathecal methotrexate, and prophylactic cranial irradiation. The same induction was repeated 3 months from the original treatment. Maintenance therapy continued for 2 years with 6-MP and vincristine. Patients with initially bulky tumor masses or white blood cell (WBC) counts > 25,000/μL underwent a cytoreductive prephase, similar to the LMB trials, consisting of vincristine and prednisone prior to induction. The B-NHL83 and B-NHL-86 protocols, which enrolled 24 and 35 evaluable patients, respectively, also included a cytoreductive prephase similar to the French LMB protocols consisting of cyclophosphamide and prednisone. B-NHL3 employed six alternating 5-day cycles – A and B – consisting of intermediate dose methotrexate, fractionated cyclophosphamide, VM26 and cytarabine in the A cycles with the B cycles consisting of the same drugs with the substitution of doxorubicin for VM26, and the omission of cytarabine. B-NHL86 also consisted of six alternating 5-day cycles as in B-NHL83 with the main modifications being the substitution of

Table 13.4 Key chemotherapy regimens, outcomes, and toxicities in adult Burkitt lymphoma/leukemia.

Trial	Number	Outcomes	Toxicity
B-NHL 83 [94]	24	CR: 63% 4-year OS: 51% 8-year OS: 49%	Grade 3/4 neutropenia: 39% Grade 3/4 thrombocytopenia: 50% Grade 3/4 anemia: 33% Grade 3/4 mucositis: 0%
B-NHL 86 [94]	35	CR: 74% 4-year OS: 51% 8-year OS: 49%	Grade 3/4 neutropenia: 81% Grade 3/4 thrombocytopenia: 35% Grade 3/4 anemia: 42% Grade 3/4 mucositis: 20% of cycles
LMB 95 [95]	72	CR: 72% 2-year EFS: 65% 2-year OS: 70%	Febrile Neutropenia: 42% of COPADM courses, 26% of CYM courses, 32% of CYVE courses Severe infection: 18% of COPADM courses, 8% of CYM courses 20% of CYVE courses Platelet transfusion: 17% of COPADM courses, 27% of CYM courses 56% of CYVE courses Red cell transfusion: 48% of COPADM courses, 45% of CYM courses 72% of CYVE courses
CODOX-M/IVAC (Magrath) [96]	41	CR: 95% 2-year EFS: 92%	Grade 4 neutropenia: 98% of all cycles A administered and 100% of all cycles B. Grade 3/4 thrombocytopenia: 48.8% of all cycles A and 100% of all cycles B (96.3% were grade 4). Grades 3 and 4 mucositis: 29% and 20.0%, respectively, of cycles A administered Neuropathy: 26 patients
United Kingdom Lymphoma Group (UKLG) [97]	52	CR: 77% 2-year EFS: 65% 2-year OS: 73% By subgroup: 2-year, EFS and OS 83% and 81.5%, respectively, while those same rates were 56% and 70% in the high-risk group.	Grade 3–4 WBC: 100% Grade 3–4 platelets: 100% High risk patients: Grade 3–4 mucositis: ~50% Low-risk patients: Grade 3–4 mucositis ~40%
Modified CODOX-M/ IVAC (Lacasce) [98]	14	CR: 86% 2-year PFS: 64% 2-year OS: 71%	Grade 3–4 neutropenia: 74% of cycles A; 100% of cycles B Grade 3–4 thrombocytopenia: 36% of cycles A; 100% of cycles B Febrile neutropenia: 17% of cycles A; 43% of cycles B Grade 3–4 mucositis: 1 case
Modified CODOX-M/ IVAC (UKLG) [99]	128 (58 with Burkitt lymphoma)	2-year PFS: 64% among Burkitt lymphoma subgroup	Grade 3–4 WBC: 99% Neutropenic fever: 80% Grade 3–4 platelets: 86% Grade 3–4 mucositis: 45% Grade 3–4 neuropathy 8%
Hyper-CVAD [100]	26	Median survival: 16 months 3-year OS: 49%	Deaths during induction: 19%

(continued)

Table 13.4 (continued)

Trial	Number	Outcomes	Toxicity
Rituximab-HyperCVAD [101]	31	CR: 86%; PR 11% 3-year OS: 89% 3-year EFS: 80% 3-year DFS: 88%	Grade 3–4 myelosuppression: 100% Febrile episodes during course 1: 45% patients; for subsequent courses, 25% after odd-numbered courses, 40% after even-numbered courses 20% of patients required vincristine dose reduction or omission due to peripheral neuropathy or ileus 14% of patients developed tumor lysis syndrome
CALGB 9251 [102]	54	CR: 80% PR: 9% 6-year OS and FFS: approximately 50%	Grade 3–4 neutropenia: 94% Grade 3–4 thrombocytopenia: 90% Grade 3–4 infection: 71% Grade 3–4 mucositis: 66%
DA-EPOCH (HIV-positive Burkitt lymphoma) [103]	39 (7 with Burkitt lymphoma)	CR: 74% PR: 13% $CD4^+ > 100/mm^3$: 87% $CD4^+ < 100/mm^3$: 56% Median follow-up 53 months: PFS 73%, OS 60% $CD4^+ > 100/mm^3$: OS 87% $CD4^+ < 100/mm^3$: OS 16%	$ANC < 500/mm^3$: 30% cycles With fever: 13% cycles Grade 3–4 anemia: 38% cycles "Serious stomatitis" < 3% cycles

Abbreviations: *IV* intravenous, *CNS* central nervous system, *CR* complete response, *OS* overall survival, *EFS* event-free survival, *DFS* disease-free survival, *FFS* failure-free survival, *ANC* absolute neutrophil count, *WBC* white blood cell, *COPADM* cyclophosphamide, vincristine, prednisone, doxorubicin, high-dose methotrexate, *CYM* cytarabine, high-dose methotrexate, *CYVE* infusional cytarabine, high-dose cytarabine, and VP16, *CODOX-M/IVAC* cyclophosphamide, vincristine, doxorubicin, methotrexate alternating with ifosfamide, VP16, cytarabine, *Hyper-CVAD* hyperfractionated cyclophosphamide, vincristine, doxorubicin, dexamethasone alternating with cytarabine and high-dose methotrexate, *CALGB* Cancer and Leukemia Group B, *DA-EPOCH* dose-adjusted infusional etoposide, infusional vincristine, infusional doxorubicin, cyclophosphamide, prednisone

ifosfamide for cyclophosphamide, the escalation of the methotrexate dose, the addition of vincristine to day 1 of each cycle, and a more intense use of leucovorin rescue. Patients treated on the B-NHL83 and B-NHL86 protocols had dramatically improved outcomes when compared to patients on the ALL 01/81 study. The CR rate was 44% among the ALL 01/81 patients compared to 63% and 74% in the latter two studies, respectively. All patients on the ALL 01/81 protocol died within 1.5 years, while OS rates in the latter two studies were 49% and 51% at 4 and 8 years.

The CODOX-M/IVAC regimen was designed by Magrath et al. and is often referred to eponymously (Table 13.4) [96]. Forty-one patients (20 adults and 21 children) were categorized as low or high risk, low risk being defined as a single extra-abdominal mass or completely resected abdominal disease with normal LDH and high risk being defined as all other cases. Low-risk patients received three courses of cycle A (CODOX-M), consisting of cyclophosphamide, adriamycin, vincristine (without dose capping on days 1 and 8 in cycle 1 and days 1, 8, and 15 in cycle 3), high-dose methotrexate, leucovorin rescue, intrathecal cytarabine on days 1 and 3, and intrathecal methotrexate on day 15. Patients with high-risk disease were treated with alternating courses of cycles A and B (IVAC) for a total of 4 cycles. Cycle B consisted of ifosfamide with mesna to prevent hemorrhagic cystitis, etoposide, high-dose cytarabine, and intrathecal methotrexate on day 5. Patients with CNS involvement at presentation received more intensive intrathecal chemotherapy. Patients with high-risk disease were randomized to receive GM-CSF support, as well. Ninety-five percent of patients

Table 13.5 Chemotherapy dosing of key current regimens in adult Burkitt lymphoma and leukemia*

Trial	Chemotherapy drugs, doses, and schedule

LMB 95 [95]	*Treatment groups as follows (refer to text for description of risk groups):*
	 Group A (low risk): COPAD x 3
	 Group B (intermediate risk): COP → COPADM1 → COPADM2 → CYM1 → CYM2 → m1
	 Group C (high risk): COP → COPADM1 → COPADM2 → CYVE1 → CYVE2 → m1 → cranial RT for CNS+ disease → m2 → m3 → m4
	 Prephase (COP):
	   Cyclophosphamide 0.3 g/m^2 IV, day 1
	   Vincristine 1 mg/m^2 (capped at 2 mg), IV, day 1
	   Prednisone 60 mg/m^2 orally or IV, daily, days 1–7
	   Intrathecal methotrexate (with hydrocortisone) 15 mg, day 1
	   Intrathecal cytarabine (with hydrocortisone) 40 mg, days 3 and 5 for high-risk group C patients only
	 Induction (COPADM1), start day 8
	   Vincristine 1.4 mg/m^2 (capped at 2 mg), IV, day 1
	   High-dose methotrexate 3 g/m^2, IV, over 3 h, day 1, with Leucovorin rescue in Group B; for dose adaptation for Group C patients, refer to text
	   Intrathecal methotrexate (with hydrocortisone) 15 mg, days 2 and 6
	   Intrathecal cytarabine (with hydrocortisone) 40 mg, day 4, in high-risk group C patients only
	   Doxorubicin 60 mg/m^2 IV day 2
	   Cyclophosphamide 0.5 g/m^2 in 2 fractions, IV, days 2, 3, 4
	   Prednisone 60 mg/m^2, IV or orally, daily, days 1–6
	 Induction (COPADM2)
	   Same as COPADM1 with the following additions:
	   Vincristine 1.4 mg/m^2 (capped at 2 mg) on day 6
	   Cyclophophamide increased to 1 g/m^2 in 2 fractions, IV, days 2, 3, 4
	   Group A patients received COPADM1 without high-dose methotrexate and additional dose of vincristine 1.4 mg/m^2 (capped at 2 mg) on day 6
	 Consolidation, Group B patients (CYM):
	   High-dose methotrexate 3 g/m^2, IV, over 3 h, day 1, with Leucovorin rescue
	   Intrathecal methotrexate (with hydrocortisone) 15 mg, day 2
	   Cytarabine 100 mg/m^2, continuous infusion, days 2–6
	   Intrathecal cytarabine (with hydrocortisone) 30 mg, day 6
	 Consolidation, Group C patients (CYVE):
	   Cytarabine 50 mg/m^2, continuous 12-h infusion, days 1–5
	   High-dose cytarabine 3 g/m^2 daily, IV over 3 h, days 2–5
	   VP16 200 mg/m^2 IV daily, days 2–5
	 Maintenance (m1)
	   Vincristine 1.4 mg/m^2 (capped at 2 mg), on day 1
	   Group B: high-dose methotrexate 3 g/m^2 IV over 3 h, day 1, with Leucovorin resuce
	   Prednisone 60 mg/m^2 orally daily days 1–5
	   Intrathecal methotrexate (with hydrocortisone) 15 mg day 2 (Group C also intrathecal cytarabine (with hydrocortisone) 40 mg, day 2)
	   Cyclophosphamide 0.5 g/m^2 IV daily, days 1–2
	   Doxorubicin 60 mg/m^2 IV day 2
	 Maintenance (m2 or m4)
	   VP16 150 mg/m^2 IV daily, days 28–30
	   Cytarabine 100 mg/m^2 SC (in two fractions) days 28–32
	 Maintenance (m3)
	   Same as m1 but without high-dose methotrexate or intrathecal chemotherapy

(continued)

Table 13.5 (continued)

Trial	Chemotherapy drugs, doses, and schedule
CODOX-M/IVAC (Magrath) [96]	Treatment groups as follows (refer to text for description of risk groups):
	High-risk: A → B → A → B
	Low-risk: A → A → A
	For high-risk patients:
	Regimen A, CODOX-M:
	Cyclophosphamide 800 mg/m^2 IV, over 30 min, day 1 then 200 mg/m^2 IV over 15 min daily, days 2–5
	Doxorubicin 40 mg/m^2, IV, day 1
	Vincristine 1.5 mg/m^2 (no maximum dose), IV, daily on days 1, 8 for cycle 1 and daily on days 1, 8, 15 for cycle 3
	Methotrexate 1,200 mg/m^2 IV over 1 h on day 10 followed immediately by 240 mg/m^2/h by continuous infusion over 23 h on day 10, with leucovorin rescue
	Filgrastim 5 mcg/kg daily sq from day 13 until ANC > 1,000/mm^3
	Regimen B, IVAC:
	Ifosfamide 1,500 mg/m^2 + mesna 360 mg/m^2 IV over 1 h daily, days 1–5
	Mesna 360 mg/m^2 IV over 15 minutes every 3 h × 6 doses 3 h after each ifosfamide + mesna administration
	Etoposide 60 mg/m^2 daily IV over 1 h daily, days 1–5
	Cytarabine 2,000 mg/m^2 IV over 3 h every 12 h × 4 doses, days 1 and 2
	Filgrastim 5 mcg/kg daily starting on day 13 as in regimen B
	Intrathecal therapy based on CNS status at presentation:
	No CNS disease at presentation:
	Regimen A
	Cytarabine 70 mg on days 1 and 3
	Methotrexate 12 mg on day 15
	Regimen B
	Methotrexate 12 mg on day 5
	CNS disease at presentation: Intrathecal therapy for the **first** cycle A and cycle B were modified as indicated below; intrathecal therapy for the second cycle A and cycle B were identical to those for patients with no CNS disease at presentation:
	Regimen A
	Cytarabine 70 mg on days 1,3, and 5
	Methotrexate 12 mg on days 15 and 17
	Regimen B
	Cytarabine 70 mg on days 7 and 9
	Methotrexate 12 mg on day 5
	For low-risk patients, modifications to regimen A as follows:
	Vincristine given only on days 1 and 8 of each cycle
	Intrathecal cytarabine 70 mg on day 1; intrathecal methotrexate 12 mg on day 3
	Following the initial treatment cycle, subsequent cycles commenced when ANC > 1,000/μL
UKLG [97]	Same as original Magrath, except Regimen A modified with the exclusion of day 15 IV vincristine during cycle 3
Modified CODOX-M (Lacasce) [98]	CODOX-M:
	Cyclophosphamide: 800 mg/m^2, IV, daily, days 1–2
	Vincristine 1.4 mg/m^2 (**maximum dose 2 mg**), IV, days 1 and 10
	Doxorubicin 50 mg/m^2 IV, day 1
	Methotrexate 3 g/m^2, IV, day 10 with leucovorin rescue

(continued)

Table 13.5 (continued)

Trial	Chemotherapy drugs, doses, and schedule
	Intrathecal methotrexate 12 mg and intrathecal cytarabine 50 mg on day 1 (with additional intrathecal cytarabine 50 mg on day 3 in high-risk patients)
	Filgrastim days 1–6 and 12–13
	IVAC:
	Ifosfamide 1,500 mg/m^2 daily, IV, days 1–5
	Mesna, days 1–5
	Etoposide 60 mg/m^2 daily, IV, days 1–5
	Cytarabine 2,000 mg/m^2, IV, every 12 h for 4 doses, days 1–2
	Intrathecal methotrexate 12 mg day 5
	Filgrastim support, days 6–13
	Main departures from original CODOX-M/IVAC in bold
	Additional intrathecal therapy for patients with CNS disease as follows:
	First cycle A: additional cytarabine 50 mg on day 5 and methotrexate 12 mg on day 10
	First cycle B: additional cytarabine 50 mg on days 3 and 5
Modified CODOX-M/IVAC (UKLG) [99]	CODOX-M:
	Cyclophosphamide: 800 mg/m^2 IV, day 1 and 200 mg/m^2 daily, IV, days 2–5
	Vincristine 1.5 mg/m^2 IV days 1 and 8 (capped at 2 mg)
	Doxorubicin 40 mg/m^2 IV day 1
	Methotrexate, age 65 or younger, 300 mg/m^2 IV over 1 h, day 10 followed by 2,700 mg/m^2 IV over 23 h; age greater than 65, 100 mg/m^2 IV over 1 h, day 10 followed by 900 mg/m^2 IV over 23 h, with Leucovorin rescue
	Intrathecal cytarabine 70 mg days 1 and 3
	Intrathecal methotrexate 12 mg day 15
	Filgrastim day 13 daily until granulocyte count $> 1 \times 10^9$/L then discontinue
	IVAC:
	Etoposide 60 mg/m^2 IV, daily, days 1–5
	Ifosfamide, age 65 or younger: 1.5 g/m^2 IV daily, days 1–5 with mesna 300 mg/m^2 IV followed by mesna 300 mg/m^2 q4 h × 2 doses; age greater than 65: 1 g/m^2 IV daily, days 1–5 with mesna 200 mg/m^2 IV followed by mesna 200 mg/m^2 q4 h x 2 doses
	Cytarabine, age 65 or younger 2 g/m^2, age greater than 65: 1 g/m^2, both q 12 h × 4 doses
	Intrathecal methotrexate 12 mg day 5
	Filgrastim day 7 daily until granulocyte count $> 1.0 \times 10^9$/L
	Main departures from original CODOX-M/IVAC in bold
	Additional intrathecal therapy for patients with CNS disease as follows:
	During CODOX-M cycles: additional cytarabine 70 mg on day 5 and methotrexate 12 mg on day 17
	During IVAC cycles: additional cytarabine 70 mg on days 7 and 9
Hyper-CVAD/MA [100]	Odd cycles (1, 3, 5, 7):
	Cyclophosphamide 300 mg/m^2 intravenously (IV) over 2 h every 12 h for six doses on days 1–3, with mesna 600 mg/m^2/day IV via continuous infusion on days 1–3 beginning 1 h before cyclophosphamide and completed by 12 h after the last dose of cyclophosphamide
	Vincristine 2 mg IV on days 4 and 11
	Doxorubicin 50 mg/m^2 IV over 2 h via central venous catheter on day 4
	Dexamethasone 40 mg daily either orally or IV on days 1–4 and days 11–14
	Even cycles (2, 4, 6, 8):
	Methotrexate 1 g/m^2 IV over 24 h on day 1 with leucovorin rescue
	Cytarabine 3 g/m^2 (1 g/m^2 for age ≥ 60) over 2 h every 12 h for four doses on days 2 and 3
	Filgrastim support with each cycle

(continued)

Table 13.5 (continued)

Trial	Chemotherapy drugs, doses, and schedule
	Intrathecal therapy:
	For patients with no CNS involvement at presentation:
	Intrathecal methotrexate 12 mg on day 2 of each cycle
	Intrathecal cytarabine 100 mg on day 7 of each cycle
	For patients with CNS involvement at presentation:
	Intrathecal therapy was administered twice weekly until the CSF cell count was normalized and the cytologic examination was negative for evidence of malignant cells; the program was then resumed as for prophylactic therapy.
	Cycle length 21 days
Rituximab-Hyper-CVAD [101]	Similar to Hyper-CVAD protocol with the addition of rituximab 375 mg/m^2 given IV on days 1 and 11 of odd-numbered cycles and on days 2 and 8 of even-numbered cycles, for 8 doses total over the first 4 cycles.
CALGB 9251 [102]	Cycle 1:
	Cyclophosphamide 200 mg/m^2 IV daily, days 1–5
	Prednisone 60 mg/m^2 po daily, days 1–7
	Cycles 2, 4, 6:
	Ifosfamide 800 mg/m^2 IV daily, days 1–5
	Mesna 200 mg/m^2 IV daily, 0, 4, and 8 h after ifosfamide
	Methotrexate 150 mg/m^2 IV for 30 min then 1.35 g/m^2 IV for 23.5 h, with leucovorin rescue
	Vincristine 2 mg IV day 1
	Cytarabine 150 mg/m^2/day by continuous infusion on days 4 and 5
	Etoposide 80 mg/m^2 IV over 1 hr on days 4 and 5
	Dexamethasone 10 mg/m^2 orally days 1 through 5
	Intrathecal methotrexate 15 mg, cytarabine 40 mg, and hydrocortisone 50 mg on days 1 and 5
	Cycles 3, 5, 7
	Cyclophosphamide 200 mg/m^2/day on days 1–5
	Methotrexate 150 mg/m^2 IV over 30 minutes, then 1.35 g/m^2 IV over 23.5 h, with leucovorin rescue
	Vincristine 2 mg IV day 1
	Doxorubicin 25 mg/m^2 IV bolus on days 4 and 5
	Dexamethasone 10 mg/m^2 orally days 1–5
	Intrathecal methotrexate 15 mg, cytarabine 40 mg, and hydrocortisone 50 mg on days 1 and 5
	Cranial irradiation was originally included but modified during the protocol, reserved for those patients with marrow or CNS disease, beginning after the completion of chemotherapy. The number of doses of intrathecal chemotherapy was reduced from two with each of cycles 2–7 to one with each cycle (12 doses reduced to 6 doses).
	Cycle length 21 days
DA-EPOCH (HIV-positive Burkitt lymphoma) [103]	Etoposide 50 mg/m^2/day CIVI, days 1–4 (96 h)
	Doxorubicin 10 mg/m^2/day CIVI days 1–4 (96 h)
	Vincristine 0.4 mg/m^2/day (no maximum dose) CIVI days 1–4 (96 h)
	Cyclophosphamide (cycle 1)
	CD4+ cells ≥100/mm^3: 375 mg/m^2 IV, day 5
	CD4+ cells < 100/mm^3: 187 mg/m^2/IV, day 5
	Dose adjustment for cyclophosphamide after cycle 1:
	nadir ANC > 500/μL: ↑187 mg above previous cycle
	nadir ANC < 500/μL or platelets < 25,000/μL: ↓187 mg below previous cycle
	Prednisone 60 mg/m^2/day PO days 1–5
	Filgrastim 5 μg/kg/day SC from day 6 until ANC > 5,000/μL (past nadir)

Table 13.5 (continued)

Trial	Chemotherapy drugs, doses, and schedule
	Intrathecal therapy:
	For patients with no CNS disease:
	Intrathecal methotrexate 12 mg days 1 and 5 of cycles 3–6
	For patients with CNS disease:
	Treatment began with methotrexate alone and if no response was seen, was escalated to methotrexate/cytarabine as described below.
	Treatment phase: Intrathecal or intraventricular methotrexate or methotrexate/cytarabine/prednisone twice weekly for 2 weeks beyond negative CSF cytology and flow cytometry, for a minimum of 4 weeks followed by
	Consolidation phase: intrathecal therapy once weekly for 6 weeks followed by
	Maintenance phase: intrathecal therapy once monthly for 6 months
	Cycle length 21 days

*Chemotherapy regimens should also include prophylactic therapy with antifungal, anti-*Pneumocystis carinii* pneumonia, and antiviral drugs

Abbreviations: *po* orally, *IV* intravenous, *CNS* central nervous system, *BID* twice daily, *CIVI* continuous intravenous infusion, *SC* subcutaneously

attained a CR. EFS was 92% at 2 years, with no events occurring beyond 2 years and no significant difference in EFS between the pediatric and adult patients. The most pronounced toxicities were cytopenias, neuropathy, and mucositis, as described in Table 13.4.

The United Kingdom Lymphoma Group (UKLG) evaluated 52 patients treated using the Magrath regimen in a larger, international, multicenter phase II trial [97]. Low-risk disease was required to fit all of the following criteria: normal LDH, WHO performance status of 0 or 1, Ann Arbor stage I–II, and no tumor mass >10 cm in size. Patients who did not fulfill all four markers were characterized as having high-risk disease. As in the initial study by Magrath et al., low-risk patients received three courses of cycle A, while high-risk patients received alternating rounds of cycles A and B for four cycles total. Seventy-seven percent of patients achieved a CR. Among all patients, 2-year EFS was approximately 65%, and 2-year OS was 73%. In the low-risk subgroup, EFS and OS were 83% and 82%, respectively, while those same rates were 60% and 70% in the high-risk group.

These studies of the CODOX-M/IVAC regimen focused on children (in the initial study by Magrath et al.) and adults, with the median age of patients in the original Magrath et al. study being 25 years and that of patients in the UKLG study being 35 years. LaCasce et al. studied a modified CODOX-M/IVAC regimen in a phase II trial of older adults to assess efficacy and treatment-related toxicities in this population. Fourteen patients, with a median age of 47 years, were enrolled. Major departures from the original CODOX-M (cycle A) design included a reduction in the cyclophosphamide course to 800 mg/m^2 on days 1 and 2, capping the vincristine dose at 2 mg, reducing the intrathecal cytarabine dose, reducing the methotrexate dose to 3 g/m^2, and increasing the doxorubicin dose to 50 mg/m^2 to maintain dose intensity. The IVAC (cycle B) dosing was without any dramatic changes. Three patients had low-risk disease and 11 had high-risk disease. Eighty-six percent of all patients – all low-risk patients and 9/11 high-risk patients – achieved a CR. Two-year progression-free survival (PFS) for all patients was 64%, and OS was 71%. There were no treatment-related deaths and no cases of grade 3 or 4 neuropathy and only one case of grade 3 or 4 mucositis – rates considerably lower than in the original Magrath protocol. As in the original Magrath study, however, grade 3 or 4 cytopenias were still prominent. The authors concluded that this modified regimen was effective, with outcomes similar to previous trials of more intense dosing in younger patients, and well-tolerated [98]. The UKLG has also completed a study of CODOX-M/IVAC with a reduced methotrexate dose (3 g/m^2 in patients 65 and younger, 1 g/m^2 in patients older than 65) with the aim of reducing toxicity while maintaining efficacy [99]. Both Burkitt lymphoma ($n = 58$) and DLBCL ($n = 70$) patients were enrolled. Efficacy outcomes were comparable to prior studies with a 2-year PFS of 64% among Burkitt lymphoma patients, and toxicities were less than in prior studies. The authors concluded that in the absence of a randomized clinical trial that the lower methotrexate dose in this trial seemed reasonable for use in future trials.

The hyper-CVAD regimen has been evaluated by investigators at M.D. Anderson Cancer Center [100]. Twenty-six consecutive newly diagnosed adult patients with B-ALL received this regimen consisting of eight total cycles alternating between odd- and even-numbered cycles. Odd cycles delivered hyper-fractionated cyclophosphamide with mesna to prevent hemorrhagic cystitis, vincristine, doxorubicin, and dexamethasone. Even cycles comprised methotrexate and cytarabine. Intrathecal chemotherapy was included in both cycles. CR was obtained in 21 of 26 patients (81%) with 12 of 21 patients in continuous remission at a median follow-up of 3.5 years. The 3-year OS rate was 49% with age, anemia, and peripheral blasts identified as independent poor prognostic factors. The overall median age of patients in this trial was 58 with the median age for patients under age 60 (14 patients, 54%) of 38 years. The 3-year OS for patients under age 60 was 77%, while in patients over age 60 (12 patients, 46%) was 17% ($p < 0.01$).

The Cancer and Leukemia Group B (CALGB) evaluated a high-intensity regimen in 30 patients with SNCCL and 24 with L3 ALL (Table 13.4) [102]. Cycle 1 consisted of cyclophosphamide and prednisone; cycles 2, 4, and 6 contained ifosfamide, mesna, methotrexate, vincristine, cytarabine, etoposide and dexamethasone, along with intrathecal methotrexate and cytarabine; cycles 3, 5, and 7 contained cyclophosphamide, methotrexate, doxorubicin, dexamethasone, and vincristine, along with intrathecal cytarabine and methotrexate. Prophylactic cranial irradiation was administered between cycles 3 and 4. Overall, 43 of 54 patients (80%) achieved a CR (18 of 24 patients with L3 ALL and 25 of 30 patients with SNCCL) with 28 patients alive (52%) and in continuous CR at a median follow-up of 5.1 years. Cytopenias and neurologic toxicities were the primary adverse events.

Role of Rituximab

The monoclonal anti-CD20 antibody rituximab was approved for use in the USA in 1997 for relapsed/refractory indolent lymphoma and has contributed to improved EFS and OS in prospective trials in various B-cell lymphomas, including follicular lymphoma and DLBCL [106, 107]. Its precise mechanism of action has not yet been clearly defined, but involves complement-mediated and antibody-mediated cellular cytotoxicity mechanisms [108]. Rituximab theoretically should be clinically active in Burkitt lymphoma and leukemia as these diseases are characterized by strong surface expression of CD20. In vitro data have shown that rituximab is effective in Burkitt lymphoma cell lines with cell death that occurs through autophagy with caspase-independent apoptosis and phosphorylation of AKT [109, 110]. Further, rituximab was shown to induce Fas-related apoptosis with inhibition of nuclear factor kappa of B cells (NF-KB) activity and p38 mitogen-activated protein kinase (MAPK) signaling and rituximab sensitized Burkitt lymphoma cells to chemotherapeutic drugs through downregulation of the anti-apoptotic proteins Bcl-2 and Bcl-x$_L$ [111, 112].

Thomas et al. from the M.D. Anderson Cancer Center studied the addition of rituximab to hyper-CVAD in Burkitt lymphoma and B-ALL and found that this addition was well tolerated [101]. Rituximab was given on days 1 and 11 of the odd-numbered cycles and on days 2 and 8 of the even-numbered cycles for a total of 8 doses during the initial 4 cycles. Outcomes among the 31 patients treated with rituximab were compared to historical controls from the 48 patients treated by the same group with hyper-CVAD alone. The percentage of CRs was similar in both groups, approximately 85%. However, the patients treated with rituximab had a markedly lower relapse rate (7%) compared to the group treated with hyper-CVAD alone (34%, $p = 0.008$). Three-year EFS and DFS rates were also significantly improved in the rituximab group, with those differences even more pronounced in a comparison of elderly patients. For example, 3-year OS was 89% in the rituximab (R)-hyper-CVAD group compared to 53% in the historical hyper-CVAD alone group, $p < 0.01$. Three-year DFS was 88% in the R-hyper-CVAD group, compared to 60% in the hyper-CVAD along group, $p = 0.03$. Prospective randomized trials would be needed to definitively prove rituximab's benefit, although this will be difficult to complete due to the rarity of this disease in adults. Other clinical trials incorporating rituximab into the Magrath regimen [60, 113, 114] (in HIV-negative and HIV-positive patients) and the CALGB regimen [115] are ongoing.

Therapy of HIV-Related Burkitt Lymphoma/Leukemia

Historically, caution has been applied in using dose-intense regimens for the treatment of HIV-positive patients with Burkitt lymphoma/leukemia given their underlying immunosuppression and fear of infectious complications. With the more commonplace use of HAART, however, the survival of HIV-positive patients, in general, has increased, while infectious complications and hesitation to use intensive chemotherapy have decreased [9]. Among all patients with HIV-related NHL, the most important prognostic factors have been International Prognostic Index (IPI) score and the CD4 count [116]. It is important to note that the impact of HAART has likely contributed to improved survival of HIV-related NHL, although this impact appears to be isolated primarily to DLBCL (Figs. 13.7 and 13.8) [9, 74, 117, 118]. This observation should be interpreted with caution due to the retrospective nature of the studies and the fact that Burkitt lymphoma patients did not receive the most dose-intensive regimens available, although the data strongly imply that improved therapeutic strategies are warranted for HIV-related Burkitt lymphoma.

Dose intensive regimens regimens utilized in immunocompetent Burkitt lymphoma/leukemia have been evaluated in HIV-positive patients showing acceptable toxicity and comparable efficacy compared with HIV-negative patients, although these studies have been small. Wang et al. performed a retrospective analysis that included 14 HIV-positive patients treated at Memorial Sloan-Kettering Cancer Center [119]. Eight patients received CODOX-M/IVAC while the remaining patients received less intensive regimens, such as CHOP. CR rates and 2-year EFS rates were similar between the two groups (approximately 60–70%), although the higher proportion of high-risk features in the CODOX-M/IVAC group likely impacted the outcomes in that group. HIV-negative patients were also included in that analysis; the rate of infectious complications among HIV-negative and positive patients treated with CODOX-M/IVAC appeared equal.

Cortes et al. from M.D. Anderson evaluated the hyper-CVAD regimen in 13 patients with HIV-related Burkitt lymphoma. Sixty-four percent of patients received concomitant HAART during chemotherapy. Ninety-two percent of patients achieved a CR, while the 2-year OS was 48% [120]. The Spanish PETHEMA group conducted the LAL3/97 study of HIV-positive and negative Burkitt lymphoma patients treated with a regimen based on the GMALL B-ALL protocol (described above) [121]. Fourteen patients (28%) were HIV-positive, and half received HAART. There was no statistically significant difference in outcome between HIV-positive and negative patients, with CR rates of 71% and 77% in the HIV-positive and negative groups, respectively, and 2-year OS rates of 43% and 55%, respectively.

Dose-adjusted (DA)-EPOCH (etoposide, prednisone, vincristine, cyclophosphamide, doxorubicin) has also been studied in HIV-related Burkitt lymphoma. Little et al. evaluated this regimen,

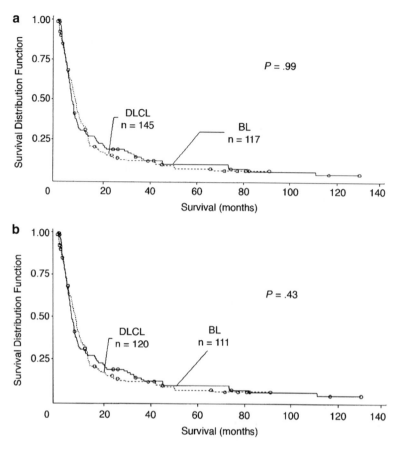

Fig. 13.7 Survival of patients with HIV-related diffuse large B cell lymphoma versus Burkitt lymphoma in the Pre-HAART Era. (**a**) Survival of all patients and (**b**) survival of patients treated with curative intent by pathologic type (pre-HAART era). (Reprinted with permission. © 2008 American Society of Clinical Oncology. All rights reserved. Lim et al. [117])

containing six cycles of 96-hour infusional etoposide, infusional vincristine, and infusional doxorubicin, and bolus cyclophosphamide, in 39 HIV-positive patients with newly diagnosed aggressive B-cell lymphoma (31 cases of DLBCL, 7 cases of Burkitt lymphoma, and 1 case of primary effusion lymphoma) [103]. The cyclophosphamide dose of the initial cycle was determined by patients' CD4 cell counts, and the cyclophosphamide dosing for subsequent cycles was either escalated or decreased based on the nadir absolute neutrophil count (ANC) during the previous 3-week cycle. HAART was suspended during treatment but was reinstituted upon completion of the sixth and final chemotherapy cycle. CNS prophylaxis was administered to the last 17 enrolled patients. Eighteen percent of patients had CNS involvement at treatment initiation. Among the seven patients with Burkitt lymphoma, OS at 53 months was 43%.

In France, as the LMB regimen had been established as the standard of care, the LMB86 protocol was evaluated prospectively in 63 patients with HIV-related St. Jude Stage IV Burkitt lymphoma/leukemia by Galicier et al. [73]. At diagnosis, the median CD4 cell count was $239 \times 10^6/L$; 80% of patients had bone marrow involvement, and 76% had CNS involvement. Forty-four patients (70%) achieved a CR; the estimated 2-year OS was 47%. Seven treatment-related deaths occurred.

The role of rituximab in the treatment of HIV-positive patients is unclear and has not yet been firmly delineated. The AIDS Malignancies Consortium conducted a randomized trial of CHOP

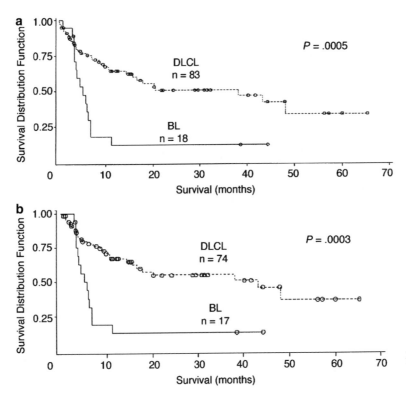

Fig. 13.8 Survival of patients with HIV-related diffuse large B cell lymphoma versus Burkitt lymphoma in the post-HAART Era. (**a**) Survival of all patients and (**b**) survival of patients treated with curative intent by pathologic type (HAART era). (Reprinted with permission. © 2008. American Society of Clinical Oncology. All rights reserved. Lim et al. [117])

versus R-CHOP in 150 HIV-positive patients with NHL [122]. No significant difference was found between the two groups in time to progression, progression-free survival, or OS. The lack of benefit from the addition of rituximab was possibly due to increased infectious complications in the ritux-imab-containing arm, an observation that raised concerns regarding the use of rituximab in HIV-positive patients. However, this increased risk may be limited primarily to patients with CD4 counts less than 50/μL. Additionally, these results are not entirely applicable to patients with Burkitt lymphoma, as the CHOP regimen represents suboptimal chemotherapy for this disease.

The PETHEMA group recently published an interim analysis that compared consecutively identified HIV-positive and negative patients treated with the rituximab-containing GMALL B-ALL/NHL2002 regimen [123]. Nineteen (53%) of the total 36 analyzed patients were HIV-positive. CR rates were 88% and 84%, respectively, for HIV-negative and -positive patients. While HIV-positive patients had more toxicities (grade 3–4 mucositis 27% vs. 7% of cycles, $p = 0.0005$, and severe infectious episodes 26% vs. 8%, $p = 0.0025$), no statistically significant differences between HIV-negative and positive patients in 2-year OS (82% vs. 73%, respectively) or 2-year DFS (93% vs. 87%, respectively) were observed, leading to the conclusion that intensive chemoimmunotherapy may be administered safely to HIV-positive patients.

Additionally, Spina et al. pooled the results of three phase II trials investigating the combination of rituximab with infusional cyclophosphamide, doxorubicin, and etoposide (R-CDE) in 74 patients with HIV-related B cell lymphoma, 28% of whom had Burkitt lymphoma [124]. Response and survival rates were not evaluated by lymphoma histology, but 70% of all patients achieved a CR. The estimated 2-year failure-free survival (FFS) and OS rates were 59% and 64%, respectively.

Fourteen percent of patients developed opportunistic infections, and 23% of patients developed non-opportunistic infections, supporting other researchers' concerns regarding the inclusion of rituximab in regimens for HIV-positive patients.

DA-EPOCH combined with rituximab was evaluated in a study of six HIV-positive and 13 HIV-negative patients with newly diagnosed Burkitt lymphoma [125]. All patients achieved a CR, while at a median follow-up of 29 months, OS and PFS rates were both 100%. Neutropenic fever occurred in 16% of patients. Additionally, the AIDS Malignancy Consortium has reported the results of a randomized phase II trial of EPOCH with either concurrent (with each EPOCH cycle) or sequential (weekly for 6 weeks after EPOCH completion) rituximab in 106 patients with HIV-related aggressive B-cell lymphoma (25% of patients in the concurrent group had Burkitt lymphoma vs. 15% in the sequential arm, with the remainder having primarily DLBCL) [126]. Concurrent administration was not believed to be associated with increased toxicity and was believed to improve the likelihood of a CR.

Tumor Lysis Syndrome

Due to the rapid doubling time of Burkitt lymphoma and leukemia cells, patients undergoing treatment are particularly susceptible to the development of tumor lysis syndrome (TLS), characterized by hyperuricemia, hyperkalemia, hyperphosphatemia, hypocalcemia, and renal failure – metabolic disturbances all related to the rapid destruction of tumor cells. Renal failure, in particular, is often related to renal urate deposition. Critical preventive measures include aggressive hydration and control of hyperuricemia with agents such as allopurinol, a xanthine oxidase inhibitor, and rasburicase, a recombinant urate oxidase catalyzing the breakdown of uric acid into allantoin, which is comparatively more water-soluble [127, 128].

According to 2008 Guidelines for Management of Pediatric and Adult Tumor Lysis Syndrome, patients with Burkitt lymphoma are at high risk of TLS [128]. Such high-risk patients with hyperuricemia associated with TLS at the time of treatment initiation were recommended to receive rasburicase, as were pediatric patients at high risk of TLS development, regardless of uric acid level. Of note, while rasburicase is approved by the Food and Drug Administration for use in pediatric patients, its use in adult patients is off-label in the USA. Support for the use of rasburicase stems from trials conducted mainly in pediatric populations. Goldman et al. conducted a randomized trial of 52 pediatric patients with either leukemia or lymphoma at high risk for TLS development, defined as (1) Murphy stage III or IV NHL, (2) (ALL) with a peripheral WBC count of 25,000/μL or higher at presentation, or (3) any childhood lymphoma or leukemia with a uric acid level of 8 mg/dL or higher at the time of study entry [129]. Patients were randomized to receive either oral allopurinol 300 mg/m^2 (or 10 mg/kg) divided every 8 h vs. intravenous rasburicase 0.20 mg/kg over 30 min daily, both for 5–7 days. The study's main objective was to compare the decrease in plasma uric acid levels by the two uric acid–lowering agents during the first 5 days of cytoreductive chemotherapy. The primary efficacy end point was the area under the serial plasma uric acid concentration curves (AUC) from the start of study drug until 96 h. Patients receiving rasburicase exhibited a more rapid decline in plasma uric acid levels, as well as lower absolute levels, during the course of induction therapy. Five patients with advanced Burkitt lymphoma and leukemia were in the rasburicase group, while four were in the allopurinol group. Among lymphoma/leukemia subtypes, these patients had the greatest reduction in exposure to plasma uric acid with rasburicase when comparing the two treatment arms. The number of patients enrolled was not large enough to detect an intergroup difference in renal failure development or the need for hemodialysis. Additionally, the Groupe d'Etude des Lymphomes de l'Adulte (GELA) Trial on Rasburicase Activity, which enrolled 100 patients with aggressive NHL (one with Burkitt lymphoma), established the safety and efficacy of rasburicase

0.20 mg/kg/d intravenously for 3–7 days in lowering uric acid levels. Rasburicase should be avoided in patients with glucose-6-phosphate dehydrogenase deficiency due to a risk of hemolytic anemia. Further investigation into the optimum rasburicase dose has been performed, with a retrospective study from our institution suggesting that a single dose of 3 mg may be as efficacious as FDA-approved doses [130].

Newly diagnosed patients may present in acute renal failure attributed to TLS. In these circumstances, a short course of attenuated chemotherapy containing cyclophosphamide and prednisone, similar to that incorporated in the prephase of the LMB89 [91] pediatric protocol and the B-NHL83 and B-NHL86 [94] adult protocols described above, may improve renal function and performance status to allow the necessary initiation of more intensive induction chemotherapy.

Relapsed/Refractory Disease and the Role of Stem Cell Transplant

The optimal therapy for patients who fail to achieve a complete response with initial therapy or for patients with relapsed disease is unclear. Griffin et al. evaluated the R-ICE regimen (rituximab, ifosfamide, carboplatin, etoposide) with intrathecal chemotherapy in 20 patients with one of the following: recurrent/refractory DLBCL (six patients), Burkitt lymphoma (12 patients), and B-ALL (two patients) [131]. The authors did not report prior treatments of the patient population, so the number of patients who previously received ifosfamide or etoposide, as in the Magrath regimen, is unclear. Among the 14 patients with either Burkitt lymphoma or B-ALL, 64% had responses with 4 CRs and 5 PRs. Four patients with Burkitt lymphoma or B-ALL survived without disease and proceeded to stem cell transplantation (3 autologous, 1 allogeneic). This regimen appeared to have activity in this pediatric population, although the small patient number precluded definitive conclusions. In general, salvage chemotherapy has provided disappointing results in adult patients and no standard or optimal regimen exists [18].

Stem cell transplant has been evaluated in the setting of refractory or relapsed disease, as well as in first CR. In a retrospective analysis from the European Group for Blood and Marrow Transplantation, Sweetenham and colleagues reported 70 patients in first remission and 47 patients with relapsed disease [132]. Among those patients transplanted in the first complete remission, 3-year actuarial OS was 72%, compared to 37% for patients in chemotherapy-sensitive relapse and 7% for patients with chemotherapy-resistant relapse. Investigators at City of Hope transplanted 10 Burkitt lymphoma/Burkitt-like lymphoma patients in the first remission and reported a 60% 3-year DFS [133]. In the setting of relapsed/refractory disease, they reported a 5-year DFS of 30% for patients transplanted during induction failure and 34% for relapsed patients [134].

The data regarding allogeneic transplant in Burkitt lymphoma/leukemia are limited. Bureo et al. reported their experience with autologous and allogeneic transplant in 46 pediatric patients with high-grade NHL transplanted in six Spanish centers [135]. Fourteen patients underwent allogeneic BMT and 32 autologous BMT (46% lymphoblastic lymphoma, 41% BL, and 13% diffuse large cell lymphoma). More than 60% of patients were in second or third CR with 28% in first CR and 11% with active disease (4/5 with active chemotherapy-sensitive disease). Overall EFS was 58% with a median follow-up of 33 months. EFS was similar for allogeneic BMT and autologous patients. The European Bone Marrow Transplantation Lymphoma Registry reported its experience with allogeneic transplant in Burkitt lymphoma in a retrospective analysis of 71 patients treated between 1982 and 1998 [136]. Transplantation was done in 38.5% of patients in first CR; 24.6% in second or higher CR; 17% were not in CR but had chemotherapy-sensitive disease, and 20% had chemotherapy-resistant disease. Median OS was 4.7 months, and actuarial 4-year OS was 37% and actuarial 4-year PFS 35%. Procedure-related mortality at 4 years was 31%. In their analysis, the authors matched the patients who had undergone allogeneic transplant to similar patients from the registry who had received autologous transplants. Relapse rates were equivalent in the allogeneic and autologous groups, while treatment-related mortality (TRM) rates were worse in the allogeneic group. Among allogeneic transplant patients, the development of acute graft-versus-host disease had no effect on survival. This phenomenon, coupled with the equivalent relapse rates between autologous and allogeneic transplant recipients, has lessened enthusiasm regarding a potential graft-versus-leukemia/lymphoma effect in this disease.

Novel Therapies

Novel agents that have shown clinical activity in other hematologic malignancies have been evaluated mainly in laboratory investigations in Burkitt lymphoma and leukemia. *C-myc's* role in epigenetic regulation [137, 138] has prompted investigation into the potential of epigenetic modification in Burkitt lymphoma and leukemia therapy. Histone deactylase inhibitors, such as depsipeptide, have shown intriguing results in preclinical studies [139]. The proteasome inhibitor bortezomib, currently approved for use in multiple myeloma and mantle cell lymphoma, has been shown in preclinical studies to interfere with the expression of some EBV latency genes, as well as the expression of a number of proteins inhibiting apoptosis [140]. In addition, cellular strategies directed against EBV-encoded proteins are being examined, as well as therapeutics that target the different pathways downstream of LMP2A as discussed before, including mTOR, RAS, and AKT [43].

Conclusion

Burkitt lymphoma and leukemia are highly aggressive B-lymphocyte malignancies characterized by the chromosomal translocations involving the *c-myc* oncogene. Clinical trials over the past two decades have demonstrated that its highly aggressive nature requires dose-intense chemotherapy to provide the best chance of cure. This treatment strategy has resulted in long-term disease-free survival rates of approximately 60–70% for patients less than 50–60 years of age. The advent of rituximab over the past decade has offered a potential therapeutic advance in this disease, although further clinical study is warranted. Close attention to TLS prevention and monitoring are critical to prevent treatment-related mortality and morbidity. Stem cell transplant does not have a clear role in the up-front management of this disease, although it represents an option for select patients with relapsed and refractory disease. Continued preclinical research is needed to continue to unravel the biologic importance of EBV and *c-myc* and continued collaborative clinical studies are needed to examine the integration of monoclonal antibodies and other novel therapeutics with standard therapy as well as to improve the outcomes of older individuals with Burkitt lymphoma and leukemia.

References

1. Burkitt, D. (1958). A sarcoma involving the jaws in African children. *The British Journal of Surgery, 46*, 218–223.
2. Swerdlow, S. H., Campo, E., Harris, N. L., et al. (2008). *WHO classification of tumours of hematopoietic and lymphoid tissues*. Lyon: IARC.
3. Harris, N. L., Jaffe, E. S., Stein, H., et al. (1994). A revised European-American classification of lymphoid neoplasms: A proposal from the International Lymphoma Study Group. *Blood, 84*, 1361–1392.
4. Harris, N. L., Jaffe, E. S., Diebold, J., et al. (1999). World Health Organization classification of neoplastic diseases of the hematopoietic and lymphoid tissues: Report of the Clinical Advisory Committee meeting-Airlie House, Virginia, November 1997. *Journal of Clinical Oncology, 17*, 3835–3849.

5. Bennett, J. M., Catovsky, D., Daniel, M. T., et al. (1976). Proposals for the classification of the acute leukaemias. French-American-British (FAB) co-operative group. *British Journal Haematology, 33*, 451–458.
6. A clinical evaluation of the International Lymphoma Study Group classification of non-Hodgkin's lymphoma. The Non-Hodgkin's Lymphoma Classification Project. *Blood* 89, 3909–3918, 1997.
7. Morton, L. M., Wang, S. S., Devesa, S. S., et al. (2006). Lymphoma incidence patterns by WHO subtype in the United States, 1992–2001. *Blood, 107*, 265–276.
8. Orem, J., Mbidde, E. K., Lambert, B., et al. (2007). Burkitt's lymphoma in Africa, a review of the epidemiology and etiology. *African Health Sciences, 7*, 166–175.
9. Blinder, V. S., Chadburn, A., Furman, R. R., et al. (2008). Improving outcomes for patients with Burkitt lymphoma and HIV. *AIDS Patient Care and STDs, 22*, 175–187.
10. Cote, T. R., Biggar, R. J., Rosenberg, P. S., et al. (1997). Non-Hodgkin's lymphoma among people with AIDS: Incidence, presentation and public health burden. AIDS/Cancer Study Group. *International Journal of Cancer, 73*, 645–650.
11. Biggar, R. J., Chaturvedi, A. K., Goedert, J. J., et al. (2007). AIDS-related cancer and severity of immunosuppression in persons with AIDS. *Journal of the National Cancer Institute, 99*, 962–972.
12. Oster, S. K., Ho, C. S., Soucie, E. L., et al. (2002). The myc oncogene: MarvelouslY Complex. *Advances in Cancer Research, 84*, 81–154.
13. Li, Z., Van Calcar, S., Qu, C., et al. (2003). A global transcriptional regulatory role for c-Myc in Burkitt's lymphoma cells. *Proceedings of the National Academy of Sciences of the United States of America, 100*, 8164–8169.
14. Hecht, J. L., & Aster, J. C. (2000). Molecular biology of Burkitt's lymphoma. *Journal of Clinical Oncology, 18*, 3707–3721.
15. Vita, M., & Henriksson, M. (2006). The Myc oncoprotein as a therapeutic target for human cancer. *Seminars in Cancer Biology, 16*, 318–330.
16. Neri, A., Barriga, F., Knowles, D. M., et al. (1988). Different regions of the immunoglobulin heavy-chain locus are involved in chromosomal translocations in distinct pathogenetic forms of Burkitt lymphoma. *Proceedings of the National Academy of Sciences of the United States of America, 85*, 2748–2752.
17. Gerbitz, A., Mautner, J., Geltinger, C., et al. (1999). Deregulation of the proto-oncogene c-myc through t(8;22) translocation in Burkitt's lymphoma. *Oncogene, 18*, 1745–1753.
18. Blum, K. A., Lozanski, G., & Byrd, J. C. (2004). Adult Burkitt leukemia and lymphoma. *Blood, 104*, 3009–3020.
19. Shiramizu, B., Barriga, F., Neequaye, J., et al. (1991). Patterns of chromosomal breakpoint locations in Burkitt's lymphoma: Relevance to geography and Epstein-Barr virus association. *Blood, 77*, 1516–1526.
20. Gutierrez, M. I., Bhatia, K., Barriga, F., et al. (1992). Molecular epidemiology of Burkitt's lymphoma from South America: Differences in breakpoint location and Epstein-Barr virus association from tumors in other world regions. *Blood, 79*, 3261–3266.
21. Bhatia, K., Spangler, G., Gaidano, G., et al. (1994). Mutations in the coding region of c-myc occur frequently in acquired immunodeficiency syndrome-associated lymphomas. *Blood, 84*, 883–888.
22. Thorley-Lawson, D. A., & Gross, A. (2004). Persistence of the Epstein-Barr virus and the origins of associated lymphomas. *The New England Journal of Medicine, 350*, 1328–1337.
23. van den Bosch, C. A. (2004). Is endemic Burkitt's lymphoma an alliance between three infections and a tumour promoter? *The Lancet Oncology, 5*, 738–746.
24. Kutok, J. L., & Wang, F. (2006). Spectrum of Epstein-Barr virus-associated diseases. *Annual Review of Pathology, 1*, 375–404.
25. Brady, G., MacArthur, G. J., & Farrell, P. J. (2007). Epstein-Barr virus and Burkitt lymphoma. *Journal of Clinical Pathology, 60*, 1397–1402.
26. Epstein, M. A., Achong, B. G., & Barr, Y. M. (1964). Virus particles in cultured lymphoblasts from Burkitt's lymphoma. *Lancet, 1*, 702–703.
27. Wright, D. H. (1999). What is Burkitt's lymphoma and when is it endemic? *Blood, 93*, 758.
28. Anwar, N., Kingma, D. W., Bloch, A. R., et al. (1995). The investigation of Epstein-Barr viral sequences in 41 cases of Burkitt's lymphoma from Egypt: Epidemiologic correlations. *Cancer, 76*, 1245–1252.
29. Klumb, C. E., Hassan, R., De Oliveira, D. E., et al. (2004). Geographic variation in Epstein-Barr virus-associated Burkitt's lymphoma in children from Brazil. *International Journal of Cancer, 108*, 66–70.
30. Kennedy, G., Komano, J., & Sugden, B. (2003). Epstein-Barr virus provides a survival factor to Burkitt's lymphomas. *Proceedings of the National Academy of Sciences of the United States of America, 100*, 14269–14274.
31. Humme, S., Reisbach, G., Feederle, R., et al. (2003). The EBV nuclear antigen 1 (EBNA1) enhances B cell immortalization several thousandfold. *Proceedings of the National Academy of Sciences of the United States of America, 100*, 10989–10994.
32. Komano, J., Maruo, S., Kurozumi, K., et al. (1999). Oncogenic role of Epstein-Barr virus-encoded RNAs in Burkitt's lymphoma cell line Akata. *Journal of Virology, 73*, 9827–9831.

33. Niller, H. H., Salamon, D., Ilg, K., et al. (2003). The in vivo binding site for oncoprotein c-Myc in the promoter for Epstein-Barr virus (EBV) encoding RNA (EBER) 1 suggests a specific role for EBV in lymphomagenesis. *Medical Science Monitor, 9*, HY1–HY9.

34. Caldwell, R. G., Wilson, J. B., Anderson, S. J., et al. (1998). Epstein-Barr virus LMP2A drives B cell development and survival in the absence of normal B cell receptor signals. *Immunity, 9*, 405–411.

35. Spanopoulou, E., Roman, C. A., Corcoran, L. M., et al. (1994). Functional immunoglobulin transgenes guide ordered B-cell differentiation in Rag-1-deficient mice. *Genes & Development, 8*, 1030–1042.

36. Mombaerts, P., Iacomini, J., Johnson, R. S., et al. (1992). RAG-1-deficient mice have no mature B and T lymphocytes. *Cell, 68*, 869–877.

37. Fruehling, S., & Longnecker, R. (1997). The immunoreceptor tyrosine-based activation motif of Epstein-Barr virus LMP2A is essential for blocking BCR-mediated signal transduction. *Virology, 235*, 241–251.

38. Fruehling, S., Swart, R., Dolwick, K. M., et al. (1998). Tyrosine 112 of latent membrane protein 2A is essential for protein tyrosine kinase loading and regulation of Epstein-Barr virus latency. *Journal of Virology, 72*, 7796–7806.

39. Ikeda, A., Merchant, M., Lev, L., et al. (2004). Latent membrane protein 2A, a viral B cell receptor homologue, induces CD5+ B-1 cell development. *Journal of Immunology, 172*, 5329–5337.

40. Engels, N., Merchant, M., Pappu, R., et al. (2001). Epstein-Barr virus latent membrane protein 2A (LMP2A) employs the SLP-65 signaling module. *The Journal of Experimental Medicine, 194*, 255–264.

41. Fukuda, M., & Longnecker, R. (2004). Latent membrane protein 2A inhibits transforming growth factor-beta 1-induced apoptosis through the phosphatidylinositol 3-kinase/Akt pathway. *Journal of Virology, 78*, 1697–1705.

42. Merchant, M., & Longnecker, R. (2001). LMP2A survival and developmental signals are transmitted through Btk-dependent and Btk-independent pathways. *Virology, 291*, 46–54.

43. Portis, T., & Longnecker, R. (2004). Epstein-Barr virus (EBV) LMP2A mediates B-lymphocyte survival through constitutive activation of the Ras/PI3K/Akt pathway. *Oncogene, 23*, 8619–8628.

44. Swart, R., Ruf, I. K., Sample, J., et al. (2000). Latent membrane protein 2A-mediated effects on the phosphatidylinositol 3-Kinase/Akt pathway. *Journal of Virology, 74*, 10838–10845.

45. Moody, C. A., Scott, R. S., Amirghahari, N., et al. (2005). Modulation of the cell growth regulator mTOR by Epstein-Barr virus-encoded LMP2A. *Journal of Virology, 79*, 5499–5506.

46. Haluska, F. G., Finver, S., Tsujimoto, Y., et al. (1986). The t(8; 14) chromosomal translocation occurring in B-cell malignancies results from mistakes in V-D-J joining. *Nature, 324*, 158–161.

47. Haluska, F. G., Tsujimoto, Y., & Croce, C. M. (1987). The t(8;14) chromosome translocation of the Burkitt lymphoma cell line Daudi occurred during immunoglobulin gene rearrangement and involved the heavy chain diversity region. *Proceedings of the National Academy of Sciences of the United States of America, 84*, 6835–6839.

48. Tamaru, J., Hummel, M., Marafioti, T., et al. (1995). Burkitt's lymphomas express VH genes with a moderate number of antigen-selected somatic mutations. *The American Journal of Pathology, 147*, 1398–1407.

49. Bellan, C., Lazzi, S., Hummel, M., et al. (2005). Immunoglobulin gene analysis reveals 2 distinct cells of origin for EBV-positive and EBV-negative Burkitt lymphomas. *Blood, 106*, 1031–1036.

50. Dave, S. S., Fu, K., Wright, G. W., et al. (2006). Molecular diagnosis of Burkitt's lymphoma. *The New England Journal of Medicine, 354*, 2431–2442.

51. Hummel, M., Bentink, S., Berger, H., et al. (2006). A biologic definition of Burkitt's lymphoma from transcriptional and genomic profiling. *The New England Journal of Medicine, 354*, 2419–2430.

52. Wright, G. H. (1971). *Burkitt's Lymphoma: A review of the pathology, immunology and possible aetiological factors*. New York: Appleton-Century-Crofts.

53. Perkins, A. S., & Friedberg, J. W. (2008). Burkitt lymphoma in adults. *Hematology American Society of Hematology Educcation Program, 2008*, 341–348.

54. Raphael, M., Gentilhomme, O., Tulliez, M., et al. (1991). Histopathologic features of high-grade non-Hodgkin's lymphomas in acquired immunodeficiency syndrome. The French Study Group of Pathology for Human Immunodeficiency Virus-Associated Tumors. *Archives of Pathology & Laboratory Medicine, 115*, 15–20.

55. Nakamura, N., Nakamine, H., Tamaru, J., et al. (2002). The distinction between Burkitt lymphoma and diffuse large B-Cell lymphoma with c-myc rearrangement. *Modern Pathology, 15*, 771–776.

56. Haralambieva, E., Boerma, E. J., van Imhoff, G. W., et al. (2005). Clinical, immunophenotypic, and genetic analysis of adult lymphomas with morphologic features of Burkitt lymphoma. *The American Journal of Surgical Pathology, 29*, 1086–1094.

57. Einerson, R. R., Law, M. E., Blair, H. E., et al. (2006). Novel FISH probes designed to detect IGK-MYC and IGL-MYC rearrangements in B-cell lineage malignancy identify a new breakpoint cluster region designated BVR2. *Leukemia, 20*, 1790–1799.

58. Leucci, E., Cocco, M., Onnis, A., et al. (2008). MYC translocation-negative classical Burkitt lymphoma cases: An alternative pathogenetic mechanism involving miRNA deregulation. *The Journal of Pathology, 216*, 440–450.

59. He, L., He, X., Lim, L. P., et al. (2007). A microRNA component of the p53 tumour suppressor network. *Nature, 447*, 1130–1134.
60. Savage, K. J., Johnson, N. A., Ben-Neriah, S., et al. (2009). MYC gene rearrangements are associated with a poor prognosis in diffuse large B-cell lymphoma patients treated with R-CHOP chemotherapy. *Blood, 114*, 3533–3537.
61. Berglund, M., Thunberg, U., Amini, R. M., et al. (2005). Evaluation of immunophenotype in diffuse large B-cell lymphoma and its impact on prognosis. *Modern Pathology, 18*, 1113–1120.
62. Colomo, L., Lopez-Guillermo, A., Perales, M., et al. (2003). Clinical impact of the differentiation profile assessed by immunophenotyping in patients with diffuse large B-cell lymphoma. *Blood, 101*, 78–84.
63. Gascoyne, R. D., Adomat, S. A., Krajewski, S., et al. (1997). Prognostic significance of Bcl-2 protein expression and Bcl-2 gene rearrangement in diffuse aggressive non-Hodgkin's lymphoma. *Blood, 90*, 244–251.
64. McClure, R. F., Remstein, E. D., Macon, W. R., et al. (2005). Adult B-cell lymphomas with burkitt-like morphology are phenotypically and genotypically heterogeneous with aggressive clinical behavior. *The American Journal of Surgical Pathology, 29*, 1652–1660.
65. Colomo, L., Loong, F., Rives, S., et al. (2004). Diffuse large B-cell lymphomas with plasmablastic differentiation represent a heterogeneous group of disease entities. *The American Journal of Surgical Pathology, 28*, 736–747.
66. Le Gouill, S., Talmant, P., Touzeau, C., et al. (2007). The clinical presentation and prognosis of diffuse large B-cell lymphoma with t(14;18) and 8q24/c-MYC rearrangement. *Haematologica, 92*, 1335–1342.
67. Kanungo, A., Medeiros, L. J., Abruzzo, L. V., et al. (2006). Lymphoid neoplasms associated with concurrent t(14;18) and 8q24/c-MYC translocation generally have a poor prognosis. *Modern Pathology, 19*, 25–33.
68. O'Conor, G. T. (1963). Significant aspects of childhood lymphoma in Africa. *Cancer Research, 23*, 1514–1518.
69. Armitage, J. O., & Weisenburger, D. D. (1998). New approach to classifying non-Hodgkin's lymphomas: Clinical features of the major histologic subtypes. Non-Hodgkin's Lymphoma Classification Project. *Journal of Clinical Oncology, 16*, 2780–2795.
70. Jaffe, E. S., Harris, N. L., Stein, H., et al. (2001). *World Health Organization classification of tumours*. Lyon: IARC.
71. Davi, F., Delecluse, H. J., Guiet, P., et al. (1998). Burkitt-like lymphomas in AIDS patients: Characterization within a series of 103 human immunodeficiency virus-associated non-Hodgkin's lymphomas. Burkitt's Lymphoma Study Group. *Journal of Clinical Oncology, 16*, 3788–3795.
72. Salzburg, J., Burkhardt, B., Zimmermann, M., et al. (2007). Prevalence, clinical pattern, and outcome of CNS involvement in childhood and adolescent non-Hodgkin's lymphoma differ by non-Hodgkin's lymphoma subtype: A Berlin-Frankfurt-Munster Group Report. *Journal of Clinical Oncology, 25*, 3915–3922.
73. Galicier, L., Fieschi, C., Borie, R., et al. (2007). Intensive chemotherapy regimen (LMB86) for St Jude stage IV AIDS-related Burkitt lymphoma/leukemia: A prospective study. *Blood, 110*, 2846–2854.
74. Ostronoff, M., Soussain, C., Zambon, E., et al. (1992). Burkitt's lymphoma in adults: A retrospective study of 46 cases. *Nouvelle Revue Française d'Hématologie, 34*, 389–397.
75. Wright, D. H., & Pike, P. A. (1968). Bone marrow involvement in Burkitt's tumour. *British Journal Haematology, 15*, 409–416.
76. Magrath, I. T., & Sariban, E. (1985). Clinical features of Burkitt's lymphoma in the USA. *IARC Sci Publ, 60*, 119–127.
77. van der Burg, M., Barendregt, B. H., van Wering, E. R., et al. (2001). The presence of somatic mutations in immunoglobulin genes of B cell acute lymphoblastic leukemia (ALL-L3) supports assignment as Burkitt's leukemia-lymphoma rather than B-lineage ALL. *Leukemia, 15*, 1141–1143.
78. Lister, T. A., Crowther, D., Sutcliffe, S. B., et al. (1989). Report of a committee convened to discuss the evaluation and staging of patients with Hodgkin's disease: Cotswolds meeting. *Journal of Clinical Oncology, 7*, 1630–1636.
79. Murphy, S. B. (1978). Childhood non-Hodgkin's lymphoma. *The New England Journal of Medicine, 299*, 1446–1448.
80. www.nccn.org
81. Lubel, J. S., Testro, A. G., & Angus, P. W. (2007). Hepatitis B virus reactivation following immunosuppressive therapy: Guidelines for prevention and management. *Internal Medicine Journal, 37*, 705–712.
82. Saab, S., Dong, M. H., Joseph, T. A., et al. (2007). Hepatitis B prophylaxis in patients undergoing chemotherapy for lymphoma: A decision analysis model. *Hepatology, 46*, 1049–1056.
83. Ziegler, J. L. (1972). Chemotherapy of Burkitt's lymphoma. *Cancer, 30*, 1534–1540.
84. Anderson, J. R., Jenkin, R. D., Wilson, J. F., et al. (1993). Long-term follow-up of patients treated with COMP or LSA2L2 therapy for childhood non-Hodgkin's lymphoma: A report of CCG-551 from the Childrens Cancer Group. *Journal of Clinical Oncology, 11*, 1024–1032.
85. Ziegler, J. L. (1977). Treatment results of 54 American patients with Burkitt's lymphoma are similar to the African experience. *The New England Journal of Medicine, 297*, 75–80.

86. Murphy, S. B., Bowman, W. P., Abromowitch, M., et al. (1986). Results of treatment of advanced-stage Burkitt's lymphoma and B cell (SIg+) acute lymphoblastic leukemia with high-dose fractionated cyclophosphamide and coordinated high-dose methotrexate and cytarabine. *Journal of Clinical Oncology, 4*, 1732–1739.

87. Bowman, W. P., Shuster, J. J., Cook, B., et al. (1996). Improved survival for children with B-cell acute lympho-blastic leukemia and stage IV small noncleaved-cell lymphoma: A pediatric oncology group study. *Journal of Clinical Oncology, 14*, 1252–1261.

88. Schwenn, M. R., Blattner, S. R., Lynch, E., et al. (1991). HiC-COM: A 2-month intensive chemotherapy regimen for children with stage III and IV Burkitt's lymphoma and B-cell acute lymphoblastic leukemia. *Journal of Clinical Oncology, 9*, 133–138.

89. Reiter, A., Schrappe, M., Ludwig, W. D., et al. (1992). Favorable outcome of B-cell acute lymphoblastic leuke-mia in childhood: A report of three consecutive studies of the BFM group. *Blood, 80*, 2471–2478.

90. Soussain, C., Patte, C., Ostronoff, M., et al. (1995). Small noncleaved cell lymphoma and leukemia in adults. A retrospective study of 65 adults treated with the LMB pediatric protocols. *Blood, 85*, 664–674.

91. Patte, C., Auperin, A., Michon, J., et al. (2001). The Societe Francaise d'Oncologie Pediatrique LMB89 proto-col: Highly effective multiagent chemotherapy tailored to the tumor burden and initial response in 561 unse-lected children with B-cell lymphomas and L3 leukemia. *Blood, 97*(11), 3370–3379.

92. Patte, C., Auperin, A., Gerrard, M., et al. (2007). Results of the randomized international FAB/LMB96 trial for intermediate risk B-cell non-Hodgkin lymphoma in children and adolescents: It is possible to reduce treatment for the early responding patients. *Blood, 109*, 2773–2780.

93. Cairo, M. S., Gerrard, M., Sposto, R., et al. (2007). Results of a randomized international study of high-risk central nervous system B non-Hodgkin lymphoma and B acute lymphoblastic leukemia in children and adoles-cents. *Blood, 109*, 2736–2743.

94. Hoelzer, D., Ludwig, W. D., Thiel, E., et al. (1996). Improved outcome in adult B-cell acute lymphoblastic leukemia. *Blood, 87*, 495–508.

95. Divine, M., Casassus, P., Koscielny, S., et al. (2005). Burkitt lymphoma in adults: A prospective study of 72 patients treated with an adapted pediatric LMB protocol. *Annals of Oncology, 16*, 1928–1935.

96. Magrath, I., Adde, M., Shad, A., et al. (1996). Adults and children with small non-cleaved-cell lymphoma have a similar excellent outcome when treated with the same chemotherapy regimen. *Journal of Clinical Oncology, 14*, 925–934.

97. Mead, G. M., Sydes, M. R., Walewski, J., et al. (2002). An international evaluation of CODOX-M and CODOX-M alternating with IVAC in adult Burkitt's lymphoma: Results of United Kingdom Lymphoma Group LY06 study. *Annals of Oncology, 13*, 1264–1274.

98. Lacasce, A., Howard, O., Lib, S., et al. (2004). Modified magrath regimens for adults with Burkitt and Burkitt-like lymphomas: Preserved efficacy with decreased toxicity. *Leukaemia & Lymphoma, 45*, 761–767.

99. Mead, G. M., Barrans, S. L., Qian, W., et al. (2008). A prospective clinicopathologic study of dose-modified CODOX-M/IVAC in patients with sporadic Burkitt lymphoma defined using cytogenetic and immunopheno-typic criteria (MRC/NCRI LY10 trial). *Blood, 112*, 2248–2260.

100. Thomas, D. A., Cortes, J., O'Brien, S., et al. (1999). Hyper-CVAD program in Burkitt's-type adult acute lym-phoblastic leukemia. *Journal of Clinical Oncology, 17*, 2461–2470.

101. Thomas, D. A., Faderl, S., O'Brien, S., et al. (2006). Chemoimmunotherapy with hyper-CVAD plus rituximab for the treatment of adult Burkitt and Burkitt-type lymphoma or acute lymphoblastic leukemia. *Cancer, 106*, 1569–1580.

102. Lee, E. J., Petroni, G. R., Schiffer, C. A., et al. (2001). Brief-duration high-intensity chemotherapy for patients with small noncleaved-cell lymphoma or FAB L3 acute lymphocytic leukemia: Results of cancer and leukemia group B study 9251. *Journal of Clinical Oncology, 19*, 4014–4022.

103. Little, R. F., Pittaluga, S., Grant, N., et al. (2003). Highly effective treatment of acquired immunodeficiency syndrome-related lymphoma with dose-adjusted EPOCH: Impact of antiretroviral therapy suspension and tumor biology. *Blood, 101*, 4653–4659.

104. Bernstein, J. I., Coleman, C. N., Strickler, J. G., et al. (1986). Combined modality therapy for adults with small noncleaved cell lymphoma (Burkitt's and non-Burkitt's types). *Journal of Clinical Oncology, 4*, 847–858.

105. McMaster, M. L., Greer, J. P., Greco, F. A., et al. (1991). Effective treatment of small-noncleaved-cell lym-phoma with high-intensity, brief-duration chemotherapy. *Journal of Clinical Oncology, 9*, 941–946.

106. Feugier, P., Van Hoof, A., Sebban, C., et al. (2005). Long-term results of the R-CHOP study in the treatment of elderly patients with diffuse large B-cell lymphoma: A study by the Groupe d'Etude des Lymphomes de l'Adulte. *Journal of Clinical Oncology, 23*, 4117–4126.

107. Marcus, R., Imrie, K., Solal-Celigny, P., et al. (2008). Phase III study of R-CVP compared with cyclophosph-amide, vincristine, and prednisone alone in patients with previously untreated advanced follicular lymphoma. *Journal of Clinical Oncology, 26*, 4579–4586.

108. Glennie, M. J., French, R. R., Cragg, M. S., et al. (2007). Mechanisms of killing by anti-CD20 monoclonal antibodies. *Molecular Immunology, 44*, 3823–3837.

109. Turzanski, J., Daniels, I., & Haynes, A. P. (2009). Involvement of macroautophagy in the caspase-independent killing of Burkitt lymphoma cell lines by rituximab. *British Journal of Haematology, 145*(1), 137–140.
110. Daniels, I., Abulayha, A. M., Thomson, B. J., et al. (2006). Caspase-independent killing of Burkitt lymphoma cell lines by rituximab. *Apoptosis, 11*, 1013–1023.
111. Vega, M. I., Huerta-Yepez, S., Jazirehi, A. R., et al. (2005). Rituximab (chimeric anti-CD20) sensitizes B-NHL cell lines to Fas-induced apoptosis. *Oncogene, 24*, 8114–8127.
112. Jazirehi, A. R., Huerta-Yepez, S., Cheng, G., et al. (2005). Rituximab (chimeric anti-CD20 monoclonal antibody) inhibits the constitutive nuclear factor-{kappa}B signaling pathway in non-Hodgkin's lymphoma B-cell lines: Role in sensitization to chemotherapeutic drug-induced apoptosis. *Cancer Research, 65*, 264–276.
113. http://www.clinicaltrials.gov/ct2/show/NCT00392990?term=rituximab+and+burkitt%27s+lymphoma&rank=6
114. http://www.clinicaltrials.gov/ct2/show/NCT00388193?term=rituximab+and+burkitt%27s+lymphoma&rank=4
115. http://clinicaltrials.gov/ct2/show/NCT00039130?cond=%22Burkitt+Lymphoma%22&rank=6
116. Bower, M., Gazzard, B., Mandalia, S., et al. (2005). A prognostic index for systemic AIDS-related non-Hodgkin lymphoma treated in the era of highly active antiretroviral therapy. *Annals of Internal Medicine, 143*, 265–273.
117. Lim, S. T., Karim, R., Nathwani, B. N., et al. (2005). AIDS-related Burkitt's lymphoma versus diffuse large-cell lymphoma in the pre-highly active antiretroviral therapy (HAART) and HAART eras: Significant differences in survival with standard chemotherapy. *Journal of Clinical Oncology, 23*, 4430–4438.
118. Spina, M., Simonelli, C., Talamini, R., et al. (2005). Patients with HIV with Burkitt's lymphoma have a worse outcome than those with diffuse large-cell lymphoma also in the highly active antiretroviral therapy era. *Journal of Clinical Oncology, 23*, 8132–8133. author reply 8133-4.
119. Wang, E. S., Straus, D. J., Teruya-Feldstein, J., et al. (2003). Intensive chemotherapy with cyclophosphamide, doxorubicin, high-dose methotrexate/ifosfamide, etoposide, and high-dose cytarabine (CODOX-M/IVAC) for human immunodeficiency virus-associated Burkitt lymphoma. *Cancer, 98*, 1196–1205.
120. Cortes, J., Thomas, D., Rios, A., et al. (2002). Hyperfractionated cyclophosphamide, vincristine, doxorubicin, and dexamethasone and highly active antiretroviral therapy for patients with acquired immunodeficiency syndrome-related Burkitt lymphoma/leukemia. *Cancer, 94*, 1492–1499.
121. Oriol, A., Ribera, J. M., Esteve, J., et al. (2003). Lack of influence of human immunodeficiency virus infection status in the response to therapy and survival of adult patients with mature B-cell lymphoma or leukemia. Results of the PETHEMA-LAL3/97 study. *Haematologica, 88*, 445–453.
122. Kaplan, L. D., Lee, J. Y., Ambinder, R. F., et al. (2005). Rituximab does not improve clinical outcome in a randomized phase 3 trial of CHOP with or without rituximab in patients with HIV-associated non-Hodgkin lymphoma: AIDS-Malignancies Consortium Trial 010. *Blood, 106*, 1538–1543.
123. Oriol, A., Ribera, J. M., Bergua, J., et al. (2008). High-dose chemotherapy and immunotherapy in adult Burkitt lymphoma: Comparison of results in human immunodeficiency virus-infected and noninfected patients. *Cancer, 113*, 117–125.
124. Spina, M., Jaeger, U., Sparano, J. A., et al. (2005). Rituximab plus infusional cyclophosphamide, doxorubicin, and etoposide in HIV-associated non-Hodgkin lymphoma: Pooled results from 3 phase 2 trials. *Blood, 105*, 1891–1897.
125. Dunleavy, K., Healey-Bird, B. R., Pittaluga, S., et al. (2007). Efficacy and toxicity of dose-adjusted EPOCH-Rituximab in adults with newly diagnosed Burkitt lymphoma. *JCO, 25*, 8035.
126. Levine, A. M., Lee, J., Kaplan, L., et al. (2008). Efficacy and toxicity of concurrent rituximab plus infusional EPOCH in HIV-associated lymphoma: AIDS Malignancy Consortium Trial 034. *JCO, 26*, 8527.
127. Hummel, M., Reiter, S., Adam, K., et al. (2008). Effective treatment and prophylaxis of hyperuricemia and impaired renal function in tumor lysis syndrome with low doses of rasburicase. *European Journal of Haematology, 80*, 331–336.
128. Coiffier, B., Altman, A., Pui, C. H., et al. (2008). Guidelines for the management of pediatric and adult tumor lysis syndrome: An evidence-based review. *Journal of Clinical Oncology, 26*, 2767–2778.
129. Goldman, S. C., Holcenberg, J. S., Finklestein, J. Z., et al. (2001). A randomized comparison between rasburicase and allopurinol in children with lymphoma or leukemia at high risk for tumor lysis. *Blood, 97*, 2998–3003.
130. Trifilio, S., Gordon, L., Singhal, S., et al. (2006). Reduced-dose rasburicase (recombinant xanthine oxidase) in adult cancer patients with hyperuricemia. *Bone Marrow Transplantation, 37*, 997–1001.
131. Griffin, T. C., Weitzman, S., Weinstein, H., et al. (2008). A study of rituximab and ifosfamide, carboplatin, and etoposide chemotherapy in children with recurrent/refractory B-cell (CD20+) non-Hodgkin lymphoma and mature B-cell acute lymphoblastic leukemia: A report from the Children's Oncology Group. *Pediatric Blood Cancer, 52*(2), 177–181.
132. Sweetenham, J. W., Pearce, R., Taghipour, G., et al. (1996). Adult Burkitt's and Burkitt-like non-Hodgkin's lymphoma–outcome for patients treated with high-dose therapy and autologous stem-cell transplantation in first remission or at relapse: Results from the European Group for Blood and Marrow Transplantation. *Journal of Clinical Oncology, 14*, 2465–2472.

133. Nademanee, A., Molina, A., O'Donnell, M. R., et al. (1997). Results of high-dose therapy and autologous bone marrow/stem cell transplantation during remission in poor-risk intermediate- and high-grade lymphoma: International index high and high-intermediate risk group. *Blood, 90,* 3844–3852.

134. Nademanee, A., Molina, A., Dagis, A., et al. (2000). Autologous stem-cell transplantation for poor-risk and relapsed intermediate- and high-grade non-Hodgkin's lymphoma. *Clinical Lymphoma, 1,* 46–54.

135. Bureo, E., Ortega, J. J., Munoz, A., et al. (1995). Bone marrow transplantation in 46 pediatric patients with non-Hodgkin's lymphoma. Spanish Working Party for Bone Marrow Transplantation in Children. *Bone Marrow Transplantation, 15,* 353–359.

136. Peniket, A. J., Ruiz de Elvira, M. C., Taghipour, G., et al. (2003). An EBMT registry matched study of allogeneic stem cell transplants for lymphoma: Allogeneic transplantation is associated with a lower relapse rate but a higher procedure-related mortality rate than autologous transplantation. *Bone Marrow Transplantation, 31,* 667–678.

137. McMahon, S. B., Wood, M. A., & Cole, M. D. (2000). The essential cofactor TRRAP recruits the histone acetyltransferase hGCN5 to c-Myc. *Molecular and Cellular Biology, 20,* 556–562.

138. Patel, J. H., Du, Y., Ard, P. G., et al. (2004). The c-MYC oncoprotein is a substrate of the acetyltransferases hGCN5/PCAF and TIP60. *Molecular and Cellular Biology, 24,* 10826–10834.

139. Kano, Y., Akutsu, M., Tsunoda, S., et al. (2007). Cytotoxic effects of histone deacetylase inhibitor FK228 (depsipeptide, formally named FR901228) in combination with conventional anti-leukemia/lymphoma agents against human leukemia/lymphoma cell lines. *Investigational New Drugs, 25,* 31–40.

140. Zou, P., Kawada, J., Pesnicak, L., et al. (2007). Bortezomib induces apoptosis of Epstein-Barr virus (EBV)-transformed B cells and prolongs survival of mice inoculated with EBV-transformed B cells. *Journal of Virology, 81,* 10029–10036.

Chapter 14
Treatment of Acute Lymphoblastic Leukemia in Young Adults

Nicolas Boissel, Françoise Huguet, and Hervé Dombret

Introduction

Acute lymphoblastic leukemia (ALL) in adult and children are contrasting diseases in terms of characteristics but mostly, in terms of outcome. During the last 40 years, progress in the treatment of childhood ALL has dramatically improved the cure rate in children [1]. These advances have been obtained through a stepwise improvement of protocols including the use of a multiagent chemotherapeutic regimen, strategies to reduce extramedullary relapse, the intensification of post-remission therapy, and the use of extensive maintenance therapy. Most of these breakthroughs have been validated through successive randomized trials. During the same period, improvement of adult protocols has been real but more modest [2]. Over the last decade, 5-year overall survival for children with ALL was around 80% while reaching only 30–40% in adults [3, 4]. A partial explanation for this disparity is the difference in characteristics between adults and children with ALL [5]. Adults display a higher frequency of unfavorable features including the presence of the Philadelphia chromosome (Ph) and a higher WBC at diagnosis [6]. Favorable features, such as hyperdiploidy and translocation t(12;21), are found in children but rarely in adults [7]. However, even within identical biological subtypes, outcomes observed in adult protocols are inferior to those obtained in children [6, 8, 9]. Differences in drug metabolism, treatment-related morbidity, and treatment compliance have been reported as potential explanations for these discrepancies [10–13].

Adolescents and young adults (AYA) aged 15–30 years constitute a transition population between children and older adults. At this age, the incidence of acute myeloid leukemia (AML) slowly increases and the incidence of ALL progressively decreases with comparable rates (around 7/1,000,000/year) (Fig. 14.1) [14]. The incidence of ALL decreases until age 35–40 years and rises again in older patients. In most centers, young adults older than 20 years are treated with adult protocols that have been designed to treat and thus to be tolerated by patients up to 60 years of age. For personal, familial, social and/or economical reasons, adolescents aged 15–20 years with inaugural symptoms of ALL may first be seen by family physicians, internists, or emergency physicians from adult or pediatric institutions. This initial diversity leads to a wide pattern of subsequent referral. Several North American studies have repeatedly shown that only one-third of adolescents aged 15–19 years diagnosed with cancer are referred to pediatric hospitals, as compared to more than 80% in younger children [15, 16]. In these pediatric hospitals, treatment may significantly differ from adult centers. In pediatric ALL protocols, patients older than 10 years of age are usually considered "higher risk" and thus more intensively treated. In contrast, older adolescents, 20–30 years of age, treated in

N. Boissel (✉)
Hematology Department, EA 3518, Saint-Louis Hospital, Paris Diderot University,
1 avenue Claude Vellefaux, 75010 Paris, France
e-mail: nicolas.boissel@sls.aphp.fr

A.S. Advani and H.M. Lazarus (eds.), *Adult Acute Lymphocytic Leukemia*, Contemporary Hematology,
DOI 10.1007/978-1-60761-707-5_14, © Springer Science+Business Media, LLC 2011

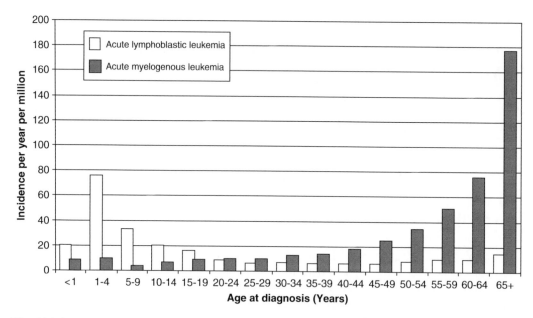

Fig. 14.1 Age-specific incidence rate of ALL and AML (Surveillance, Epidemiology, and End Results (SEER) Program 2000–2005)

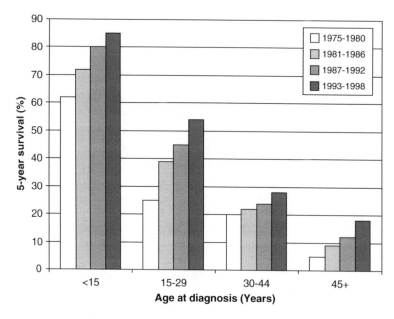

Fig. 14.2 Five-year survival rate for ALL by era, SEER [14]

adult trials are *a priori* considered as standard- or low-risk patients. In many countries, this situation has led to a paradox that adolescents with ALL may thus be considered either as children with high-risk disease or as adults with low-risk disease. In both situations, due to this unique incidence distribution of ALL, AYA represent a minority of patients included in clinical trials. Nevertheless, improvement in outcome observed in this population during the last decades is real, even if less impressive than that reported in children (Fig. 14.2) [14, 17, 18]. This chapter will summarize the point of view of adult physicians on the progresses made in the management of AYA with ALL.

Adolescents with ALL : Young Adults or Old Children?

Adolescent ALL Characteristics

This discrepancy in therapeutic strategies for adolescent patients has led to a number of retrospective studies comparing the outcome of patients treated in pediatric *vs.* adult clinical trials. In a preliminary study presented at the ASH meeting in 1990, the pediatric French acute lymphoblastic leukemia (FRALLE) and the adult acute lymphoblastic leukemia (LALA) groups demonstrated the advantage of a pediatric therapeutic regimen compared to an adult therapeutic regimen in a cohort of French patients aged 15–20 years [19]. In the past 10 years, this initial observation has been confirmed by half a dozen retrospective studies in the United States and Europe, with studies demonstrating a significantly better outcome for adolescents treated on pediatric trials (Fig. 14.3) [20–25]. As reported in Table 14.1, gains up to 11% in complete remission (CR) rates, 9–41% in overall survival, and 16–35% in event-free survival were reported for patients treated on pediatric trials. Of note, this difference in outcome was not reported by the Finnish study that compared patients aged 10–16 years treated in Nordic Society for Paediatric Hematology and Oncology (NOPHO) trials to AYA aged 17–25 years treated in adult Finnish Leukemia Group protocols [26].

In all these studies, pediatric and adult cohorts were relatively well matched with respect to clinical and biological characteristics, except for age (Table 14.1). Adolescents treated on pediatric trials were significantly younger than adolescents treated on adult trials. In AYA patients, immunophenotype and cytogenetic features differed from both adult ALL and pediatric ALL patients. The incidence of T-cell ALL (T-ALL) was increased (11–30%), slightly above the 20% observed in adult ALL population [3]. The frequency of Ph-positive ALL in AYA patients was low (1–8%), but higher than that observed in childhood ALL [3]. In these cohorts, a translocation t(4;11) was found in less than 3% of cases, very similar to the frequency observed in children older than 1 year [27]. Hyperdiploidy, a favorable prognostic feature found in 25% of children and 5–10% of adults, was found in 20% of adolescent patients [1].

Dose Intensity

Differences in drugs and dose intensity may be the major reason for the differences in outcome for AYA patients treated on pediatric *vs.* adult trials (Table 14.2). Pediatric protocols are mainly based on the Berlin-Frankfurt-Munich (BFM) schedule; use more non-myelotoxic drugs like vincristine, steroids, and asparaginase; and include reinforced delayed intensification (Table 14.2). Adult regimens include higher doses of myelotoxic drugs like anthracycline, cytarabine, cyclophosphamide, and etoposide; and more patients proceed to allogeneic (ASCT)/autologous stem cell transplantation (autoSCT) (Table 14.2). In the French study, adolescents treated in the pediatric FRALLE-93 protocol received five times more steroids, three times more vincristine, and 20 times more asparaginase than adolescents concomitantly treated in the adult LALA-94 trial [20]. The period of treatment administration was also shorter in the pediatric trial (24 months vs. 30 months). The pediatric BFM-based FRALLE-93 induction regimen includes asparaginase and 50% more steroids than the adult LALA-94 induction regimen. This difference probably impacted the CR rate, which was significantly higher in the pediatric protocol (94% vs. 83%, $p = .04$). In the US study comparing the outcome of adolescents aged 16–21 years treated on the pediatric Children's Cancer Group (CCG)-1882/1901 protocols or on the adult Cancer And Leukemia Group B (CALGB)-8811/9111/9311/9511/19802 protocols, pediatric patients received more vincristine, steroids, and asparaginase [25]. Similar findings have been demonstrated when comparing pediatric and adult therapeutic regimens in the studies from the Netherlands, Sweden, and the United Kingdom [21, 23, 24].

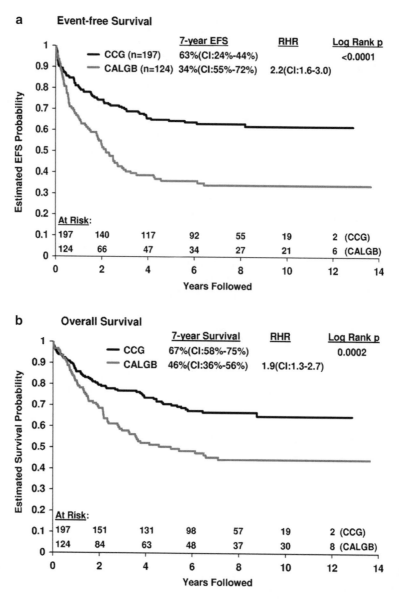

Fig. 14.3 Comparison of the outcome of adolescents concomitantly treated in the pediatric CCG and adult CALGB trials. Event-free survival (**a**) and overall survival (**b**) are shown (*RHR* relative hard rate for CALGB patient; *CI* confidence interval) [25]

The efficacy of non-myelotoxic drugs has been demonstrated in the setting of pediatric randomized trials. A study from Dana-Farber Cancer Institute (DFCI) demonstrated an improved response to increased steroid exposure in patients aged 1–18 years. Dexamethasone, more widely used by pediatricians, has been shown to reduce the risk of CNS and bone marrow relapse in two randomized trials from the CCG and the Medical Research Council (MRC). Higher doses of asparaginase have also been shown to benefit children aged 9–18 years despite some increase in related toxicity [28]. In a study of the Pediatric Oncoly Group, repeated doses of asparaginase during the early phase of therapy significantly improved the outcome of T-ALL [29]. At the present time, no randomized trial on the role of asparaginase has been performed in adults [30]. Nevertheless, the degree

Table 14.1 Characteristics and outcome of adolescents among pediatric and adult trials in comparative studies

	Years	Age (years)	Pts n	ALL characteristics (%)				CR (%)	EFS		OS		Reference
				T-ALL	Ph+	t(4;11)	Hyperdiploid		(years)	(%)	(years)	(%)	
FRALLE 93	1993–1999	15–20	77	30	1	2	9	94	5	67	5	78	[20]
LALA 94	1994–2000	15–20	100	28	3	1	21	83	5	41	5	45	
DCOG ALL 6–9	1985–1999	15–18	47	26	2	0	29	98	5	69	5	79	[21]
HOVON ALL-5/18	1985–1999	15–18	44	27	4	0.5	23	91	5	34	5	38	
UKALL 97/99	1997–2002	15–17	61	22	8	NA	NA	98	5	65	5	71	[23]
UKALL XII/E2993	1997–2002	15–17	67	11	3	NA	NA	94	5	49	5	56	
NOPHO92	1992–2000	15–18	36	NA	NA	NA	NA	NA	5	74	NA	NA	[24]
Adult ALL group	1994–2000	15–20	23	NA	NA	NA	NA	NA	5	39	NA	NA	
CCG	1989–1995	16–20	197	16	3	3	NA	90	7	63	7	67	[25]
CALGB	1988–2001	16–20	124	25	6	2	NA	90	7	34	7	46	
AEIOP 95/2000	1996–2003	14–18	150	NA	NA	NA	NA	94	NA	NA	2	80	[22]
GIMEMA	1996–2003	14–18	95	NA	NA	NA	NA	89	NA	NA	2	71	

NA not available

Table 14.2 Differences in dose intensity among pediatric and adult trials in comparative studies

	VCR (mg/m²)	PDN (mg/m²)	DEXA (mg/m²)	ASPA (U/m²)	DNR/DXR (mg/m²)	AraC (mg/m²)	Delayed intensification	ASCT (%)	Reference
FRALLE 93	19 inf	4,340	140	180,000	280/75	960	Yes	17	[20]
LALA 94	6 inf	840	320 TD	9,000	150/96	2,900	No	9	
DCOG ALL 6–9	48	0	1,000	101,000	NA	NA	Yes	4	[21]
HOVON ALL-5/18	6,8	1,800	0	70,000	NA	24,000	Yes, AML-like (ALL-18)	25	
UKALL 97	32	6,080	900	108,000	180/0	2,700	Yes (randomized)	13	[23]
UKALL XII/E2993	14	3,180	280	120,000	340/0	2,925	No	30	[24]
NOPHO92	30TD	4,260	220	420,000	120/120	1,800	Yes	NA	
Adult ALL group	16TD	3,720	0	0	390/0	31,200	No	NA	
CCG 1,882	8TD+22.5	7,695[a]	210	90,000	100/75	1,800	Yes	3	[25]
CALGB	22TD	8,640	140	48,000	135–240/90	1,200	Yes	1	

VCR vincristine; *PDN* prednisone; *DEXA* dexamethasone; *ASPA* asparaginase; *DNR* daunorubicin; *DXR* doxorubicin; *AraC* cytarabine; *ASCT* allogeneic stem cell transplantation; *NA* not available; *TD* total dose; *inf* infusion

[a] Average (2 years consolidation for girls, 3 years for boys)

of asparagine depletion with pegylated asparaginase therapy does correlate with outcome in adult ALL patients [31]. In addition to the choice and the cumulative dose of drugs, one of the major concepts that improved the outcome of children with ALL is the use of delayed intensification. Initially proposed by the BFM study group, the benefit of this strategy has been demonstrated by the CCG in patients older than 10 years of age and in slow early responders [32–34].

Conversely, all adult protocols but one, (LALA-94), administrated higher doses of anthracycline. Relatively high doses of cytarabine (up to 31,200 mg/m^2) were also administered in adult protocols. The association of anthracycline with high-dose cytarabine, as is used in AML protocols, is often chosen as intensive consolidation in adults with ALL. Only the adult CALGB trial scheduled a pediatric-like delayed intensification. More generally, one may schematically oppose previous pediatric and adult trials to consider ALL therapy by more continuous exposure to non-myelotoxic agents in children and shorter but more myelosuppressive cycles in adults. In adult trials, more patients also receive ASCT in first CR.

Allogeneic Transplantation (ASCT)

These pediatric *vs.* adult retrospective studies also revealed a heterogeneous attitude concerning ASCT. It first appeared that the rate of allogeneic transplantation was highly variable within adult or pediatric protocols (Table 14.2). When comparing adult to pediatric protocols, higher rates of ASCT were commonly observed in adult trials. The rate of ASCT was 1–30% in adult trials compared to 3–17% in pediatric trials. In the French experience, a higher rate of transplanted adolescents were observed in the pediatric FRALLE-93 trial than in the adult LALA-94 (17% vs. 9% respectively) [20]. In the Dutch experience, 25% of adult adolescents treated in the Dutch Hemato-Oncology Association (HOVON) protocols underwent ASCT, but only 4% in the Dutch Childhood Oncology Group (DCOG) trials [21]. In the MRC, 30% of adults adolescents were allografted but only 13% in the pediatric cohort [23]. When reported, the indication for alloSCT differed in two major points: (1) adult protocols retain wide criteria for ASCT in first CR based on initial characteristics of the disease; (2) pediatric protocols tend to reserve transplant for patients with Ph-positive ALL or those who are slow early responders [35, 36].

Adherence to Treatment

Comparisons of adult and pediatric results in adolescents with ALL highlighted that the problem of adherence to treatment should be examined from different angles. Patient compliance to treatment is a well-recognized difficulty that widely impairs the care of the adolescent and young adult population. Specific adolescent behaviors have been identified. A developed sense of independency and of invincibility may keep the patient away from his or her physician and the therapeutic schedule. The difficulties in communication between adolescents and their parents add some confusion about who is in charge of the administration of the medication [37]. This lack of communication may also lead to delays in reporting secondary effects or psychological/social difficulties [38]. The Society of International Oncology (SIOP) Working Committee on Psychosocial Issues in Pediatric Oncology has made several recommendations to prevent noncompliance [39]. Risk factors for poor compliance, such as low socioeconomic status, lack of social support, cultural and linguistic barriers, or poor parental involvement should be identified and taken into account early in the treatment.

On the other hand, adherence to treatment also concerns the physician in charge. Discrepancies in therapy management between adult physicians and pediatricians have been pointed out by Schiffer when dissecting the reasons for the difference in outcome: "A consequence of better regimens? Better doctors? Both?" [40]. This editorial emphasizes the complexity of ALL protocols and the way "pediatricians administer these treatments with a military precision on the basis of a near-religious conviction about the necessity of maintaining prescribed dose and schedule come hell, high water, birthdays, Bastille Day, or Christmas." [40] Few data are available to illustrate this widely observed point of view. In both childhood and adult ALL, a short delay between remission induction and consolidation has been evidenced as an important prognostic factor [41, 42]. In the French comparison, despite similar induction intensities, a significantly longer recovery interval between CR time and day 1 of first post-remission course was allowed for patients treated in the adult LALA protocol (7 days vs. 2 days in the pediatric FRALLE) [20]. A longer allowed recovery time interval between courses was also noticed in the DCOG/HOVON comparison [21]. In the MRC pediatric UKALL X and adult UKALL XA trials, protocol deviations were reported in 2.5% of pediatric cases and 22% of adult cases [6]. Interestingly, the majority of deviations in the UKALL XA concerned the administration of more therapy than scheduled by the randomization, half of these cases concerning ASCT or autoSCT. Nearly all these comments arise from retrospective studies and call for prospective observation and evaluation in specific designed trials.

Outcome of AYA in Adult Protocols

Most adult trials include patients older than 15–18 years of age but do not specifically consider the outcome of AYA. Considering patients with a broad range of age, often up to 60 years or older, these trials have to deal with heterogeneous diseases but also heterogeneous tolerance to chemotherapy. For these reasons, adult protocols frequently favored less intensive upfront approaches and broad indications of either ASCT or autoSCT, particularly in younger patients. This lack of stratification on age makes it difficult to identify optimized therapy in younger patients. Table 14.3 summarizes the results of adult protocols reported during the last decade that specifically detailed the outcome of AYA [6, 43–50]. The age cutoff that defined the frontier between younger and older adults vary among these protocols from 30 to 45 years and does not necessarily correspond to a reasonable definition of AYA population. In these trials, the outcome of younger adults is clearly better than older patients. It is remarkable that the long-term survival rate of AYA with ALL has reached and even gone beyond 50%.

Prognostic Factors and Risk Assessment

Conversely to other hematological malignancies or to pediatric ALL [51, 52], there is no consensual risk stratification in adult ALL. Many classifications are used including patient age, disease characteristics at diagnosis, and response to treatment. Age is probably one of the most important prognostic factors in ALL. Excluding infants, cure rates gradually decrease with age. In adults, as illustrated in Table 14.3, long-term survival progressively decreases from 40% to 50% in patients below 30 years of age to less than 20% in patients above 60 years of age [6, 47, 49]. The impact of age on the prognosis of adult ALL is a composite of other more or less well-described factors that also fluctuate among age: the characteristics of the disease (immunophenotype, cytogenetic, molecular markers), the presence of comorbidities, and the variation of pharmacodynamic parameters. As previously underlined, AYA are thus considered a standard risk in the majority of adult protocols and there are few data to support that age is a strong prognostic factor in this population up to 30 years old. Among other well-reported factors associated with outcome, a high white blood cell (WBC) count

Table 14.3 Treatment results from selected clinical trials involving AYA with ALL

	Age range (years)	Years	N (pts)	Ph+	Early death (%)	CR (%)	DFS		OS		Reference
								% or time		% or time	
Adult trials											
SWOG 8417/19	15+	1985–1991	353	Y	15	62	med.	18 m	med.	18 m	[43]
	15–34		201		6	71	–	–	med.	27 m	
	35–49		67		14	60	–	–	med.	17 m	
	≥50		85		37	41	–	–	med.	5 m	
MRC UKALL XA	15+	1985–1992	617	Y	–	88	5 years	28%	–	–	[6, 44]
	15–19		200		–	97	10 years	35%	10	60%	
	20–39		228		–	89	10 years	29%	10	43%	
	40+		189		–	77	10 years	15%	10	19%	
GIMEMA ALL0288	12+		769	Y	7	82	9 years	29%	9	27%	[45]
	12–20		288		–	87	8 years	38%	8	34%	
	21–30		187		–	83	8 years	32%	8 years	36%	
JALSG ALL93	15–60	1993–1997	263	Y	6	78	6 years	30%	6 years	33%	[46]
	15–29		130		–	84	6 years	34%	6 years	48%	
	30–60		133		–	72	6 years	26%	6 years	21%	
CALGB 9111	15+	1991–1993	185	Y	8	85	3 years	40%	3 years	43%	[47]
	15–29		73		–	90	3 years	46%	3 years	57%	
	30–59		77		–	84	3 years	43%	3 years	40%	
	60+		35		–	77	3 years	19%	3 years	17%	
GOELAL02	15–59	1994–1998	198	Y	2	86	med.	28 m	med.	29 m	[48]
	15–34		110		–	94	med.	37.2 m	med.	50.5 m	
	35–59		88		–	75	med.	14.8 m	med.	15.5 m	
HyperCVAD	14+	1992–2000	288	Y	5	92	–	–	5 years	38%	[49]
	14–39		147		–	95	–	–	5 years	51%	
	40–59		82		–	94	–	–	5 years	30%	
	60+		59		15	80	–	–	5 years	17%	
Hybrid trials											
GRAALL-2003	15–60	2003–2005	225	N	6	94	2 years	59%	2 years	58%	[50]
	15–45		172		4	95	2 years	61%	2 years	60%	
	46–60		53		13	87	2 years	53%	2 years	47%	
GMALL 07/03	15–60	2003–2006	713	Y	5	89	–	–	5 years	54%	[99]
	15–35		NA		–	90	–	–	5 years	64%	

(continued)

Table 14.3 (continued)

	Age range (years)	Years	N (pts)	Ph+	Early death (%)	CR (%)	DFS time	DFS % or time	OS time	OS % or time	Reference
Pediatric trials											
PETHEMA ALL-96	15–30	1996–2005	81	N	1	98	6 years	61%	6 years	69%	[100]
(standard-risk)	15–18		35		3	94	6 years	60%	6 years	77%	
	19–30		46		0	100	6 years	63%	6 years	63%	
DFCI 00-01	18–50	NA	75	Y	1	84	–	–	2 years	77.1%	[102]
USCH (A-BFM)	19–57	NA	34	NA	–	97	3 years	EFS: 61%	–	–	[103]
FRALLE 2000B/T	16–57	2001–2007	28	N	0	82	4 years	90%	4 years	83%	[101]

Y yes; *N* no; *med.* median; *NA* not available

at diagnosis is a poor prognostic feature reported by many pediatric and adult trials, especially in patients with B-cell precursor (BCP)-ALL. In adults, WBC count does not necessarily correlate with age [6]. Therefore, it does not confer a particular prognosis to AYA when compared to older adults.

Immunologic, cytogenetic, and molecular characterization of the disease is helpful in understanding the profile of ALL in AYA. As mentioned above, there is an increased frequency of T-ALL in patients aged 10–40 years. Conversely to what was reported in children, the outcome of adult patients with T-ALL is generally considered superior to that of BCP-ALL [1, 53, 54]. This difference is less obvious since Ph-positive ALL is separately treated and analyzed [50, 55]. In the AYA population, Ph-positive ALL is less frequent than in the general adult population [6, 56]. Considered by most of pediatric and adult trials as a high-risk feature, the presence of the t(9;22)(q34;q11) translocation and/or *BCR-ABL* rearrangement requires individualized treatment with tyrosine kinase inhibitors. Pro-B-ALL is associated with the t(4;11) translocation. Both of these features are associated with a poor outcome in children and adults and are typically considered as criteria to proceed to ASCT [54, 57, 58]. In AYA, the t(4;11) is a rare event, with a frequency lower than the 10% reported in the adult population [6].

Immature T-ALL is uncommon in children below 10 years of age, but the frequency of this subgroup increases with age with an incidence of 22% in patients aged 11–20 years and 38% in adult patients above 20 years of age [59]. Immature T-ALL has been identified by many groups to be associated with a poor outcome [60–63]. Patients with either early or mature T-ALL are considered as high-risk patients in the German Multicenter Study Group for Adult ALL (GMALL) and thus candidates for alloSCT. Much progress has been accomplished in the last decade to understand the physiopathology and the prognosis of T-ALL [64]. Approximately half of adult patients with T-ALL have the *SIL-TAL1* or *CALM-AF10* fusion transcript or demonstrate deregulated expression of *HOX11* or *HOX11L2* [59]. In T-ALL patients treated on the pediatric FRALLE and the adult LALA trials, the frequency of *HOX11L2* and *SIL-TAL1* among T-ALL decreased with age, whereas the frequency of *HOX11* steadily increased [59]. Immature T-ALL with the *CALM-AF10* fusion transcript has been reported to be a feature of AYA (median age 25 years), and has been suggested to be associated with a poor outcome and early resistance to standard induction regimen [65]. Salvage therapy inspired from AML regimens may be of interest in this population of immature T-ALL [62]. More recently, the activation of the *NOTCH1* pathway has been implicated in T-ALL leukemogenesis. Both *NOTCH1* and *FBXW7* mutations have been implicated in more than 50% of T-ALL [66, 67]. Both mutations have been associated with a favorable outcome in pediatric and adult ALL, but no relation with age has been identified [68–70].

Early response to therapy is a composite marker of the intrinsic sensitivity of the disease and of the pharmacodynamics of the patient [3]. Response to prednisone and early bone marrow response are important prognostic factors widely validated in childhood trials but infrequently used in adult trials [45, 50, 71]. In the Italian Group for Adult Hematologic Diseases (GIMEMA) ALL 0288 trial, which included patients aged 12–59 years, response to prednisone was a strong age-independent prognostic factor for OS and DFS [45]. The quality of remission may be assessed by evaluating minimal residual disease (MRD). Evidence that the level of MRD is strongly predictive of outcome initially arose from pediatric studies [72–74]. The value of MRD in adults was initially confirmed using transcript-fusion-based MRD in Ph-positive ALL [75, 76] More recently, the prognostic value of MRD has been confirmed in adult studies [55, 77, 78]. In the Polish Adult Leukemia Group (PALG) ALL 4-2002 study, standard-risk AYA patients were defined by age <35 years, WBC <30 K/L, absence of an unfavorable immunophenotype, and achieving CR after 1 cycle. MRD was assessed by flow cytometry at different time points. In these standard-risk patients, a persistent MRD < 0.1% after induction and consolidation identified patients with a very low risk of relapse (11% vs. 75% for others). In the ongoing GMALL study, MRD is assessed by PCR. Patients with high levels of MRD ($>10^{-4}$) after induction and first consolidation are eligible for ASCT in the first CR [79]. The majority of ongoing trials in adult Ph-negative ALL in Europe prospectively use MRD for risk stratification [80].

Remission Induction

The majority of induction regimens have arisen from the BFM program and consist of the sequential administration of four to five drugs: steroids, vincristine, anthracycline, cyclophosphamide, and asparaginase. As mentioned above, higher doses of anthracycline mainly daunorubicin, are used in adult protocols in comparison to the original BFM schedule. The benefit of anthracycline dose reinforcement has been suggested but remains matter of debate [81, 82]. The majority of these protocols include repeated administration of asparaginase in their induction therapy, but only half of them reintroduce asparaginase in their post-remission regimen. Remarkably, the hyper-CVAD regimen developed at the M. D. Anderson Cancer Center did not include any asparaginase in the treatment schedule and provided comparable results in terms of CR rate and long-term survival [49]. The early use of cyclophosphamide during induction has been suggested to benefit patients with T-ALL and may be of interest in the AYA population, at least in this subgroup of ALL [49, 53]. In the GIMEMA ALL 0288 trial, the addition of cyclophosphamide was randomized during a conventional four-drug induction. Addition of cyclophosphamide increased the CR rate in multivariate analysis [45]. The French Group for Research on Adult Acute Lymphoblastic Leukemia (GRAALL)-2003 protocol included the hyper-C sequence, a repeated administration of cyclophosphamide, developed by M.D. Anderson in a BFM-based induction regimen for patients with slow early prednisone or bone marrow response [50]. The notable improvement in CR rate led the GRAALL to randomize this hyper-C sequence in its current GRAALL-2005 trial.

CR rates reported in these protocols are comparable to those observed in other adult protocols (78–94%) [4, 83]. In AYA, CR rates are typically 84–97%, higher than those observed in older patients. Early toxicity is less than 10% and, when reported, even lower in younger patients. In the more recent protocols, few patients have failed induction therapy. In the hyper-CVAD regimen, CR was achieved in 99% of patients aged <30 years and in 80% of patients older than 60 years with 15% induction deaths [49]. The same observation was reported in the GRAALL-2003 [50]. A 94% CR rate and 4% early deaths were observed in patients aged <45 years. Given the high CR rates achieved with current induction therapy, there are rare cases of refractory disease in AYA patients. Therefore, efforts must be now oriented toward improving the supportive care, evaluating the quality of this remission and optimizing the post-remission therapy.

Post-remission Therapy

Post-remission therapy is based on the intensive administration of chemotherapy derived from either pediatric protocols or historical randomized trials that often failed to demonstrate any benefit in the adult population. The fact that post-remission intensification improves the outcome of patients was demonstrated in randomized pediatric trials. However, mainly non-randomized trials have provided the same evidence in adults. It is once more intriguing than such therapy may be less efficient as the patient becomes an adult. This discrepancy may be due to different parameters: (1) the lower frequency of patients in adult protocols, (2) the difference in ALL characteristics, (3) the differences in adherence to treatment, and (4) the excess of toxicity of reinforced schedules in older adults. The GMALL group reported an improvement in outcome after introduction in the 01/81 and 02/84 trials of a late intensification based on the same drugs used during induction [84]. The CALGB reported improved remission duration and survival in comparison to historical studies after administration of two blocks of early intensification and a 8-week late intensification [53]. The MRC randomized in two similar and concomitant pediatric (<15 years, UKALL X) and adult (≥15 years, UKALL XA) protocols the administration of AML-style early (5 weeks) and late (20 weeks) intensifications [44, 85]. The pediatric UKALL X demonstrated a marked improved outcome in children receiving both intensifications. However, in the adult protocol, only relapse-free survival and not overall survival was improved. As mentioned above, there were significant differences in adherence to treatment between both protocols. In UKALL XA, an increased risk of death in CR for each additional intensification was also reported. When looking at different age ranges, the rate of CR death was around 3% in young adults (15–39 years) and 17% in patients beyond 40 years of age [6]. However, the rate of patients alive in continuous CR was very similar in patients aged 10–14 years, 15–19 years, and 20–39 years (55, 52, and 56% respectively) and decreased in older patients (29%). In the Spanish Program for the Study and Treatment of Hematological Malignances (PETHEMA) ALL-89 trial, the randomized administration of a late 6-week intensification did not modify the outcome of patients [86]. In the more recent GRAALL-2003 experience, the benefit of the reinforced strategy that comprised a late intensification was mainly seen in patients beyond 45 years of age [50]. The rate of relapse risk did not significantly differ between younger and older patients (2 years cumulative incidence (CI) of relapse: 25% vs. 20% for patients >45 years) but the rate of death in CR was significantly lower in younger patients (2 years-CI of death in CR: 2% vs. 15% for patients >45 years). These observations underscore the fact that post-remission reinforced strategies that may benefit AYA patients should be more cautiously applied in older patients.

Allogeneic Stem Cell Transplantation (ASCT)

The indication for ASCT in adult ALL is still a matter of debate. Most clinical trials have been based on donor availability, the so-called "biological randomization". Early studies have logically focused on patients with high-risk disease. Conflicting data have been published with variable definitions of high-risk disease and a wide diversity of chemotherapy administrated in patients with no donor [87–89]. Criteria to define high-risk patients differed between these studies but were based on patient age, phenotypic and cytogenetic characteristics of the disease, and the resistance of the disease after one induction course. The interpretation of these results in the population of AYA is thus difficult since age >35 years is one of the common high-risk factors used in these adult studies. Two French groups reported three protocols (LALA-87/94 and GOELAL-02) with an improved outcome for high-risk patients with ASCT when a HLA-compatible donor was available [48, 90, 91]. These results were not confirmed by the more recent PETHEMA ALL-93 and European Organisation for Research and Treatment of Cancer (EORTC) ALL-3 studies [92, 93]. Two meta-analyses concluded there was an advantage to ASCT in patients with high-risk ALL and that this procedure was cost-effective [94, 95]. The results of the International ALL Trial (MRC UKALL XII/ECOG E2993) were recently published [96]. This is the largest randomized trial evaluating the role of ASCT in first CR. More than 1,900 adult patients were enrolled in this trial. A matched sibling ASCT improved the overall survival of patients with standard-risk ALL, defined by age ≤35 years and low WBC count at presentation (<100 G/L for BCP-ALL or <30 G/L for T-ALL) and the absence of the Ph. In standard-risk patients, 5-year overall survival was 62% in patients with a donor compared with 52% in patients without a donor ($p = .02$). No benefit was observed in high-risk patients, probably due to a higher transplant-related mortality (39% vs. 20% in standard-risk patients) that counterbalanced the reduction in relapse risk.

Autologous Stem Cell Transplantation (autoSCT)

The place of autoSCT in post-remission therapy is even more difficult to assess in AYA patients. The LALA, the EORTC, and the PETHEMA groups reported in five trials conducted in the last two decades equivalent results for patients treated with chemotherapy or autologous transplantation

[91–93, 97]. In a meta-analysis of three trials, the LALA group suggested a lower incidence of relapse in autografted patients. However, this did not translate into better disease-free and overall survivals [98]. The recent International ALL Trial MRC UKALL XII/ECOG E2993) randomized 456 patients to autoSCT vs. chemotherapy [96]. AutoSCT was inferior to chemotherapy alone, including in AYA patients with standard-risk ALL. Given the long-term toxicities of autoSCT in comparison to chemotherapy alone, it appears difficult to recommend this procedure in any subgroup of AYA with ALL in first CR.

Current Therapeutic Options for ALL in AYA

Following the results of recent retrospective studies of ALL therapy in adolescents, different therapeutic approaches have been adopted. More adolescents, at least up until 18 years of age, are enrolled in pediatric protocols. For older patients, two approaches are currently taken: (1) the use of pediatric-inspired "hybrid" protocols, (2) the use of pediatric protocols. There are few data on the respective feasibility and results of both of these therapeutic approaches.

Treating AYA in "Hybrid" Protocols

Hybrid protocols, adapting features from adult regimens but maintaining a pediatric-inspired backbone, might be the first step toward more intensive pediatric trials in adults or AYA. The GMALL 07/2003 is a MRD-based risk stratification trial that includes an 8-drug induction, five blocks of consolidation, a reinduction and a maintenance therapy [99]. An ASCT is indicated for patients with high-risk initial characteristics, late CR, or with persistent elevated MRD. As shown in Table 14.3, the CR rate in AYA was 90%, similar to the rate observed in the whole adult population. In this cohort of 713 patients with a median age of 34 years (range: 15–55 years), the 5-year overall survival was 54%. The 5-year overall survival was 64% for AYA (<35 years) and 67% in standard risk AYA. The GRAALL-2003 trial proposed a risk-adapted strategy with a reinforcement of induction with a hyper-C sequence in poor early responders, and an ASCT in high-risk patients [50]. The 5-drug induction regimen was followed by six blocks of consolidation with high-dose methotrexate, a reinduction, three more blocks, and maintenance therapy. As already mentioned, age impacted the tolerance but not the relapse risk after chemotherapy. The overall survival at 3.5 years for patients younger than 35 years of age was 70% in comparison to 44% in the previous LALA-94 protocol (Fig. 14.4).

Treating AYA According to Pediatric Trials

The rationale of this approach is the relative homogeneity of ALL characteristics between patients 10 and 30 years of age. Ph-positive ALL occurs in a minority of patients, and patients with Ph-positive ALL should be treated on specific trials that combine conventional chemotherapy and tyrosine kinase inhibitors to optimize control of the disease prior to proceeding to ASCT. The PETHEMA reported the outcome of 81 AYA patients aged 15–30 years with standard-risk ALL (WBC ≤30 K/L and absence of the t(9;22), t(1;19), or 11q23 abnormalities) treated in the ALL-96 trial [100]. The CR rate was 98%, and there was one toxic death during induction. Young adults experienced more hematological toxicity than adolescents, with increased episodes of neutropenia and longer treatment delays during consolidation and maintenance. The outcome of AYA was similar in this relatively small cohort with 6-year overall survivals of 77% and 63%, respectively. The Hôtel

B-ALL and in pediatric patients [125, 126]. The target gene for this deletion has not yet been identified. Deletions of 9p21 (targets *INK4/ARF*) are frequent and have been mentioned somewhere else in this chapter. Finally, *MYB*, a transcription factor involved in proliferation, survival, and differentiation of hematopoietic cells and that when overexpressed leads to leukemogenesis in mice has been found duplicated in 8% of T-ALL [127, 128].

Mutations that give way to constitutively active oncogenes have also been described in T-ALL, and are another mechanism of transformation of T-lymphocyte precursors cooperating in a multi-hit model. For example, *NOTCH1* encodes a heterodimeric transmembrane receptor with an intracellular fragment that translocates to the nucleus upon ligand binding and forms part of a transcription activation complex that targets MYC among other proteins. It regulates cell fate in multiple tissues, hematopoietic stem cell self-renewal, and regulates commitment of common lymphoid progenitors (CLP) to T-lineage, and T-cell development. In the rare t(7;9) *NOTCH1* is juxtaposed to *TCRB*, and results in constitutively active *NOTCH1* that lacks the N-terminus. Mice transplanted with bone marrow expressing activated *NOTCH* alleles developed T-ALL showing its oncogenic activity in T precursors [129]. Gain-of-function mutations in *NOTCH1* have emerged as the most frequent genetic event in T-ALL, and are present in 56% of pediatric T-ALL [130], and in 36–70% of adults with T-ALL [131–133]. These mutations result in constitutive activation of NOTCH1 through ligand-independent cleavage of intracellular NOTCH (result of mutations in the extracellular heterodimerization domain), increased half-life of NOTCH through truncation of the pest domain responsible for protein turnover, or both simultaneously. FBXW7 protein ubiquitin ligase mutations also lead to NOTCH1 activation, through inhibition of its degradation, and are present in 25% adult T-ALL. *NOTCH1* and *FBXW7* mutations are an independent good prognosis factor [133].

The JAK family of proteins is a family of non-receptor tyrosine kinases that associate with cytokine receptors that lack kinase activity, and activate STAT proteins. *JAK1* gain of function mutations have been described in 18% of adult T-ALL, and 3% of B-ALL and associate with older age at diagnosis and poor prognosis, and display a distinct gene expression profile [134].

Gene Expression Changes in T-ALL

Gene expression profile analysis has uncovered specific signatures in T-ALL defined by the aberrant expression of the above reviewed oncogenes, and found that the classification recapitulates particular stages of thymocyte development [118, 135]. The overexpression of transcription factors that regulate thymopoiesis is often independent of detectable alterations at their chromosome location. Thus, overexpression of *HOX11* defines T-ALL with an early cortical thymocyte as its normal counterpart and good prognosis. *HOX11* overexpression can result from translocations or be present without associated cytogenetic abnormalities [135–137]. A potential mechanism for *HOX11* overexpression is promoter demethylation [138]. Curiously, while *HOX11L2* overexpressing leukemia cases have similar GEP to cases with *HOX11*, they do not share similar clinical fates. The two other groups of T-ALL, defined by *TAL1* and *LYL1* expressions, are bad prognosis groups [135]. Leukemias with *TAL1* overexpression have a developmental arrest in the late cortical stage, and are frequently devoid of an apparent chromosome rearrangement [139]. *LYL1* overexpression may present with no chromosome rearrangements, or present with a t(7;19) rearrangement and resemble the early pro-T differentiation stage.

Likewise, high expression of *ERG* and *BAALC* have been associated with immature phenotype and a higher relapse risk in adult T-ALL. Because they are also bad markers in AML, it has been suggested they may be prognostic markers of stem cell disease [140].

Aberrant Lymphocyte Development

Among the several clues as to the etiology of ALL, a few features are especially glaring. First, many of the translocations found in the disease do not appear to be entirely leukemogenic on their own, but likely need other "hits." This is certainly of no surprise given what we know from mouse models and other leukemia (e.g., AML). In addition, there is a plethora of translocations that involve the immunoglobulin gene, or the T cell receptor. Is there a theme to these observations that reveal something about the pathogenesis of ALL?

Recombinase Activating Genes (RAG)

In the course of normal development, B and T lymphocytes undergo DNA rearrangement of the *V(D)J* genes that form the antigen binding domain of the B and T cell receptors (BCR and TCR), in order to achieve the diversity that will allow the recognition of millions of different antigens. This process comprises the generation of double strand breaks, mediated by the RAG protein complex (RAG, formed by RAG1 and RAG2), and the joining phase, mediated by the DNA-repair factors that form the non-homologous end joining (NHEJ) repair pathway [141]. RAG recognizes short conserved sequences called recombination signal sequences (RSS) that flank the *V*, *D*, and *J* genes. Sites with sequences resembling the RSS are predicted to occur as frequent as every 2Kb in the human genome [142, 143], and are called cryptic RSS [144, 145].

Translocations can arise when RAG proteins mistakenly target a cryptic RSS selecting the incorrect partner for the antigen-receptor locus during the *VDJ* rearrangement process, known as type 1 or "substrate-selection error" model (Fig. 3.2). Examples of this mechanism are the *TAL2* and *LMO2* genes involved in t(7;9) (q34;q32) and t(11;14)(p13;q11) recurrent translocations in T-ALL. These genes have a sequence closely resembling a RSS that can be targeted by RAG [142, 143, 146–148]. In the case of *SIL/TAL1* T-ALL, the rearrangement is the result of the deletion of a chromosome fragment in 1p32 flanked by 2 cryptic RSS [149]. As a variant of this mechanism, oncogene activation can result from further rearrangement, and not from the translocation per se, as has been shown to be the case in t(7;9). This translocation is present at very low levels in 60% of normal individuals. In the T-ALL cases, secondary recombination results in the *TAL2-JB2* fusion, leading to *TAL2* activation and T-ALL [148]. A recent publication attributes a RAG-mediated mechanism to the deletion of exons 3 to 6 of Ikaros in B-ALL [45].

In a second mechanism of translocation, an *IG* or *TCR* gene is fused to the broken end of an oncogene locus during the rearrangement process. The origin of the DNA break in the proto-oncogene locus may or may not be RAG-mediated. Therefore, two antigen receptor gene segments and one oncogene are involved. The oncogene accesses the post-cleavage synaptic complex (type 2 or "end donation" model [144, 150]). Examples of this mechanism include the translocations t(8;14) (q24;q11), t(10;14) (q24;q11), and t(11;14)(p13;q11) [142, 144, 151–156]. In all cases, the result is the juxtaposition of an oncogene and an *IG/TCR* locus with a strong regulatory element that results in the aberrant overexpression of the oncogene.

There is increasing evidence that genes affecting the normal differentiation of B cells may be involved in ALL. In a landmark study, the St. Jude's group studied 242 pediatric ALL cases by high-density SNP arrays [157]. This allowed them to look for deletions and amplifications in the genome. In B precursor ALL, there was an average of 3.8 copy number changes per case, with the majority being deletions. There were 54 common deletions, and these focused on genes involved in B cell differentiation, most predominately *PAX5*, *EBF1*, and *IKZF*. Indeed, fully 40% of all precursor B-ALL cases had an alteration of genes involved in B cell differentiation. Thus, a prime focus in

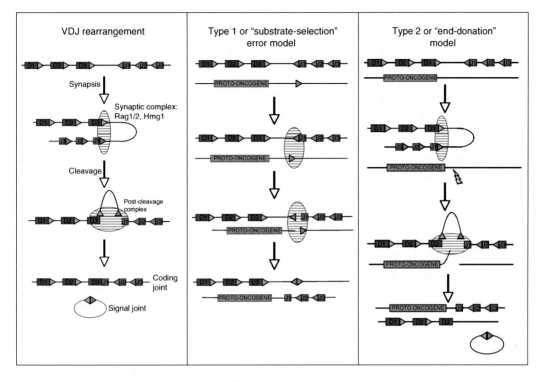

Fig. 3.2 Schematic representation of normal VDJ rearrangement and mechanism of chromosomal translocation that are RAG-mediated. In the type 1 or "substrate-selection" error model, a cryptic RSS close to a proto-oncogene is targeted by the RAG complex by mistake, and the proto-oncogene gets juxtaposed to a strong promoter from the antigen receptor loci, resulting in extopic and overexpression of the proto-oncogen. In the type 2, the initial chromosome break is not RAG-related, and the DNA broken end invades the post-cleavage complex (Adapted from [143])

ALL seems to be genetic instability, affecting differentiation and blocking cells in an early development phase; and abnormal RAG activity, which may in part be excess activity given the block in development.

Oligoclonality and Clonal Evolution

As described above, in normal B and T cell differentiation, there is a rearrangement of the immunoglobulin (*IG*) and T-cell receptor (*TCR*) genes. Thus, if ALL arises from a lymphocyte that has undergone gene rearrangement, the leukemia should have a predominant gene rearrangement. Immunoglobulin and/or *TCR* rearrangements can be detected at diagnosis in over 90% of ALL [158–160]. The junction areas between *V*, *D*, and *J* genes are unique for each clone, and can be used as leukemia fingerprints in the investigation of minimal residual disease (MRD). However, as many as 40% of leukemia have more than one rearrangement detected at diagnosis [161–163]. There are three different possibilities: (1) the presence of a monoclonal blast population with biallelic rearrangements or duplication of chromosome 14; (2) the presence of multiple leukemia subclones driven by the persistence of the recombinase machinery that can replace the VH from an existing VDJ rearrangement or mediate "open and shut" VH events; and (3) "true oligoclonality" resulting from the simultaneous transformation of multiple lymphoid precursors. Oligoclonality has implications for the development of assays for the detection of MRD, as it is uncertain the clone that will emerge at relapse, and the use of two MRD-PCR markers to decrease the incidence of false negatives is widely spread [163–165]. Although clonal evolution and clonal selection have been shown at relapse, the emergence of a completely new clone at relapse is infrequent [166–168].

Recently, genome-wide copy number abnormality (CNA) studies have shown that about 6% of relapsed leukemias are genetically distinct from the diagnostic clone, and that more than 50% of relapses arise from clonal evolution of the initial clone [169]. Specifically, Mullighan et al. investigated genetic evolution and relapse in 61 pediatric ALL cases, focusing on the detection of genomic CNAs as a measure of the leukemia "fingerprint." From these assays, the number of gene copies (increased or decreased) could be assessed and compared between paired diagnostic and relapsed samples. The results may be an underestimate of the genetic complexity of diagnostic and relapsed samples, since other types of genetic lesions (mutations, translocations) are not necessarily detected by this method. Nonetheless, the analysis details some interesting and exciting features about relapse in ALL. At diagnosis, approximately 10 CNAs were detected per case (B-cell > T-cell). More CNAs were found at relapse than diagnosis. For example, the average CNAs in B-ALL were 11 at diagnosis, compared to 14 at relapse. The bulk of these additional CNAs were new deletions. In comparing the diagnostic to relapse samples, four patterns emerge (Fig. 3.3). One pattern (<10% of cases) were relapse samples that were totally distinct from the diagnostic samples. These genetically distinct clones may have arisen from an early progenitor without detectable CNA marker, or alternatively, represent a truly different leukemia. The second pattern (<10%) is those cases that have identical CNA at diagnosis and relapse. A third category, comprising ~30% of cases, had a clear evolution from the diagnostic sample. Lastly, the remaining majority (>50%) of cases at relapse share some CNAs with the diagnostic samples, but also have additional CNAs not found in the diagnostic samples. The most likely interpretation is that in this situation, the diagnostic and relapse cases

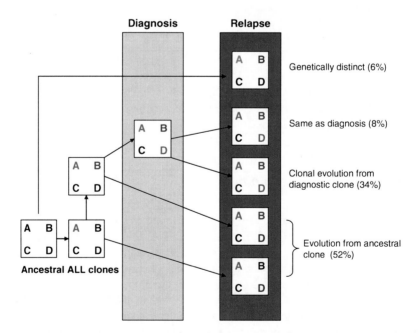

Fig. 3.3 Clonal evolution in ALL. Numerous pre-diagnostic clones ("ancestral") evolve into a malignant ALL clone, discovered at diagnosis. At relapse, there are four possibilities: (1) the detection of a genetically distinct clone; (2) the reemergence of the original clone; (3) clonal evolution from the diagnostic clone; and (4) evolution from an ancestral clone. In this cartoon, each letter ("A," "B," etc.) refers to a chromosome; each different color refers to a new genetic event (deletion, duplication, etc.) on that chromosome. Black letters are wild type (Adapted from [169])

54. Boucheix, C., David, B., Sebban, C., et al. (1994). Immunophenotype of adult acute lymphoblastic leukemia, clinical parameters, and outcome: An analysis of a prospective trial including 562 tested patients (LALA87). French Group on Therapy for Adult Acute Lymphoblastic Leukemia. *Blood, 84*(5), 1603–1612.

55. Holowiecki, J., Krawczyk-Kulis, M., Giebel, S., et al. (2008). Status of minimal residual disease after induction predicts outcome in both standard and high-risk Ph-negative adult acute lymphoblastic leukaemia. The Polish Adult Leukemia Group ALL 4-2002 MRD Study. *British Journal of Haematology, 142*(2), 227–237.

56. Secker-Walker, L. M., Craig, J. M., Hawkins, J. M., & Hoffbrand, A. V. (1991). Philadelphia positive acute lymphoblastic leukemia in adults: Age distribution, BCR breakpoint and prognostic significance. *Leukemia, 5*(3), 196–199.

57. Pui, C. H., Gaynon, P. S., Boyett, J. M., et al. (2002). Outcome of treatment in childhood acute lymphoblastic leukaemia with rearrangements of the 11q23 chromosomal region. *Lancet, 359*(9321), 1909–1915.

58. Hoelzer, D., Thiel, E., Loffler, H., et al. (1988). Prognostic factors in a multicenter study for treatment of acute lymphoblastic leukemia in adults. *Blood, 71*(1), 123–131.

59. Asnafi, V., Beldjord, K., Libura, M., et al. (2004). Age-related phenotypic and oncogenic differences in T-cell acute lymphoblastic leukemias may reflect thymic atrophy. *Blood, 104*(13), 4173–4180.

60. Thiel, E., Kranz, B. R., Raghavachar, A., et al. (1989). Prethymic phenotype and genotype of pre-T (CD7+/ER-) -cell leukemia and its clinical significance within adult acute lymphoblastic leukemia. *Blood, 73*(5), 1247–1258.

61. Gokbuget, N., & Hoelzer, D. (2006). Treatment of adult acute lymphoblastic leukemia. *Hematology, 2006*, 133–141.

62. Asnafi, V., Buzyn, A., Thomas, X., et al. (2005). Impact of TCR status and genotype on outcome in adult T-cell acute lymphoblastic leukemia: A LALA-94 study. *Blood, 105*(8), 3072–3078.

63. Vitale, A., Guarini, A., Ariola, C., et al. (2006). Adult T-cell acute lymphoblastic leukemia: Biologic profile at presentation and correlation with response to induction treatment in patients enrolled in the GIMEMA LAL 0496 protocol. *Blood, 107*(2), 473–479.

64. Meijerink, J. P., den Boer, M. L., & Pieters, R. (2009). New genetic abnormalities and treatment response in acute lymphoblastic leukemia. *Seminars in Hematology, 46*(1), 16–23.

65. Asnafi, V., Radford-Weiss, I., Dastugue, N., et al. (2003). CALM-AF10 is a common fusion transcript in T-ALL and is specific to the TCRgammadelta lineage. *Blood, 102*(3), 1000–1006.

66. Weng, A. P., Ferrando, A. A., Lee, W., et al. (2004). Activating mutations of NOTCH1 in human T cell acute lymphoblastic leukemia. *Science, 306*(5694), 269–271.

67. O'Neil, J., Grim, J., Strack, P., et al. (2007). FBW7 mutations in leukemic cells mediate NOTCH pathway activation and resistance to gamma-secretase inhibitors. *The Journal of Experimental Medicine, 204*(8), 1813–1824.

68. Breit, S., Stanulla, M., Flohr, T., et al. (2006). Activating NOTCH1 mutations predict favorable early treatment response and long-term outcome in childhood precursor T-cell lymphoblastic leukemia. *Blood, 108*(4), 1151–1157.

69. Asnafi, V., Buzyn, A., Le Noir, S., et al. (2009). NOTCH1/FBXW7 mutation identifies a large subgroup with favourable outcome in adult T-cell acute lymphoblastic leukemia (T-ALL): A GRAALL study. *Blood, 113*, 3918–3924.

70. Malyukova, A., Dohda, T., von der Lehr, N., et al. (2007). The tumor suppressor gene hCDC4 is frequently mutated in human T-cell acute lymphoblastic leukemia with functional consequences for Notch signaling. *Cancer Research, 67*(12), 5611–5616.

71. Stanulla, M., & Schrappe, M. (2009). Treatment of childhood acute lymphoblastic leukemia. *Seminars in Hematology, 46*(1), 52–63.

72. Cave, H., van der Werff ten Bosch, J., Suciu, S., et al. (1998). Clinical significance of minimal residual disease in childhood acute lymphoblastic leukemia. European Organization for Research and Treatment of Cancer – Childhood Leukemia Cooperative Group. *The New England Journal of Medicine, 339*(9), 591–598.

73. Coustan-Smith, E., Behm, F. G., Sanchez, J., et al. (1998). Immunological detection of minimal residual disease in children with acute lymphoblastic leukaemia. *Lancet, 351*(9102), 550–554.

74. van Dongen, J. J., Seriu, T., Panzer-Grumayer, E. R., et al. (1998). Prognostic value of minimal residual disease in acute lymphoblastic leukaemia in childhood. *Lancet, 352*(9142), 1731–1738.

75. Dombret, H., Gabert, J., Boiron, J. M., et al. (2002). Outcome of treatment in adults with Philadelphia chromosome-positive acute lymphoblastic leukemia – results of the prospective multicenter LALA-94 trial. *Blood, 100*(7), 2357–2366.

76. Pane, F., Cimino, G., Izzo, B., et al. (2005). Significant reduction of the hybrid BCR/ABL transcripts after induction and consolidation therapy is a powerful predictor of treatment response in adult Philadelphia-positive acute lymphoblastic leukemia. *Leukemia, 19*(4), 628–635.

77. Vidriales, M. B., Perez, J. J., Lopez-Berges, M. C., et al. (2003). Minimal residual disease in adolescent (older than 14 years) and adult acute lymphoblastic leukemias: Early immunophenotypic evaluation has high clinical value. *Blood, 101*(12), 4695–4700.

78. Bruggemann, M., Raff, T., Flohr, T., et al. (2006). Clinical significance of minimal residual disease quantification in adult patients with standard-risk acute lymphoblastic leukemia. *Blood, 107*(3), 1116–1123.
79. Gokbuget, N., Raff, R., Brugge-Mann, M., et al. (2004). Risk/MRD adapted GMALL trials in adult ALL. *Annals of Hematology, 83*(Suppl 1), S129–S131.
80. Fielding, A. (2008). The treatment of adults with acute lymphoblastic leukemia. *Hematology American Society of Hematology Education Program, 2008*, 381–389.
81. Todeschini, G., Tecchio, C., Meneghini, V., et al. (1998). Estimated 6-year event-free survival of 55% in 60 consecutive adult acute lymphoblastic leukemia patients treated with an intensive phase II protocol based on high induction dose of daunorubicin. *Leukemia, 12*(2), 144–149.
82. Mancini, M., Scappaticci, D., Cimino, G., et al. (2005). A comprehensive genetic classification of adult acute lymphoblastic leukemia (ALL): Analysis of the GIMEMA 0496 protocol. *Blood, 105*(9), 3434–3441.
83. Rowe, J. M. (2009). Optimal management of adults with ALL. *British Journal of Haematology, 144*(4), 468–483.
84. Hoelzer, D., Thiel, E., Ludwig, W. D., et al. (1993). Follow-up of the first two successive German multicentre trials for adult ALL (01/81 and 02/84). German Adult ALL Study Group. *Leukemia, 7*(Suppl 2), S130–S134.
85. Chessells, J. M., Bailey, C., & Richards, S. M. (1995). Intensification of treatment and survival in all children with lymphoblastic leukaemia: Results of UK Medical Research Council trial UKALL X. Medical Research Council Working Party on Childhood Leukaemia. *Lancet, 345*(8943), 143–148.
86. Ribera, J. M., Ortega, J. J., Oriol, A., et al. (1998). Late intensification chemotherapy has not improved the results of intensive chemotherapy in adult acute lymphoblastic leukemia. Results of a prospective multicenter randomized trial (PETHEMA ALL-89). Spanish Society of Hematology. *Haematologica, 83*(3), 222–230.
87. Stein, A., & Forman, S. J. (2008). Allogeneic transplantation for ALL in adults. *Bone Marrow Transplantation, 41*(5), 439–446.
88. Bachanova, V., & Weisdorf, D. (2008). Unrelated donor allogeneic transplantation for adult acute lymphoblastic leukemia: A review. *Bone Marrow Transplantation, 41*(5), 455–464.
89. Larson, R. (2008). Allogeneic hematopoietic cell transplantation for adults with ALL. *Bone Marrow Transplantation, 42*(Suppl 1), S18–S24.
90. Sebban, C., Lepage, E., Vernant, J. P., et al. (1994). Allogeneic bone marrow transplantation in adult acute lymphoblastic leukemia in first complete remission: A comparative study. French Group of Therapy of Adult Acute Lymphoblastic Leukemia. *Journal of Clinical Oncology, 12*(12), 2580–2587.
91. Thomas, X., Boiron, J. M., Huguet, F., et al. (2004). Outcome of treatment in adults with acute lymphoblastic leukemia: Analysis of the LALA-94 trial. *Journal of Clinical Oncology, 22*(20), 4075–4086.
92. Ribera, J. M., Oriol, A., Bethencourt, C., et al. (2005). Comparison of intensive chemotherapy, allogeneic or autologous stem cell transplantation as post-remission treatment for adult patients with high-risk acute lymphoblastic leukemia. Results of the PETHEMA ALL-93 trial. *Haematologica, 90*(10), 1346–1356.
93. Labar, B., Suciu, S., Zittoun, R., et al. (2004). Allogeneic stem cell transplantation in acute lymphoblastic leukemia and non-Hodgkin's lymphoma for patients <or=50 years old in first complete remission: Results of the EORTC ALL-3 trial. *Haematologica, 89*(7), 809–817.
94. Yanada, M., Matsuo, K., Suzuki, T., & Naoe, T. (2006). Allogeneic hematopoietic stem cell transplantation as part of postremission therapy improves survival for adult patients with high-risk acute lymphoblastic leukemia: A metaanalysis. *Cancer, 106*(12), 2657–2663.
95. Orsi, C., Bartolozzi, B., Messori, A., & Bosi, A. (2007). Event-free survival and cost-effectiveness in adult acute lymphoblastic leukaemia in first remission treated with allogeneic transplantation. *Bone Marrow Transplantation, 40*(7), 643–649.
96. Goldstone, A. H., Richards, S. M., Lazarus, H. M., et al. (2008). In adults with standard-risk acute lymphoblastic leukemia, the greatest benefit is achieved from a matched sibling allogeneic transplantation in first complete remission, and an autologous transplantation is less effective than conventional consolidation/maintenance chemotherapy in all patients: Final results of the International ALL Trial (MRC UKALL XII/ECOG E2993). *Blood, 111*(4), 1827–1833.
97. Thiebaut, A., Vernant, J. P., Degos, L., et al. (2000). Adult acute lymphocytic leukemia study testing chemotherapy and autologous and allogeneic transplantation. A follow-up report of the French protocol LALA 87. *Hematology/Oncology Clinics of North America, 14*(6), 1353–1366.
98. Dhedin, N., Dombret, H., Thomas, X., et al. (2006). Autologous stem cell transplantation in adults with acute lymphoblastic leukemia in first complete remission: Analysis of the LALA-85, -87 and -94 trials. *Leukemia, 20*(2), 336–344.
99. Gokbuget, N., Arnold, R., Bohme, A., et al. (2007). Improved outcome in high risk and very high risk ALL by risk adapted SCT and in standard risk ALL by intensive chemotherapy in 713 adult ALL patients treated according to the prospective GMALL study 07/2003. *Blood (ASH Annual Meeting Abstracts), 110*(11), 12.
100. Ribera, J. M., Oriol, A., Sanz, M. A., et al. (2008). Comparison of the results of the treatment of adolescents and young adults with standard-risk acute lymphoblastic leukemia with the Programa Espanol de Tratamiento en Hematologia pediatric-based protocol ALL-96. *Journal of Clinical Oncology, 26*(11), 1843–1849.

101. Haiat, S., Vekhoff, A., Marzac, C., et al. (2007). Improved outcome of adult acute lymphoblastic leukemia treated with a pediatric protocol: Results of a pilot study. *Blood (ASH Annual Meeting Abstracts), 110*(11), 2822.
102. DeAngelo, D. J., Dahlberg, S., Silverman, L. B., et al. (2007). A multicenter phase II study using a dose intensified pediatric regimen in adults with untreated acute lymphoblastic leukemia. *Blood (ASH Annual Meeting Abstracts), 110*(11), 587.
103. Douer, D., Watkins, K., Mark, L., et al. (2007). A dose intensified pediatric-like regimen using multiple doses of intravenous pegylated asparaginase in adults with newly diagnosed acute lymphoblastic leukemia. *Blood (ASH Annual Meeting Abstracts), 110*(11), 2823.
104. Douer, D., Yampolsky, H., Cohen, L. J., et al. (2007). Pharmacodynamics and safety of intravenous pegaspargase during remission induction in adults aged 55 years or younger with newly diagnosed acute lymphoblastic leukemia. *Blood, 109*(7), 2744–2750.
105. Rytting, M., Thomas, D., Kantarjian, H., et al. (2007). Adaptation of augmented Berlin-Frankfurt-Munster (ABFM) therapy in adolescents and young adults with acute lymphoblastic leukemia (ALL). *Blood (ASH Annual Meeting Abstracts), 110*(11), 4342.
106. Giri, N., Nair, C. N., Pai, S. K., Kurkure, P. A., Gopal, R., & Advani, S. H. (1987). Avascular necrosis of bone in acute lymphoblastic leukemia. *American Journal of Pediatric Hematology/Oncology, 9*(2), 143–145.
107. Mattano, L. A., Jr., Sather, H. N., Trigg, M. E., & Nachman, J. B. (2000). Osteonecrosis as a complication of treating acute lymphoblastic leukemia in children: A report from the children's cancer group. *Journal of Clinical Oncology, 18*(18), 3262–3272.
108. Strauss, A. J., Su, J. T., Dalton, V. M., Gelber, R. D., Sallan, S. E., & Silverman, L. B. (2001). Bony morbidity in children treated for acute lymphoblastic leukemia. *Journal of Clinical Oncology, 19*(12), 3066–3072.

Chapter 15
Philadelphia Chromosome Positive Acute Lymphoblastic Leukemia

Deborah A. Thomas, Susan O'Brien, Stefan Faderl, and Hagop Kantarjian

Biology of Philadelphia Positive ALL

The Philadelphia (Ph) chromosome [t(9,22)(q34;q11)]/*BCR-ABL1* is the most frequent karyotypic aberration in adults with acute lymphoblastic leukemia (ALL) [1]. It occurs in 20–30% of adult ALL cases overall, with the incidence rising to over 50% in patients aged 50 years or older [2]. In contrast, the Ph chromosome is relatively rare in children with ALL, with an incidence of only 1–3% [3]. Approximately two thirds of de novo ALL cases harbor one or more chromosomal aberrations in addition to t(9,22), most frequently an extra copy of der(22)t(9,22), deletion 9p, trisomy 21, trisomy 8, or monosomy 7 (or loss of 7p) [4–6]. Approximately 15% of patients with the Ph chromosome will also have the favorable feature of high hyperdiploidy (modal chromosome number 51–67 chromosomes) [1, 4, 5, 7]. Prior to the use of tyrosine kinase inhibitor (TKI)-based therapy, there was no prognostic relevance of these secondary chromosomal abnormalities. In the TKI era, the presence of abnormalities of 9p has been generally associated with worse outcome, whereas the prognostic impact of der(22)t(9,22) has not been firmly established owing to conflicting reports, likely confounded by its association with high hyperdiploidy [8, 9].

The Ph chromosome results from a reciprocal translocation that fuses the breakpoint cluster region (*BCR*) gene from chromosome 22 to the Abelson tyrosine kinase (*ABL*) gene from chromosome 9 [10–13]. This translocation ultimately results in a constitutively active tyrosine kinase protein. The location of the breakpoint within the *BCR* gene results in either the p190[bcr-abl] protein observed exclusively in Ph-positive ALL, or the p210[bcr-abl] protein common to 20–40% cases of Ph-positive ALL and nearly all cases of Ph-positive chronic myelogenous leukemia (CML) [14]. The p230[bcr-abl] protein is associated with chronic neutrophilic leukemia [15]. In vitro, the p190[bcr-abl] protein appears to have higher tyrosine kinase activity and enhanced efficiency in stimulating the proliferation of lymphoblasts [16]. Some investigators have reported improved clinical outcomes with the p190[bcr-abl] protein expression (compared with p210[bcr-abl]) whereas others have found no prognostic significance of the breakpoint [17–19]. Overexpression of the *BCR-ABL* fusion gene activates a multitude of downstream signaling pathways which induce proliferation, such as Ras/Raf/mitogen activated protein kinase (MAPK) and Jak–STAT (Janus kinase-signal transducer – transcription activator of transcription) [20–23]. Development of growth factor–independent malignant clones ensues, contributing further to the pathogenesis of the disease.

D.A. Thomas (✉)
Department of Leukemia, The University of Texas M. D. Anderson Cancer Center,
1515 Holcombe Blvd, Unit 428, Houston, TX 77030, USA
e-mail: debthomas@mdanderson.org

A.S. Advani and H.M. Lazarus (eds.), *Adult Acute Lymphocytic Leukemia*, Contemporary Hematology,
DOI 10.1007/978-1-60761-707-5_15, © Springer Science+Business Media, LLC 2011

Table 15.1 Historical chemotherapy regimens for adult de novo Ph-positive ALL

Study	Year	No.	%CR	Median EFS/CRD (mos)	% OS (X years)
CALGB 8762 [26]	1992	14	71	—	—*
GMALL 1/81, 2/84, 3/87, 4/89 [27]	1992	25	76	—	—*
CALGB 8811 [28]	1995	30	70	7	16 (3)
MRC UKALL XA [29]	1997	40	83	13	13 (3)
CALGB 8461 [30]	1999	67	82	11	12 (5)
Hyper-CVAD [31]	2000	67	90	11	16 (3)
LALA-94 [32]	2002	154	67	—	19 (3)
GMALL [19]	2002	175	68	—	13 (3)
GIMEMA 0496 [17]	2006	101	67	—	16 (7)

EFS event-free survival, *CRD* complete remission duration; *OS* overall survival, *CALGB* Cancer and Leukemia Group B, *GMALL* German Multi-Centre Acute Lymphoblastic Leukemia, *MRC* Medical Research Council, *hyper-CVAD* fractionated cyclophosphamide, vincristine, doxorubicin, dexamethasone, *GET-LALA* Groupe d'Etude et de Traitement de la Leucémie Aiguë Lymphoblastique de l'Adulte, *GIMEMA* Gruppo Italiano Malattie EMatologiche dell'Adulto
—, not reported, *Median OS for CALGB 8762 [26] 11 mos, GMALL 1/81, 2/84, 3/87, 4/89 [27] 8 months

Historical Outcomes with Chemotherapy for Ph-Positive ALL

Historically, prior to the advent of TKIs, outcome after chemotherapy for adults with newly diagnosed Ph-positive ALL was dismal. Outcomes for children with Ph-positive ALL were influenced by age, leukocyte count, and corticosteroid response with 5-year disease-free survival (DFS) rates ranging from 20% to 49% depending on the prognostic category [24, 25]. Table 15.1 lists the outcomes observed with several standard chemotherapy regimens as applied to adults. Although the complete remission (CR) rates with these conventional and intensive ALL regimens ranged from 60 to 90%, long-term DFS rates were less than 20% in the absence of allogeneic stem cell transplant (SCT) [31–33]. Median survival ranged from 7 to 15 months owing to relapse-related mortality. The improved CR rates achieved with the more intensive chemotherapy regimens did not translate into an increase in the durability of responses or improved survival (OS) [31, 34, 35]. The quality of the molecular response (determined by the log reduction in the level of BCR-ABL transcripts by polymerase chain reaction [PCR]) after frontline chemotherapy has correlated with outcome, even prior to the availability of TKIs. In a study using high-dose anthracycline-based chemotherapy, chemosensitive patients with Ph-positive ALL who achieved at least a 3-log reduction in *BCR-ABL* transcripts by quantitative real-time PCR (RT-PCR) after consolidation chemotherapy had 2-year DFS and OS rates of 27% and 48%, respectively, not dissimilar from those observed after allogeneic SCT in first CR [36]. None of the patients who had less than a 3-log reduction in *BCR-ABL* transcripts were alive at 2 years. This further emphasized the importance of achieving an optimal molecular response in order to improve outcome, providing the impetus for development of selective small molecule inhibitors of the ABL tyrosine kinase.

Historical Outcomes with Stem Cell Transplant for Ph-Positive ALL

Owing to the dismal outcomes with chemotherapy alone, allogeneic SCT in first CR was established as the only potential curative modality. However, allogeneic SCT was often feasible only in younger patients without significant comorbidities for whom a suitable donor (inclusive of all stem sources such as matched unrelated marrow) was identified prior to disease recurrence, limiting the applicability of this approach. Since the benefits of allogeneic SCT in first CR were attributed to the intense myeloablative therapy and graft-versus-leukemia effect, the high risk of transplant-related mortality (TRM) using alternative donors was accepted owing to the poor outcomes with chemotherapy alone.

The prospective multi-center French, Belgian, Swiss, and Australian Groupe d'Etude et de Traitement de la Leucémie Aiguë Lymphoblastique de l'Adulte LALA-94 trial of 154 patients with Ph-positive ALL showed that 3-year OS rates were superior if a molecular CR (absence of detectable *BCR-ABL* transcripts by PCR) was achieved (54% versus 19%) and if allogeneic SCT was performed in first CR (37% for allogeneic SCT versus 12% for chemotherapy, $p=0.02$) [32]. Investigators from the City of Hope and Stanford University reported outcomes for 79 patients with Ph-positive ALL (median age 36 years) who underwent matched-related sibling (MRS) allogeneic SCT in first CR after a conditioning regimen of fractionated total body irradiation (TBI) and high-dose etoposide between 1985 and 2005. Ten-year rates of OS, nonrelapse mortality, and relapse were 54%, 31%, and 18%, respectively [37]. Transplant-related mortality was predominantly related to infections or graft-versus-host disease.

In an initial report of outcome for the Ph-positive subset of ALL patients ($n=167$) less than 55 years of age enrolled in the frontline randomized MRC UKALL XII/ECOG E2993 trial, the 5-year relapse risk decreased from 81% with chemotherapy or autologous SCT to 32% with allogeneic SCT (conditioning regimen of TBI and etoposide) [38]. Five-year event-free (EFS) and OS rates improved from 17 to 36% and 19 to 42%, respectively, despite the high rates of TRM. In an update of this study including 267 patients with de novo Ph-positive ALL, Fielding and colleagues [9] reported improved outcomes for the 28% who received allogeneic SCT in first CR; 5-year OS rates were 44% after MRS SCT, 36% after matched unrelated donor (MUD) SCT, and 19% after chemotherapy. Treatment-related mortality was 27% after MRS SCT and 39% after MUD SCT. After accounting for differences in prognostic factors such as age and leukocyte count, and excluding chemotherapy-treated patients who were ineligible for allogeneic SCT owing to relapse or death, only relapse-free survival (RFS) remained as favorable for the allogeneic SCT group. An intention-to-treat analysis based on availability of MRS donor showed similar OS rates between the donor and no donor groups (34% versus 25%, respectively).

Although the long-term OS rates (ranging from 27% to 65%) improved after allogeneic SCT in first CR, relapse remained the primary cause of failure, with persistent detection of *BCR-ABL* transcripts by RT-PCR heralding eventual disease recurrence [33, 39–41]. In a retrospective review of 197 patients with Ph-positive ALL who underwent allogeneic SCT, the 5-year OS rates were 34% for patients in first CR, 21% for those in second or subsequent CR, and 9% for those with active disease ($p<0.0001$) [42]. Multivariate analysis identified younger age, CR status at the time of SCT, conditioning with TBI-based regimen, and an HLA-identical sibling donor as factors associated with improved OS. Although newer modalities such as nonmyeloablative reduced intensity conditioning regimens and use of stem cells derived from umbilical cord blood have broadened the applicability of allogeneic SCT, a significant proportion of patients with Ph-positive ALL remain ineligible for this potentially curative modality and are in need of novel therapeutic approaches [43].

Imatinib Mesylate for Previously Treated Ph-Positive ALL

Imatinib mesylate (Gleevec/Glivec; Novartis Pharmaceuticals, Basel, Switzerland) is an oral selective inhibitor of the ABL, c-kit and platelet-derived growth factor receptor (PDGFR) tyrosine kinases [44–46]. Imatinib binds to the inactive moiety of the BCR-ABL kinase while partially blocking the adenosine triphosphate (ATP) binding site, preventing a conformational switch to the activated form of the oncoprotein. The activity of single agent imatinib was initially investigated in patients with relapsed or refractory Ph-positive ALL. A phase I clinical trial of imatinib administered at doses ranging from 300 to 1,000 mg daily demonstrated a 70% hematological response rate with a 20% CR rate [47]. A phase II trial of intermediate dose imatinib (600 mg) yielded a CR rate of 29% [48]. The estimated median time to progression and OS were 2.2 and 4.9 months, respectively, with durable responses in only a minority of cases. The degree of reduction in the level of peripheral blood and bone marrow *BCR-ABL* transcripts by PCR correlated with response and predicted time to progression [49]. Other predictors of failure to imatinib included higher leukocyte count, presence of circulating blasts, short duration of prior CR, and presence of der(22)t(9,22) [50]. Relapse in the central nervous system (CNS) was not uncommon, as imatinib concentrations in the cerebrospinal fluid (CSF) only reach 1–2% of detectable serum levels, in part related to the high expression of P-glycoprotein in the CNS, emphasizing the need for concurrent CNS prophylaxis [51–53]. Toxicity profile was similar to that observed in the trials of single agent imatinib for Ph-positive CML, and included transient myelosuppression, fluid retention syndrome, nausea, muscle cramps, rash, and transient elevations in hepatic transaminases [54].

Imatinib-Based Chemotherapy Regimens for De Novo Ph-Positive ALL

Although monotherapy with imatinib was tolerable and exhibited modest activity in the setting of recurrent or refractory disease, the durability of responses was suboptimal. In vitro data suggested either additive (doxorubicin, cyclophosphamide, cytarabine, etoposide) or synergistic (vincristine) cytotoxic effects in Ph-positive cell lines when imatinib was given in combination with standard chemotherapeutics [55–57]. Imatinib was thus incorporated into combination chemotherapy regimens typically used for de novo Ph-positive ALL, either concurrently (simultaneous administration of imatinib with chemotherapy) or sequentially (alternating "blocks" of therapy with imatinib with "blocks" of chemotherapy). A synopsis of these imatinib-based chemotherapy regimens is provided in Table 15.2, divided according to the age groups for which these programs were designed. Outcomes for the elderly subset after frontline imatinib-based therapy are discussed in detail in a subsequent section.

Imatinib-Based Chemotherapy Regimens for Younger De Novo Ph Positive ALL

The first report of a clinical trial of this nature included 20 patients with de novo or minimally treated Ph-positive ALL (no age restrictions) [58]. Imatinib 400 mg was given concurrently with the first 14 days of each of the eight intensive induction-consolidation cycles of the hyper-CVAD regimen (fractionated cyclophosphamide, vincristine, doxorubicin, and dexamethasone alternating with high-dose methotrexate and cytarabine) followed by continuous dosing during maintenance phase chemotherapy. Allogeneic SCT was performed in first CR as feasible. In the first report with relatively short follow-up, the CR rate was 96% with a 2-year DFS rate of 85%. The molecular CR rate (confirmed by nested PCR) approached 60%. There was no significant additional toxicity with the combination compared with hyper-CVAD alone.

The regimen was therefore modified with dose escalation of the imatinib to 600 mg during the first 14 days of induction therapy followed by continuous dosing beginning with day 1 of the first cycle of consolidation chemotherapy (high-dose methotrexate and cytarabine). For the maintenance phase, the imatinib was dose-escalated further as tolerated to a maximum dose of

Table 15.2 Imatinib-based chemotherapy regimens for de novo Ph-positive ALL

Subtype	Chemotherapy regimen	Imatinib dosing I	Post-I	M	No.	Med age (range) (years)	% CR	% Rel	% DFS (years)	% Survival (years)
Adults (all ages)										
Thomas [58–60]	Hyper-CVAD	C	C	C	39	51 (17–84)	93	22	68 (3)	55 (3)
Adults (age < 65 years)										
Yanada [61]	JALSG ALL202	C	A	C	80	48 (15–63)	96	26	60 (1)	76 (1)
Hatta [62]					103	45 (15–64)	97	25	51 (3)	58 (3)
Lee [63]	Modified linker	C	C	C	20	37 (15–67)	95	32	62 (2)	59 (2)
Wassmann [64]	GMALL									
	Alternating	None	A	NR	47	46 (21–65)	NA	NR	52 (2)	36 (2)
	Concurrent	None	C	NR	45	41 (19–63)	NA	NR	61 (2)	43 (2)
de Labarthe [65]	GRAAPH-2003	None	C	NR	45	45 (16–59)	96	19	51 (1.5)	65 (1.5)
Tanguy-Schmidt [66]									43 (4)	52 (4)
Elderly (> 55 years)										
Ottmann [67]	GMALL									
	Chemo	None	C	C	28	68 (54–79)	50	41	29 (1.5)	35 (1.5)
	Imatinib	Only	C	C	27		96	54	57 (1.5)	41 (1.5)
Vignetti [68]	GIMEMA	+ Pred	Only	Only	30	69 (61–83)	100	48	48 (1)	74 (1)
Delannoy [69]	GRAALL AFR09	None	C	A	30	66 (58–78)	72	60	58 (1)	66 (1)

I induction, *M* maintenance, *C* concurrent, *A* alternating, *NR* not reported, *NA* not applicable, *JALSG* Japan Adult Leukemia Study Group, *GMALL* German Multi-Centre Acute Lymphoblastic Leukemia, *hyper-CVAD* fractionated cyclophosphamide, vincristine, doxorubicin, dexamethasone, *GRAAPH* Group for Research on Adult Acute Lymphoblastic Leukemia, *GIMEMA* Gruppo Italiano Malattie EMatologiche dell'Adulto, *GRAALL* Group for Research in Adult, Acute Lymphoblastic Leukemia, *Chemo* chemotherapy, [I]Only[/I] imatinib only, *Pred* prednisone

800 mg administered concurrently with vincristine and prednisone every 4 weeks for 24 months (interrupted by two intensifications of hyper-CVAD and imatinib months 6 and 13). The imatinib was continued indefinitely thereafter at the best tolerated daily dose (not below 300 mg). An interim update of outcome for the 54 patients with de novo or minimally treated Ph-positive ALL treated with the hyper-CVAD and imatinib regimen was subsequently reported [59]. Overall CR rate was 93% for patients with active disease; overall 3-year rates of CR duration and OS were 68% and 55%, respectively (Fig. 15.1a, b). Sixteen patients (33%) underwent allogeneic SCT in first CR within a median of 5 months from the start of therapy (range, 1–13 months). In the de novo group, the 3-year OS rates were similar with or without allogeneic SCT (66% versus 49%, $p=0.36$). The 3-year CR duration rate was 84% for the patients who achieved molecular CR with the chemotherapy regimen (2 of 16 had allogeneic SCT) compared with 64% for those who did not (14 of 35 had allogeneic SCT), $p=0.1$. Overall rates of CR duration and OS were not influenced by molecular CR status (Fig. 15.1c). With a median follow-up of 52 months (range, 19–83+), 22% of the patients relapsed within a median time of 15 months from the start of therapy, including two after allogeneic SCT (the latter without imatinib maintenance). None of the cases harbored the T315I ABL kinase domain (KD) mutation at the time of disease recurrence.

The Japanese Adult Leukemia Study Group (JALSG) reported a CR rate of 96% and molecular CR rate of 71% in 80 patients with de novo Ph-positive ALL younger than 65 years of age after therapy with an imatinib-based chemotherapy regimen. An induction phase of concurrent imatinib and chemotherapy (cyclophosphamide, daunorubicin, vincristine, prednisone) was followed by consolidation chemotherapy consisting of blocks of single agent imatinib alternating with blocks of high-dose methotrexate and cytarabine for 8 total cycles followed by 2 years of maintenance

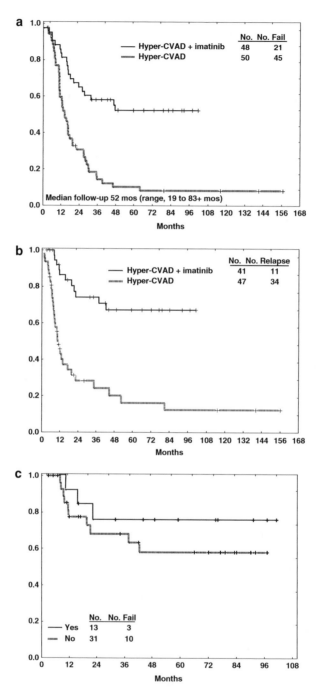

Fig. 15.1 Outcomes for de novo Ph-positive ALL with the hyper-CVAD and imatinib regimen compared with the historical experience with hyper-CVAD alone are depicted with respect to overall survival (**a**) and CR duration (**b**). Achievement of molecular CR after therapy with hyper-CVAD and imatinib did not influence CR duration (**c**)

therapy with imatinib, vincristine, and prednisone [70]. Thirty-nine patients underwent allogeneic SCT in first CR. Short-term EFS and OS rates were 60% and 76%, respectively, and were significantly superior to the historical experience. There appeared to be no difference in OS rates with or without allogeneic SCT (73% versus 85%, p = NS) in the initial analysis. An update of this study included 103 patients with newly diagnosed Ph-positive ALL (Table 15.2) [62]. The CR rate was 97%, and the 3-year OS rate was 58%. Allogeneic SCT was performed in first CR in 54 of the 74 patients (73%) under 55 years of age. Relapse occurred in 18 of 20 (90%) patients who did not undergo allogeneic SCT in first CR, as opposed to 7 of 54 (13%) patients who did, translating into 3-year OS rates of 75% versus 36% (p not reported). Allogeneic SCT was performed in first CR for 8 of the 25 patients (32%) over 55 years of age with the majority undergoing reduced intensity conditioning. Within this elderly group, 3-year OS rates were 75% with allogeneic SCT versus 43% (p not reported) without SCT.

Lee and colleagues [63] also reported favorable outcomes for 20 patients with newly diagnosed Ph-positive ALL (median age 37 years) after incorporating imatinib (600 mg days 1–14 of induction followed by 400 mg days 1–14 of each consolidation cycle) into a conventional ʟ-asparaginase-based ALL regimen. After the first 12 patients were treated, the dosing schema was modified to a continuous schedule of imatinib. The CR rate was 95%; 15 patients (75%) proceeded to allogeneic SCT in first CR. The CR duration and OS outcomes were superior compared with their historical experience. The use of concurrent imatinib and ʟ-asparaginase often resulted in transient hyperbilirubinemia requiring dose interruptions or dose modifications.

In the Group for Research on Adult Acute Lymphoblastic Leukemia (GRAAPH) 2003 study, imatinib was not commenced until consolidation chemotherapy with high-dose cytarabine and mitoxantrone (HAM) in good early responders (corticosteroid sensitivity and chemosensitivity) or during induction in conjunction with dexamethasone and vincristine in poor early responders. Imatinib was given continuously thereafter until allogeneic SCT [65]. In the early report, the rates of CR, DFS, and OS were significantly improved compared with the historical experience (Table 15.2). All eligible patients with an available matched donor underwent allogeneic SCT. Autologous SCT was performed in the setting of good molecular response if no donor was identified. An update of this trial with a longer median follow-up of 46 months was recently reported [66]. Outcomes with 4-year DFS and OS rates were improved compared with the LALA-94 regimen (43% versus 20%, $p=0.002$ and 52% versus 20%, $p=0.0001$, respectively). In the allogeneic SCT ($n=22$), autologous SCT ($n=10$), and no SCT groups, the 4-year OS rates were 55%, 80%, and 25%, respectively, with differences between the allogeneic and autologous SCT groups in part related to 7 deaths in CR (32%) after allogeneic SCT.

The optimal dosing schema for imatinib (alternating versus concurrently with chemotherapy) was not well delineated by these studies since outcomes were improved across a variety of regimens. Wassmann et al. [64] analyzed the outcomes of two sequential cohorts of patients with de novo Ph-positive ALL treated according to German Multi-Centre Acute Lymphoblastic Leukemia (GMALL) protocols. First, a treatment regimen consisting of blocks of chemotherapy alternating with single agent imatinib was designed owing to concerns of potential overlapping toxicity. Once the feasibility and tolerance of concurrent imatinib and chemotherapy was demonstrated by other investigators, a concurrent regimen was implemented. The superiority of the latter approach was evidenced by a higher molecular CR rate (52% versus 19%, $p = 0.01$) prior to consolidation chemotherapy, although this did not translate into significant improvements in EFS or OS compared with the alternating regimen. Allogeneic SCT was successfully employed in over 70% of the cases regardless of the dosing schema of imatinib, significantly higher than the historical transplantation rate of 50% for the LALA and GMALL multicenter group cooperative trials, potentially masking the effect of achievement of molecular CR after TKI-based therapy on outcome (since most patients achieve molecular CR after allogeneic SCT).

The prognostic relevance of molecular CR in the context of TKI-based therapy has not yet been firmly established. Yanada et al. [71] showed that achievement of molecular CR was not associated with improved RFS; however, an increase in the level of *BCR-ABL* transcripts by PCR during hematologic CR was predictive for disease recurrence in patients who had not undergone allogeneic SCT. Prospective monitoring of the levels of *BCR-ABL* transcripts by PCR should be conducted with ABL sequencing for KD mutations performed if significant increments are observed.

The addition of imatinib to frontline chemotherapy has significantly improved the outcome for younger patients with newly diagnosed Ph-positive ALL. Nearly all investigators have reported superior RFS and OS rates with imatinib-based therapy compared with their historical experience, despite variations in the delivery of imatinib and relatively short follow-up. These advances are in part related to the increased durability of responses and the improved rates of allogeneic SCT in first CR. Interim therapy with single agent imatinib has also been used as a bridge to allogeneic SCT after completion of frontline therapy with imatinib plus chemotherapy [72]. This approach also reduced the relapse rate prior to allogeneic SCT without an apparent worsening in the acute transplantation-related morbidity or mortality in comparison to historical controls.

Perspectives on Allogeneic Stem Cell Transplant in the TKI-Era

The exact role of allogeneic SCT for de novo Ph-positive ALL in the TKI era continues to be defined, with the feasibility of this modality still driven by availability of a suitable donor, absence of significant comorbidities, and ability to sustain a durable CR. Advances in SCT such as the application of nonmyeloablative reduced intensity conditioning regimens to older patients or those with comorbidities prohibiting traditional myeloablative regimens, in addition to increased availability of umbilical cord blood as a source of stem cells, have allowed allogeneic SCT to be applied in a more systematic fashion [43].

The incorporation of imatinib into frontline therapy regimens for Ph-positive ALL has also improved the rate of allogeneic SCT in first CR compared with the historical experience [58, 64, 65, 70]. This success is in part related to (1) an increase in the proportion of sustained remissions, offering additional time for identification of a suitable donor, and to (2) an improvement in the quality of the remissions (e.g., lower levels of *BCR-ABL* transcripts by PCR after imatinib-based therapy) resulting in a lower pre-transplantation tumor burden.

Two of the early nonrandomized studies of imatinib-based chemotherapy for de novo Ph-positive ALL applied allogeneic SCT in first CR as standard of care when feasible. In the early analyses of these imatinib-based regimens, survival outcomes with or without allogeneic SCT were similar, despite the selection biases favoring SCT [58, 60, 65, 70]. In 2007, Fielding et al. [73] evaluated the effects of incorporation of imatinib (600 mg) into the MRC UKALLXII/ECOGE2993 regimen for the de novo Ph-positive ALL subset, initially into the postinduction phase until 2 years after allogeneic SCT (first implemented in 2003), then earlier into the induction phase (applied in 2005). Although the CR rates improved from 83% to 91% with administration of imatinib in phase 2 of the induction, the 3-year OS rates were similar between the imatinib ($n=153$) and no imatinib ($n=267$) groups (23% versus 26%, $p=$NS), with the analysis confined only to those patients with at least 6 months of follow-up. The rate of allogeneic SCT in first CR was also similar between the two groups (58% versus 61%, respectively, $p=$NS). Further follow-up may be required prior to definitive conclusions regarding the effect, or lack thereof, of imatinib on RFS and OS in this study.

Although the initial reports of frontline imatinib-based chemotherapy suggested that outcomes were similar with or without allogeneic SCT in first CR, long-term updates of these studies (e.g., hyper-CVAD and imatinib, JALSG ALL202, and GRAAPH-2003) provide emerging data that allogeneic SCT improves outcome for Ph-positive ALL in the TKI-era [59, 62, 66]. Additional experience and longer follow-up of these studies should clarify whether allogeneic SCT can be deferred in a select group of Ph-positive ALL patients otherwise eligible for this modality, although interpretations may be confounded by the interventional or prophylactic use of TKI therapy in the post transplant setting.

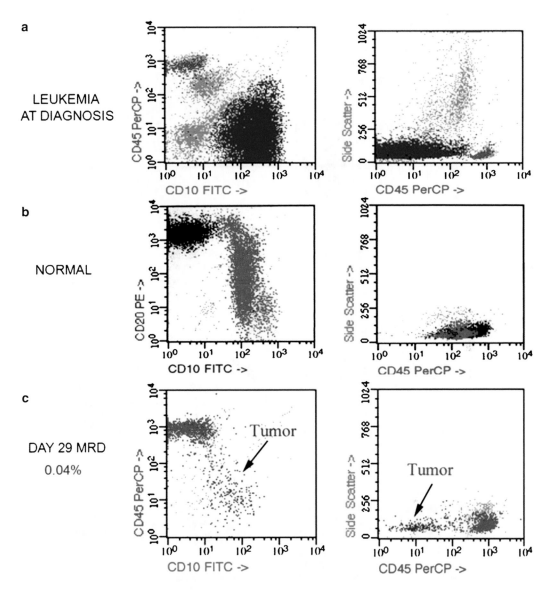

Fig. 4.1 Multiparameter flow cytometry identifies aberrant leukemic phenotypes. (**a**) Comparison of multiple antigen pairs demonstrates aberrant leukemic phenotypes, e.g., CD10+ CD45−, occupying a position in which normal cells are not seen (gray arrow, compare to **b**). (**c**) These aberrant phenotypes allow for the identification of MRD cells after therapy

CD45 and CD20 [36, 40, 45, 46]. For example, prednisone has been shown to reduce CD10 and CD34 expression in leukemic blasts in vitro [47]. Fortunately, these altered phenotypes are still sufficiently different from that of normal B cells and B cell precursors that MRD can still be detected in nearly all cases [40]. In T-ALL, as with pre-B ALL, treatment of patients results in maturation-like changes in leukemic T cell phenotypes which limits the usefulness of many of the most valuable immature markers like TdT and CD99, and makes flow-based detection of T-ALL MRD more difficult than that of pre-B ALL [48]. Finally, a small subset (2–5%) of leukemic cells cannot be detected using standard 3–4 antigen detection. Fortunately, the latest flow cytometry technologies allow for the measurement of 6–12 distinct fluorochromes simultaneously. Adding

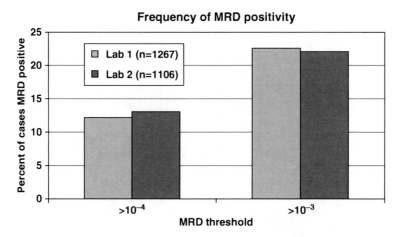

Fig. 4.2 Comparison of flow cytometry–based MRD measurements. Two independent central reference labs for the Children's Oncology Group received more than 1000 samples each from the same study cohort and performed identical multiparameter flow cytometry on each sample. The percentages of samples whose MRD were identified as positive, using cutoffs of either 10^{-4} or 10^{-3} did not differ between the labs

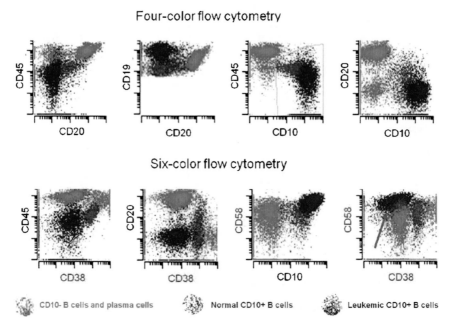

Fig. 4.3 Flow cytometry using 6 colors improves detection of MRD. Standard 4-color flow cytometry cannot always clearly separate the aberrant leukemia population from normal human B cells. Six-color flow can more easily identify the aberrant population for accurate quantitation, in this case based on underexpression of CD38 and overexpression of CD58 (arrow), in a case where CD10 and CD45 both show overlap with normal B cell precursors

more markers in the same tube can help resolve abnormal populations that are incompletely resolved with fewer antigens (see example in Fig. 4.3). This technology, though less accessible currently, holds promise for improving MRD detection in the future.

Comparing PCR to Flow Cytometry–Based MRD

Each approach to measuring MRD has its advantages and disadvantages. For example, PCR-based techniques have greater sensitivity in most cases, allowing quantifiable thresholds in the range of 10^{-5}. However, PCR-based approaches are time and labor intensive and are non-informative in up to 10% or more of patients. In addition, the time required to produce reagents needed for these studies makes it difficult to design clinical trials with very early intervention based on MRD results. However, once reagents are prepared, monitoring of patients at many points over time becomes relatively easy and inexpensive. In comparison, flow-based MRD measurements are rapid and relatively cost-efficient, and potentially more quantitative. However, they are not as sensitive as PCR-based methods, and require experience to be able to distinguish low-level abnormal populations from background normal cells. (Table 4.1).

The ideal MRD platform would provide a simple, precise, reproducible, and cost-effective technology that could be standardized in multiple institutions, have sensitivity consistently greater than 10^{-4}, and be achievable in nearly all patients. Neither PCR nor flow cytometry yet fulfills these qualifications completely. Several studies have shown that in general both technologies are highly comparable, though as expected PCR-based assays often have higher sensitivity [49–52]. Therefore, selection of an MRD approach may primarily depend on the intended use. For example, PCR-based MRD can identify some patients with no detectable leukemia with a very high degree of sensitivity (10^{-5} or even better) and such patients have an excellent outcome. Studies whose intention is to de-intensify therapy for very low risk patients may choose PCR-based MRD for its higher sensitivity in most cases. However, flow cytometry performed very early in therapy may serve the same purpose. In Brazil, for example, flow-based MRD has been used to identify relatively low-risk patients who may receive lower intensity therapy in areas of limited resources and supportive care [53]. On the other hand, either approach can identify high-risk populations with slow clearance and/or residual disease. If treatment is to be intensified very early in the course of therapy, the rapidity of flow cytometry may make it preferable. Some groups have advocated using both technologies concurrently to minimize false-negative and false-positive results, while allowing accurate MRD assessment in nearly all patients [50, 51, 54]. However, this obviously increases cost substantially. Moreover, it is not clear that the MRD levels from these techniques are interchangeable; even though there is excellent correlation between flow and PCR-based methods overall, individual patients are often classified differently with respect to risk assignment [55].

Table 4.1 Comparison of PCR-based and flow-based MRD assays

	Translocation PCR	Antigen receptor PCR	Flow cytometry
Sensitivity	10^{-5}–10^{-6}	10^{-5}–10^{-6}	10^{-3}–10^{-4}
Applicability	40–50% of cases	70–90% of cases	90–95% of cases
Turn-around time	Moderate	Slower	Rapid
Cost per time point	+	+++	++
Cost per multiple time points	++	+++	+++
Pitfalls	Limited application	Time and cost	Limited sensitivity
	RNA stability	Clonal evolution	Phenotypic drift
	Contamination	Contamination	Less well standardized

The Prognostic Significance of MRD

The use of MRD as a measure of therapeutic response in patients with ALL is now generally well accepted [12, 17, 56–63]. Indeed, many studies have shown the profound prognostic significance of MRD in ALL (Table 4.2) [24, 54, 64–70].

Early studies established that PCR and flow-based measurements could extend the lower end of the scale of leukemia burden [9, 10, 12, 13, 29, 71]. Indeed, as improved peripheral blood and bone marrow response predicted better outcome, so too did lower MRD correlate with improved outcome. Over the past decade, we have made great progress both in understanding the role of MRD as well as advancing the technology to measure it. The St. Jude's group initially demonstrated that flow cytometry can be used to identify patients at low risk for relapse (i.e., 90% RFS) using a single MRD measurement at day 43 of therapy [64]. Subsequently, this group demonstrated that measuring an earlier bone marrow MRD at day 19 of induction ($<10^{-4}$) identified a subset with even better survival of 94% RFS [72]. The COG, in a study of nearly 2000 children, showed that increasing levels of MRD at end of induction are associated with progressively worse outcome, with 88% 5 year EFS for patients with MRD $< 10^{-4}$ in their day 29 bone marrow sample, down to 30% 5 year EFS for those with $>10^{-2}$ (1%) residual disease (Fig. 4.4) [68]. Thus, measurement of MRD within about the first month of therapy can identify subgroups with either very good or very poor outcome depending on the level of MRD detected. DFCI and PALG demonstrated that a single MRD measurement at end induction doesn't need to be very sensitive to identify a very high risk group; patients with end induction MRD $>10^{-3}$ had a relapse-free survival of only 19–28% [67, 69]. The recent COG study also found that a very early measurement of MRD in peripheral blood (day 8) also predicts outcome, retaining prognostic ability independent of day 29 bone marrow MRD (Fig. 4.4) [68]. In the same study, bone marrow MRD measured later in treatment (end consolida-

Table 4.2 MRD predicts outcome in ALL in multiple studies

Study group	Group	Tech.	Time points	Thresholds	Findings
St. Jude [64, 72]	Child	Flow	Mid-induction d19	D19 $< 10^{-4}$	94% RFS
			End induction d43	D19 $> 10^{-4}$	67% RFS
			Continuation Wk14+32	D43 $< 10^{-4}$	90% RFS
				D43 $> 10^{-4}$	57% RFS
				Wk14 $> 10^{-4}$	31% RFS
				Wk32 $> 10^{-4}$	14% RFS
GMALL [66]	Adult	PCR	Mid-induction d11, d24	LR: D11/24 $< 10^{-4}$	100% RFS
			Mid-consolidation wk16	IR: other	53% RFS
				HR: Wk16 $> 10^{-4}$	6% RFS
DFCI [67]	Child	PCR	End induction d30	D30 $< 10^{-3}$	88% RFS
				D30 $> 10^{-3}$	28% RFS
COG [68]	Child	Flow	End induction d29	NCI-SR D29 $< 10^{-4}$	89–95% EFS
				NCI-SR D29 $> 10^{-4}$	59–64% EFS
				NCI-HR D29 $< 10^{-4}$	72–79% EFS
				NCI-HR D29 $> 10^{-4}$	33–34% EFS
PALG [69]	Child	Flow	End induction wk4	Wk4 $< 10^{-3}$	74% RFS
				Wk4 $> 10^{-3}$	19% RFS
I-BFM-SG (24)	Child	PCR	End induction d33	SR: D33/78 $< 10^{-4}$	93% EFS
			End consolidation d78	IR: Other	74% EFS
				HR: D78 $> 10^{-3}$	16% EFS

EFS event-free survival, *RFS* relapse-free survival, *D* day from diagnosis, *Wk* week from diagnosis, *LR* low risk, *SR* standard risk, *IR* intermediate risk, *HR* high risk, *NCI* National Cancer Institute risk criteria, *GMALL* German Multicenter Adult ALL, *DFCI* Dana Farber Cancer Institute, *COG* Children's Oncology Group, *PALG* Polish Adult Leukemia Group, *I-BFM-SG* International Berlin-Frankfurt-Munster Study Group

Second Generation Tyrosine Kinase Inhibitors for Ph-Positive ALL

The second-generation TKIs dasatinib (BMS-354825; SPRYCEL; Bristol-Myers Squibb, New York, NY) and nilotinib (AMN107, Novartis Pharmaceuticals, Basel, Switzerland) are increasingly potent inhibitors of ABL. These TKIs and several of the more recently developed multitargeted agents are in active clinical investigation; each inhibits c-kit, PDGFR, FLT3, and other kinases with varying potency (Table 15.4).

Dasatinib

Dasatinib is a dual Src and ABL inhibitor with 325-fold more potency in vitro than imatinib against wild-type BCR-ABL; it also inhibits the c-kit, PDGFR, and ephrin A receptor kinases [104]. Unlike imatinib, it binds to both the inactive and active forms of the BCR-ABL protein. Also, the intracellular uptake of dasatinib is not dependent on OCT-1 activity, although it is a substrate for efflux proteins [105, 106]. Dasatinib has demonstrated in vitro efficacy against all imatinib-resistant KD mutations tested, with the exception of T315I and F317L (Fig. 15.2) [104]. Table 15.5 outlines the

Table 15.4 Spectrum of activity of BCR-ABL inhibitors

Drug	Kinases inhibited
Imatinib	BCR-ABL, c-kit, platelet derived growth factor receptor (PDGFR)
Dasatinib	BCR-ABL, Src family kinases, c-kit, ephrin receptor kinases, PDGFR
Nilotinib	BCR-ABL, c-kit, PDGFR
Bosutinib	BCR-ABL, Src family kinases
INNO-406	BCR-ABL, Lyn kinase
BIRB-796	BCR-ABL, p38 mitogen-activated protein (MAP) kinase
XL228	BCR-ABL, Src family kinases, IGF1-R
PHA739358	BCR-ABL, aurora kinases
AP24534	BCR-ABL, FLT3, FGF1-R
DCC2036	BCR-ABL

Table 15.5 Dasatinib-based chemotherapy regimens for Ph-positive ALL

Study	Regimen	Dasatinib dosing	No.	Med age (range) (yrs)	% CR	% Relapse	% DFS (yrs)	% Survival (yrs)
Imatinib-failures								
Ottmann [107]	START	70 mg twice daily	36	46 (15–85)	33	NR	32 (1)	NR
Jabbour [108]	Hyper-CVAD	100 mg days 1–14	14	43 (21–69)	71	29	NR	NR
Newly diagnosed or minimally treated								
Ravandi [109]	Hyper-CVAD	100 mg once daily days 1–14	35	53 (21–79)	94	15	59 (2)	64 (2)
Rousselot [110]	EWALL Ph-01	140 mg daily induction, then 100 mg daily	21	71 (61–83)	95	5	NR	NR
Foa [111]	GIMEMA LAL1205	70 mg twice daily days 1–84 (+ prednisone)	34	54 (24–76)	100	26	NR	81 (1)

START Src/Abl Tyrosine Kinase Inhibition Activity: Research Trials of Dasatinib, *hyper-CVAD* fractionated cyclophosphamide, vincristine, doxorubicin, dexamethasone, *EWALL* European Working Group on Adult ALL, *GIMEMA* Gruppo Italiano Malattie EMatologiche dell'Adulto, *NR* not reported
Refer to the text for the details of the chemotherapy regimens

clinical outcomes observed with dasatinib administered either as monotherapy or in combination with chemotherapy for imatinib-resistant or newly diagnosed Ph-positive ALL.

In a phase I trial of dasatinib for imatinib-resistant Ph-positive ALL, a hematological response rate of 80% was observed in 10 patients [112, 113]. In the Src/Abl Tyrosine Kinase Inhibition Activity: Research Trials of Dasatinib (START) phase II study where 36 patients (median age 46 years) with imatinib-resistant Ph-positive ALL were treated with single agent dasatinib 70 mg twice daily, the CR rate was 31% (Table 15.5) [107]. However, the major cytogenetic response rate was nearly double that at 57%, with the difference related to the myelosuppressive effects of dasatinib prohibiting sufficient recovery of cytopenias to satisfy CR response criteria. Although a high proportion of patients with P- and A-loop ABL KD mutations responded to dasatinib, all patients with a baseline T315I mutation failed therapy. Adverse events including myelosuppression, diarrhea, and peripheral edema were often amenable to dose modifications. The unique toxicity of pleural effusions occurred in 5–20% of the cases, and has been attributed to dasatinib's potent inhibition of PDGFR. More recent data suggested that administering dasatinib once daily produced similar response rates with an improved toxicity profile, particularly with respect to myelosuppression and pleural effusions [114]. Based on the efficacy demonstrated in these and other clinical trials, dasatinib was granted approval by the US Food and Drug Administration (FDA) for the treatment of all phases of CML and Ph-positive ALL resistant or intolerant to imatinib.

Unlike imatinib, dasatinib has activity against leukemia cell lines which express high levels of PgP, and may therefore offer CNS protection. Indeed, treatment with dasatinib has been associated with durable regression of CNS disease in mouse models [115]. Stabilization and regression of CNS disease was also noted in a small series of patients treated with dasatinib-based therapy for CNS relapse [115]. Further corroboration of the CNS effect of dasatinib stems from the identification of dasatinib-resistant ABL KD mutations in the CSF [115]. However, there is insufficient data to support modification of the current standard practice to administer CNS prophylaxis (such as intrathecal chemotherapy) in the context of dasatinib-based therapy.

Use of dasatinib in the frontline setting is now being explored. In the GIMEMA LAL 1205 trial, dasatinib 70 mg twice daily was administered for 12 weeks in conjunction with prednisone and intrathecal chemotherapy for CNS prophylaxis to 48 adults with de novo Ph-positive ALL (median age 54 years, range 24–76 years) [111]. The CR rate was 100% in 34 evaluable patients. After a median follow-up of 11 months, the OS rate at 10 months was 81%. Nine patients (26%) relapsed, including 5 with T315I and 1 with E255K ABL KD mutations. The log reduction of *BCR-ABL* transcripts by PCR during the induction period had prognostic relevance. Details of continuation therapy were not provided; therefore an analysis of the impact of dasatinib monotherapy on outcome will be hampered by the heterogeneity of subsequent treatment approaches.

Two trials have reported the use of dasatinib in combination with chemotherapy for newly diagnosed Ph-positive ALL. Preliminary results of a dasatinib-based frontline chemotherapy regimen for patients older than 55 years of age were reported by the European Working Group on Adult ALL (EWALL) [110]. Dasatinib was administered 140 mg daily during the induction (vincristine, dexamethasone), then 100 mg daily during the subsequent consolidation (methotrexate and L-asparaginase alternating with high-dose cytarabine for six cycles) and maintenance chemotherapy phases. The CR rate was 95% in 22 patients. No observations could be made regarding the durability of responses since the median follow-up was less than 6 months.

Based on the success of the hyper-CVAD and imatinib regimen in de novo Ph-positive ALL and activity of the hyper-CVAD and dasatinib regimen in imatinib-resistant Ph-positive ALL, the frontline regimen was modified to incorporate dasatinib 50 mg twice daily days 1–14 of each intensive cycle in lieu of the imatinib (Table 15.5). [108, 109] Thirty-five patients were treated with a median age of 53 years (range, 21–79 years). The rates of CR, molecular CR, relapse and estimated 3-year OS were 94%, 61%, 15%, and 64%, respectively, after a median follow-up of 14 months (longest 37 months). Comparison to the prior experience with the hyper-CVAD and imatinib regimen [59] showed similar CRD, DFS, and OS outcomes, albeit with shorter follow-up. Based on these findings, recent modifications to the hyper-CVAD and dasatinib regimen included (1) change in dasatinib dosing from twice daily to once daily with continuous administration of 70 mg daily starting with consolidation chemotherapy, and (2) incorporation of the anti-CD20 monoclonal antibody rituximab if the baseline lymphoblast CD20 expression was at least 20% (based on the favorable experience with hyper-CVAD and rituximab in Ph-negative B-lymphoblastic leukemia) [116].

Nilotinib

Nilotinib is an aminopyrimidine derivative of imatinib which inhibits c-kit and PDGFR like its parent compound (Table 15.4) [117]. However, it is 20- to 50-fold more potent as an ABL kinase inhibitor, and retains much of this potency against imatinib-resistant cell lines [118, 119]. Phase I and II clinical trials of nilotinib in imatinib-resistant Ph-positive ALL demonstrate hematological responses in 30–35% of the cases [120]. Dose-dependent adverse events included myelosuppression, transient indirect hyperbilirubinemia, pruritis, and rash. Certain ABL KD mutations involving the P-loop (e.g., Y253F/H or E255K/V) are resistant to nilotinib. Currently, this agent is only approved by the FDA for imatinib-resistant or intolerant chronic phase CML.

Later Generation ABL Tyrosine Kinase Inhibitors

Development of third- or fourth-generation novel TKIs which target specific ABL KD mutations remains the focus of developmental therapeutics in this disease (Table 15.4). Several of these agents have dual activity against the Src/ABL kinases, and are currently being investigated in clinical trials (e.g., bosutinib or SKI-606 [121, 122], INNO-406 [123]); however, neither of these agents have activity against the T315I KD mutation. The differential selectivity, or lack thereof, of other tyrosine kinases besides ABL, as in the case of bosutinib (which does not inhibit c-kit or PDGFR) may improve clinical outcome simply by altering the safety profile.

Targeting the T315I ABL Kinase Domain Mutation

Several other agents targeting the T315I KD mutation are in preclinical or clinical stages of development: (1) dual specific Abl/Src kinase inhibitors such as AP23464 [124], (2) ABL, Src, and PDGFR inhibitors such as ON012380 with activity in T315I mutated cell lines, and (3) pyrimidine Src/Abl inhibitors such as PD166326 [125]. Combination TKI therapy may prove worthy of further study as in vitro data suggest that the combination of imatinib with nilotinib and/or dual Src/Abl inhibitors such as dasatinib or AP23464 further enhance the ability of imatinib to prevent autophosphorylation of wild-type BCR-ABL [126, 127]. Carefully designed clinical trials of such TKI combinations will require frequent monitoring of *BCR-ABL* transcripts by PCR and ABL KD mutations owing to potential for selection of TKI-specific mutations.

Role of Monoclonal Antibodies in Ph-Positive ALL

The expression of CD20 (at least 20%) occurs in approximately 40% of B-lymphoblastic leukemia and appears to be associated with worse outcome [128, 129]. In the MRC UKALLXII/ECOG2993 trial, Ph-negative B-lymphoblastic leukemia cases with low levels of CD20 expression and high levels of CD22 expression had superior OS rates [130]. The prognostic significance of CD20 expression prior to frontline treatment with hyper-CVAD, hyper-CVAD with imatinib, or hyper-CVAD with dasatinib was evaluated in 126 patients with de novo or minimally treated Ph-positive ALL [131]. There was no difference in outcome by CD20 expression for Ph-positive ALL cases treated with chemotherapy alone. In contrast to the experience in Ph-negative B-lymphoblastic leukemia, the rates of DFS and OS were superior for CD20-positive subgroups treated with TKI-based chemotherapy, particularly for dasatinib, suggesting there are beneficial off-target effects of TKIs which should be exploited further. An example is the potential induction of a leukemia-specific response characterized by clonal T-cell large granular lymphocytosis, which has been associated with favorable survival outcomes in the setting of TKI therapy with either imatinib or dasatinib [132, 133]. Use of monoclonal antibodies directed against CD20, CD22, or CD52 (e.g., rituximab or ofatumumab, epratuzumab, or alemtuzumab, respectively) may further improve the outcome of Ph-positive ALL when administered in conjunction with TKI-based therapy, particularly given the encouraging data in Ph-negative B-lymphoblastic leukemia [116, 134].

Future Directions

Long-term efficacy of the newer TKIs continues to be explored, with clinical trials incorporating dasatinib into chemotherapy regimens for de novo and imatinib-resistant Ph-positive ALL underway. Development of novel third- and fourth- generation TKIs which target several pathways involved in the pathogenesis of Ph-positive ALL may further improve outcome and potentially circumvent resistance mechanisms. However, long-term control of Ph-positive ALL with TKI monotherapy will likely not be feasible owing to the high rate of genomic instability, which can foster development of multiple ABL KD mutations. These mutations, in turn, will be selected or de-selected depending on the spectrum of sensitivity and inherent resistance to the specific TKI. Rationally designed clinical trials of combination TKI therapy with or without chemotherapy should be explored based on preclinical models suggesting additive or synergistic effects.

Conclusions

Ph-positive ALL was previously the most unfavorable subtype of adult ALL; however, with the advent of TKI therapy, prognosis has improved such that outcomes are superior to those for some of the other high risk subsets of B-lymphoblastic leukemia. Emerging data have established that the standard of care for de novo Ph-positive ALL should be TKI-based therapy with imatinib, but potentially with dasatinib or later-generation TKIs after further maturation of the data. The concurrent use of imatinib with chemotherapy appears superior from an efficacy perspective and feasible from a safety perspective. However, new challenges have emerged with respect to the induction of resistance to imatinib via ABL KD mutations. The development of novel TKIs with increased potency for ABL inhibition and their ongoing incorporation into frontline therapy should further improve outcome, although resurgence or emergence of novel ABL KD mutations will likely remain a therapeutic challenge.

Strategies designed to optimize the achievement of a complete molecular response to TKI-based chemotherapy while circumventing development of resistance will be paramount to ensuring eradication of the disease. Assessments for ABL KD mutations should be routinely incorporated into the monitoring schema in order to better define the implications for therapeutic interventions. The role of allogeneic SCT in first CR continues to be redefined as emerging long-term data suggests that improvements in outcome are incurred with this modality in the TKI era. An optimal potentially curative strategy for the treatment of the younger patient with de novo Ph-positive ALL involves the integration of multi-modality therapy, including frontline TKI-based multi-agent chemotherapy followed by allogeneic SCT in first CR (as feasible or as indicated) with consideration for post transplantation "maintenance" regimen of TKI monotherapy on an investigational clinical trial. For the elderly patient with de novo Ph-positive ALL, the optimal chemotherapy regimen or even role for chemotherapy remains to be delineated, particularly owing to relative intolerance compared with younger counterparts. Reduced intensity allogeneic SCT in first CR should be considered in the older patient with Ph-positive ALL whenever feasible, owing to the relatively high rates of disease recurrence with TKI-based therapy and encouraging outcomes reported to date with this intervention. Novel strategies to circumvent resistance such as combination TKI therapy, incorporation of therapeutic agents targeting other interrelated downstream signaling pathways of BCR-ABL, and integration of monoclonal antibody therapy should be systematically explored in Ph-positive ALL.

References

1. Faderl, S., Kantarjian, H. M., Talpaz, M., & Estrov, Z. (1998). Clinical significance of cytogenetic abnormalities in adult acute lymphoblastic leukemia. *Blood, 91*(11), 3995–4019.
2. Larson, R. A. (2006). Management of acute lymphoblastic leukemia in older patients. *Seminars in Hematology, 43*(2), 126–133.
3. Schultz, K. R., Pullen, D. J., Sather, H. N., et al. (2007). Risk- and response-based classification of childhood B-precursor acute lymphoblastic leukemia: A combined analysis of prognostic markers from the Pediatric Oncology Group (POG) and Children's Cancer Group (CCG). *Blood, 109*(3), 926–935.
4. Heerema, N. A., Harbott, J., Galimberti, S., et al. (2004). Secondary cytogenetic aberrations in childhood Philadelphia chromosome positive acute lymphoblastic leukemia are nonrandom and may be associated with outcome. *Leukemia, 18*(4), 693–702.
5. Wetzler, M., Dodge, R. K., Mrozek, K., et al. (2004). Additional cytogenetic abnormalities in adults with Philadelphia chromosome-positive acute lymphoblastic leukaemia: A study of the Cancer and Leukaemia Group B. *British Journal Haematology, 124*(3), 275–288.
6. Rieder, H., Ludwig, W. D., Gassmann, W., et al. (1996). Prognostic significance of additional chromosome abnormalities in adult patients with Philadelphia chromosome positive acute lymphoblastic leukaemia. *British Journal Haematology, 95*(4), 678–691.
7. Moorman, A. V., Harrison, C. J., Buck, G. A., et al. (2007). Karyotype is an independent prognostic factor in adult acute lymphoblastic leukemia (ALL): Analysis of cytogenetic data from patients treated on the Medical Research Council (MRC) UKALLXII/Eastern Cooperative Oncology Group (ECOG) 2993 trial. *Blood, 109*(8), 3189–3197.
8. Yanada, M., Takeuchi, J., Sugiura, I., et al. (2008). Karyotype at diagnosis is the major prognostic factor predicting relapse-free survival for patients with Philadelphia chromosome-positive acute lymphoblastic leukemia treated with imatinib-combined chemotherapy. *Haematologica, 93*(2), 287–290.
9. Fielding, A. K., Rowe, J. M., Richards, S. M., et al. (2009). Prospective outcome data on 267 unselected adult patients with Philadelphia chromosome-positive acute lymphoblastic leukemia confirms superiority of allogeneic transplantation over chemotherapy in the pre-imatinib era: Results from the International ALL Trial MRC UKALLXII/ECOG2993. *Blood, 113*(19), 4489–4496.
10. Rowley, J. D. (1973). Letter: A new consistent chromosomal abnormality in chronic myelogenous leukaemia identified by quinacrine fluorescence and Giemsa staining. *Nature, 243*(5405), 290–293.
11. Daley, G. Q., Van Etten, R. A., & Baltimore, D. (1990). Induction of chronic myelogenous leukemia in mice by the P210bcr/abl gene of the Philadelphia chromosome. *Science, 247*(4944), 824–830.
12. Heisterkamp, N., Jenster, G., ten Hoeve, J., Zovich, D., Pattengale, P. K., & Groffen, J. (1990). Acute leukaemia in bcr/abl transgenic mice. *Nature, 344*(6263), 251–253.
13. Lugo, T. G., Pendergast, A. M., Muller, A. J., & Witte, O. N. (1990). Tyrosine kinase activity and transformation potency of bcr-abl oncogene products. *Science, 247*(4946), 1079–1082.
14. Voncken, J. W., Kaartinen, V., Pattengale, P. K., Germeraad, W. T., Groffen, J., & Heisterkamp, N. (1995). BCR/ABL P210 and P190 cause distinct leukemia in transgenic mice. *Blood, 86*(12), 4603–4611.

15. Melo, J. V. (1996). The diversity of BCR-ABL fusion proteins and their relationship to leukemia phenotype. *Blood, 88*(7), 2375–2384.
16. Li, S., Ilaria, R. L., Jr., Million, R. P., Daley, G. Q., & Van Etten, R. A. (1999). The P190, P210, and P230 forms of the BCR/ABL oncogene induce a similar chronic myeloid leukemia-like syndrome in mice but have different lymphoid leukemogenic activity. *The Journal of Experimental Medicine, 189*(9), 1399–1412.
17. Cimino, G., Pane, F., Elia, L., et al. (2006). The role of BCR/ABL isoforms in the presentation and outcome of patients with Philadelphia-positive acute lymphoblastic leukemia: A seven-year update of the GIMEMA 0496 trial. *Haematologica, 91*(3), 377–380.
18. Kantarjian, H. M., Talpaz, M., Dhingra, K., et al. (1991). Significance of the P210 versus P190 molecular abnormalities in adults with Philadelphia chromosome-positive acute leukemia. *Blood, 78*(9), 2411–2418.
19. Gleissner, B., Gokbuget, N., Bartram, C. R., et al. (2002). Leading prognostic relevance of the BCR-ABL translocation in adult acute B-lineage lymphoblastic leukemia: A prospective study of the German Multicenter Trial Group and confirmed polymerase chain reaction analysis. *Blood, 99*(5), 1536–1543.
20. Tauchi, T., Okabe, S., Miyazawa, K., & Ohyashiki, K. (1998). The tetramerization domain-independent Ras activation by BCR-ABL oncoprotein in hematopoietic cells. *International Journal of Oncology, 12*(6), 1269–1276.
21. Skorski, T., Kanakaraj, P., Nieborowska-Skorska, M., et al. (1995). Phosphatidylinositol-3 kinase activity is regulated by BCR/ABL and is required for the growth of Philadelphia chromosome-positive cells. *Blood, 86*(2), 726–736.
22. Chai, S. K., Nichols, G. L., & Rothman, P. (1997). Constitutive activation of JAKs and STATs in BCR-Abl-expressing cell lines and peripheral blood cells derived from leukemic patients. *Journal of Immunology, 159*(10), 4720–4728.
23. Ilaria, R. L., Jr., & Van Etten, R. A. (1996). P210 and P190(BCR/ABL) induce the tyrosine phosphorylation and DNA binding activity of multiple specific STAT family members. *The Journal of Biological Chemistry, 271*(49), 31704–31710.
24. Schrappe, M., Arico, M., Harbott, J., et al. (1998). Philadelphia chromosome-positive (Ph+) childhood acute lymphoblastic leukemia: Good initial steroid response allows early prediction of a favorable treatment outcome. *Blood, 92*(8), 2730–2741.
25. Arico, M., Valsecchi, M. G., Camitta, B., et al. (2000). Outcome of treatment in children with Philadelphia chromosome-positive acute lymphoblastic leukemia. *The New England Journal of Medicine, 342*(14), 998–1006.
26. Westbrook, C. A., Hooberman, A. L., Spino, C., et al. (1992). Clinical significance of the BCR-ABL fusion gene in adult acute lymphoblastic leukemia: A Cancer and Leukemia Group B study (8762). *Blood, 80*(12), 2983–2990.
27. Gotz, G., Weh, H. J., Walter, T. A., et al. (1992). Clinical and prognostic significance of the Philadelphia chromosome in adult patients with acute lymphoblastic leukemia. *Annals of Hematology, 64*(2), 97–100.
28. Larson, R. A., Dodge, R. K., Burns, C. P., et al. (1995). A five-drug remission induction regimen with intensive consolidation for adults with acute lymphoblastic leukemia: Cancer and Leukemia Group B study 8811. *Blood, 85*(8), 2025–2037.
29. Secker-Walker, L. M., Prentice, H. G., Durrant, J., Richards, S., Hall, E., & Harrison, G. (1997). Cytogenetics adds independent prognostic information in adults with acute lymphoblastic leukaemia on MRC trial UKALL XA. MRC Adult Leukaemia Working Party. *British Journal Haematology, 96*(3), 601–610.
30. Wetzler, M., Dodge, R. K., Mrozek, K., et al. (1999). Prospective karyotype analysis in adult acute lymphoblastic leukemia: The Cancer and Leukemia Group B experience. *Blood, 93*(11), 3983–3993.
31. Faderl, S., Kantarjian, H. M., Thomas, D. A., et al. (2000). Outcome of Philadelphia chromosome-positive adult acute lymphoblastic leukemia. *Leukaemia & Lymphoma, 36*(3–4), 263–273.
32. Dombret, H., Gabert, J., Boiron, J. M., et al. (2002). Outcome of treatment in adults with Philadelphia chromosome-positive acute lymphoblastic leukemia–results of the prospective multicenter LALA-94 trial. *Blood, 100*(7), 2357–2366.
33. Radich, J. P. (2001). Philadelphia chromosome-positive acute lymphocytic leukemia. *Hematology/Oncology Clinics of North America, 15*(1), 21–36.
34. Kantarjian, H. M., O'Brien, S., Smith, T. L., et al. (2000). Results of treatment with hyper-CVAD, a dose-intensive regimen, in adult acute lymphocytic leukemia. *Journal of Clinical Oncology, 18*(3), 547–561.
35. Kantarjian, H., Thomas, D., O'Brien, S., et al. (2004). Long-term follow-up results of hyperfractionated cyclophosphamide, vincristine, doxorubicin, and dexamethasone (Hyper-CVAD), a dose-intensive regimen, in adult acute lymphocytic leukemia. *Cancer, 101*(12), 2788–2801.
36. Pane, F., Cimino, G., Izzo, B., et al. (2005). Significant reduction of the hybrid BCR/ABL transcripts after induction and consolidation therapy is a powerful predictor of treatment response in adult Philadelphia-positive acute lymphoblastic leukemia. *Leukemia, 19*(4), 628–635.
37. Laport, G. G., Alvarnas, J. C., Palmer, J. M., et al. (2008). Long-term remission of Philadelphia chromosome-positive acute lymphoblastic leukemia after allogeneic hematopoietic cell transplantation from matched sibling donors: A 20-year experience with the fractionated total body irradiation-etoposide regimen. *Blood, 112*(3), 903–909.

38. Goldstone, A. H., Prentice, H. G., Durrant, J., et al. (2001). Allogeneic transplant (related or unrelated donor) is the preferred treatment for adult Philadelphia chromosome positive (Ph+) acute lymphoblastic leukemia (ALL). Results from the international ALL trial (MRC UKALLXII/ECOG E2993) [abstract 3556]. *Blood, 98*, 856a.

39. Barrett, A. J., Horowitz, M. M., Ash, R. C., et al. (1992). Bone marrow transplantation for Philadelphia chromosome-positive acute lymphoblastic leukemia. *Blood, 79*(11), 3067–3070.

40. Chao, N. J., Blume, K. G., Forman, S. J., & Snyder, D. S. (1995). Long-term follow-up of allogeneic bone marrow recipients for Philadelphia chromosome-positive acute lymphoblastic leukemia. *Blood, 85*(11), 3353–3354.

41. Avivi, I., & Goldstone, A. H. (2003). Bone marrow transplant in Ph + ALL patients. *Bone Marrow Transplantation, 31*(8), 623–632.

42. Yanada, M., Naoe, T., Iida, H., et al. (2005). Myeloablative allogeneic hematopoietic stem cell transplantation for Philadelphia chromosome-positive acute lymphoblastic leukemia in adults: Significant roles of total body irradiation and chronic graft-versus-host disease. *Bone Marrow Transplantation, 36*(10), 867–872.

43. Marks, D. I., Aversa, F., & Lazarus, H. M. (2006). Alternative donor transplants for adult acute lymphoblastic leukaemia: A comparison of the three major options. *Bone Marrow Transplantation, 38*(7), 467–475.

44. Schindler, T., Bornmann, W., Pellicena, P., Miller, W. T., Clarkson, B., & Kuriyan, J. (2000). Structural mechanism for STI-571 inhibition of abelson tyrosine kinase. *Science, 289*(5486), 1938–1942.

45. Heinrich, M. C., Blanke, C. D., Druker, B. J., & Corless, C. L. (2002). Inhibition of KIT tyrosine kinase activity: A novel molecular approach to the treatment of KIT-positive malignancies. *Journal of Clinical Oncology, 20*(6), 1692–1703.

46. Apperley, J. F., Gardembas, M., Melo, J. V., et al. (2002). Response to imatinib mesylate in patients with chronic myeloproliferative diseases with rearrangements of the platelet-derived growth factor receptor beta. *The New England Journal of Medicine, 347*(7), 481–487.

47. Druker, B. J., Sawyers, C. L., Kantarjian, H., et al. (2001). Activity of a specific inhibitor of the BCR-ABL tyrosine kinase in the blast crisis of chronic myeloid leukemia and acute lymphoblastic leukemia with the Philadelphia chromosome. *The New England Journal of Medicine, 344*(14), 1038–1042.

48. Ottmann, O. G., Druker, B. J., Sawyers, C. L., et al. (2002). A phase 2 study of imatinib in patients with relapsed or refractory Philadelphia chromosome-positive acute lymphoid leukemias. *Blood, 100*(6), 1965–1971.

49. Scheuring, U. J., Pfeifer, H., Wassmann, B., et al. (2003). Early minimal residual disease (MRD) analysis during treatment of Philadelphia chromosome/Bcr-Abl-positive acute lymphoblastic leukemia with the Abl-tyrosine kinase inhibitor imatinib (STI571). *Blood, 101*(1), 85–90.

50. Wassmann, B., Pfeifer, H., Scheuring, U. J., et al. (2004). Early prediction of response in patients with relapsed or refractory Philadelphia chromosome-positive acute lymphoblastic leukemia (Ph + ALL) treated with imatinib. *Blood, 103*(4), 1495–1498.

51. Pfeifer, H., Wassmann, B., Hofmann, W. K., et al. (2003). Risk and prognosis of central nervous system leukemia in patients with Philadelphia chromosome-positive acute leukemias treated with imatinib mesylate. *Clinical Cancer Research, 9*(13), 4674–4681.

52. Leis, J. F., Stepan, D. E., Curtin, P. T., et al. (2004). Central nervous system failure in patients with chronic myelogenous leukemia lymphoid blast crisis and Philadelphia chromosome positive acute lymphoblastic leukemia treated with imatinib (STI-571). *Leukaemia & Lymphoma, 45*(4), 695–698.

53. Takayama, N., Sato, N., O'Brien, S. G., Ikeda, Y., & Okamoto, S. (2002). Imatinib mesylate has limited activity against the central nervous system involvement of Philadelphia chromosome-positive acute lymphoblastic leukaemia due to poor penetration into cerebrospinal fluid. *British Journal Haematology, 119*(1), 106–108.

54. Atallah, E., Kantarjian, H., & Cortes, J. (2007). Emerging safety issues with imatinib and other Abl tyrosine kinase inhibitors. *Clinical Lymphoma & Myeloma, 7*(Suppl 3), S105–S112.

55. Thiesing, J. T., Ohno-Jones, S., Kolibaba, K. S., & Druker, B. J. (2000). Efficacy of STI571, an abl tyrosine kinase inhibitor, in conjunction with other antileukemic agents against bcr-abl-positive cells. *Blood, 96*(9), 3195–3199.

56. Kano, Y., Akutsu, M., Tsunoda, S., et al. (2001). In vitro cytotoxic effects of a tyrosine kinase inhibitor STI571 in combination with commonly used antileukemic agents. *Blood, 97*(7), 1999–2007.

57. Topaly, J., Zeller, W. J., & Fruehauf, S. (2001). Synergistic activity of the new ABL-specific tyrosine kinase inhibitor STI571 and chemotherapeutic drugs on BCR-ABL-positive chronic myelogenous leukemia cells. *Leukemia, 15*(3), 342–347.

58. Thomas, D. A., Faderl, S., Cortes, J., et al. (2004). Treatment of Philadelphia chromosome-positive acute lymphocytic leukemia with hyper-CVAD and imatinib mesylate. *Blood, 103*(12), 4396–4407.

59. Thomas, D. A., Kantarjian, H. M., Cortes, J., et al. (2008). Outcome after frontline therapy with the hyper-CVAD and imatinib mesylate regimen for adults with de novo or minimally treated Philadelphia chromosome (Ph) positive acute lymphoblastic leukemia (ALL) [abstract 2931]. *Blood, 112*(11), 1008.

60. Thomas, D. A., Kantarjian, H. M., Cortes, J., et al. (2006). Outcome with the hyper-CVAD and imatinib mesylate regimen as frontline therapy for adult Philadelphia (Ph) positive acute lymphocytic leukemia (ALL) [abstract 284]. *Blood, 108*(11), 87a.

61. Yanada, M., & Naoe, T. (2006). Imatinib combined chemotherapy for Philadelphia chromosome-positive acute lymphoblastic leukemia: Major challenges in current practice. *Leukaemia & Lymphoma, 47*(9), 1747–1753.
62. Hatta, Y., Mizuta, S., Ohtake, S., et al. (2009). Promising outcome of imatinib-combined chemotherapy followed by allogeneic hematopoietic stem cell transplantation for Philadelphia chromosome-positive acute lymphoblastic leukemia: Results of the Japan Adult Leukemia Study Group (JALSG) Ph+ALL202 regimen [abstract 3090]. *Blood, 114*(22), 1201.
63. Lee, K. H., Lee, J. H., Choi, S. J., et al. (2005). Clinical effect of imatinib added to intensive combination chemotherapy for newly diagnosed Philadelphia chromosome-positive acute lymphoblastic leukemia. *Leukemia, 19*(9), 1509–1516.
64. Wassmann, B., Pfeifer, H., Goekbuget, N., et al. (2006). Alternating versus concurrent schedules of imatinib and chemotherapy as front-line therapy for Philadelphia-positive acute lymphoblastic leukemia (Ph+ALL). *Blood, 108*(5), 1469–1477.
65. de Labarthe, A., Rousselot, P., Huguet-Rigal, F., et al. (2007). Imatinib combined with induction or consolidation chemotherapy in patients with de novo Philadelphia chromosome-positive acute lymphoblastic leukemia: Results of the GRAAPH-2003 study. *Blood, 109*(4), 1408–1413.
66. Tanguy-Schmidt, A., de Labarthe, A., Rousselot, P., et al. (2009). Long-term results of the imatinib GRAAPH-2003 study in newly-diagnosed patients with de novo Philadelphia chromosome-positive acute lymphoblastic leukemia [abstract 3080]. *Blood, 114*(22), 1198.
67. Ottmann, O. G., Wassmann, B., Pfeifer, H., et al. (2007). Imatinib compared with chemotherapy as front-line treatment of elderly patients with Philadelphia chromosome-positive acute lymphoblastic leukemia (Ph+ALL). *Cancer, 109*(10), 2068–2076.
68. Vignetti, M., Fazi, P., Cimino, G., et al. (2007). Imatinib plus steroids induces complete remissions and prolonged survival in elderly Philadelphia chromosome-positive patients with acute lymphoblastic leukemia without additional chemotherapy: Results of the Gruppo Italiano Malattie Ematologiche dell'Adulto (GIMEMA) LAL0201-B protocol. *Blood, 109*(9), 3676–3678.
69. Delannoy, A., Delabesse, E., Lheriter, V., et al. (2006). Imatinib and methylprednisolone alternated with chemotherapy improve the outcome of elderly patients with Philadelphia-positive acute lymphoblastic leukemia: Results of the GRAALL AFR09 study. *Leukemia, 20*(9), 1526–1532.
70. Yanada, M., Takeuchi, J., Sugiura, I., et al. (2006). High complete remission rate and promising outcome by combination of imatinib and chemotherapy for newly diagnosed BCR-ABL-positive acute lymphoblastic leukemia: A phase II study by the Japan Adult Leukemia Study Group. *Journal of Clinical Oncology, 24*(3), 460–466.
71. Yanada, M., Sugiura, I., Takeuchi, J., et al. (2008). Prospective monitoring of BCR-ABL1 transcript levels in patients with Philadelphia chromosome-positive acute lymphoblastic leukaemia undergoing imatinib-combined chemotherapy. *British Journal Haematology, 143*(4), 503–510.
72. Lee, S., Kim, Y. J., Min, C. K., et al. (2005). The effect of first-line imatinib interim therapy on the outcome of allogeneic stem cell transplantation in adults with newly diagnosed Philadelphia chromosome-positive acute lymphoblastic leukemia. *Blood, 105*(9), 3449–3457.
73. Fielding, A. K., Richards, S. M., Lazarus, H. M., et al. (2007). Does imatinib change the outcome in Philapdelphia chromosome positive acute lymphoblastic leukaemia in adults? Data from the UKALLXII/ECOG2993 study [abstract 8]. *Blood, 110*(11), 10a.
74. Radich, J., Gehly, G., Lee, A., et al. (1997). Detection of bcr-abl transcripts in Philadelphia chromosome-positive acute lymphoblastic leukemia after marrow transplantation. *Blood, 89*(7), 2602–2609.
75. Wassmann, B., Pfeifer, H., Stadler, M., et al. (2005). Early molecular response to posttransplantation imatinib determines outcome in MRD+Philadelphia-positive acute lymphoblastic leukemia (Ph+ALL). *Blood, 106*(2), 458–463.
76. Anderlini, P., Sheth, S., Hicks, K., Ippoliti, C., Giralt, S., & Champlin, R. E. (2004). Re: Imatinib mesylate administration in the first 100 days after stem cell transplantation. *Biology of Blood and Marrow Transplantation, 10*(12), 883–884.
77. Carpenter, P. A., Snyder, D. S., Flowers, M. E., et al. (2007). Prophylactic administration of imatinib after hematopoietic cell transplantation for high-risk Philadelphia chromosome-positive leukemia. *Blood, 109*(7), 2791–2793.
78. Pfeifer, H., Wassmann, B., Pavlova, A., et al. (2007). Kinase domain mutations of BCR-ABL frequently precede imatinib-based therapy and give rise to relapse in patients with de novo Philadelphia-positive acute lymphoblastic leukemia (Ph+ALL). *Blood, 110*(2), 727–734.
79. Vignetti, M., Fazi, P., Cimino, G., et al. (2007). Imatinib plus steroids induces complete remissions and prolonged survival in elderly Philadelphia chromosome-positive acute lymphoblastic leukemia patients without additional chemotherapy: Results of the GIMEMA LAL0201-B protocol. *Blood, 109*(9), 3676–3678.
80. Gorre, M. E., Mohammed, M., Ellwood, K., et al. (2001). Clinical resistance to STI-571 cancer therapy caused by BCR-ABL gene mutation or amplification. *Science, 293*(5531), 876–880.

81. Wendel, H. G., de Stanchina, E., Cepero, E., et al. (2006). Loss of p53 impedes the antileukemic response to BCR-ABL inhibition. *Proceedings of the National Academy of Sciences of the United States of America, 103*(19), 7444–7449.

82. Iacobucci, I., Lonetti, A., Messa, F., et al. (2008). Expression of spliced oncogenic Ikaros isoforms in Philadelphia-positive acute lymphoblastic leukemia patients treated with tyrosine kinase inhibitors: Implications for a new mechanism of resistance. *Blood, 112*(9), 3847–3855.

83. Donato, N. J., Wu, J. Y., Stapley, J., et al. (2003). BCR-ABL independence and LYN kinase overexpression in chronic myelogenous leukemia cells selected for resistance to STI571. *Blood, 101*(2), 690–698.

84. Gambacorti-Passerini, C., Barni, R., le Coutre, P., et al. (2000). Role of alpha1 acid glycoprotein in the in vivo resistance of human BCR-ABL(+) leukemic cells to the abl inhibitor STI571. *Journal of the National Cancer Institute, 92*(20), 1641–1650.

85. Illmer, T., Schaich, M., Platzbecker, U., et al. (2004). P-glycoprotein-mediated drug efflux is a resistance mechanism of chronic myelogenous leukemia cells to treatment with imatinib mesylate. *Leukemia, 18*(3), 401–408.

86. Mahon, F. X., Belloc, F., Lagarde, V., et al. (2003). MDR1 gene overexpression confers resistance to imatinib mesylate in leukemia cell line models. *Blood, 101*(6), 2368–2373.

87. White, D. L., Saunders, V. A., Dang, P., et al. (2007). Most CML patients who have a suboptimal response to imatinib have low OCT-1 activity: Higher doses of imatinib may overcome the negative impact of low OCT-1 activity. *Blood, 110*(12), 4064–4072.

88. Crossman, L. C., Druker, B. J., Deininger, M. W., Pirmohamed, M., Wang, L., & Clark, R. E. (2005). hOCT 1 and resistance to imatinib. *Blood, 106*(3), 1133–1134. author reply 4.

89. Geay, J. F., Buet, D., Zhang, Y., et al. (2005). p210BCR-ABL inhibits SDF-1 chemotactic response via alteration of CXCR4 signaling and down-regulation of CXCR4 expression. *Cancer Research, 65*(7), 2676–2683.

90. Graham, S. M., Jorgensen, H. G., Allan, E., et al. (2002). Primitive, quiescent, Philadelphia-positive stem cells from patients with chronic myeloid leukemia are insensitive to STI571 in vitro. *Blood, 99*(1), 319–325.

91. Marin, D., Bazeos, A., Mahon, F. X., et al. (2010). Adherence is the critical factor for achieving molecular responses in patients with chronic myeloid leukemia who achieve complete cytogenetic responses on imatinib. *J Clin Oncol, 28*(14), 2381–2388.

92. Thomas, D. A. (2007). Philadelphia chromosome positive acute lymphocytic leukemia: A new era of challenges. *Hematology Am Soc Hematol Educ Program*, 435–443.

93. Azam, M., Latek, R. R., & Daley, G. Q. (2003). Mechanisms of autoinhibition and STI-571/imatinib resistance revealed by mutagenesis of BCR-ABL. *Cell, 112*(6), 831–843.

94. Hochhaus, A., Kreil, S., Corbin, A. S., et al. (2002). Molecular and chromosomal mechanisms of resistance to imatinib (STI571) therapy. *Leukemia, 16*(11), 2190–2196.

95. Shah, N. P., Nicoll, J. M., Nagar, B., et al. (2002). Multiple BCR-ABL kinase domain mutations confer polyclonal resistance to the tyrosine kinase inhibitor imatinib (STI571) in chronic phase and blast crisis chronic myeloid leukemia. *Cancer Cell, 2*(2), 117–125.

96. Soverini, S., Martinelli, G., Colarossi, S., et al. (2007). Second-line treatment with dasatinib in patients resistant to imatinib can select novel inhibitor-specific BCR-ABL mutants in Ph + ALL. *The Lancet Oncology, 8*(3), 273–274.

97. Golemovic, M., Verstovsek, S., Giles, F., et al. (2005). AMN107, a novel aminopyrimidine inhibitor of Bcr-Abl, has in vitro activity against imatinib-resistant chronic myeloid leukemia. *Clinical Cancer Research, 11*(13), 4941–4947.

98. Cobb, B. S., & Smale, S. T. (2005). Ikaros-family proteins: In search of molecular functions during lymphocyte development. *Current Topics in Microbiology and Immunology, 290*, 29–47.

99. Mulligan, C. G., Miller, C. B., Radtke, I., et al. (2008). BCR-ABL1 lymphoblastic leukaemia is characterized by the deletion of Ikaros. *Nature, 453*(7191), 110–114.

100. Mulligan, C. G., Su, X., Zhang, J., et al. (2009). Deletion of IKZF1 and prognosis in acute lymphoblastic leukemia. *The New England Journal of Medicine, 360*(5), 470–480.

101. Thomas, J., Wang, L., Clark, R. E., & Pirmohamed, M. (2004). Active transport of imatinib into and out of cells: Implications for drug resistance. *Blood, 104*(12), 3739–3745.

102. Hu, Y., Liu, Y., Pelletier, S., et al. (2004). Requirement of Src kinases Lyn, Hck and Fgr for BCR-ABL1-induced B-lymphoblastic leukemia but not chronic myeloid leukemia. *Nature Genetics, 36*(5), 453–461.

103. Hu, Y., Swerdlow, S., Duffy, T. M., Weinmann, R., Lee, F. Y., & Li, S. (2006). Targeting multiple kinase pathways in leukemic progenitors and stem cells is essential for improved treatment of Ph + leukemia in mice. *Proceedings of the National Academy of Sciences of the United States of America, 103*(45), 16870–16875.

104. Shah, N. P., Tran, C., Lee, F. Y., Chen, P., Norris, D., & Sawyers, C. L. (2004). Overriding imatinib resistance with a novel ABL kinase inhibitor. *Science, 305*(5682), 399–401.

105. Giannoudis, A., Davies, A., Lucas, C. M., Harris, R. J., Pirmohamed, M., & Clark, R. E. (2008). Effective dasatinib uptake may occur without human organic cation transporter 1 (hOCT1): Implications for the treatment of imatinib-resistant chronic myeloid leukemia. *Blood, 112*(8), 3348–3354.

106. Hiwase, D. K., Saunders, V., Hewett, D., et al. (2008). Dasatinib cellular uptake and efflux in chronic myeloid leukemia cells: Therapeutic implications. *Clinical Cancer Research, 14*(12), 3881–3888.

107. Ottmann, O., Dombret, H., Martinelli, G., et al. (2007). Dasatinib induces rapid hematologic and cytogenetic responses in adult patients with Philadelphia chromosome positive acute lymphoblastic leukemia with resistance or intolerance to imatinib: Interim results of a phase 2 study. *Blood, 110*(7), 2309–2315.

108. Jabbour, E., O'Brien, S., Thomas, D. A., et al. (2008). Combination of the hyper-CVAD regimen with dasatinib is effective in patients with relapsed Philadelphia chromosome (Ph) positive acute lymphoblastic leukemia (ALL) and lymphoid blast phase chronic meyloid leukemia (CML-LB) [abstract 2919]. *Blood, 112*(11), 1004.

109. Ravandi, F., O'Brien, S., Thomas, D., et al. First report of phase II study of dasatinib with hyperCVAD for the frontline treatment of patients with Philadelphia chromosome positive (Ph+) acute lymphoblastic leukemia. *Blood*; E-published.

110. Rousselot, P., Cayuela, J.-M., Recher, C., et al. (2008). Dasatinib (Sprycel®) and chemotherapy for first-line treatment in elderly patients with de novo Philadelphia positive ALL: Results of the first 22 patients included in the EWALL-Ph-01 trial (on behalf of the European Working Group on Adult ALL (EWALL)) [abstract 2920]. *Blood, 112*(11), 1004.

111. Foà, R., Vitale, A., Guarini, A., et al. (2008). Line treatment of adult Ph+ acute lymphoblastic leukemia (ALL) patients. Final results of the GIMEMA LAL1205 study [abstract 305]. *Blood, 112*(11), 305.

112. Talpaz, M., Shah, N. P., Kantarjian, H., et al. (2006). Dasatinib in imatinib-resistant Philadelphia chromosome-positive leukemias. *The New England Journal of Medicine, 354*(24), 2531–2541.

113. Coutre, S. G. M., Dombret, H., et al. (2006). Dasatinib (D) in patients (pts) with chronic myelogenous leukemia (CML) in lymphoid blast crisis (LB-CML) or Philadelphia-chromosome positive acute lymphoblastic leukemia (Ph+ALL) who are imatinib (IM)-resistant (IM-R) or intolerant (IM-I): The CA180015 "START-L" study [abstract 6528]. *Journal of Clinical Oncology, 24*, 344s.

114. Larson, R. A., Ottmann, O. G., Shah, N. P., et al. (2008). Dasatinib 140 mg once daily (QD) has equivalent efficacy and improved safety compared with 70 mg twice daily (BID) in patients with imatinib-resistant or -intolerant Philadelphia chromosome-positive acute lymphoblastic leukemia (Ph+ALL): 2-Year data from CA180-035 [abstract 2926]. *Blood, 112*(11), 1006.

115. Porkka, K., Koskenvesa, P., Lundan, T., et al. (2008). Dasatinib crosses the blood-brain barrier and is an efficient therapy for central nervous system Philadelphia chromosome-positive leukemia. *Blood, 112*(4), 1005–1012.

116. Thomas, D. A., Kantarjian, H. M., Faderl, S., et al. (2009). Chemoimmunotherapy with a modified hyper-CVAD and rituximab regimen improves outcome for patients with de novo Philadelphia negative precursor B-Cell acute lymphoblastic leukemia (ALL) [abstract 836]. *Blood, 114*(22), 344.

117. Jabbour, E., Cortes, J., Giles, F., O'Brien, S., & Kantarijan, H. (2007). Drug evaluation: Nilotinib – A novel Bcr-Abl tyrosine kinase inhibitor for the treatment of chronic myelocytic leukemia and beyond. *IDrugs, 10*(7), 468–479.

118. O'Hare, T., Walters, D. K., Stoffregen, E. P., et al. (2005). In vitro activity of Bcr-Abl inhibitors AMN107 and BMS-354825 against clinically relevant imatinib-resistant Abl kinase domain mutants. *Cancer Research, 65*(11), 4500–4505.

119. Weisberg, E., Manley, P. W., Breitenstein, W., et al. (2005). Characterization of AMN107, a selective inhibitor of native and mutant Bcr-Abl. *Cancer Cell, 7*(2), 129–141.

120. Kantarjian, H., Giles, F., Wunderle, L., et al. (2006). Nilotinib in imatinib-resistant CML and Philadelphia chromosome-positive ALL. *The New England Journal of Medicine, 354*(24), 2542–2551.

121. Cortes, J., Kantarjian, H. M., Baccarani, M., et al. (2006). A phase 1/2 study of SKI-606, a dual inhibitor of Src and Abl kinases, in adult patients with Philadelphia chromosome positive (Ph) chronic myelogenous leukemia (CML) or acute lymphocytic leukemia (ALL) relapsed, refractory or intolerant of imatinib [abstract 168]. *Blood, 108*(11), 54a.

122. Gambacorti-Passerini, C., Brummendorf, T., Kantarjian, H., et al. (2007). Bosutinib (SKI-606) exhibits clinical activity in patients with Philadelphia chromosome positive CML or ALL who failed imatinib [abstract 7006]. *Proceedings of the American Society of Clinical Oncology, 25*, 18S.

123. Kimura, S., Naito, H., Segawa, H., et al. (2005). NS-187, a potent and selective dual Bcr-Abl/Lyn tyrosine kinase inhibitor, is a novel agent for imatinib-resistant leukemia. *Blood, 106*(12), 3948–3954.

124. O'Hare, T., Pollock, R., Stoffregen, E. P., et al. (2004). Inhibition of wild-type and mutant Bcr-Abl by AP23464, a potent ATP-based oncogenic protein kinase inhibitor: Implications for CML. *Blood, 104*(8), 2532–2539.

125. Swords, R., Alvarado, Y., & Giles, F. (2007). Novel Abl kinase inhibitors in chronic myeloid leukemia in blastic phase and Philadelphia chromosome-positive acute lymphoblastic leukemia. *Clinical Lymphoma & Myeloma, 7*(Suppl 3), S113–S119.

126. Weisberg, E., Catley, L., Wright, R. D., et al. (2007). Beneficial effects of combining nilotinib and imatinib in preclinical models of BCR-ABL+leukemias. *Blood, 109*(5), 2112–2120.

127. O'Hare, T., Walters, D. K., Stoffregen, E. P., et al. (2005). Combined Abl inhibitor therapy for minimizing drug resistance in chronic myeloid leukemia: Src/Abl inhibitors are compatible with imatinib. *Clinical Cancer Research, 11*(19 Pt 1), 6987–6993.

128. Thomas, D. A., O'Brien, S., Jorgensen, J. L., et al. (2009). Prognostic significance of CD20 expression in adults with de novo precursor B-lineage acute lymphoblastic leukemia. *Blood, 113*(25), 6330–6337.
129. Maury, S., Huguet, F., Leguay, T., et al. (2010). Adverse prognostic significance of CD20 expression in adults with Philadelphia chromosome-negative B-cell precursor acute lymphoblastic leukemia. *Haematologica, 95*(2), 324–328.
130. Paietta, E., Li, X., Richards, S., et al. (2008). Implications for the use of monoclonal antibodies in future adult ALL trials: Analysis of antigen expression in 505 B-Lineage (B-Lin) ALL patients (pts) on the MRC UKALLXII/ECOG2993 Intergroup trial [abstract 1907]. *Blood, 112*(11), 666.
131. Santos, F. P. S., O'Brien, S., Thomas, D. A., et al. (2009). Prognostic impact of CD20 and CD25 expression in patients with Philadelphia-positive (Ph+) acute lymphoblastic leukemia (ALL) [abstract 984]. *Blood, 114*(22), 408.
132. Riva, G., Luppi, M., Barozzi, P., et al. (2010). Emergence of BCR-ABL-specific cytotoxic T cells in the bone marrow of patients with Ph + acute lymphoblastic leukemia during long-term imatinib mesylate treatment. *Blood, 115*(8), 1512–1518.
133. Mustjoki, S., Ekblom, M., Arstila, T. P., et al. (2009). Clonal expansion of T/NK-cells during tyrosine kinase inhibitor dasatinib therapy. *Leukemia, 23*(8), 1398–1405.
134. Stock, W., Sanford, B., Lozanski, G., et al. (2009). Alemtuzumab can be incorporated Into front-line therapy of adult acute lymphoblastic leukemia (ALL): Final phase I results of a Cancer and Leukemia Group B Study (CALGB 10102) [abstract 838]. *Blood, 114*(22), 345.

Chapter 16
Molecular Therapies

Camille N. Abboud

Introduction

Unfortunately the advances made in the management of pediatric acute lymphoblastic leukemia (ALL) have not been matched in adult ALL. Only 30–40% of adult patients with ALL will achieve long-term disease-free survival with current agents and regimens, despite very high (~90%) initial complete response (CR) rates [1, 2]. Most patients will relapse within 12–24 months of their initial CR; many relapse while they are still receiving maintenance therapy [1, 3, 4]. Salvage regimens offer CR rates of ~30% or higher, but disease-free intervals are brief [5]. Five year overall survival following relapse is a dismal ~7% with currently available strategies [6]. Though allogeneic stem cell transplantation improves long term survival, graft-versus-leukemia effects are relatively modest [1–3]. This is illustrated by two lines of evidence: (1) a report from the International Bone Marrow Transplant Registry, which found similar relapse rates in matched sibling and syngeneic transplants and (2) reports detailing the lack of efficacy of donor lymphocyte infusions for relapsed ALL after allogeneic transplantation [2, 4]. There is clearly a need for novel agents and combinations of agents in the management of adult ALL across all phases of disease.

Despite this need, very few new agents have been introduced in the past decade for the management of adult ALL [5]. The development of new drugs has been hindered by the rarity of ALL and the complexity of existing treatment algorithms. Encouragingly, targeted therapies have already yielded dramatic success stories in ALL. Imatinib has improved response rates and disease-free survival through targeted inhibition of the ABL-kinase in Philadelphia chromosome positive ALL [7, 8]. And unlike normal myeloid precursors, ALL blasts lack asparagine synthetase and are dependent on exogenous asparagine. L-asparaginase enzymatically depletes asparagine. This addition to ALL regimens has lead to improvements in clinical outcomes [5]. But given the molecular and genetic heterogeneity of ALL, it is unlikely that a single agent will produce durable remissions or cures in a majority of patients. Targeted therapies are likely to follow the therapeutic model of imatinib, which has profoundly impacted the management of Philadelphia chromosome positive ALL, but must be given in conjunction with other therapies to prevent rapid disease relapse [7, 9]. This chapter will explore novel genetic, molecular, and immunologic targets in ALL and discuss early clinical results when available. We anticipate that maximum clinical impact from targeted therapeutics will occur when they are combined with multiple active agents to manipulate diverse pathways. In our conclusions, we will propose rational ways to incorporate some of these agents into existing treatment schemes.

C.N. Abboud (✉)
Section of Leukemia and Bone Marrow Transplantation, Division of Oncology, Washington University in Saint Louis, 660 South Euclid, Saint Louis, MO, USA 63110
e-mail: CABBOUD@im.wustl.edu

A.S. Advani and H.M. Lazarus (eds.), *Adult Acute Lymphocytic Leukemia*, Contemporary Hematology,
DOI 10.1007/978-1-60761-707-5_16, © Springer Science+Business Media, LLC 2011

Epigenetic Therapy

Chromosomal abnormalities are common in ALL. These abnormalities are diverse, occurring as balanced and unbalanced translocations, deletions, duplications, inversions, and numerical abnormalities of either single or multiple chromosomes [10]. Some examples of common karotypic changes and their frequencies in adult ALL include t(9;22) (11–34%), t(4;11) (3–7%), del(9p) (5–15%), hyperdiploidy (defined as >50 chromosomes) (2–9%) and hypodiploidy (defined as <46 chromosomes) (4–9%) [11–14]. Trisomy 8 and monosomy 7 are often associated with t(9;22) [15, 16]. Higher resolution platforms such as high-resolution array comparative genomic hybridization (aCGH) reveal even greater heterogeneity in ALL chromosomes. When combined with conventional cytogenetics, aCGH increases the yield of abnormalities found from 52 to 94% of patients [17]. These physical, irreversible changes in the DNA contribute to disease by either creating new fusion genes or dysregulation of intact genes [18, 19].

Though helpful in defining prognosis and identifying some genes involved in leukemogenesis, cytogenetic changes fall short of explaining the diverse changes in mRNA expression seen in ALL with gene expression profiling [20, 21]. Dysregulation of microRNA and epigenetic changes in promoter methylation and histone acetylation are likely to contribute to the aberrant activation and silencing of genes in ALL [22]. Epigenetic changes, unlike most chromosomal abnormalities, may be reversible. Both hypomethylating agents and histone deacetylase inhibitors are in clinical development in ALL and other diseases.

Methylation

DNA methylation occurs only at cytosine bases that are located 5′ to guanosine. These di-nucleotide pairs are clustered within the human genome in the promoter regions of about half of the genes in so-called *CpG islands* (CGIs) [23–25]. The majority of these CGIs are unmethylated in normal tissues. CGI methylation is observed in normal physiologic processes including X-chromosome inactivation, genetic imprinting and tissue-specific regulation of gene expression [26]. Methylation is conserved in daughter cells [27]. Aberrant promoter hypermethylation has also been widely described in human malignancies and is associated with the silencing of the downstream gene.

Clinical experience with hypomethylating agents has rapidly expanded in the last 5 years. Decitabine and azacitidine have both been approved for the treatment of myelodysplastic syndrome [28]. The former has also shown significant activity in elderly patients with acute myeloid leukemia [29–31]. The latter has been able to extend survival in high-risk MDS patients and induce global hypomethylation in responding patients [32, 33].

Initial studies in ALL suggest that methylation status varies with age and lineage. Older ALL patients have a higher number of methylated loci and more frequent methylation of members of the p53 cascade [34]. Similarly, there is differential methylation of several loci (*SYK-1, ASPP-1, sFRP-2, sFRP-5,* and *WIF-1*) between T- and B-ALL as well as the total number of methylated loci in hand curated lists [35]. However, most methylation studies published in ALL have limited their focus to the methylation status of one, or just a handful of genes, resulting in potentially significant bias [36–49]. Nevertheless, methylation changes appear to be a common phenomenon in ALL with 70–90% of cases demonstrating hypermethylation at one cancer-related loci, and 25–40% demonstrating 3 or more hypermethylated loci [34, 35, 40, 42, 50–52]. Potential targets of leukemogenic methylation changes include: CALCA, *ER, MDR1 p15, p57,* and *p21.* Several of these genes are involved in the p53 pathway, which though commonly mutated in human malignancies, is rarely mutated in ALL [41–49, 53]. These methylation changes appear to be specific to the malignant lymphocytes in ALL, as normal tissues from ALL patients and lymphocytes from healthy controls lack hypermethylation at these loci [52]. Recently, unbiased platforms to investigate genome-wide methylation have been developed (e.g., the Illumnia human methylation array 27). Such platforms allow the user to look across the methylome and investigate changes in over 27,000 well-annotated loci. When coupled with mRNA profiling this technology may allow for an unbiased survey of the methylome in ALL and help to identify novel genes and pathways whose altered expression contribute to disease progression, drug-resistance, and the maintenance of minimal residual disease. Results from such unbiased platforms will be critical to confirm previous findings and to contextualize the ALL specific methylome in relationship to ALL pathophysiology.

To help understand what contribution the methylation pattern of various genes may have on ALL, Roman-Gomez interrogated the methylation status of 15 genes chosen based on a literature search in 251 patients with ALL [34]. Methylation did not correlate with clinical variables or complete remission rates. The authors did find that increased methylation at these loci correlated with a significant decrease in both disease-free and overall survival. A genome-wide methylation study was conducted by the investigators at M.D. Anderson Cancer Center [54]. Using a novel amplification and array approach they identified over 400 potential targets that were evenly distributed across the autosomes. These genes clustered in 18 molecular pathways. A subset of these genes were then validated as being methylated in ALL cell lines and primary patient samples. The authors were able to manipulate the expression of these genes with hypomethylating agents. Although there was no overlap between their 15 validated genes and those described by Roman-Gomez, they too observed worse overall survival in patients with increased CpG island methylation.

Given the discrepancy between separate studies, methylation-dependent pathways have yet to yield clear targets for ALL therapy. However, increasing levels of promoter methylation have been consistently associated with an inferior prognosis. In addition in vitro, hypomethylating agents may be able to alter gene expression in ALL. Preclinical data suggests that hypomethylating agents may sensitize other leukemias to treatments such as ATRA [55–57]. Hypomethylating agents are currently being incorporated in the management of AML in the maintenance setting after autologous stem cell transplantation [58]. Therefore, it may be reasonable to incorporate them into ALL regimens in a similar fashion.

Histone Acetylation

The acetylation of histones adds another layer of complexity to the regulation of transcription. Acetylation neutralizes the charge of the lysine residues and allows the nucleosome to unfold and expose the associated DNA. This physical change in the DNA structure alters gene expression by allowing RNA-polymerases to access the DNA. Low levels of acetylation, and hence condensation of the DNA complex, are generally associated with transcriptional silencing [59–63]. Like many biologic processes, the acetylation status of a particular lysine residue is the result of the balance of two opposing enzymes: histone acetyltransferases (HAT) and histone deacetylases (HDACs). Acetylation is clearly altered in several human malignancies and patients with inherited syndromes altering their capacity to acetylate or deacetylate are associated with an increased risk of cancer [64–69].

Like hypermethylation, oncogenic acetylation changes are potentially sensitive to small molecule therapy. Clinical studies with HDAC inhibitors are ongoing in many solid and hematologic malignancies and one, vorinostat, has been FDA approved for the treatment of relapsed cutaneous T-cell lymphoma [70, 71].

Several HDAC inhibitors are in preclinical and early clinical development in ALL. Romanski et al. treated four different PR-B ALL cell lines with HDAC inhibitors [72].

Using LAQ824, which inhibits histone H3 and H4 deacetylation, thus inducing hyperacetylation, they were able to inhibit the proliferation of the cells and increase apoptosis in both caspase-dependent and caspase-independent manners [73]. They also showed that LAQ824 decreased the expression of the anti-apoptotic gene Bcl-2 and disrupted the mitochondrial membrane potential. In a similar fashion, LBH589 was evaluated by Scuto et al. in two Philadelphia-chromosome-negative human ALL cell lines [74]. They were again able to show that the HDAC inhibitor was able to induce cell-cycle arrest, apoptosis, and histone hyperacetylation. In addition, changes in acetylation lead to the increase in mRNA expression of several genes that are pro-apoptotic and involved in DNA damage repair: *FANCG*, *FOXO3A*, *GADD45A*, *GADD45B*, and *GADD45G*, by up to a 45-fold induction.

Hypomethylating agents and HDAC inhibitors alter gene expression through separate mechanisms, raising the possibility of synergy by combining therapies [75]. Preclinical evidence suggests that combination therapy with a hypomethylating agent and an HDAC inhibitor enhances the antineoplastic action of each [76].

There is compelling evidence for the inclusion of epigenetic modifying agents in the treatment of ALL. This class of therapeutics is generally well tolerated and targets pathways unrelated to traditional chemotherapeutics. A major challenge will be rationally designing clinical trials that incorporate these agents with combination chemotherapy to achieve maximum benefit.

Molecular Targets

Mammalian Target of Rapamycin (mTOR)

Signaling through the mammalian target of rapamycin (mTOR) pathway is complex [77]. Depending on the stimuli the mTOR catalytic subunit can form a heterotrimeric protein kinase with mLST8 and either raptor (mTORC1) or rictor (mTORC2) [78]. When stimulated by nutrients or growth factors, mTOR will form mTORC1, which contributes to the cellular regulation of protein synthesis, ribosome biogenesis and autophagy. Through these pathways mTORC1 regulates cellular *growth* (in contrast to regulating cellular division). mTORC1 also may either stimulate or suppress PI3K-Akt signaling. The role of mTORC2 has been less well elucidated but it also appears to be involved in signaling through the PI3K-Akt pathway and regulation of the cytoskeleton [79–81]. Furthermore, mTORC1 and 2 interact with various other pathways implicated in malignant pathogenesis. mTORC1 positivity regulates cyclin D1 transcription and translation in many cancer cells, including mantle cell lymphoma (MCL) [82–84]. However, some evidence suggests that the observed activity of mTOR inhibitors in MCL is due to the inhibition of Akt rather than cyclin D1 [85]. Inhibiting both mTORC1 and mTORC2 leads to the inhibition of the translation of and the activation of HIF1-alpha (hypoxia-induced factor 1-alpha) and consequently the down-regulation of VEGF production [86–88]. This molecular avenue has been therapeutically exploited in the management of renal cell cancer with the mTOR inhibitor temsirolimus [89]. Due to the above described pleotropic effects of mTOR signaling on vital cellular functions, preclinical and clinical investigators have taken an interest in studying mTOR in ALL.

Preclinical investigations of mTOR inhibitors in ALL have been conducted along several lines. B-cell development is tightly regulated by a host of factors and disruption of various pathways, alone or in combination, may lead to malignant transformation. Rapamycin (the prototypic mTOR inhibitor) inhibits the growth of precursor B-ALL cell lines in vitro and induces apoptotic cell death. The cell lines are rescued by exogenous IL-7. Furthermore a murine model of pre-B leukemia/lymphoma showed extended survival when treated with rapamycin [90]. Another group performed similar experiments in Pre-B ALL with a novel mTOR inhibitor (CCI-779) and found similar antileukemic activity in both cell lines and xenograft models [91].

Aside from the direct anti-leukemic effects of mTOR inhibitors, they may also syngerize with other agents already employed in the management of ALL. High expression of dihydrofolate reductase (DHFR) in ALL blasts correlates with methotrexate resistance [92, 93]. Cyclin D1 is involved in DHFR synthesis [94]. mTOR inhibitors increase the degradation of cyclin D1. Following this line of logic, Teachey et al. tested the combination of an mTOR inhibitor and methotrexate in ALL cell lines and xenotransplant models [95]. They were able to demonstrate a synergism between mTOR inhibition and methotrexate, providing a strong rationale for taking this combination into the clinic.

Furthermore, mTOR signaling is involved in the angiogenic phenotype, which is common to most bone marrow malignancies [96, 97]. Blocking mTOR decreases bone marrow endothelial responses to growth factors and mitogenic stimuli. When combined with an inhibitor of NF-kappa B, mTOR inhibitors synergize to significantly abrogate proliferative responses in bone marrow endothelial cells [98]. By rationally combining agents with strong preclinical data into relatively complex regimens, effective regimens may be composed. One may envision a salvage regimen of high-dose methotrexate combined with sirolimus (an mTOR inhibitor) and bortezomib (an NF-kappa B inhibitor). A regimen such as this may be particularly useful for T-cell ALL as discussed below in the section on Notch signaling.

Angiogenesis

Angiogenesis is normally tightly regulated and only occurs in adults during wound healing, menstruation, and tissue repair [99]. Over 20 agents have been identified, which modulate angiogenesis. The balance of pro- and anti-angiogenic signals determines the process of neovascularization [100]. Of these agents, vascular endothelial growth factor (VEGF) and basic fibroblast growth factor (BFGF) are the two most potent positive regulators of angiogenesis [101–103]. The VEGF family is composed of seven ligands, VEGF-A thru –F and placenta growth factor, and three receptors, VEGFR-1 thru 3. This system plays a crucial role in the arborization of capillaries as well as promotes endothelial cell survival, proliferation, and migration. It also modulates vascular permeability and the expression of adhesion molecules on the surface of endothelial cells [104, 105]. These growth factors may also behave in an auto- or paracrine fashion in the bone marrow microenvironment and may stimulate receptors on both normal and malignant blasts, promoting survival and proliferation [106–108].

There have been conflicting reports regarding the significance of the VEGF pathways in ALL. Stachel et al. reported that children with Pre-B ALL with higher levels of pretreatment VEGF mRNA were more prone to late relapses ($p = 0.043$) [109]. Others have shown that VEGF-A levels at the end of induction chemotherapy for standard-risk ALL predict 6-year event free survival [110]. Another group reported that the expression of VEGFR1 and/or -2 on blasts in adults with ALL predicted shorter survival while increased expression of the ligand was found to predict longer survival [111]. A further study showed an increase in bone marrow microvascular density and urinary BFGF in newly diagnosed children with ALL compared to controls, but others have failed to confirm this observation [96, 112, 113]. Taken in sum, this data likely reflects the heterogeneity of ALL.

Unlike in AML where both VEGF monoclonal antibodies and tyrosine kinase inhibitors are being tested, there are currently no trials testing the anti-angiogenic agents in ALL [114]. Trials incorporating these agents will have to be well designed and take into account the ambiguity described above, while prospectively defining biologic predictors of response.

Hedgehog Signaling

Similar to the relationship described above between the inhibition of mTOR signaling and methotrexate sensitization, the Hedgehog (Hh) signaling system may be involved in the resistance of ALL cells to glucocorticoids. Hh signaling programs are involved in cellular proliferation, differentiation, survival and growth in embryonic development [115]. There are three isoforms of Hh in humans: Sonic, Indian, and Desert, of which Sonic has been the most extensively studied. Hh pathways modulate the transcription factors of the Gli family. Gli is normally only active in precursor cells, making this pathway an attractive therapeutic target [116–118]. Inappropriate activation of Hh has been implicated in the development of several malignancies including the brain, muscle, and skin [119, 120].

Interestingly, members of the Sonic Hh signaling pathway are involved in thymocyte development and contribute to the differentiation from double-negative to double-positive T-cells [121]. Transcripts for Sonic Hh and its downstream effectors, Patched and Smoothed, have been demonstrated in primitive and mature CD19+, CD33+, and CD3+ populations [122, 123]. Sonic Hh also can induce the anti-apoptotic protein Bcl-2 [124]. In vitro experiments with human T-ALL cell lines have shown that Sonic Hh activity is inversely correlated with glucocorticoid sensitivity and that blocking Sonic Hh signaling pathways leads to cell cycle arrest and apoptosis [125]. Therefore, combining Sonic Hh inhibition with glucocorticoid therapy may improve glucocorticoid-induced cell cycle arrest via synergistic Bcl-2 induction. Hh antagonists such as GDC-0449 are in early phase clinical trials [114, 126].

This discussion is not meant to imply that the Sonic Hh pathway is the principle cause of glucocorticoid resistance in ALL, but to suggest that this pathway may contribute to leukemogenesis and that due to the restriction of Sonic Hh activity to malignant and embryonic tissues, these pathways may contain "druggable" targets with limited off-target effects. We refer the interested reader to Tissing's excellent review of glucocorticoid resistance in ALL for a more complete discussion of this issue [127].

Survivin

Survivin is involved in multiple pathways in cellular homeostasis including cell division, apoptotic, and nonapoptotic cell death and acts as a stress-response factor ensuring ongoing proliferation and survival in the face of environmental stressors [128]. Survivin is a member of the inhibitor of apoptosis family (IAP) and is known to interact with cyclin-dependent kinase 1, Aurora kinase B and protein kinase A. The activation of the NF-kappa-B pathway increases the transcription of survivin [129]. Physiologically, it is expressed at low levels during mitosis and is undetectable in most adult tissues. In contrast, it is over-expressed in most human cancers with clearly aberrant expression during interphase. Similar to Sonic Hh, this specificity implies that the pathway may be antagonized with a relatively wide therapeutic window. Mice with survivin conditionally knocked out in thymocytes display impaired cellular proliferation, cell cycle arrest, mitotic spindle defects, and apoptosis. Hematopoietic-specific survivin deletion leads to bone-marrow ablation with a loss of progenitors and erythropoiesis defects [130–132]. Given its essential role in cellular housekeeping functions and aberrant expression in malignancies, survivin is an attractive target for novel therapeutics.

Survivin is consistently over-expressed in adult T-cell leukemia (90% of tested samples) and in T-ALL cell lines. Increased expression of survivin transcripts predicts shorter patient survival in adult T-ALL [133, 134]. Similarly, survivin has been found to be over-expressed in ~65% of pediatric precursor B-cell ALL. Survivin expression was not found to be associated with any established risk factors but was prognostic of 3-year relapse-free, event-free, and overall survival [135]. This is a very similar pattern to what is seen with methylation and implies that both represent novel aspects of ALL biology.

Sodium arsenite has been shown to decrease both survivin mRNA and protein levels in patient samples of adult T-ALL and induce apoptosis and inhibit cell growth [129]. Early clinical studies with the survivin inhibitor terameprocol (EM-1421) in leukemias, including ALL, are underway [114, 136].

NOTCH1 Signaling

NOTCH1 came to attention in T-ALL as the partner gene in the t(7;9) translocation [137]. Though rare, the translocation is found in <1% of T-ALLs; it inspired interest since it encodes a transmembrane receptor that is involved in determining T-cell fate [138]. After ligation and heterodimerization the intracellular segment of NOTCH is cleaved by gamma-secretase and translocates into the nucleus where it forms a transcription factor complex which includes members of the Mastermind family [139–142]. Following up on this observation, investigators found that gamma-secretase inhibitors (GSI) induced cell cycle arrest in some T-ALL cell lines and that over 50% of children and adolescents with T-ALL have at least one somatic mutation in *NOTCH1*. No B-ALL ($n = 89$) patient samples were found to have *NOTCH1* mutations [143]. Animal models have subsequently shown that forced intracellular expression of Notch1 and 3 are sufficient to produce a short latency, aggressive T-cell leukemia [144–146].

Fortunately, GSI have already been developed as potential drugs for Alzheimer's disease, and have been rapidly assessed in preclinical models of T-ALL [147]. In vitro studies have shown that GSIs can induce cell cycle arrest in a proportion of T-ALL cell lines after several days and apoptosis after 14 days of incubation [143]. Although encouraging, these results are not akin to the successes seen with imatinib in BCR-ABL-dependent leukemia. The modest activity of GSIs questions the level of dependence of T-ALL cell lines and primary leukemias on NOTCH signaling. The mutations may be involved in early T-ALL leukemogenesis, but their relevance is diminished with progression of disease. Following up of these results, others have studied GSIs in combination with dexamethasone and vincristine in T-ALL cell cultures. De Keersmaecker et al. were able to demonstrate synergy between dexamethasone and GSIs but not between GSIs and vincristine [148]. In addition to combining GSIs with traditional chemotherapy, investigators have dissected downstream pathways in NOTCH signaling that may lend themselves to novel combination therapies.

Notch1 induces transcription of several members of the NF-kappaB pathway. Investigators found that pharmacologic inhibition of NF-kappaB induced apoptosis in Notch1-dependent human T-ALL cell lines. They followed up this observation with mouse bone marrow transplant experiments in which intracellular Notch1 was overexpressed in a genetic background of attenuated NF-kappaB signaling. This weakening of NF-kappa B leads to an increased latency and reduced severity of disease [149]. These studies suggest a role for the combined use of GSI and NF-kappaB inhibitors in the management of NOTCH1 mutated T-ALL. A follow-up phase I Children's Oncology Group study found little activity of single agent bortezomib in pediatric refractory ALL, though all cases were of the pre-B phenotype [150]. Interestingly Avellino et al. reported significant activity with rapamycin, citing its ability to inhibit both mTOR and NF-kappaB signaling, in the majority of primary ALL samples, including 7 out of 10 T-lineage samples and 7 out of 15 B-lineage samples [151]. Rapamycin also increased the anthracyclines induced apoptosis in ALL (cells are normally rescued by NF-kappaB-dependent mechanisms). These results may help explain the synergy seen between pegylated liposomal doxorubicin and bortezomib in multiple myeloma [152].

Chan et al. have also shown that the mTOR pathway is a direct target of Notch signaling in T-cell ALL [149]. In follow-up experiments to this proteomic observation, they demonstrated that the combination of GSIs, an mTOR inhibitor, and NF-kappaB inhibitor was highly synergistic against T-cell ALL cell lines. These results argue for aggressive, novel combination regimens in T-cell ALL with both new and old drugs.

Toll-like Receptor Signaling

Despite the relatively modest graft-versus-leukemia effects and a failure of donor lymphocyte infusions to generate a robust graft-versus-leukemia effect, allogeneic stem cell transplantations have repetitively demonstrated superiority to chemotherapy or autologous transplantations in high risk patients [3, 153, 154]. Interestingly, outcomes in ALL after allogeneic transplantation correlate with the degree of graft-versus-host disease [155, 156]. A major focus of transplantation research continues to be aimed at attempting to unravel the GVL and GVHD effects of allogeneic transplantation. Unfortunately, attempts to augment the host response to ALL cells without the use of stem cell transplantation (e.g., interferon) have been unsuccessful [157].

Toll-like receptors (TLRs) may offer a novel avenue to modulate the immune system. TLRs are evolutionarily conserved transmembrane proteins that act as members of the innate immune system. TLRs are expressed on antigen-presenting cells. To date, 10 members of the TLR family have been described. The extracellular domain of the TLRs recognize conserved elements on infectious agents and stimulate the innate immunity as well as provide co-stimulatory molecules that promote strong T-helper type 1 responses [158]. In early preclinical work, investigators have demonstrated that ligation of TLR2 and 9 leads to increased allogeneic T-cell activation by ALL cells [159]. These results, though, remain relatively immature and will require further vetting before moving TLR agonists forward in clinical trials of ALL. But the early results are intriguing and they may eventually find application in augmentation of donor lymphocyte infusions in ALL. As TLR small molecule therapy has already been developed, and is currently being tested in other malignancies, opportunities exist to rapidly assess their activity in ALL [160].

Other Pathways and Targets

Traditional medicinal-chemistry approaches have been yielding important results. Recent advances in nucleoside purine analogues have lead to the FDA approval of nelarabine and clofarabine for relapsed and refractory disease [161–163]. The pipeline of nucleoside analogues (e.g., forodesine, troxacitabine, sapacitabine, CP-4055, 3′-C-ethynylcytidine, and 5-azapyrimidines) is currently rich and likely to yield important results [162]. Integration of these new chemotherapeutics with novel targeted therapies and older, complex drugs regiments will be an important future endeavor.

Other pathways, agents, and targets have also been studied recently in ALL. Much of the human data for these agents come from phase I trials in mixed populations of advanced AML and ALL. Similar to the pathways previously discussed, therapeutic blockade of any of these targets, will likely be most beneficial when combined with cytotoxic chemotherapy or other targeted agents. In addition to some patients with AML, adults with ALL and the t(4;11) translocation may overexpress the FLT-3 kinase [164]. There is some preclinical evidence to support FLT-3 inhibition in ALL, though single-agent inhibition of FLT-3 has demonstrated little activity in AML [165]. Flavopiridol is a cyclin-dependent kinase inhibitor that has shown modest single-agent activity in ALL (12.5%) [166]. Similarly, heat-shock protein antagonists and BCL2 targeted therapy have been explored [167, 168].

The role of the microenvironment is being actively explored in multiple hematological malignancies; this may ultimately prove important in ALL pathophysiology and therapy [169–172].

Monoclonal Antibodies

The phenomenal success of rituximab therapy in the treatment of non-Hodgkin's lymphomas has led to exploration of monoclonal antibody (Mab) therapy in a variety of hematologic malignancies, including ALL. At present, multiple monoclonal antibodies have been developed (often for the treatment of other diseases) and applied to ALL therapy. Antigens targeted by these Mabs include CD19, CD20, CD22, CD33, and CD52 [173]. Each of these cell surface proteins is expressed in only a subset of ALL; a result of fluctuation in antigen expression during normal T- and B-cell development and differentiation. Mabs activate various pathways leading to targeted cell death including: antibody-dependent cell-mediated cytotoxicity via interaction with phagocyte Fc receptors; compliment activation leading to activation of the MAC complex; and dimerization of transmembrane proteins leading to intracellular signaling and apoptosis. Individual Mabs may activate multiple pathways simultaneous, or only a single pathway. In addition, Mabs may be conjugated to a toxin (e.g., gemtuzumab ozogamicin) or a radioactive isotope (e.g., Bexxar: I [131]-tositumomab; Zevalin: (90)Yttrium-iritumomab tiuxetan), thus increasing the spectrum of clinically useful mechanisms leading to Mab directed cell death.

CD20 is the target of multiple clinically important monoclonal antibodies including rituximab, tositumomab, and ibritumomab tiuxetan. In addition, a litany of new anti-CD20 Mabs are in development, each with a subtle theoretical improvement over rituximab, including recognition of novel CD20 peri-membrane epitopes, which may increase complement activation, and complete antibody humanization [173]. CD20 is expressed predominantly in pre-B and mature B cells, with low expression in lymphoblasts and CD34+ cells, limiting the probable efficacy of anti-CD20 Mabs to precursor B-cell ALL, Burkitt's, CLL, and other non-Hodgkin's B-cell lymphomas (NHL). Clinical experience treating ALL with anti-CD20 Mabs has been limited to Burkitt's lymphoma and Burkitt-like B-ALL. In a phase II clinical trial, Thomas et al. found that rituximab did not increase toxicity when combined with Hyper-CVAD [174]. Within this cohort, the 14 patients with Burkitt-like B-ALL had a 3-year overall survival of 77%, an improvement over their historical controls. This study is encouraging and we can expect further exploration with rituximab and other anti-CD20 Mabs in subsets of CD20+ pre-B ALL.

CD22 is targeted by epratuzumab, which has been clinically investigated in the treatment of ALL, NHL, and inflammatory disorders. CD22, like CD20, is expressed during differentiation to pre-B-cells and nearly 90% of childhood pre-B ALL express this antigen [175]. An initial single-arm, dose tolerability study was published by Raetz et al., combining epratuzumab therapy with standard re-induction therapy in relapsed pediatric pre-B ALL [175]. In general, epratuzumab was well tolerated, but dose limiting toxicity occurred in two patients with seizures or transaminitis. Of the 15 patients treated, 14 had undetectable levels of CD22+ lymphoblasts 24 h after epratuzumab therapy and 9 patients achieved CR without evidence of minimal residual disease, suggesting an encouraging leukemia-specific effect of epratuzumab.

CD19 is more widely expressed during B-cell maturation than either CD20 or CD22 [176]. It appears early during B-cell differentiation, but is not expressed on mature plasma cells or peripheral circulating B-cells [177], making it an ideal therapeutic target in ALL. However, the development of effective Mabs has proven difficult. In 2003, CALGB published the results of trial 9311, combining chemotherapy with a blocked ricin anti-CD19 immunoconjugate [178]. Responses were only modest and molecular monitoring before and after the immunoconjugate showed a disappointingly inconsistent change in the number of leukemic cells remaining. This immunoconjugate has also been

Table 16.1 Proposed schema for integrating novel agents into ALL regimens

Class of agent	ALL phenotype	Phase of disease	Rationale	Potential specific agents	Common toxicities
Hypomethylating agents	B-ALL and T-ALL	Maintenance after chemotherapy or transplant	Alters gene expression, unlikely to be able to control aggressive disease and associated cytopenias may preclude combinations with cytotoxic agents	Decitabine, azacitidine	Hematologic, nausea, diarrhea [70]
HDAC inhibitors	B-ALL and T-ALL	Any phase	Alters gene expression without overlapping myelosuppression with cytotoxic agents	Vorinostat, LBH589	Diarrhea, dysgeusia, weight loss, fatigue, hyperglycemia, hematologic, thrombosis [70]
mTOR inhibitor	B-ALL, preferably T-ALL	Induction or salvage with high-dose methotrexate; maintence with POMP	Synergistic with methotrexate, GSIs and NF-kappa B inhibitors	Temsirolimus (IV) during intense chemotherapy and everolimus (oral) with maintenance therapy	Rash, hyperglycemia, hyperlipidemia, hematologic, interstitial lung disease [70]
Sonic Hedgehog antagonist	T-ALL	Induction or salvage concurrent with dexamethasone or prednisone	Synergistic with glucocorticoids	GDC-0449	Hyponatremia, fatigue [125]
Survivin Inhibitors	B-ALL and T-ALL	As part of combination regimes in any phase of disease	Potenitally synergistic with NF-kappa B inhibitors	Terameprocol (EM-1421)	Metabolic acidosis at high dose [135]
Gamma-secretase inhibitors (GSIs)	T-ALL	Any phase combined with cytotoxic chemotherapy and/or mTOR inhibitors	Synergistic in vitro with mTOR and NF-kappa B inhibitors	LY-411575	Rash, bowel obstruction [188]
NF-kappa B inhibitors	B-ALL, preferably T-ALL	Any phase combined with mTOR inhibitors, GSIs and/or anthracyclines	Synergistic in vitro with mTOR inhibitors, anthracyclines and GSIs	Bortezomib	Peripheral neuropathy, nausea, diarrhea, fatigue, hematologic [71]
Toll-like receptor agonists	B-ALL and T-ALL	Augmenting the graft-versus-leukemia effects of allogeneic stem cell transplants and donor lymphocyte infusions	Enhance the immune response to alloantigens on ALL	PF-3512676	Flu-like symptoms, neutropenia [189]

explored in chronic lymphocytic leukemia, where it is well tolerated, but demonstrated limited single-agent efficacy [179].

CD52 is widely expressed on both malignant B lymphocytes and T lymphoblasts, but not on CD34+ cells [180]. One series reported 66% of ALL tumors expressing CD52, suggesting this antigen could be a potential therapeutic target [181]. Alemtuzumab has been widely studied and approved for the treatment of chronic lymphocytic leukemia, but experience remains limited in the treatment of ALL. Tibes et al. treated 15 patients with relapsed AML (9 patients) or ALL (6 patients) with 30 mg alemtuzumab three times a week for 4–12 weeks. No complete responses were observed, 10 patients progressed on therapy and only 2 patients received more than 1 month of therapy. Treatment was complicated by cytopenias and infections. This study suggested a limited value of alemtuzumab for single agent therapy, and the CALGB is current exploring its value in the treatment of minimal residual disease.

CD33 is expressed on 90% of AML blasts and the conjugated Mab gemtuzumab ozogamicin was developed to exploit this early hematopoietic antigen ozogamicin [182]. CD33 is also expressed in 15% of ALL blasts at diagnosis [183]. Although gemtuzumab ozogamicin has demonstrated significant efficacy in relapsed acute promyelocytic leukemia, where CD33 is highly expressed [184], and in relapsed AML [185], its use in both pediatric and adult ALL has thus far been limited to case reports [186, 187]. These small series highlight the potential of this modified Mab for further evaluation in selected ALL patients.

Although Mab clinical experience is limited in ALL, extensive experience in CLL, NHL, breast cancer and other malignancies suggests that this class of therapeutics is likely to prove valuable once appropriate ALL antigens and epitopes can be identified. Mechanisms of anti-leukemic Mab effects are still being evaluated in the laboratory, even for Mabs with broad clinical experience, such as rituximab. Rational Mab drug design will ultimately require knowledge of antigen expression during leukemogenesis, in conjunction with exploitation of leukemic response to specific epitope binding.

Conclusions

The need to improve outcomes across all phases of illness in adult ALL is clear. Relapse rates remain high and salvage regimens often lead to disappointing results. There are many drugs and pathways currently being investigated in ALL. There are relative few patients and these novel strategies need to be prioritized for clinical trials based on the strength of their preclinical evidence. Also, rational integration of these new agents, into what are already very complex treatment algorithms for ALL, will be essential. Where and how these agents will best synergize with current multi-drug therapies remains to be seen. The clear answer is through well designed clinical trials. Table 16.1 offers suggestions as to where to incorporate some of these agents into ALL clinical trials. In a disease as aggressive and heterogeneous as ALL it is unlikely that any of these will represent a *silver-bullet*, it is more likely that each additional agent will result in incremental improvements in current therapies.

References

1. Lamanna, N., von Hassel, M., Weiss, M., et al. (2008). Relapsed acute lymphoblastic leukemia. In E. H. Estey, S. H. Faderl, & H. M. Kantarjian (Eds.), *Acute leukemia* (pp. 275–279). New York: Springer.
2. Kolb, H. J., Schattenberg, A., Goldman, J. M., et al. (1995). Graft-versus-leukemia effect of donor lymphocyte transfusions in marrow grafted patients. *Blood, 86,* 2041–2050.
3. Passweg, J. R., Tiberghien, P., Cahn, J. Y., et al. (1998). Graft-versus-leukemia effects in T lineage and B lineage acute lymphoblastic leukemia. *Bone Marrow Transplantation, 21,* 153–158.

4. Gale, R. P., Horowitz, M. M., Ash, R. C., et al. (1994). Identical-twin bone marrow transplants for leukemia. *Annals of Internal Medicine, 120*, 646–652.

5. Larson, R. A., Yu, D., Sanford, B. L., et al. (2008). Recent clinical trials in acute lymphoblastic leukemia by the Cancer and Leukemia group B. In S. Faderl, H. M. Kantarjian, & E. H. Estey (Eds.), *Acute leukemias* (pp. 137–144). New York: Springer.

6. Fielding, A. K., Richards, S. M., Chopra, R., et al. (2007). Outcome of 609 adults after relapse of acute lymphoblastic leukemia (ALL); an MRC UKALL12/ECOG 2993 study. *Blood, 109*, 944–950.

7. Thomas, D. A., Faderl, S., Cortes, J., et al. (2004). Treatment of Philadelphia chromosome-positive acute lymphocytic leukemia with hyper-CVAD and imatinib mesylate. *Blood, 103*, 4396–4407.

8. Towatari, M., Yanada, M., Usui, N., et al. (2004). Combination of intensive chemotherapy and imatinib can rapidly induce high-quality complete remission for a majority of patients with newly diagnosed BCR-ABL-positive acute lymphoblastic leukemia. *Blood, 104*, 3507–3512.

9. Sala-Torra, O., & Radich, J. P. (2008). Philadelphia chromosome-positive acute lymphoblastic leukemia. In S. Faderl, H. M. Kantarjian, & E. H. Estey (Eds.), *Acute leukemias* (pp. 177–189). New York: Springer.

10. Wetlzer, M., & Kryzstof, M. (2008). Molecular biology and genetics. In S. Faderl, H. M. Kantarjian, & E. H. Estey (Eds.), *Acute leukemias* (pp. 95–108). New York: Springer.

11. Bloomfield, C. D., Secker-Walker, L. M., Goldman, A. I., et al. (1989). Six-year follow-up of the clinical significance of karyotype in acute lymphoblastic leukemia. *Cancer Genetics and Cytogenetics, 40*, 171–185.

12. Fenaux, P., Lai, J. L., Morel, P., et al. (1989). Cytogenetics and their prognostic value in childhood and adult acute lymphoblastic leukemia (ALL) excluding L3. *Hematological Oncology, 7*, 307–317.

13. A Collaborative Study of the Group Francais de Cytogenetique Hematologique. (1996). Cytogenetic abnormalities in adult acute lymphoblastic leukemia: Correlations with hematologic findings outcome. *Blood, 87*, 3135–3142.

14. Secker-Walker, L. M., Prentice, H. G., Durrant, J., et al. (1997). Cytogenetics adds independent prognostic information in adults with acute lymphoblastic leukaemia on MRC trial UKALL XA. MRC Adult Leukaemia Working Party. *British Journal Haematology, 96*, 601–610.

15. Garipidou, V., Yamada, T., Prentice, H. G., et al. (1990). Trisomy 8 in acute lymphoblastic leukemia (ALL): A case report and update of the literature. *Leukemia, 4*, 717–719.

16. Wetzler, M., Dodge, R. K., Mrozek, K., et al. (1999). Prospective karyotype analysis in adult acute lymphoblastic leukemia: The cancer and leukemia Group B experience. *Blood, 93*, 3983–3993.

17. Vranova, V., Mentzlova, D., Oltova, A., et al. (2008). Efficacy of high-resolution comparative genomic hybridization (HR-CGH) in detection of chromosomal abnormalities in children with acute leukaemia. *Neoplasma, 55*, 23–30.

18. Pui, C. H., & Evans, W. E. (1998). Acute lymphoblastic leukemia. *The New England Journal of Medicine, 339*, 605–615.

19. Faderl, S., Kantarjian, H. M., Talpaz, M., et al. (1998). Clinical significance of cytogenetic abnormalities in adult acute lymphoblastic leukemia. *Blood, 91*, 3995–4019.

20. Chiaretti, S., Li, X., Gentleman, R., et al. (2004). Gene expression profile of adult T-cell acute lymphocytic leukemia identifies distinct subsets of patients with different response to therapy and survival. *Blood, 103*, 2771–2778.

21. Holleman, A., Cheok, M. H., den Boer, M. L., et al. (2004). Gene-expression patterns in drug-resistant acute lymphoblastic leukemia cells and response to treatment. *The New England Journal of Medicine, 351*, 533–542.

22. Mi, S., Lu, J., Sun, M., et al. (2007). MicroRNA expression signatures accurately discriminate acute lymphoblastic leukemia from acute myeloid leukemia. *Proceedings of the National Academy of Sciences of the United States of America, 104*, 19971–19976.

23. Bird, A. (2002). DNA methylation patterns and epigenetic memory. *Genes & Development, 16*, 6–21.

24. Jones, P. A., & Baylin, S. B. (2002). The fundamental role of epigenetic events in cancer. *Nature Reviews. Genetics, 3*, 415–428.

25. Herman, J. G., & Baylin, S. B. (2003). Gene silencing in cancer in association with promoter hypermethylation. *The New England Journal of Medicine, 349*, 2042–2054.

26. Roman-Gomez, J., Jimenez-Velasco, A., Barrios, M., et al. (2007). Poor prognosis in acute lymphoblastic leukemia may relate to promoter hypermethylation of cancer-related genes. *Leukaemia & Lymphoma, 48*, 1269–1282.

27. Laird, P. W. (2003). The power and the promise of DNA methylation markers. *Nature Reviews. Cancer, 3*, 253–266.

28. Silverman, L. R., & Mufti, G. J. (2005). Methylation inhibitor therapy in the treatment of myelodysplastic syndrome. *Nature Clinical Practice. Oncology, 2*(Suppl 1), S12–S23.

29. Cashen, A., Schiller, G. J., Larsen, J. S., et al. (2006). Phase II study of low-dose decitabine for the front-line treatment of older patients with acute myeloid leukemia (AML). *Blood (ASH Annual Meeting Abstracts), 108*, 1984.

30. Cashen, A. F., Schiller, G. J., O'Donnell, M. R., et al. (2008). Preliminary results of a multicenter phase II trial of 5-day decitabine as front-line therapy for elderly patients with acute myeloid leukemia (AML). *Blood (ASH Annual Meeting Abstracts), 112*, 560.

31. Blum, W. G., Klisovic, R., Liu, S., et al. (2009) Efficacy of a novel schedule of decitabine in previously untreated AML, age 60 or older. ASCO annual meeting 2009, Orlando, p. 7010.

32. Silverman, L. R., Demakos, E. P., Peterson, B. L., et al. (2002). Randomized controlled trial of azacitidine in patients with the myelodysplastic syndrome: A study of the cancer and leukemia group B. *Journal of Clinical Oncology, 20*, 2429–2440.

33. Fenaux, P., Mufti, G. J., Hellstrom-Lindberg, E., et al. (2009). Efficacy of azacitidine compared with that of conventional care regimens in the treatment of higher-risk myelodysplastic syndromes: A randomized, open-label, phase III study. *The Lancet Oncology, 10*, 223–232.

34. Roman-Gomez, J., Jimenez-Velasco, A., Castillejo, J. A., et al. (2004). Promoter hypermethylation of cancer-related genes: A strong independent prognostic factor in acute lymphoblastic leukemia. *Blood, 104*, 2492–2498.

35. Roman-Gomez, J., Jimenez-Velasco, A., Agirre, X., et al. (2005). Lack of CpG island methylator phenotype defines a clinical subtype of T-cell acute lymphoblastic leukemia associated with good prognosis. *Journal of Clinical Oncology, 23*, 7043–7049.

36. Kawano, S., Miller, C. W., Gombart, A. F., et al. (1999). Loss of p73 gene expression in leukemias/lymphomas due to hypermethylation. *Blood, 94*, 1113–1120.

37. Melki, J. R., Vincent, P. C., Brown, R. D., et al. (2000). Hypermethylation of E-cadherin in leukemia. *Blood, 95*, 3208–3213.

38. Wong, I. H., Ng, M. H., Huang, D. P., et al. (2000). Aberrant p15 promoter methylation in adult and childhood acute leukemias of nearly all morphologic subtypes: Potential prognostic implications. *Blood, 95*, 1942–1949.

39. Roman, J., Castillejo, J. A., Jimenez, A., et al. (2001). Hypermethylation of the calcitonin gene in acute lympho-blastic leukaemia is associated with unfavourable clinical outcome. *British Journal of Haematology, 113*, 329–338.

40. Garcia-Manero, G., Daniel, J., Smith, T. L., et al. (2002). DNA methylation of multiple promoter-associated CpG islands in adult acute lymphocytic leukemia. *Clinical Cancer Research, 8*, 2217–2224.

41. Roman-Gomez, J., Castillejo, J. A., Jimenez, A., et al. (2002). 5′ CpG island hypermethylation is associated with transcriptional silencing of the p21(CIP1/WAF1/SDI1) gene and confers poor prognosis in acute lymphoblastic leukemia. *Blood, 99*, 2291–2296.

42. Shen, L., Toyota, M., Kondo, Y., et al. (2003). Aberrant DNA methylation of p57KIP2 identifies a cell-cycle regulatory pathway with prognostic impact in adult acute lymphocytic leukemia. *Blood, 101*, 4131–4136.

43. Agirre, X., Vizmanos, J. L., Calasanz, M. J., et al. (2003). Methylation of CpG dinucleotides and/or CCWGG motifs at the promoter of TP53 correlates with decreased gene expression in a subset of acute lymphoblastic leukemia patients. *Oncogene, 22*, 1070–1072.

44. Roman-Gomez, J., Jimenez-Velasco, A., Agirre, X., et al. (2004). The normal epithelial cell-specific 1 (NES1) gene, a candidate tumor suppressor gene on chromosome 19q13.3-4, is downregulated by hypermethylation in acute lymphoblastic leukemia. *Leukemia, 18*, 362–365.

45. Roman-Gomez, J., Jimenez-Velasco, A., Agirre, X., et al. (2004). Transcriptional silencing of the Dickkopfs-3 (Dkk-3) gene by CpG hypermethylation in acute lymphoblastic leukaemia. *British Journal of Cancer, 91*, 707–713.

46. Jimenez-Velasco, A., Roman-Gomez, J., Agirre, X., et al. (2005). Downregulation of the large tumor suppressor 2 (LATS2/KPM) gene is associated with poor prognosis in acute lymphoblastic leukemia. *Leukemia, 19*, 2347–2350.

47. Agirre, X., Roman-Gomez, J., Vazquez, I., et al. (2006). Abnormal methylation of the common PARK2 and PACRG promoter is associated with downregulation of gene expression in acute lymphoblastic leukemia and chronic myeloid leukemia. *International Journal of Cancer, 118*, 1945–1953.

48. Agirre, X., Roman-Gomez, J., Jimenez-Velasco, A., et al. (2006). ASPP1, a common activator of TP53, is inactivated by aberrant methylation of its promoter in acute lymphoblastic leukemia. *Oncogene, 25*, 1862–1870.

49. San Jose-Eneriz, E., Agirre, X., Roman-Gomez, J., et al. (2006). Downregulation of DBC1 expression in acute lymphoblastic leukaemia is mediated by aberrant methylation of its promoter. *British Journal Haematology, 134*, 137–144.

50. Roman-Gomez, J., Jimenez-Velasco, A., Agirre, X., et al. (2006). CpG island methylator phenotype redefines the prognostic effect of t(12;21) in childhood acute lymphoblastic leukemia. *Clinical Cancer Research, 12*, 4845–4850.

51. Gutierrez, M. I., Siraj, A. K., Bhargava, M., et al. (2003). Concurrent methylation of multiple genes in childhood ALL: Correlation with phenotype and molecular subgroup. *Leukemia, 17*, 1845–1850.

52. Takahashi, T., Shivapurkar, N., Reddy, J., et al. (2004). DNA methylation profiles of lymphoid and hematopoietic malignancies. *Clinical Cancer Research, 10*, 2928–2935.

53. Ponder, B. A. (2001). Cancer genetics. *Nature, 411*, 336–341.
54. Kuang, S. Q., Tong, W. G., Yang, H., et al. (2008). Genome-wide identification of aberrantly methylated promoter associated CpG islands in acute lymphocytic leukemia. *Leukemia, 22*, 1529–1538.
55. Ruter, B., Wijermans, P. W., & Lubbert, M. (2004). DNA methylation as a therapeutic target in hematologic disorders: Recent results in older patients with myelodysplasia and acute myeloid leukemia. *International Journal of Hematology, 80*, 128–135.
56. Avramis, V. I., Mecum, R. A., Nyce, J., et al. (1989). Pharmacodynamic and DNA methylation studies of high-dose 1-beta-D-arabinofuranosyl cytosine before and after in vivo 5-azacytidine treatment in pediatric patients with refractory acute lymphocytic leukemia. *Cancer Chemotherapy and Pharmacology, 24*, 203–210.
57. Youssef, E. M., Chen, X. Q., Higuchi, E., et al. (2004). Hypermethylation and silencing of the putative tumor suppressor Tazarotene-induced gene 1 in human cancers. *Cancer Research, 64*, 2411–2417.
58. CALGB-8461 and CALGB-20602. (2008). Accessed on September 5, 2008, www.clinicaltrials.gov
59. Cheung, P., Allis, C. D., & Sassone-Corsi, P. (2000). Signaling to chromatin through histone modifications. *Cell, 103*, 263–271.
60. Jenuwein, T., & Allis, C. D. (2001). Translating the histone code. *Science, 293*, 1074–1080.
61. Wolffe, A. P., & Pruss, D. (1996). Deviant nucleosomes: The functional specialization of chromatin. *Trends in Genetics, 12*, 58–62.
62. Turner, B. M. (2000). Histone acetylation and an epigenetic code. *Bioessays, 22*, 836–845.
63. Strahl, B. D., & Allis, C. D. (2000). The language of covalent histone modifications. *Nature, 403*, 41–45.
64. Mahlknecht, U., & Hoelzer, D. (2000). Histone acetylation modifiers in the pathogenesis of malignant disease. *Molecular Medicine, 6*, 623–644.
65. Cress, W. D., & Seto, E. (2000). Histone deacetylases, transcriptional control, and cancer. *Journal of Cellular Physiology, 184*, 1–16.
66. Marks, P., Rifkind, R. A., Richon, V. M., et al. (2001). Histone deacetylases and cancer: Causes and therapies. *Nature Reviews. Cancer, 1*, 194–202.
67. Murata, T., Kurokawa, R., Krones, A., et al. (2001). Defect of histone acetyltransferase activity of the nuclear transcriptional coactivator CBP in Rubinstein-Taybi syndrome. *Human Molecular Genetics, 10*, 1071–1076.
68. Lin, R. J., Nagy, L., Inoue, S., et al. (1998). Role of the histone deacetylase complex in acute promyelocytic leukaemia. *Nature, 391*, 811–814.
69. Urnov, F. D., & Wolffe, A. P. (2000). Chromatin organisation and human disease. *Emerging Therapeutic Targets, 4*, 665–685.
70. www.zolinza.com, Accessed September 5, 2008.
71. Gold Standard, Clinical pharmacology (Internet database). Gold Standard, Tampa.
72. Romanski, A., Bacic, B., Bug, G., et al. (2004). Use of a novel histone deacetylase inhibitor to induce apoptosis in cell lines of acute lymphoblastic leukemia. *Haematologica, 89*, 419–426.
73. Catley, L., Weisberg, E., Tai, Y. T., et al. (2003). NVP-LAQ824 is a potent novel histone deacetylase inhibitor with significant activity against multiple myeloma. *Blood, 102*, 2615–2622.
74. Scuto, A., Kirschbaum, M., Kowolik, C., et al. (2008). The novel histone deacetylase inhibitor, LBH589, induces expression of DNA damage response genes and apoptosis in Ph- acute lymphoblastic leukemia cells. *Blood, 111*, 5093–5100.
75. Shaker, S., Bernstein, M., Momparler, L. F., et al. (2003). Preclinical evaluation of antineoplastic activity of inhibitors of DNA methylation (5-aza-2′-deoxycytidine) and histone deacetylation (trichostatin A, depsipeptide) in combination against myeloid leukemic cells. *Leukemia Research, 27*, 437–444.
76. Lemaire, M., Momparler, L. F., Farinha, N. J., et al. (2004). Enhancement of antineoplastic action of 5-aza-2′-deoxycytidine by phenylbutyrate on L1210 leukemic cells. *Leukaemia & Lymphoma, 45*, 147–154.
77. Sarbassov, D. D., Ali, S. M., & Sabatini, D. M. (2005). Growing roles for the mTOR pathway. *Current Opinion in Cell Biology, 17*, 596–603.
78. Sabatini, D. M. (2006). mTOR and cancer: Insights into a complex relationship. *Nature Reviews. Cancer, 6*, 729–734.
79. Sarbassov, D. D., Guertin, D. A., Ali, S. M., et al. (2005). Phosphorylation and regulation of Akt/PKB by the rictor-mTOR complex. *Science, 307*, 1098–1101.
80. Hresko, R. C., & Mueckler, M. (2005). mTOR.RICTOR is the Ser473 kinase for Akt/protein kinase B in 3T3-L1 adipocytes. *The Journal of Biological Chemistry, 280*, 40406–40416.
81. Sarbassov, D. D., Ali, S. M., Kim, D. H., et al. (2004). Rictor, a novel binding partner of mTOR, defines a rapamycin-insensitive and raptor-independent pathway that regulates the cytoskeleton. *Current Biology, 14*, 1296–1302.
82. Muise-Helmericks, R. C., Grimes, H. L., Bellacosa, A., et al. (1998). Cyclin D expression is controlled post-transcriptionally via a phosphatidylinositol 3-kinase/Akt-dependent pathway. *The Journal of Biological Chemistry, 273*, 29864–29872.

83. Gao, N., Flynn, D. C., Zhang, Z., et al. (2004). G1 cell cycle progression and the expression of G1 cyclins are regulated by PI3K/AKT/mTOR/p70S6K1 signaling in human ovarian cancer cells. *American Journal of Physiology. Cell Physiology, 287*, C281–C291.

84. Law, M., Forrester, E., Chytil, A., et al. (2006). Rapamycin disrupts cyclin/cyclin-dependent kinase/p21/proliferating cell nuclear antigen complexes and cyclin D1 reverses rapamycin action by stabilizing these complexes. *Cancer Research, 66*, 1070–1080.

85. Rudelius, M., Pittaluga, S., Nishizuka, S., et al. (2006). Constitutive activation of Akt contributes to the pathogenesis and survival of mantle cell lymphoma. *Blood, 108*, 1668–1676.

86. Hudson, C. C., Liu, M., Chiang, G. G., et al. (2002). Regulation of hypoxia-inducible factor 1alpha expression and function by the mammalian target of rapamycin. *Molecular and Cellular Biology, 22*, 7004–7014.

87. Del Bufalo, D., Ciuffreda, L., Trisciuoglio, D., et al. (2006). Antiangiogenic potential of the Mammalian target of rapamycin inhibitor temsirolimus. *Cancer Research, 66*, 5549–5554.

88. Thomas, G. V., Tran, C., Mellinghoff, I. K., et al. (2006). Hypoxia-inducible factor determines sensitivity to inhibitors of mTOR in kidney cancer. *Natural Medicines, 12*, 122–127.

89. Hudes, G., Carducci, M., Tomczak, P., et al. (2007). Temsirolimus, interferon alfa, or both for advanced renal-cell carcinoma. *The New England Journal of Medicine, 356*, 2271–2281.

90. Brown, V. I., Fang, J., Alcorn, K., et al. (2003). Rapamycin is active against B-precursor leukemia in vitro and in vivo, an effect that is modulated by IL-7-mediated signaling. *Proceedings of the National Academy of Sciences of the United States of America, 100*, 15113–15118.

91. Teachey, D. T., Obzut, D. A., Cooperman, J., et al. (2006). The mTOR inhibitor CCI-779 induces apoptosis and inhibits growth in preclinical models of primary adult human ALL. *Blood, 107*, 1149–1155.

92. Zhang, C. Y., Feng, Y. X., Yu, Y., et al. (2006). The molecular mechanism of resistance to methotrexate in mouse methotrexate-resistant cells by cancer drug resistance and metabolism SuperArray. *Basic & Clinical Pharmacology & Toxicology, 99*, 141–145.

93. Serra, M., Reverter-Branchat, G., Maurici, D., et al. (2004). Analysis of dihydrofolate reductase and reduced folate carrier gene status in relation to methotrexate resistance in osteosarcoma cells. *Annals of Oncology, 15*, 151–160.

94. Ewen, M. E., Sluss, H. K., Sherr, C. J., et al. (1993). Functional interactions of the retinoblastoma protein with mammalian D-type cyclins. *Cell, 73*, 487–497.

95. Teachey, D. T., Sheen, C., Hall, J., et al. (2008). mTOR inhibitors are synergistic with methotrexate: An effective combination to treat acute lymphoblastic leukemia. *Blood, 112*, 2020–2023.

96. Perez-Atayde, A. R., Sallan, S. E., Tedrow, U., et al. (1997). Spectrum of tumor angiogenesis in the bone marrow of children with acute lymphoblastic leukemia. *The American Journal of Pathology, 150*, 815–821.

97. Gunsilius, E. (2003). Evidence from a leukemia model for maintenance of vascular endothelium by bone-marrow-derived endothelial cells. *Advances in Experimental Medicine and Biology, 522*, 17–24.

98. Costa, L. F., Balcells, M., Edelman, E. R., et al. (2006). Proangiogenic stimulation of bone marrow endothelium engages mTOR and is inhibited by simultaneous blockade of mTOR and NF-kappaB. *Blood, 107*, 285–292.

99. Ribatti, D., Nico, B., Crivellato, E., et al. (2007). The history of the angiogenic switch concept. *Leukemia, 21*, 44–52.

100. Mangi, M. H., & Newland, A. C. (2000). Angiogenesis and angiogenic mediators in haematological malignancies. *British Journal Haematology, 111*, 43–51.

101. Dvorak, H. F. (2002). Vascular permeability factor/vascular endothelial growth factor: A critical cytokine in tumor angiogenesis and a potential target for diagnosis and therapy. *Journal of Clinical Oncology, 20*, 4368–4380.

102. Montesano, R., Vassalli, J. D., Baird, A., et al. (1986). Basic fibroblast growth factor induces angiogenesis in vitro. *Proceedings of the National Academy of Sciences of the United States of America, 83*, 7297–7301.

103. Basilico, C., & Moscatelli, D. (1992). The FGF family of growth factors and oncogenes. *Advances in Cancer Research, 59*, 115–165.

104. Nagy, J. A., & Senger, D. R. (2006). VEGF-A, cytoskeletal dynamics, and the pathological vascular phenotype. *Experimental Cell Research, 312*, 538–548.

105. Hicklin, D. J., & Ellis, L. M. (2005). Role of the vascular endothelial growth factor pathway in tumor growth and angiogenesis. *Journal of Clinical Oncology, 23*, 1011–1027.

106. Moore, M. A. (1990). Haemopoietic growth factor interactions: In vitro and in vivo preclinical evaluation. *Cancer Surveys, 9*, 7–80.

107. Kittler, E. L., McGrath, H., Temeles, D., et al. (1992). Biologic significance of constitutive and subliminal growth factor production by bone marrow stroma. *Blood, 79*, 3168–3178.

108. Cluitmans, F. H., Esendam, B. H., Landegent, J. E., et al. (1995). Constitutive in vivo cytokine and hematopoietic growth factor gene expression in the bone marrow and peripheral blood of healthy individuals. *Blood, 85*, 2038–2044.

109. Stachel, D., Albert, M., Meilbeck, R., et al. (2007). Expression of angiogenic factors in childhood B-cell precursor acute lymphoblastic leukemia. *Oncology Reports, 17*, 147–152.
110. Avramis, I. A., Panosyan, E. H., Dorey, F., et al. (2006). Correlation between high vascular endothelial growth factor-A serum levels and treatment outcome in patients with standard-risk acute lymphoblastic leukemia: A report from Children's Oncology Group Study CCG-1962. *Clinical Cancer Research, 12*, 6978–6984.
111. Faderl, S., Do, K. A., Johnson, M. M., et al. (2005). Angiogenic factors may have a different prognostic role in adult acute lymphoblastic leukemia. *Blood, 106*, 4303–4307.
112. Yetgin, S., Yenicesu, I., Cetin, M., & Tuncer, M. (2001). Clinical importance of serum vascular endothelial and basic fibroblast growth factors in children with acute lymphoblastic leukemia. *Leukaemia & Lymphoma, 42*, 83–88.
113. Pule, M. A., Gullmann, C., Dennis, D., et al. (2002). Increased angiogenesis in bone marrow of children with acute lymphoblastic leukaemia has no prognostic significance. *British Journal Haematology, 118*, 991–998.
114. www.clinicaltrials.gov, Accessed on August 21, 2008.
115. Ruiz i Altaba, A., Sanchez, P., et al. (2002). Gli and hedgehog in cancer: Tumours, embryos and stem cells. *Nature Reviews. Cancer, 2*, 361–372.
116. Ingham, P. W., & McMahon, A. P. (2001). Hedgehog signaling in animal development: Paradigms and principles. *Genes & Development, 15*, 3059–3087.
117. Ruiz i Altaba, A., Palma, V., & Dahmane, N. (2002). Hedgehog-Gli signalling and the growth of the brain. *Nature Reviews. Neuroscience, 3*, 24–33.
118. Felsher, D. W., & Bishop, J. M. (1999). Reversible tumorigenesis by MYC in hematopoietic lineages. *Molecular Cell, 4*, 199–207.
119. Ruiz i Altaba, A. (1999). Gli proteins and Hedgehog signaling: Development and cancer. *Trends in Genetics, 15*, 418–425.
120. Corcoran, R. B., & Scott, M. P. (2001). A mouse model for medulloblastoma and basal cell nevus syndrome. *Journal of Neurooncology, 53*, 307–318.
121. Varas, A., Hager-Theodorides, A. L., Sacedon, R., et al. (2003). The role of morphogens in T-cell development. *Trends in Immunology, 24*, 197–206.
122. Stewart, G. A., Lowrey, J. A., Wakelin, S. J., et al. (2002). Sonic hedgehog signaling modulates activation of and cytokine production by human peripheral CD4+ T cells. *Journal of Immunology, 169*, 5451–5457.
123. Lowrey, J. A., Stewart, G. A., Lindey, S., et al. (2002). Sonic hedgehog promotes cell cycle progression in activated peripheral CD4(+) T lymphocytes. *Journal of Immunology, 169*, 1869–1875.
124. Regl, G., Kasper, M., Schnidar, H., et al. (2004). Activation of the BCL2 promoter in response to Hedgehog/GLI signal transduction is predominantly mediated by GLI2. *Cancer Research, 64*, 7724–7731.
125. Ji, Z., Mei, F. C., Johnson, B. H., et al. (2007). Protein kinase A, not Epac, suppresses hedgehog activity and regulates glucocorticoid sensitivity in acute lymphoblastic leukemia cells. *The Journal of Biological Chemistry, 282*, 37370–37377.
126. Lo Russo, P. M., Rudin, C., Borad, M., et al. (2008). A first-in-human, first-in-class, phase (ph) I study of systemic Hedgehog (Hh) pathway antagonist, GDC-0449, in patients (pts) with advanced solid tumors. In: ASCO Annual Meeting. *Journal of Clinical Oncology, 26*(3516), 157.
127. Tissing, W. J., Meijerink, J. P., den Boer, M. L., et al. (2003). Molecular determinants of glucocorticoid sensitivity and resistance in acute lymphoblastic leukemia. *Leukemia, 17*, 17–25.
128. Altieri, D. C. (2008). Survivin, cancer networks and pathway-directed drug discovery. *Nature Reviews. Cancer, 8*, 61–70.
129. Che, X. F., Zheng, C. L., Owatari, S., et al. (2006). Overexpression of survivin in primary ATL cells and sodium arsenite induces apoptosis by down-regulating survivin expression in ATL cell lines. *Blood, 107*, 4880–4887.
130. Xing, Z., Conway, E. M., Kang, C., et al. (2004). Essential role of survivin, an inhibitor of apoptosis protein, in T cell development, maturation, and homeostasis. *The Journal of Experimental Medicine, 199*, 69–80.
131. Leung, C. G., Xu, Y., Mularski, B., et al. (2007). Requirements for survivin in terminal differentiation of erythroid cells and maintenance of hematopoietic stem and progenitor cells. *The Journal of Experimental Medicine, 204*, 1603–1611.
132. Okada, H., Bakal, C., Shahinian, A., et al. (2004). Survivin loss in thymocytes triggers p53-mediated growth arrest and p53-independent cell death. *The Journal of Experimental Medicine, 199*, 399–410.
133. Nakayama, K., & Kamihira, S. (2002). Survivin an important determinant for prognosis in adult T-cell leukemia: A novel biomarker in practical hemato-oncology. *Leukaemia & Lymphoma, 43*, 2249–2255.
134. Sugahara, K., Uemura, A., Harasawa, H., et al. (2004). Clinical relevance of survivin as a biomarker in neoplasms, especially in adult T-cell leukemias and acute leukemias. *International Journal of Hematology, 80*, 52–58.
135. Troeger, A., Siepermann, M., Escherich, G., et al. (2007). Survivin and its prognostic significance in pediatric acute B-cell precursor lymphoblastic leukemia. *Haematologica, 92*, 1043–1050.

136. Goel, S., Burris, H., Mendelson, et al. (2007). ASCO Annual Meeting. *Journal of Clinical Oncology, 25*(3584), 158.
137. Ellisen, L. W., Bird, J., West, D. C., et al. (1991). TAN-1, the human homolog of the drosophila notch gene, is broken by chromosomal translocations in T lymphoblastic neoplasms. *Cell, 66,* 649–661.
138. Radtke, F., Wilson, A., Stark, G., et al. (1999). Deficient T cell fate specification in mice with an induced inactivation of Notch1. *Immunity, 10,* 547–558.
139. Rand, M. D., Grimm, L. M., Artavanis-Tsakonas, S., et al. (2000). Calcium depletion dissociates and activates heterodimeric notch receptors. *Molecular and Cellular Biology, 20,* 1825–1835.
140. Sanchez-Irizarry, C., Carpenter, A. C., Weng, A. P., et al. (2004). Notch subunit heterodimerization and prevention of ligand-independent proteolytic activation depend, respectively, on a novel domain and the LNR repeats. *Molecular and Cellular Biology, 24,* 9265–9273.
141. Francis, R., McGrath, G., Zhang, J., et al. (2002). aph-1 and pen-2 are required for Notch pathway signaling, gamma-secretase cleavage of betaAPP, and presenilin protein accumulation. *Developmental Cell, 3,* 85–97.
142. Wallberg, A. E., Pedersen, K., Lendahl, U., & Roeder, R. G. (2002). p300 and PCAF act cooperatively to mediate transcriptional activation from chromatin templates by notch intracellular domains in vitro. *Molecular and Cellular Biology, 22,* 7812–7819.
143. Weng, A. P., Ferrando, A. A., Lee, W., et al. (2004). Activating mutations of NOTCH1 in human T cell acute lymphoblastic leukemia. *Science, 306,* 269–271.
144. Vilimas, T., Mascarenhas, J., Palomero, T., et al. (2007). Targeting the NF-kappaB signaling pathway in Notch1-induced T-cell leukemia. *Natural Medicines, 13,* 70–77.
145. Pear, W. S., Aster, J. C., Scott, M. L., et al. (1996). Exclusive development of T cell neoplasms in mice transplanted with bone marrow expressing activated Notch alleles. *The Journal of Experimental Medicine, 183,* 2283–2291.
146. Rohn, J. L., Lauring, A. S., Linenberger, M. L., & Overbaugh, J. (1996). Transduction of Notch2 in feline leukemia virus-induced thymic lymphoma. *Journal of Virology, 70,* 8071–8080.
147. Wong, G. T., Manfra, D., Poulet, F. M., et al. (2004). Chronic treatment with the gamma-secretase inhibitor LY-411, 575 inhibits beta-amyloid peptide production and alters lymphopoiesis and intestinal cell differentiation. *The Journal of Biological Chemistry, 279,* 12876–12882.
148. De Keersmaecker, K., Lahortiga, I., Mentens, N., et al. (2008). In vitro validation of gamma-secretase inhibitors alone or in combination with other anti-cancer drugs for the treatment of T-cell acute lymphoblastic leukemia. *Haematologica, 93,* 533–542.
149. Chan, S. M., Weng, A. P., Tibshirani, R., et al. (2007). Notch signals positively regulate activity of the mTOR pathway in T-cell acute lymphoblastic leukemia. *Blood, 110,* 278–286.
150. Horton, T. M., Pati, D., Plon, S. E., et al. (2007). A phase 1 study of the proteasome inhibitor bortezomib in pediatric patients with refractory leukemia: A children's oncology group study. *Clinical Cancer Research, 13,* 1516–1522.
151. Avellino, R., Romano, S., Parasole, R., et al. (2005). Rapamycin stimulates apoptosis of childhood acute lymphoblastic leukemia cells. *Blood, 106,* 1400–1406.
152. Sonneveld, P., Hajek, R., Nagler, A., et al. (2008). Combined pegylated liposomal doxorubicin and bortezomib is highly effective in patients with recurrent or refractory multiple myeloma who received prior thalidomide/lenalidomide therapy. *Cancer, 112,* 1529–1537.
153. Sebban, C., Lepage, E., Vernant, J. P., et al. (1994). Allogeneic bone marrow transplantation in adult acute lymphoblastic leukemia in first complete remission: A comparative study. French Group of therapy of adult acute lymphoblastic leukemia. *Journal of Clinical Oncology, 12,* 2580–2587.
154. Goldstone, A. H., Richards, S. M., Lazarus, H. M., et al. (2008). In adults with standard-risk acute lymphoblastic leukemia, the greatest benefit is achieved from a matched sibling allogeneic transplantation in first complete remission, and an autologous transplantation is less effective than conventional consolidation/maintenance chemotherapy in all patients: Final results of the International ALL trial (MRC UKALL XII/ECOG E2993). *Blood, 111,* 1827–1833.
155. Sullivan, K. M., Weiden, P. L., Storb, R., et al. (1989). Influence of acute and chronic graft-versus-host disease on relapse and survival after bone marrow transplantation from HLA-identical siblings as treatment of acute and chronic leukemia. *Blood, 73,* 1720–1728.
156. Horowitz, M. M., Gale, R. P., Sondel, P. M., et al. (1990). Graft-versus-leukemia reactions after bone marrow transplantation. *Blood, 75,* 555–562.
157. Delannoy, A., Cazin, B., Thomas, X., et al. (2002). Treatment of acute lymphoblastic leukemia in the elderly: An evaluation of interferon alpha given as a single agent after complete remission. *Leukaemia & Lymphoma, 43,* 75–81.
158. Takeda, K., Kaisho, T., & Akira, S. (2003). Toll-like receptors. *Annual Review of Immunology, 21,* 335–376.

159. Corthals, S. L., Wynne, K., She, K., et al. (2006). Differential immune effects mediated by Toll-like receptors stimulation in precursor B-cell acute lymphoblastic leukaemia. *British Journal of Haematology, 132*, 452–458.

160. Manegold, C., Gravenor, D., Woytowitz, D., et al. (2008). Randomized phase II trial of a toll-like receptor 9 agonist oligodeoxynucleotide, PF-3512676, in combination with first-line taxane plus platinum chemotherapy for advanced-stage non-small-cell lung cancer. *Journal of Clinical Oncology, 26*, 3979–3986.

161. Korycka, A., Lech-Maranda, E., & Robak, T. (2008). Novel purine nucleoside analogues for hematological malignancies. *Recent Patents on Anticancer Drug Discovery, 3*, 123–136.

162. Galmarini, C. M., Popowycz, F., & Joseph, B. (2008). Cytotoxic nucleoside analogues: Different strategies to improve their clinical efficacy. *Current Medicinal Chemistry, 15*, 1072–1082.

163. Larson, R. A. (2007). Three new drugs for acute lymphoblastic leukemia: Nelarabine, clofarabine, and forodesine. *Seminars in Oncology, 34*, S13–S20.

164. Torelli, G. F., Guarini, A., Porzia, A., et al. (2005). FLT3 inhibition in t(4;11)+ adult acute lymphoid leukaemia. *British Journal Haematology, 130*, 43–50.

165. Brown, P., Levis, M., Shurtleff, S., et al. (2005). FLT3 inhibition selectively kills childhood acute lymphoblastic leukemia cells with high levels of FLT3 expression. *Blood, 105*, 812–820.

166. Karp, J. E., Passaniti, A., Gojo, I., et al. (2005). Phase I and pharmacokinetic study of flavopiridol followed by 1-beta-D-arabinofuranosylcytosine and mitoxantrone in relapsed and refractory adult acute leukemias. *Clinical Cancer Research, 11*, 8403–8412.

167. Marcucci, G., Byrd, J. C., Dai, G., et al. (2003). Phase 1 and pharmacodynamic studies of G3139, a Bcl-2 antisense oligonucleotide, in combination with chemotherapy in refractory or relapsed acute leukemia. *Blood, 101*, 425–432.

168. Rahmani, M., Reese, E., Dai, Y., et al. (2005). Cotreatment with suberanoylanilide hydroxamic acid and 17-allylamino 17-demethoxygeldanamycin synergistically induces apoptosis in Bcr-Abl+ Cells sensitive and resistant to STI571 (imatinib mesylate) in association with down-regulation of Bcr-Abl, abrogation of signal transducer and activator of transcription 5 activity, and Bax conformational change. *Molecular Pharmacology, 67*, 1166–1176.

169. Podar, K., Chauhan, D., & Anderson, K. C. (2009). Bone marrow microenvironment and the identification of new targets for myeloma therapy. *Leukemia, 23*, 10–24.

170. Brown, V. I., Seif, A. E., Reid, G. S., et al. (2008). Novel molecular and cellular therapeutic targets in acute lymphoblastic leukemia and lymphoproliferative disease. *Immunologic Research, 42*, 84–105.

171. Ramakrishnan, A., & Deeg, H. J. (2009). A novel role for the marrow microenvironment in initiating and sustaining hematopoietic disease. *Expert Opinion on Biological Therapy, 9*, 21–28.

172. Pui, C. H., & Jeha, S. (2007). New therapeutic strategies for the treatment of acute lymphoblastic leukaemia. *Nature Reviews. Drug Discovery, 6*, 149–165.

173. Bello, C., & Sotomayor, E. M. (2007). Monoclonal antibodies for B-cell lymphomas: Rituximab and beyond. *Hematology American Society of Hematology Education Program, 2007*, 233–242.

174. Thomas, D. A., Faderl, S., O'Brien, S., et al. (2006). Chemoimmunotherapy with hyper-CVAD plus rituximab for the treatment of adult Burkitt and Burkitt-type lymphoma or acute lymphoblastic leukemia. *Cancer, 106*, 1569–1580.

175. Raetz, E. A., Cairo, M. S., Borowitz, M. J., et al. (2008). Chemoimmunotherapy reinduction with epratuzumab in children with acute lymphoblastic leukemia in marrow relapse: A Children's Oncology Group Pilot Study. *Journal of Clinical Oncology, 26*, 3756–3762.

176. Uckun, F. M., Jaszcz, W., Ambrus, J. L., et al. (1988). Detailed studies on expression and function of CD19 surface determinant by using B43 monoclonal antibody and the clinical potential of anti-CD19 immunotoxins. *Blood, 71*, 13–29.

177. Anderson, K. C., Bates, M. P., Slaughenhoupt, B. L., et al. (1984). Expression of human B cell-associated antigens on leukemias and lymphomas: A model of human B cell differentiation. *Blood, 63*, 1424–1433.

178. Szatrowski, T. P., Dodge, R. K., Reynolds, C., et al. (2003). Lineage specific treatment of adult patients with acute lymphoblastic leukemia in first remission with anti-B4-blocked ricin or high-dose cytarabine: Cancer and Leukemia Group B Study 9311. *Cancer, 97*, 1471–1480.

179. Tsimberidou, A. M., Giles, F. J., Kantarjian, H. M., et al. (2003). Anti-B4 blocked ricin post chemotherapy in patients with chronic lymphocytic leukemia–long-term follow-up of a monoclonal antibody-based approach to residual disease. *Leukaemia & Lymphoma, 44*, 1719–1725.

180. Frampton, J. E., & Wagstaff, A. J. (2003). Alemtuzumab. *Drugs, 63*, 1229–1243. discussion 45-6.

181. Gilleece, M. H., & Dexter, T. M. (1993). Effect of Campath-1H antibody on human hematopoietic progenitors in vitro. *Blood, 82*, 807–812.

182. Dinndorf, P. A., Andrews, R. G., Benjamin, D., et al. (1986). Expression of normal myeloid-associated antigens by acute leukemia cells. *Blood, 67*, 1048–1053.

183. Pui, C. H., Rubnitz, J. E., Hancock, M. L., et al. (1998). Reappraisal of the clinical and biologic significance of myeloid-associated antigen expression in childhood acute lymphoblastic leukemia. *Journal of Clinical Oncology, 16*, 3768–3773.

184. Lo-Coco, F., Cimino, G., Breccia, M., et al. (2004). Gemtuzumab ozogamicin (Mylotarg) as a single agent for molecularly relapsed acute promyelocytic leukemia. *Blood, 104*, 1995–1999.

185. Sievers, E. L. (2001). Efficacy and safety of gemtuzumab ozogamicin in patients with CD33-positive acute myeloid leukaemia in first relapse. *Expert Opinion on Biological Therapy, 1*, 893–901.

186. Chevallier, P., Mahe, B., Garand, R., et al. (2008). Combination of chemotherapy and gemtuzumab ozogamicin in adult Philadelphia positive acute lymphoblastic leukemia patient harboring CD33 expression. *International Journal of Hematology, 88*, 209–211.

187. Cotter, M., Rooney, S., O'Marcaigh, A., et al. (2003). Successful use of gemtuzumab ozogamicin in a child with relapsed CD33-positive acute lymphoblastic leukaemia. *British Journal Haematology, 122*, 687–688.

188. Fleisher, A. S., Raman, R., Siemers, E. R., et al. (2008). Phase 2 safety trial targeting amyloid beta production with a gamma-secretase inhibitor in Alzheimer disease. *Archives of Neurology, 65*, 1031–1038.

189. Leonard, J. P., Link, B. K., Emmanouilides, C., et al. (2007). Phase I trial of toll-like receptor 9 agonist PF-3512676 with and following rituximab in patients with recurrent indolent and aggressive non Hodgkin's lymphoma. *Clinical Cancer Research, 13*, 6168–6174.

Chapter 17
Treatment of Relapsed Acute Lymphoblastic Leukemia

Daniel J. DeAngelo

Introduction

Tremendous progress has been made in the treatment of childhood acute lymphoblastic leukemia (ALL). Currently, pediatric patients with ALL have a complete remission rate (CR) of 95% with estimated 5-year event-free survival (EFS) rates of 80–85% [1]. Pediatric patients are typically risk stratified based on patients' age, white cell count, and immunophenotype. High-risk patients have inferior outcomes as compared to standard-risk patients with a 5-year EFS of 75% and a 5-year DFS of 78%. Because standard-risk patients perform remarkably well, efforts have been made to reduce their therapy, including both systemic and central nervous system (CNS) therapy, in order to avoid unnecessary late complications.

The results of adult patients with ALL have not kept pace with their pediatric counterparts. The Cancer and Leukemia Group B (CALGB) initiated a five-drug induction regimen starting with protocol 8811 [2]. In addition to prednisone, daunorubicin, vincristine, cyclophosphamide, and asparaginase were added both during induction as well as during early intensification. A subsequent study (CALGB 9111) randomized patients to the addition of filgrastim (G-CSF), which resulted in a statistically significant improvement in the CR rate to 87% compared with 77% in the placebo arm [3]. However, no improvements were seen in the 3-year DFS rate of 41% or the overall survival (OS) rate of 43%. Current CALGB trials that are using a modular A-B-C regimen (protocols 19802 and 10102) [4], characterized by dose-intensive daunorubicin followed by a high-dose methotrexate and cytarabine consolidation therapy remain disappointing, with CR rates of approximately 80% range and a median overall survival of only 19 months. This disappointing median OS is due entirely to post-remission relapses. Other common adult ALL regimens include hyper-CVAD, which consists of alternating cycles of cyclophosphamide, vincristine, doxorubicin, and dexamethasone, with cycles of methotrexate and cytarabine [5]. Complete remission rates with hyper-CVAD approach 90%; however, the 5-year DFS and OS rate remain unacceptably low at 38%.

In spite of the high CR rates in both pediatric and adult patients with ALL, relapse is an almost insurmountable problem for most individuals. The higher rates of relapse in adult patients with ALL is likely attributable to higher risk disease, for example, more adult patients have adverse cytogenetics such as the Philadelphia chromosome, as well as poor toleration of the intense and prolonged chemotherapy protocols. Salvage chemotherapy regimens have shown only modest activity in patients with relapsed or refractory ALL with a short median-remission duration of only 2–7 months [6–8].

D.J. DeAngelo (✉)
Harvard Medical School, Dana-Farber Cancer Institute, 44 Binney Street,
Boston, MA 02115, USA
e-mail: ddeangelo@partners.org

A.S. Advani and H.M. Lazarus (eds.), *Adult Acute Lymphocytic Leukemia*, Contemporary Hematology,
DOI 10.1007/978-1-60761-707-5_17, © Springer Science+Business Media, LLC 2011

Table 17.1 New agents in ALL

Nucleoside analogues	
Clofarabine (Clolar)	Approved for pediatric patients with relapsed refractory ALL
Nelarabine (Arranon)	Only active in T-cell lymphoblastic leukemia or lymphoma
Purine synthetase inhibitors	
Forodesine (BCX-1777)	Only active in T-cell lymphoblastic leukemia or lymphoma
Liposomal preparations	
Liposomal vincristine (Marquibo)	Less neurotoxicity as compared to standard vincristine
Liposomal daunorubicin	
Liposomal cytarabine	Can be administered every 2 weeks
Monoclonal antibodies	
Rituximab (Rituxan; anti CD-20)	May improve outcomes in CD20-positive pre-B-ALL
Epratuzumab (anti-CD22)	CD22 expressed on the surface of most pre-B-ALL cells
Alemtuzumab (Campath; anti-CD52)	May be important in minimizing minimal residual disease (MRD)
Asparaginase	
PEG-asparaginase (Oncospar)	Increased serum half-life as compared to other asparaginase products
Erwinia asparaginase	Short half-life, but can be administered in patients with allergies to either native or PEG-asparaginase
Tyrosine kinase inhibitors	
Imatinib (Gleevec; STI571)	Used in patients with BCR-ABL-positive disease
Dasatinib (Sprycel; BMS354825)	
Nilotinib (Tasigna; AMN107)	
Bosutinib (SKI066)	
INNO-406	
Aurora kinase inhibitors	
AP24534	Pan-ABL inhibitor still in clinical trials
MK-0457 (VX-680)	Limited by severe myelosuppression
PHA-739538	A multi-kinase aurora inhibitor still in clinical trials
XL-228	A multi-kinase inhibitor still in clinical trials
Methotrexate analogues	
Talotrexin (PT-525)	
Pralotrexate	Higher response rates seen in patients with T-cell lymphomas
Other	
Notch inhibitors	Notch-1, an important pathway in T-lymphoblastic disorders. Clinical trials are ongoing.
Histone deacetylase inhibitors	
Heat shock protein 90 inhibitors	

The outcome is particularly poor in patients who relapse while on therapy or with CR duration of less than 24 months. In this group of patients, long-term survival is less than 5%. Although salvage therapy for adult and pediatric ALL patients continues to yield poor results, it remains an area of active research with the hope that the discovery of novel agents will have the ability to improve the outcome of the poor-risk group of patients (Table 17.1).

Strategies for the Treatment of Patients with Relapsed ALL

The success of long-term outcomes for patients with relapsed or refractory ALL involves the ability to obtain a complete remission (CR). However, for the majority of adults, in spite of the ability to achieve a CR, these are seldom durable in patients with refractory or relapsed disease [6, 8].

Table 17.2 Summary of treatment results using high-dose cytarabine in relapsed/refractory ALL

Regimen	N Studies	N Patients	CR rate (range) (%)
HDAC/Mi	8	217	50 (23–84)
HDAC/Mi + other	3	98	73 (70–80)
HDAC/VP + other	4	129	49 (17–76)
HDAC/ASP	4	47	36 (20–45)
HDAC/IDA	7	331	56 (18–64)
HDAC/FLU ± IDA	6	87	50 (30–83)

HDAC high-dose cytarabine, *Mi* mitoxantrone, *VP* vincristine and prednisone, *ASP* asparaginase, *IDA* idarubicin, *FLU* fludarabine

Therefore, the ability to achieve a CR and to have the opportunity to obtain a hematopoietic stem-cell transplant (SCT) remains a reasonable goal for most patients. The chance to achieve CR with second-line therapy is typically short unless hematopoietic SCT can be performed during the remission period. A variety of treatment regimens have been developed for patients with relapsed or refractory ALL [9, 10]. Most successful regimens involve either high-dose cytarabine as a single agent or in combination with other agents such as anthracyclines or epipodophyllotoxins [11–13]. The remission rate with high-dose cytarabine is slightly less than 30%, whereas single-dose anthracyclines or epipodophyllotoxins result in remission rates in the 10–15% range.

The most widely studied drug in relapsed ALL is high-dose cytarabine (Table 17.2). This has evolved from several small pilot studies that resulted in a remission rate of approximately 30–40%. Higher CR rates have been noted with combination regimens. The most commonly used regimen includes high-dose cytarabine with mitoxantrone [11, 12, 14]. Several small phase II studies have suggested remission rates in the 20–80% range. In addition to mitoxantrone, other drugs have been combined with high-dose cytarabine including amsacrine, etoposide, asparaginase, and idarubicin, with a wide range of remission rates that likely are more attributed to patient selection rather than dose intensity.

Other regimens include high-dose methotrexate followed by rescue with folinic acid with or without the addition of asparaginase. Remission rates are in the 22% range; however, this combination has fallen out of favor given the use of these agents in the treatment of patients with de novo ALL.

Epipodophyllotoxins have also been explored in combination therapy. As single agents, they have very low remission rates but seem to synergize with cytarabine as well as with anthracyclines. Combining teniposide at a dose of 165 mg/m^2 with cytarabine at 200 or 300 mg/m^2 was pioneered in early childhood studies resulting in CR rates in the 16–42% range in adults [13]. Etoposide has also been explored in several combination regimens with CR rates of 17–76% as well as in combination with high-dose Cytarabine with remission rates in the 11–33% range. The use of high-dose etoposide has been employed in several conditioning regimens for hematopoietic SCT. However, the data using high-dose etoposide in lieu of SCT are sparse.

Salvage Chemotherapy

Single-agent chemotherapy with the exception of the nucleoside analogues is typically not employed in patients with relapsed or refractory ALL. Single-agent regimens include nucleoside analogues such as clofarabine or nelarabine, cytarabine typically in high dose, anthracyclines, purine antimetabolites, methotrexate, epipodophyllotoxins such as etoposide, and L-asparaginase. The CR rates are divergent and range from 0% to 70%, typically influenced by the heterogeneity of the patient population as well as the dosing schedule of the various agents.

Combination chemotherapy regimens are more commonly used for the treatment of patients with relapsed ALL (Table 17.3). Numerous regimens have been developed and studied typically in non-randomized trials. Again, the heterogeneity of the study group and the variants in the dosing schedule make comparison difficult between such regimens. Typically, combinations include vinca alkaloids with steroids with or without the addition of an anthracycline. The hallmark of vincristine and prednisone, for example, offers patients a 20–30% remission rate. This remission rate can be increased to approximately 40% with the addition of an anthracycline such as doxorubicin or daunorubicin [15–17]. Asparaginase-based regimens have been developed predominantly by Capizzi [18]. L-asparaginase inhibits protein synthesis by depletion of the essential amino acid asparagine. High doses have been reported to increase the probability of remission in untreated patients with ALL. Synergistic activity was observed when high-dose asparaginase was used in combination with methotrexate [18–21]. Response rates in a variety of studies range from 33% to 79%. In addition, anthracyclines, daunorubicin and doxorubicin, vinca alkaloids, and corticosteroids have also been combined with L-asparaginase with the rate of CR ranging from 64% to 69%. Esterhay reported encouraging results with the MOAD regimen (methotrexate, vincristine, asparaginase, and dexamethasone) in untreated and previously treated patients with ALL. Courses were administered every 10 days, and the methotrexate dose increased by 50% up until a maximum dose of 225 mg/m^2 based on toxicity measurements. A remission rate of 79% in previously treated patients was observed with a median CR duration of 7.5 months and a median survival of 11.2 months. Patients were treated with consolidation phases in which vincristine and dexamethasone were eliminated, and six courses were administered in 10-day cycles. The use of asparaginase is not without toxicity. Typical side effects include allergic reactions, pancreatitis, hepatotoxicity, hyperglycemia, hypercoagulability, and neurotoxicity.

Table 17.3 Salvage chemotherapy regimens in relapsed or refractory adult ALL

Study	Induction chemotherapy	Complete remission (%)	Median remission duration/(months)
Miscellaneous single agents and combinations			
Paciucci et al. [81]	Mitoxantrone	50	5
Paciucci et al. [82]	Mitoxantrone + VP	57	5.5
Peterson and Bloomfield [83]	High-dose MTX + V	33	1.5
Ryan et al. [84]	Doxorubicin + ifosfamide	89	–
Vincristine-steroids-anthracyclines			
Elias et al. [15]	Doxorubicin + VP	40	7
Kantarjian et al. [16]	VAD	39	6.5
Koller et al. [17]	Hyper-CVAD	44	12
Asparaginase-base (without cytarabine)			
Aguayo et al. [19]	MTX + VP + pegylated Asp	22	3.7
Bassan et al. [85]	Asp + DNR + VP	88	8
Bostrom et al. [86]	Asp + DNR + VP	65	6
Esterhay et al. [20]	MOAD	79	7.5
Terebelo et al. [21]	MOAP	25	5.0
Woodruff et al. [87]	OPAL	69	4
Yap et al. [88]	Asp + MTX	58	4
	Asp + MTX + Ifosfamide	55	3.3

VAD vincristine, doxorubicin, and dexamethasone; *VP* vincristine and prednisone; *BMT* bone marrow transplantation; *hyper-CVAD* fractionated cyclophosphamide VAD; *DNR* daunorubicin; *MOAD* methotrexate, vincristine, asparaginase, and dexamethasone; *MAOP* methotrexate, vincristine, asparaginase, and prednisone; *OPAL* vincristine, prednisone, doxorubicin, and asparaginase; *MTX* methotrexate; *P* prednisone; *D* dexamethasone; *V* vincristine; *Asp* asparaginase

High-dose cytarabine regimens have been used as a single agent or in combination with anthracyclines with CR rates ranging from 17% to 70% [9–12, 14]. Cytarabine requires intra-cellular phosphorylation to Ara-CTP for activity. Ara-CTP is retained within the intracellular compartment and increased intracellular levels have been associated with improved remission as well as remission duration. The addition of double nucleoside analogues such as fludarabine may enhance the formation of intracellular Ara-CTP and therefore may increase activity. Unfortunately, randomized trials are few, and the addition of fludarabine to high-dose cytarabine is not typically employed.

Stem-Cell Transplantation

The duration of second remission is typically less than 6 months in adult patients with relapsed or refractory ALL [6]. There are, however, a few long-term survivors and most of these patients have undergone hematopoietic SCT, thereby reaffirming that the goal, although often difficult to obtain, is for patients to achieve a remission in order to pursue hematopoietic SCT. Therefore, the duration of the second CR must be of sufficient duration to afford the patient an opportunity to undergo SCT.

The overall survival rates in highly selected patients who receive an allogeneic transplant in second CR approach 30–40% (Table 17.4). These rates, however, are not supported by large pro-spective studies of patients with relapsed ALL. Overall survival rates for adult patients with relapsed ALL reported either from the MD Anderson or from the recent ECOG2993 study are less than 10% [6, 8]. Nevertheless, most long-term survivors had achieved a second CR and were able to proceed to an allogeneic SCT, thus supporting the observation that not only is a second CR impor-tant, but it must be of significant duration to allow SCT. This strategy led to the approval of both clofarabine as well as nelarabine in patients with relapsed ALL [22, 23].

Studies comparing chemotherapy to SCT following initial relapse suggest that children with a particularly long first remission may have favorable results with chemotherapy, reserving allogeneic transplantation for third remission. The Berlin-Frankfurt-Munster Relapse Study demonstrated excellent long-term EFS with chemotherapy if there are no circulating blasts; however, it requires

Table 17.4 Allogeneic stem cell transplantation for the treatment of acute lymphoblastic leukemia beyond first remission

Study	Donor	Remission status	Treatment	No.	Actuarial DFS (%)	Relapse (%)
MSKCC [89]	Family-member	Second	*HFTBI/Cy*	12	42	25
		Third or relapse		16	23	64
EGBMT [90]	Family-member	Second	Varied	96	~40	34
		Third or more		39	~12	73
Seattle [91]	Family-member	Second	Cy/SFTBI or Cy/FTBI	57	40	42
IBMTR [92]	Family-member	Second	Varied	391	40	45
GITMO [93]	Family-member	Second	Varied	57	41	–
Minnesota/ DFCI[94]	Unrelated donor	Second	Varied, primarily Cy/ FTBI	106	42	17
		Third		79	23	47
		Fourth		14	31	73
		Relapse		83	16	60
Scandinavia [95]	Family-member	Second	Varied	37	39	76
	Unrelated			28	54	40

Cy cyclophosphamide, *DFCI* Dana-Farber Cancer Institute, *IBMTR* International Bone Marrow Transplant Registry, *EGBMT* European Group for Bone Marrow Transplantation, *GITMO* Gruppo Italiano Trapianti di Midolio Osseo, *MSKCC* Memorial Sloan-Kettering Cancer Center, *FTBI* total-body irradiation, *F* fractionated, *HF* hyperfractionated, *SF* single fraction

2 years of continued therapy. Similarly, a retrospective analysis from the Nordic group recommended transplantation for children who had relapsed on therapy or within 6 months of stopping primary therapy but could find no advantage in transplanting children with late relapses. However, other numerous studies suggest that children with ALL in second remission fare significantly better if they received an allogeneic transplant as compared to chemotherapy alone.

The results observed for pediatric patients with ALL in remission transplanted with an unrelated donor are encouraging, but the long-term effects of the increased incidences of acute or chronic GVHD is unknown. The site of relapse is also important since chemotherapy plus CNS-directed therapy resulted in EFS of greater than 80% for late isolated CNS relapse. However, transplantation for isolated CNS disease can provide excellent results in children as well. Comparable data for adult patients are lacking.

Results of marrow transplantation are difficult to interpret as they reflect heterogeneity in conditioning regimens, risk groups, and time of relapse. Disease-free survival rates of 22–62% have been reported, with relapse rates of 13–62%. The lowest relapse rates are seen after hyperfractionated total-body irradiation with or without etoposide in the conditioning regimen. TBI and cyclophosphamide are thought to be a superior conditioning regimen to busulfan and cyclophosphamide for HLA-identical transplantation in children with ALL.

HLA-identical sibling transplants in children and adults with advanced ALL result in about 20% 5-year leukemia-free survival. Although seemingly better than chemotherapy, these studies represent highly selected patients and the results may not be generalizable. Similar results have been reported in adults never achieving remission with induction chemotherapy. In patients with very high-risk disease, leukemia relapse is the major cause of treatment failure, with an actuarial relapse risk of about 60%.

Prognostic Factors

The most significant prognostic factor for treatment response in relapsed patients with ALL is the duration of first remission. Patients with long first remissions (longer than 18 months) have a higher CR rate than those patients with short previous remissions [24, 25]. This data has also been further explored from the MD Anderson series as well as from the MRC UK ALL 12/ECOG 2993 study. In the MD Anderson series of 314 patients, age less than 40 years, performance status of less than 2, and a first CR remission duration of greater than 12 months was associated with a higher CR rate. Adverse prognostic features also included high white blood count, hypoalbuminemia, as well as elevated liver function tests. The MRC study included 609 patients who had relapsed after obtaining an initial remission. Factors that influenced survival from relapse included age and, most importantly, time from diagnosis. Patients who relapsed 2 years from their initial diagnosis had a 5-year survival of 11% as compared to 5% for those patients who relapsed less than 2 years.

Not surprisingly, the risk of relapse is associated with high-risk features at the time of diagnosis. These include elevated white blood count of greater than 30 K/L, age greater than 40, abnormal cytogenetics including the presence of the Philadelphia chromosome, as well as the presence of a translocation involving the mixed-lineage leukemia gene on 11q23. Other features at presentation that influence outcome include the presence of CNS involvement.

Clinical complete remission is typically defined based on morphologic and hematologic criteria. Minimal residual disease (MRD) has been used either by conventional cytogenetics, fluorescent in situ hybridization, or flow cytometric analysis, and when present increases the risk of disease recurrence. In addition, molecular analysis using immunoglobulin heavy chain or T-cell receptor rearrangements can also predict disease recurrence.

Biologic Features

The biologic features of patients with recurrent acute lymphoblastic leukemia are often similar to their initial clone [26]. Occasionally, clonal evolution can be observed. However, rare reports of a completely different karyotype have also been observed, raising the possibility of a second leukemic hit rather than clonal evolution. In a study of 53 adult patients aged 16–80, 9 of 32 patients had evidence of clonal evolution, and 12 of 32 (37%) had a different karyotype. The remainder of the patients had identical cytogenetic analyzes at relapse as they did at their initial diagnosis. Interestingly, the presence of clonal evolution was an adverse feature for survival, and the acquisition of unfavorable karyotypes was seen. These included abnormalities of chromosome 7 and structural changes involving chromosome 1 or 17p. Interestingly, patients who presented with a diploid karyotype seemed to recur with a diploid karyotype with a low incidence of clonal evolution.

Immunophenotypic changes at relapse occurred in 7 out of 29 cases (24%) with the acquisition of new T-cell markers or myeloid markers being most commonly observed. Mutations involving p53 have also been shown to be present in patients with relapsed ALL, but p53 mutations have been most commonly seen in patients with pre-T-cell ALL.

Clonal Evolution of Relapsed Leukemia

In most cases of relapsed ALL, there is a clear clonal relationship between the diagnostic karyotype and that of the original karyotype at the time of diagnosis. Clear relationships have been established in approximately 94% of patients with pre-B-ALL and in 71% of patients with T-cell ALL. The analysis has been principally performed using patterns of genomic copy number abnormalities (CNA). Comparing CNAs from relapsed to diagnostic samples, it is clear that CNAs were either present at low levels at the time of diagnosis and then selected for at relapse, or CNAs were newly acquired on the basis of new genomic alterations after patients received initial induction therapy. By analyzing the differences between diagnostic and relapsed samples on the basis of CNAs, it is clear that only a minority of cases have no change in their genomic copy number abnormalities. In the rest of the cases, either a secondary leukemic clone or a leukemia that arose from an ancestral clone is present. In one study, approximately 6% of cases had a genetically distinct leukemia arguing that it may have arisen from an ancestral clone prior to the time of diagnosis. In 8% of cases, there were no differences in the CNAs between the diagnostic and the relapsed sample, whereas in 34% of cases, relapsed disease represented a clear clonal evolution from the diagnostic sample. In addition, in approximately 50% of the cases, the relapsed clone was derived from an ancestral pre-diagnostic leukemia precursor and was distinct from the clone that predominated at the time of diagnosis. Notably, only a few genes that are involved in drug import, metabolism, export, or response, for example, the glucocorticoid receptor, are common examples of single-class CNAs. The diversity of genes that are targeted by relapse-associated CNAs with the presence of a relapse clone represented a minor subpopulation at the time of diagnosis that however escapes chemotherapy-induced apoptosis. This represents an extremely formidable challenge to the development of more effective therapies for relapsed ALL.

CNS Relapse

CNS relapse typically occurs 1–3 years from diagnosis and may present as an isolated CNS relapse or with systemic disease. Patients often present with symptoms or signs of increased intracranial pressure, which include headache, diplopia, nausea, vomiting, and papilledema. CNS relapses may also be accompanied by cranial nerve findings resulting in cranial nerve dysfunction. Diagnosis requires lumbar puncture and includes a pleocytosis of greater than four cells per microliter and unequivocal blasts upon microscopic examination. This is also usually associated with elevation of the CSF protein. A substantial number of patients with an apparently isolated CNS relapse by conventional microscopic criteria will have involvement in the bone marrow by PCR or other methods of detecting minimal residual disease. For patients with CNS disease, treatment should employ intrathecal therapy. Blasts are usually cleared with weekly or twice-weekly intrathecal therapy using single-agent methotrexate. Other approaches such as single-agent cytarabine, triple intrathecal therapy with methotrexate, cytarabine, and hydrocortisone or pegylated cytarabine can also be used.

Given the fact that most patients with isolated CNS relapse will have evidence of systemic disease manifested by minimal residual disease (MRD), systemic re-induction is typically recommended. Most of the data derives from the pediatric literature and studies from the Children's Cancer Group (CCG). Of 3,712 children treated between 1983 and 1988, 220 had isolated CNS relapse. After relapse, the 6-year event-free survival was 37%. A recent pediatric oncology group (POG trial) obtained an impressive 4-year event-free survival of 71% for 83 children with isolated CNS relapse. Children received vincristine, dexamethasone, and daunorubicin as induction, followed by high-dose cytarabine and asparaginase at consolidation, and then received alternating methotrexate, 6-mercaptopurine, and cyclophosphamide etoposide for intensification. After completion of intensive chemotherapy, patients then received cranial and spinal radiation and 18 months of maintenance therapy focusing on antimetabolites. All patients received triple intrathecal therapy in order to clear their CSF. The usual cranial dose was 24 Gy. However, increasing successes have come with the use of lower doses 18 Gy, thereby reducing significant neurotoxicity.

For patients with isolated CNS relapse, an effective treatment combination including intrathecal therapy with cranial radiation can be employed. Effective systemic therapy with high-dose cytarabine or high-dose methotrexate in combination with IT therapy is another common approach. CNS radiation can be performed on patients who are not previously radiated. It is important to note that patients with CNS relapse who undergo intensive CNS-directed therapy are at a high risk for neurotoxicity such as leukoencephalopathy.

Testicular Relapse

Testicular relapse is typically associated with painless enlargement of one of both testes. Diagnosis unfortunately requires biopsy. Among boys treated in CCG protocols between 1983 and 1988, 112 suffered isolated testicular relapse. The 6-year event-free survival for these children was 64%. Similar to systemic relapse, outcome improves with increasing duration of first remission.

Therapy consists of systemic re-induction and CNS treatment. In addition, re-induction with intensification is typically administered followed by maintenance therapy. Most patients receive bilateral testicular radiation at doses of 24 Gy.

Nucleoside Analogues

Clofarabine

Clofarabine is a novel purine analogue that acts by inhibiting ribonucleotide reductase and DNA polymerase, and is approved for the treatment of children with relapsed or refractory ALL [23, 27]. Clofarabine functions by depleting the cell of intracellular dNTPs available for DNA replication.

This results in premature DNA chain termination and the induction of apoptosis. Clofarabine is resistant to both phosphorolysis and deamination, both of which are important features of cytarabine drug resistance. Once clofarabine is actively transported across the cell membrane, it is rapidly phosphorylated to the triphosphate form and inhibits both ribonucleotide reductase and DNA polymerase.

Phase I studies performed in pediatric patients established a maximum tolerated dose of 52 mg/m^2 daily for 5 days [23]. A phase II trial demonstrated a 30% overall response rate; however, only seven out of the 12 remissions were complete (CR) and five patients had incomplete platelet recovery (CRp) [27]. The median CR duration in patients who did not undergo SCT was only 6 weeks. A phase I trial conducted in heavily pretreated adult patients established that the maximum tolerated dose on a 5-day schedule was 40 mg/m^2 [28]. Hepatotoxicity was the dose-limiting toxicity. In a subsequent phase II study with relapsed refractory patients with AML, ALL, high-risk MDS, and blast-phase chronic myeloid leukemia, the overall response rate was 48% including a 32% complete remission rate [29]. Combination studies with clofarabine and cytarabine (araC) were performed in adult patients with refractory acute leukemia [30]. The highest response rate was seen in patients with AML with an overall complete remission rate of 22%. Only two patients with ALL were included in this study and neither entered a CR. This combination therapy was taken forward in newly diagnosed patients over age 50 with AML, and an overall response rate of 60% was seen with 52% of patients achieving a CR and 80% of patients achieving a CRp [31]. Combination studies using clofarabine for the treatment of relapsed ALL are warranted.

Nelarabine

T lymphocytes and lymphoblasts show a marked sensitivity to the cytotoxic effects of deoxyguanosine. Unfortunately, the clinical use of deoxyguanosine is limited due to its rapid degradation by purine nucleoside phosphorylase (PNP) and subsequent short half-life. Ara-G, however, is resistant to degradation by PNP and is cytotoxic, particularly to T lymphoblasts at a micromolar concentration. Nelarabine (506U78: Arranon) is an ara-G prodrug that is demethylated by adenosine deaminase. Two phase II trials in adults and children have been recently reported in relapsed or refractory T-cell ALL. Nelarabine on an alternate day schedule at 1.5 g/m^2/day (days 1, 3, and 5) has a complete remission rate of 31% and an overall response rate of 41% [22]. No significant neurotoxicity was seen in this study, although neurotoxicity was the dose-limiting toxicity in previous phase I studies [32, 33]. In addition, a separate phase II study was conducted in pediatric patients, and nelarabine was safely administered at a dose of 650 mg/m^2/day for 5 consecutive days [34]. Nelarabine has considerably less activity in indolent peripheral T-cell lymphomas and virtually no significant activity in B-cell ALL.

Ribonucleotide reductase has a critical role in allowing cells to prepare for DNA synthesis by catalyzing the conversion of ribonucleotides into deoxyribonucleotides. Inhibitors of this pathway lead to the depletion of intracellular pools of deoxyribonucleotides and thus are able to inhibit DNA synthesis. Forodesine (BCX-1777) is a purine nucleoside analogue with the most promising results [35, 36]. This drug is a T-cell selective agent that has shown activity in T-cell malignancies. In 34 patients with refractory T-cell ALL, intravenous forodesine at a dose of 40 mg/m^2/day 5 days each week for a total of six cycles showed an overall response rate of 32% with a complete remission rate of 7%. A confirmatory phase II study is currently in development [37]. In addition to the intravenous formulation, an oral formulation is also available and has shown significant activity in cutaneous T-cell lymphomas.

Asparaginase Preparations

Asparaginase remains an important and universal component for the treatment of pediatric ALL. Asparaginase depletes the serum of asparagine, a nonessential amino acid on which many cells depend for normal metabolism. Normal cells compensate by synthesizing L-asparagine from aspartic acid and glutamine via the enzyme asparagine synthetase. However, malignant lymphoid cells have low levels of this synthetic enzyme and depend on intracellular pools of L-asparagine for protein synthesis. Asparaginase treatment is associated with several side effects including allergic reactions, thromboembolic events, pancreatitis, and abnormal lipid metabolism.

Three preparations of asparaginase are available. The standard asparaginase preparation is derived from *Escherichia coli*. Although usually not used as a single agent, *Escherichia coli* L-asparaginase has been combined in several multiagent chemotherapy regimens for the treatment of both adult and pediatric ALL [2–4]. Asparaginase derived from *Erwinia cartovora* is antigenically distinct and has been used effectively to treat patients who have experienced allergic reactions to the *E. coli* asparaginase preparation [38, 39]. Asparaginase derived from *Erwinia* has a shorter half-life than the enzyme derived from *E. coli*, and therefore it is typically administered in a twice-weekly regimen. Inferior 5-year EFS was recently documented in pediatric patients with ALL who received a once weekly *Erwinia* asparaginase injection as compared to the weekly *E. coli* preparation [40].

Hypersensitivity reactions to asparaginase are associated with the production of antibodies. Antibodies may also develop in patients without the usual clinical manifestations, which results in a much shortened asparaginase half-life, the so-called "silent" hypersensitivity. These latter antibodies reduce plasma asparaginase activity, which leads to a rebound of plasma asparagine levels.

E. coli asparaginase can be modified by covalently linking a polyethylene glycol conjugate to the enzyme. The binding preserves the enzymatic function of the drug but decreases its immunogenicity. PEG-asparaginase has decreased immunogenicity and a longer half-life than either of the other two asparaginase preparations. The half-life has been estimated to be greater than 14 days, and PEG-asparaginase has been used in relapsed ALL trials as well as in pediatric and adult induction ALL trials. A recent non-randomized trial by the Cancer and Leukemia Group showed that asparagine depletion with PEG-asparaginase resulted in superior DFS as well as overall survival (OS) [41]. PEG-asparaginase has also been employed in several ongoing clinical trials [42]. Its use seems to be well tolerated with a markedly decreased rate of allergic reactions and pancreatitis as well as an increase in serum asparagine depletion. PEG-asparaginase is now being incorporated into most pediatric and adult regimens.

Methotrexate Analogues

Methotrexate is a folic acid antagonist, which is used for a wide variety of cancers as well as auto-immune diseases. Methotrexate enters the cytoplasm and forms a polyglutamate complex. Both methotrexate and its polyglutamate forms are potent competitive inhibitors of dihydrofolate reductase (DHFR), and in addition, two additional enzymes within the purine synthetic pathway that also require folate coenzymes. The lack of tetrahydrofolate leads to an impairment of both purine and thymidine synthesis that results in inhibition of DNA replication.

Pralatrexate is a member of the 10-deazaaminopterins class of folate analogues that demonstrates greater antitumor effects than methotrexate against several murine tumor models as well as human tumor xenografts in mice [43]. Pralatrexate has high affinity for the reduced folate carrier type 1 (RFC-1) enzyme. RFC-1 is a fetal oncoprotein, which is expressed almost exclusively on fetal and malignant tissues. This carrier protein transports reduced natural folates into highly proliferative cells in order to meet the demands for purine and pyrimidine nucleotides for DNA synthesis. Pralatrexate has a higher response rate in patients with T-cell lymphomas as documented by a recent phase II study [44]. Dosing and scheduling of this agent are currently being investigated in numerous tumor types.

There are several other folate antagonists that are currently being tested in patients with relapsed leukemia, which include the multi-targeted anti-folate pemetrexed (LY231514) and talotrexin (Talvesta) [45]. Talotrexin is a novel nonpolyglutamatable anti-folate drug. This agent has a higher affinity to DHFR than methotrexate with a Ki of 0.35 pM, which is 15-fold lower than methotrexate. Talotrexin enters the cells via the reduced folate carrier (RFC) pathway. Ongoing phase I studies in patients with relapsed or refractory leukemia will hopefully define a maximum tolerated dose that can be taken forward in phase II studies.

Monoclonal Antibodies

The use of monoclonal antibodies for the treatment of patients with acute lymphoblastic leukemia is based on a phenotypic expression of specific antigens. For example, CD20 is expressed on more than 20% of lymphoblasts in about half of cases with pre-B-ALL. Investigators at MD Anderson have incorporated rituximab into frontline therapy using a hyper-CVAD regimen for patients who are positive for CD20 expression; thus, the use in patients with relapsed disease is unknown [46]. In their study, which included patients with Burkitt's leukemia (ALL-L3), the CR rate was 86%. The 3-year OS, EFS, and DFS rates were 89%, 80%, and 88%, respectively. In this study, rituximab was added without any appreciable increase in non-hematologic toxicity. In addition, a pilot study by the German multicenter ALL group added rituximab before each cycle of chemotherapy in patients with ALL only in patients who expressed CD20 on their lymphoblasts. In this study, all patients were over age 55 with the median age of 66. Their CR rate was 63%, and the survival after 1 year was 54% [47].

Epratuzumab appears to have more of an immunomodulatory mechanism of action as compared to the antiproliferative effects of rituximab. Epratuzumab targets CD22, which is expressed on the surface of most pre-B-ALL cells. Epratuzumab seems to be safe in patients with lymphoma and is undergoing safety and tolerability studies in patients with acute lymphoblastic leukemia. So far, the results have been encouraging when rituximab is used in combination with epratuzumab. In patients with non-Hodgkin's lymphoma, the monoclonal antibody combination resulted in a 60% response rate with no significant hematologic or non-hematologic toxicity [48].

The antigen CD52 is expressed on normal as well as malignant lymphocytes. Alemtuzumab is a monoclonal antibody directed against CD52. The majority of pre-B-ALL cases express CD52 defined as greater than 10% expression on the lymphoblasts [49]. Alemtuzumab is currently approved for the treatment of B-cell chronic lymphocytic leukemia and has single-agent activity in patients with refractory ALL [50, 51]. Currently, a dose escalation pilot study is being performed by the CALGB (10102) [52]. It appears that it is safe to administer 30 mg of subcutaneous alemtuzumab three times per week for 4 weeks between courses of intensive chemotherapy, a time when the patient is in minimal residual disease. Long-term data with regards to the efficacy and safety of this regimen are still ongoing.

Liposomal Conjugates

Vincristine is a vinca alkaloid and is extremely active in patients with ALL. Vincristine binds to tubulin, thereby causing microtubular depolymerization, metaphase arrest, and apoptosis. Unfortunately, vincristine also binds to neuronal tubulin, thereby disrupting axonal microtubules and causing neurotoxicity.

Current clinical practices cap the total dose of vincristine to 2.0 mg. This may result in under dosing patients with body surface areas larger than 1.4 m². Encapsulating vincristine into liposomes prolongs the half-life and allows a higher concentration of vinca alkaloid into the tumor as opposed to the normal neural tissue. When administered in full doses, liposomal vincristine appears to be less neurotoxic. A phase I study of liposomal vincristine was performed primarily in solid tumors [53]. A dose of 2.4 mg/m² was defined as the maximum tolerated dose with 2.0 mg/m² as the recommended phase II dose. Pain and obstipation were the dose-limiting toxicities. A subsequent phase II trial in patients with relapsed non-Hodgkin's lymphoma resulted in a 41% response rate [54]. In addition, the interval dosing of the liposomal vincristine was decreased every 14 days.

Liposomal vincristine is now being incorporated in place of the standard vincristine into regimens for patients with ALL. A recent phase II study using liposomal vincristine in patients with recurrent and refractory ALL was reported [55]. All patients received liposomal vincristine infused over 60 min at a dose of 2.0 mg/m² and repeated dosing every 14 days. There was one CR and one partial remission out of 14 patients, although five patients (36%) had transient reduction of their bone marrow leukemia infiltrates. It is difficult to assess the potential impact of this agent since single-agent vinca alkaloids are typically not administered in patients with ALL.

Both cytarabine and daunorubicin have also been incorporated into liposomes for the treatment of patients with ALL. In a study of 15 patients with ALL using liposomal daunorubicin in combination with vincristine and dexamethasone, 11 patients (73%) achieved a CR, and with a median follow-up of 20 months, the DFS and OS at 2 years were 36% and 38%, respectively [56]. Liposomal cytarabine has a pharmacokinetic advantage over the standard cytarabine preparation and based on efficacy comparisons, it is approved for use in lymphomatous meningitis [57]. It must be administered concurrently with corticosteroids in order to reduce the incidence of arachnoiditis. Given reports of increased neurotoxicity, care should be given when liposomal cytarabine is administered concurrently with systemic cytarabine [58].

Targeted Therapy

The frequency of Philadelphia-positive (Ph+) ALL is remarkably age dependent. The diagnosis of Ph+ ALL should be considered in all patients with precursor-B ALL, particularly in older patients. Furthermore, many patients with Ph+ ALL have coexpression of the myeloid markers CD13 and CD33. When imatinib is used as a single agent in patients with relapsed or refractory Ph+ ALL, approximately 60% of patients will achieve a hematologic remission, defined as clearance of peripheral blood blasts, but only 19% will achieve a CR [59]. Unfortunately, these responses are not durable with a median time to progression of only 2.2 months and an overall survival of 4.9 months. However, patients who are consolidated with SCT can have durable remissions with 51% of patients still in remission at a follow-up time of 12 months.

Currently, imatinib is typically added to standard induction chemotherapy for newly diagnosed patients with Ph+ ALL [60]. The addition of imatinib to hyper-CVAD results in a 96% CR rate. More importantly, a higher percentage of patients are able to proceed to a SCT. Similar studies conducted in Japan demonstrated a CR rate of 95% and a remarkably high rate of molecular remission with 73% of patients achieving a PCR-negative state [61]. The 1-year EFS and OS were 78% and 88%, respectively. Although randomized trials are lacking, imatinib is now being used as consolidation therapy prior to SCT. It is clear that low or undetectable BCR-ABL transcript levels prior to SCT portend a more favorable prognosis [62, 63].

In elderly patients, the use of combination chemotherapy is often prohibitive. The German ALL Group (GMALL) compared imatinib therapy to combination chemotherapy. Single-agent induction with imatinib was superior to multiagent chemotherapy with 93% of patients achieving a CR in contrast to 64% of patients allocated to the chemotherapy arm [64].

Many patients with Ph+ ALL have tyrosine kinase domain (TKD) mutations that often precede the initiation of imatinib [65]. Many of these mutations render patients refractory to imatinib therapy. Newer tyrosine kinase agents such as dasatinib (BMS-354825;Sprycel) and nilotinib (AMN-107;Tasigna) are able to bind to most TKD mutations except the T315I, which is resistant to all currently available ABL tyrosine kinase inhibitors.

Nilotinib has a similar structure to imatinib, but with a modified aminopyrimidine backbone. Its use in chronic phase and accelerated phase CML has led to its approval, and it is also currently undergoing testing in more advanced Ph+ leukemias [66]. In Ph+ ALL, nilotinib at a dose of 400 mg twice daily, achieved a complete remission in 26% of patients, and a complete cytogenetic remission in 34% of patients.

Dasatinib is a dual SRC and ABL kinase inhibitor with greater in vitro potency than imatinib, and has activity against the vast majority of TKD mutations. Similar to nilotinib, dasatinib does not inhibit the T315I mutation. In patients with relapsed Ph+ ALL who have failed imatinib, dasatinib induces a complete hematologic remission in 35% of patients, and a complete cytogenetic remission in 54% of patients [67]. Unfortunately, the median duration of response was short with a progression-free survival of 3.3 months. If one excludes patients with a T315I mutation, then the median progression-free survival was 5.7 months. Similar to imatinib, dasatinib is now being combined with chemotherapy in patients with Ph+ ALL [68].

Several other tyrosine kinase inhibitors are currently in clinical trials. Bosutinib (SKI-606) is an ABL-specific inhibitor that has little or no activity against platelet-derived growth factor receptor beta (PDGFR-β) or c-KIT and therefore would hopefully have fewer "off-target" side effects [69]. Another ABL-specific tyrosine kinase is INNO-406 [70]. INNO-406 also inhibits the LYN tyrosine kinase. It has several pharmacologic advantages in that it penetrates the CNS and therefore may be an attractive option for patients with leukemic meningitis.

As opposed to INNO-406, imatinib does not penetrate the cerebrospinal fluid (CSF) well, with CSF levels one to two orders of magnitude lower than corresponding plasma levels. In contrast, the CSF concentrations of INNO-406 in the CNS are approximately 10% of those in the plasma. INNO-406 is structurally similar to imatinib. Both are derived from 2-(phenylamino) pyrimidine, and therefore both are substrates for p-glycoprotein. This may limit its ability to completely eradicate cells with high p-glycoprotein levels. However, given the higher affinity for ABL, CSF levels of INNO-406 are sufficient to suppress the growth of Ph+ leukemia cells. Importantly, dasatinib, which is not a substrate for p-glycoprotein, also penetrates the CSF. However, there have been no detailed PK studies of dasatinib in the CNS.

The true incidence of CNS relapse in patients with Ph+ ALL has been limited by rapid systemic relapse. With the availability of newer tyrosine kinase inhibitors, CNS relapse has become more of an issue. Leis reported a CNS relapse in 5 of 24 patients on imatinib therapy [71]. Pfeifer et al. reported that CNS leukemia occurred in only 12% of patients that were treated with imatinib therapy [72].

Aurora kinases are currently being tested in patients with CML who have a T315I mutation. This mutation is resistant to all currently available ABL tyrosine kinases. The agent MK-0457, previously known as VX-680, is the most studied. However, both PHA-739538 and XL-228 are undergoing early clinical studies. The use of aurora kinases in patients with Ph+ ALL has not been adequately explored.

Other Agents

ALL that contains a translocation involving the mixed-lineage leukemia (MLL) gene on chromosome 11 (11q23) has a unique gene expression profile with high levels of expression of the receptor tyrosine kinase FLT3 [73]. Additionally, about a quarter of the patients contain FLT3 mutations within the second tyrosine kinase domain. There are several FLT3 inhibitors that have been in clinical trials for patients with FLT3-positive acute myelogenous leukemia, and significant biologic activity has been demonstrated with each of these agents [74–76]. It is possible that inhibition of FLT3 might represent a new therapeutic target for patients with relapsed ALL who have an MLL gene rearrangement.

The *NOTCH1* pathway is essential for normal T-cell development and is critical for the pathogenesis of T-cell ALL. Gain-of-function mutations within *NOTCH1* can reliably produce T-cell ALL in numerous animal models. These mutations are found in 60% of patients with T-cell ALL, both adult and pediatric [77]. This observation provided a strong rationale to test gamma-secretase inhibitors in T-cell ALL [78]. NOTCH has also been implicated in the pathogenesis of colonic goblet cells. *NOTCH1* inhibition results in colonic goblet cell hyperplasia and the development of secretory diarrhea. This pathway can be abrogated with the use of glucocorticoids, thus prompting additional trials using *NOTCH1* inhibitors [79].

Other novel genetic mutations reported in patients with T-cell ALL include the *NUP214-ABL1*. The *NUP214-ABL1* fusion is a constitutively activated tyrosine kinase that can transform Ba/F3 cells in a factor-independent model [80]. The *NUP214-ABL1* fusion is present in as many as 10% of patients with T-cell ALL, and may represent another example of a cryptic mutation that can result in the constitutive activation of a tyrosine kinase. Importantly, the *NUP214-ABL* fusion gene is inhibited by imatinib, thereby suggesting a novel therapeutic strategy for patients with relapsed T-cell ALL.

There are many other agents currently in development for the treatment of patients with relapsed or refractory ALL (Table 17.1). For example, histone deacetylase inhibitors (HDACi) are being developed in hematologic malignancies, which include SAHA (vorinostat), romidepsin, PXD101 (belinostat), MGCD0103, and LBH589 (panobinostat). Other strategies involve inhibition of the heat shock protein 90 (HSP90) enzyme and the AKT/mTOR pathway. Inhibition of the HSP90 and AKT/mTOR pathway is currently being explored in many solid tumors and hematologic malignancies. Their role in ALL is still unclear.

Conclusion

The selection of a treatment regimen for patients with relapsed ALL depends on several factors including age, performance status, availability of stem-cell donor, immunophenotype, and relapse location. Patients who relapse while on therapy tend to have a much poorer outcome and are often chemotherapy resistant. High-dose approaches may overcome chemotherapy resistance; however, even with SCT, long-term disease-free survival as well as overall survival remains limited.

For those patients who relapse off maintenance therapy, remission can be achieved using similar agents used to achieve the initial remission. These patients with late bone marrow relapse tend to respond to a repetition of the initially effective induction regimen. Again, remission duration and overall survival remain low, but the ability to pursue a hematopoietic SCT is the ultimate goal. For patients with early treatment failure or for patients with refractory disease, new drug combinations should be employed. At relapse, patients often have increased expression of multi-drug resistance phenotype and therefore have a higher chance that effective therapies may not be identified. In patients with extramedullary relapse, such as CNS or testicular relapse, treatment regimens need to focus on local, effective therapy as well as systemic chemotherapy, since the majority of patients have minimum residual disease in the bone marrow.

The outcome of patients with relapsed or refractory ALL remains an extremely difficult problem. In a series from the MD Anderson of 314 patients with either refractory or relapsed ALL, the median survival was only 5 months [8]. Only 24% of patients were alive at 1 year, and the 5-year survival was less than 3%. This data was corroborated by the MRC UKALL 12/ECOG 2993 study [6], which reported that patients with relapsed ALL had an overall survival at 5 years of only 7%. Only a highly selected group of patients were able to receive a SCT in second remission, and some of these patients are long-term survivors. Clearly, this data argues for improved treatment options for patients with relapsed or refractory ALL.

The Food and Drug Administration has recently approved two agents, clofarabine in relapsed pediatric patients with ALL, and nelarabine for use in both pediatric and adult patients with relapsed T-cell ALL. In addition, imatinib and dasatinib are currently being used in combination chemotherapy for patients with Ph+ ALL, both in combination with chemotherapy during initial induction as well as for patients with relapsed disease.

Multiple pathways and novel targets have been recently identified. Given the fact that ALL remains a rare disease, phase I studies are typically performed in patients with advanced hematologic malignancies followed subsequently by disease specific phase II studies. It is interesting that both nelarabine and clofarabine were approved based on relatively small phase II studies arguing for the difficulty in performing not only large multicenter phase II trials, but the impracticality of phase III trials.

As the specificity of the molecular targets increases, the availability of patients for these trials becomes a difficult and trying venue. For example, the use of FLT3 inhibitors in ALL would likely only benefit an extremely selected group of patients. Similarly, only patients with T-cell ALL who also have a *NOTCH1* gain-of-function mutation would likely benefit from a *Notch1* inhibitor. This would define an extremely small subpopulation of patients for confirmatory clinical trials and would make a randomized phase III trial virtually impossible.

It is unlikely that the addition of the new targeted inhibitors such as HDACs, ATK/mTOR, or HSP90 inhibitors will have significant activity as a single agent in patients with relapsed ALL. Strategies will need to be developed for combining these novel biologic agents into current multiagent chemotherapy regimens. Furthermore, the approval of these agents may prove difficult especially if randomized phase III trials are required. Nevertheless, the flurry of currently available agents for patients with relapsed ALL is encouraging. Hopefully, this will result in a significant improvement in the outcome of patients with relapsed ALL.

Acknowledgements I would like to thank Kelly Salvatore for assistance in preparing this manuscript.

References

1. Pui, C. H., Relling, M. V., & Downing, J. R. (2004). Acute lymphoblastic leukemia. *The New England Journal of Medicine, 350,* 1535–1548.
2. Larson, R. A., Dodge, R. K., Burns, C. P., Lee, E. J., Stone, R. M., Schulman, P., et al. (1995). A five-drug remission induction regimen with intensive consolidation for adults with acute lymphoblastic leukemia: Cancer and Leukemia Group B Study 8811. *Blood, 85,* 2025–2037.
3. Larson, R. A., Dodge, R. K., Linker, C. A., Stone, R. M., Powell, B. L., Lee, E. J., et al. (1998). A randomized controlled trial of filgrastim during remission induction and consolidation chemotherapy for adults with acute lymphoblastic leukemia: CALGB study 9111. *Blood, 92,* 1556–1564.
4. Stock, W., Johnson, J., Yu, D., Bennett, D., Sher, D., Stone, R. M., et al. (2005). Daunorubicin dose intensification during treatment of adult Acute Lymphoblastic Leukemia (ALL): Final results from Cancer and Leukemia Group B Study 19802 [abstract]. *Blood, 106,* 521a.
5. Kantarjian, H., Thomas, D., O'Brien, S., Cortes, J., Giles, F., Jeha, S., et al. (2004). Long-term follow-up results of hyperfractionated cyclophosphamide, vincristine, doxorubicin, and dexamethasone (Hyper-CVAD), a dose-intensive regimen, in adult acute lymphocytic leukemia. *Cancer, 101,* 2788–2801.
6. Fielding, A. K., Richards, S. M., Chopra, R., Lazarus, H. M., Litzow, M. R., Buck, G., et al. (2007). Outcome of 609 adults after relapse of acute lymphoblastic leukemia (ALL); an MRC UKALL12/ECOG 2993 study. *Blood, 109,* 944–950.

7. Le, Q. H., Thomas, X., Ecochard, R., Iwaz, J., Lheritier, V., Michallet, M., et al. (2007). Proportion of long-term event-free survivors and lifetime of adult patients not cured after a standard acute lymphoblastic leukemia therapeutic program: Adult acute lymphoblastic leukemia-94 trial. *Cancer, 109*, 2058–2067.

8. Thomas, D. A., Kantarjian, H., Smith, T. L., Koller, C., Cortes, J., O'Brien, S., et al. (1999). Primary refractory and relapsed adult acute lymphoblastic leukemia: Characteristics, treatment results, and prognosis with salvage therapy. *Cancer, 86*, 1216–1230.

9. Welborn, J. L. (1994). Impact of reinduction regimens for relapsed and refractory acute lymphoblastic leukemia in adults. *American Journal of Hematology, 45*, 341–344.

10. Bassan, R., Lerede, T., & Barbui, T. (1996). Strategies for the treatment of recurrent acute lymphoblastic leukemia in adults. *Haematologica, 81*, 20–36.

11. Hiddemann, W., Buchner, T., Heil, G., Schumacher, K., Diedrich, H., Maschmeyer, G., et al. (1990). Treatment of refractory acute lymphoblastic leukemia in adults with high dose cytosine arabinoside and mitoxantrone (HAM). *Leukemia, 4*, 637–640.

12. Kantarjian, H. M., Walters, R. L., Keating, M. J., Estey, E. H., O'Brien, S., Schachner, J., et al. (1990). Mitoxantrone and high-dose cytosine arabinoside for the treatment of refractory acute lymphocytic leukemia. *Cancer, 65*, 5–8.

13. Rivera, G., Aur, R. J., Dahl, G. V., Pratt, C. B., Wood, A., & Avery, T. L. (1980). Combined VM-26 and cytosine arabinoside in treatment of refractory childhood lymphocytic leukemia. *Cancer, 45*, 1284–1288.

14. Hoelzer, D. (1991). High-dose chemotherapy in adult acute lymphoblastic leukemia. *Seminars in Hematology, 28*, 84–89.

15. Elias, L., Shaw, M. T., & Raab, S. O. (1979). Reinduction therapy for adult acute leukemia with adriamycin, vincristine, and prednisone: A Southwest Oncology Group study. *Cancer Treatment Reports, 63*, 1413–1415.

16. Kantarjian, H. M., Walters, R. S., Keating, M. J., Barlogie, B., McCredie, K. B., & Freireich, E. J. (1989). Experience with vincristine, doxorubicin, and dexamethasone (VAD) chemotherapy in adults with refractory acute lymphocytic leukemia. *Cancer, 64*, 16–22.

17. Koller, C. A., Kantarjian, H. M., Thomas, D., O'Brien, S., Rios, M. B., Kornblau, S., et al. (1997). The hyper-CVAD regimen improves outcome in relapsed acute lymphoblastic leukemia. *Leukemia, 11*, 2039–2044.

18. Capizzi, R. L. (1993). Asparaginase, revisited. *Leukaemia & Lymphoma, 10*(Suppl), 147–150.

19. Aguayo, A., Cortes, J., Thomas, D., Pierce, S., Keating, M., & Kantarjian, H. (1999). Combination therapy with methotrexate, vincristine, polyethylene-glycol conjugated-asparaginase, and prednisone in the treatment of patients with refractory or recurrent acute lymphoblastic leukemia. *Cancer, 86*, 1203–1209.

20. Esterhay, R. J., Jr., Wiernik, P. H., Grove, W. R., Markus, S. D., & Wesley, M. N. (1982). Moderate dose methotrexate, vincristine, asparaginase, and dexamethasone for treatment of adult acute lymphocytic leukemia. *Blood, 59*, 334–345.

21. Terebelo, H. R., Anderson, K., Wiernik, P. H., Cuttner, J., Cooper, R. M., Faso, L., et al. (1986). Therapy of refractory adult acute lymphoblastic leukemia with vincristine and prednisone plus tandem methotrexate and L-asparaginase. Results of a Cancer and Leukemia Group B Study. *American Journal of Clinical Oncology, 9*, 411–415.

22. DeAngelo, D. J., Yu, D., Johnson, J. L., Coutre, S. E., Stone, R. M., Stopeck, A. T., et al. (2007). Nelarabine induces complete remissions in adults with relapsed or refractory T-lineage acute lymphoblastic leukemia or lymphoblastic lymphoma: Cancer and Leukemia Group B study 19801. *Blood, 109*, 5136–5142.

23. Jeha, S., Gandhi, V., Chan, K. W., McDonald, L., Ramirez, I., Madden, R., et al. (2004). Clofarabine, a novel nucleoside analog, is active in pediatric patients with advanced leukemia. *Blood, 103*, 784–789.

24. Gaynor, J., Chapman, D., Little, C., McKenzie, S., Miller, W., Andreeff, M., et al. (1988). A cause-specific hazard rate analysis of prognostic factors among 199 adults with acute lymphoblastic leukemia: The Memorial Hospital experience since 1969. *Journal of Clinical Oncology, 6*, 1014–1030.

25. Hoelzer, D., Thiel, E., Loffler, H., Buchner, T., Ganser, A., Heil, G., et al. (1988). Prognostic factors in a multicenter study for treatment of acute lymphoblastic leukemia in adults. *Blood, 71*, 123–131.

26. Mullighan, C. G., Phillips, L. A., Su, X., Ma, J., Miller, C. B., Shurtleff, S. A., et al. (2008). Genomic analysis of the clonal origins of relapsed acute lymphoblastic leukemia. *Science, 322*, 1377–1380.

27. Jeha, S., Gaynon, P. S., Razzouk, B. I., Franklin, J., Kadota, R., Shen, V., et al. (2006). Phase II study of clofarabine in pediatric patients with refractory or relapsed acute lymphoblastic leukemia. *Journal of Clinical Oncology, 24*, 1917–1923.

28. Kantarjian, H. M., Gandhi, V., Kozuch, P., Faderl, S., Giles, F., Cortes, J., et al. (2003). Phase I clinical and pharmacology study of clofarabine in patients with solid and hematologic cancers. *Journal of Clinical Oncology, 21*, 1167–1173.

29. Kantarjian, H., Gandhi, V., Cortes, J., Verstovsek, S., Du, M., Garcia-Manero, G., et al. (2003). Phase 2 clinical and pharmacologic study of clofarabine in patients with refractory or relapsed acute leukemia. *Blood, 102*, 2379–2386.

30. Faderl, S., Gandhi, V., O'Brien, S., Bonate, P., Cortes, J., Estey, E., et al. (2005). Results of a phase 1-2 study of clofarabine in combination with cytarabine (ara-C) in relapsed and refractory acute leukemias. *Blood, 105*, 940–947.

31. Faderl, S., Verstovsek, S., Cortes, J., Ravandi, F., Beran, M., Garcia-Manero, G., et al. (2006). Clofarabine and cytarabine combination as induction therapy for acute myeloid leukemia (AML) in patients 50 years of age or older. *Blood, 108*, 45–51.

32. Kisor, D. F., Plunkett, W., Kurtzberg, J., Mitchell, B., Hodge, J. P., Ernst, T., et al. (2000). Pharmacokinetics of nelarabine and 9-beta-D-arabinofuranosyl guanine in pediatric and adult patients during a phase I study of nelarabine for the treatment of refractory hematologic malignancies. *Journal of Clinical Oncology, 18*, 995–1003.

33. Kurtzberg, J., Ernst, T. J., Keating, M. J., Gandhi, V., Hodge, J. P., Kisor, D. F., et al. (2005). Phase I study of 506U78 administered on a consecutive 5-day schedule in children and adults with refractory hematologic malignancies. *Journal of Clinical Oncology, 23*, 3396–3403.

34. Berg, S. L., Blaney, S. M., Devidas, M., Lampkin, T. A., Murgo, A., Bernstein, M., et al. (2005). Phase II study of nelarabine (compound 506U78) in children and young adults with refractory T-cell malignancies: A report from the Children's Oncology Group. *Journal of Clinical Oncology, 23*, 3376–3382.

35. Gandhi, V., Kilpatrick, J. M., Plunkett, W., Ayres, M., Harman, L., Du, M., et al. (2005). A proof-of-principle pharmacokinetic, pharmacodynamic, and clinical study with purine nucleoside phosphorylase inhibitor immucillin-H (BCX-1777, forodesine). *Blood, 106*, 4253–4260.

36. Korycka, A., Blonski, J. Z., & Robak, T. (2007). Forodesine (BCX-1777, Immucillin H) – a new purine nucleoside analogue: Mechanism of action and potential clinical application. *Mini Reviews in Medicinal Chemistry, 7*, 976–983.

37. Furman, R. R., Gore, L., Ravandi, F., & Hoelzer, D. (2006). Forodesine IV (Bcx-1777) is clinically active in relapsed/refractory T-cell leukemia: Results of a Phase II Study (Interim Report) [abstract]. *Blood, 108*, 524a.

38. Duval, M., Suciu, S., Ferster, A., Rialland, X., Nelken, B., Lutz, P., et al. (2002). Comparison of Escherichia coli-asparaginase with Erwinia-asparaginase in the treatment of childhood lymphoid malignancies: Results of a randomized European Organisation for Research and Treatment of Cancer-Children's Leukemia Group phase 3 trial. *Blood, 99*, 2734–2739.

39. Rizzari, C., Zucchetti, M., Conter, V., Diomede, L., Bruno, A., Gavazzi, L., et al. (2000). L-asparagine depletion and L-asparaginase activity in children with acute lymphoblastic leukemia receiving i.m. or i.v. Erwinia C. or E. coli L-asparaginase as first exposure. *Annals of Oncology, 11*, 189–193.

40. Moghrabi, A., Levy, D. E., Asselin, B., Barr, R., Clavell, L., Hurwitz, C., et al. (2007). Results of the Dana-Farber Cancer Institute ALL Consortium Protocol 95-01 for children with acute lymphoblastic leukemia. *Blood, 109*, 896–904.

41. Wetzler, M., Sanford, B. L., Kurtzberg, J., DeOliveira, D., Frankel, S. R., Powell, B. L., et al. (2007). Effective asparagine depletion with pegylated asparaginase results in improved outcomes in adult acute lymphoblastic leukemia: Cancer and Leukemia Group B Study 9511. *Blood, 109*, 4164–4167.

42. Douer, D., Yampolsky, H., Cohen, L. J., Watkins, K., Levine, A. M., Periclou, A. P., et al. (2007). Pharmacodynamics and safety of intravenous pegaspargase during remission induction in adults aged 55 years or younger with newly diagnosed acute lymphoblastic leukemia. *Blood, 109*, 2744–2750.

43. O'Connor, O. A. (2006). Pralatrexate: An emerging new agent with activity in T-cell lymphomas. *Current Opinion in Oncology, 18*, 591–597.

44. O'Connor, O. A., Hamlin, P. A., Portlock, C., Moskowitz, C. H., Noy, A., Straus, D. J., et al. (2007). Pralatrexate, a novel class of antifol with high affinity for the reduced folate carrier-type 1, produces marked complete and durable remissions in a diversity of chemotherapy refractory cases of T-cell lymphoma. *British Journal Haematology, 139*, 425–428.

45. Giles, F., Rizzieri, D. A., George, S., Stock, W., Fontanilla, J., Choy, G. S., et al. (2006). A phase I study of Talvesta (Talotrexin) in relapsed or refractory leukemia or myelodysplastic syndrome [abstract]. *Blood, 108*, 556a.

46. Thomas, D. A., Faderl, S., O'Brien, S., Bueso-Ramos, C., Cortes, J., Garcia-Manero, G., et al. (2006). Chemoimmunotherapy with hyper-CVAD plus rituximab for the treatment of adult Burkitt and Burkitt-type lymphoma or acute lymphoblastic leukemia. *Cancer, 106*, 1569–1580.

47. Gokbuget, N., & Hoelzer, D. (2004). Treatment with monoclonal antibodies in acute lymphoblastic leukemia: Current knowledge and future prospects. *Annals of Hematology, 83*, 201–205.

48. Strauss, S. J., Morschhauser, F., Rech, J., Repp, R., Solal-Celigny, P., Zinzani, P. L., et al. (2006). Multicenter phase II trial of immunotherapy with the humanized anti-CD22 antibody, epratuzumab, in combination with rituximab, in refractory or recurrent non-Hodgkin's lymphoma. *Journal of Clinical Oncology, 24*, 3880–3886.

49. Rodig, S. J., Abramson, J. S., Pinkus, G. S., Treon, S. P., Dorfman, D. M., Dong, H. Y., et al. (2006). Heterogeneous CD52 expression among hematologic neoplasms: Implications for the use of alemtuzumab (CAMPATH-1H). *Clinical Cancer Research, 12*, 7174–7179.

50. Tibes, R., Keating, M. J., Ferrajoli, A., Wierda, W., Ravandi, F., Garcia-Manero, G., et al. (2006). Activity of alemtuzumab in patients with CD52-positive acute leukemia. *Cancer, 106*, 2645–2651.

51. Piccaluga, P. P., Martinelli, G., Malagola, M., Rondoni, M., Bianchini, M., Vigna, E., et al. (2004). Anti-leukemic and anti-GVHD effects of campath-1H in acute lymphoblastic leukemia relapsed after stem-cell transplantation. *Leukaemia & Lymphoma, 45*, 731–733.

52. Lozanski, G., Sanford, B., Mrozek, K., Edwards, C., Pearson, R., Bloomfield, C. D., et al. (2007). Quantitative measurement of CD52 expression and Alemtuzumab binding in Adult Acute Lymphoblastic Leukemia (ALL): Correlation with immunophenotype and cytogenetics in patients (Pts) enrolled on a Phase I/II trial from the Cancer and Leukemia Group B (CALGB 10102) [abstract]. *Blood, 10*, 704a.

53. Gelmon, K. A., Tolcher, A., Diab, A. R., Bally, M. B., Embree, L., Hudon, N., et al. (1999). Phase I study of liposomal vincristine. *Journal of Clinical Oncology, 17*, 697–705.

54. Sarris, A. H., Hagemeister, F., Romaguera, J., Rodriguez, M. A., McLaughlin, P., Tsimberidou, A. M., et al. (2000). Liposomal vincristine in relapsed non-Hodgkin's lymphomas: Early results of an ongoing phase II trial. *Annals of Oncology, 11*, 69–72.

55. Thomas, D. A., Sarris, A. H., Cortes, J., Faderl, S., O'Brien, S., Giles, F. J., et al. (2006). Phase II study of sphingosomal vincristine in patients with recurrent or refractory adult acute lymphocytic leukemia. *Cancer, 106*, 120–127.

56. Offidani, M., Corvatta, L., Centurioni, R., Leoni, F., Malerba, L., Mele, A., et al. (2003). High-dose daunorubicin as liposomal compound (Daunoxome) in elderly patients with acute lymphoblastic leukemia. *The Hematology Journal, 4*, 47–53.

57. Glantz, M. J., LaFollette, S., Jaeckle, K. A., Shapiro, W., Swinnen, L., Rozental, J. R., et al. (1999). Randomized trial of a slow-release versus a standard formulation of cytarabine for the intrathecal treatment of lymphomatous meningitis. *Journal of Clinical Oncology, 17*, 3110–3116.

58. Jabbour, E., O'Brien, S., Kantarjian, H., Garcia-Manero, G., Ferrajoli, A., Ravandi, F., et al. (2007). Neurologic complications associated with intrathecal liposomal cytarabine given prophylactically in combination with high-dose methotrexate and cytarabine to patients with acute lymphocytic leukemia. *Blood, 109*, 3214–3218.

59. Ottmann, O. G., Druker, B. J., Sawyers, C. L., Goldman, J. M., Reiffers, J., Silver, R. T., et al. (2002). A phase 2 study of imatinib in patients with relapsed or refractory Philadelphia chromosome-positive acute lymphoid leukemias. *Blood, 100*, 1965–1971.

60. Thomas, D. A., Faderl, S., Cortes, J., O'Brien, S., Giles, F. J., Kornblau, S. M., et al. (2004). Treatment of Philadelphia chromosome-positive acute lymphocytic leukemia with hyper-CVAD and imatinib mesylate. *Blood, 103*, 4396–4407.

61. Yanada, M., Takeuchi, J., Sugiura, I., Akiyama, H., Usui, N., Yagasaki, F., et al. (2006). High complete remission rate and promising outcome by combination of imatinib and chemotherapy for newly diagnosed BCR-ABL-positive acute lymphoblastic leukemia: A phase II study by the Japan Adult Leukemia Study Group. *Journal of Clinical Oncology, 24*, 460–466.

62. Carpenter, P. A., Snyder, D. S., Flowers, M. E., Sanders, J. E., Gooley, T. A., Martin, P. J., et al. (2007). Prophylactic administration of imatinib after hematopoietic cell transplantation for high-risk Philadelphia chromosome-positive leukemia. *Blood, 109*, 2791–2793.

63. Lee, S., Kim, D. W., Kim, Y. J., Chung, N. G., Kim, Y. L., Hwang, J. Y., et al. (2003). Minimal residual disease-based role of imatinib as a first-line interim therapy prior to allogeneic stem cell transplantation in Philadelphia chromosome-positive acute lymphoblastic leukemia. *Blood, 102*, 3068–3070.

64. Wassmann, B., Pfeifer, H., Goekbuget, N., Beelen, D. W., Beck, J., Stelljes, M., et al. (2006). Alternating versus concurrent schedules of imatinib and chemotherapy as front-line therapy for Philadelphia-positive acute lymphoblastic leukemia (Ph+ ALL). *Blood, 108*, 1469–1477.

65. Pfeifer, H., Wassmann, B., Pavlova, A., Wunderle, L., Oldenburg, J., Binckebanck, A., et al. (2007). Kinase domain mutations of BCR-ABL frequently precede imatinib-based therapy and give rise to relapse in patients with de novo Philadelphia-positive acute lymphoblastic leukemia (Ph+ ALL). *Blood, 110*, 727–734.

66. Ottmann, O. G., Larson, R. A., Kantarjian, H., le Coutre, P., Baccarani, M., Haque, A., et al. (2007). Nilotinib in patients with relapsed/refractory Philadelphia chromosome-positive acute lymphoblstic leukemia who are resistant or intolerant to imatinib [abstract]. *Blood, 118*, 828a.

67. Porrka, K., Simonsson, B., Dombret, H., Martinelli, G., Ottmann, O. G., Zhu, C., et al. (2007). Efficacy of dasatinib in patients with Philadelphia-chromosome-positive acute lymphoblastic leukemia who are resistant or intolerant to imatinib: 2-year follow-up data from START-L (CA180-015) [abstract]. *Blood, 118*, 826a.

68. Ravandi, F., Thomas, D., Kantarjian, H., Faderl, S., Koller, C., Brown, D., et al. (2007). Phase II study of combination of the HyperCVAD regimen with dasatinib in patients with Philadelphia chromosome (Ph) or BCR-ABL positive Acute Lymphoblastic Leukemia (ALL) and Lymphoid Blast Phase Chronic Myeloid Leukemia (CML-LB). *Blood, 110*, 828a.

69. Gambacorti-Passerini, C., Kantarjian, H., Bruemmendorf, T., Martinelli, G., Baccarani, M., Fischer, T., et al. (2007). Bosutinib (SKI-606) demonstrates clinical activity and is well tolerated among patients with AP and BP CML and Ph+ ALL [abstract]. *Blood, 118*, 225a.

70. Kantarjian, H. M., Cortes, J., le Coutre, P., Nagler, A., Pinilla, J., Hochhaus, A., et al. (2007). A phase I study of INNO-406 in patients with advanced Philadelphia (Ph+) chromosome-positive leukemias who are resistant or intolerant to imatinib and second generation tyrosine kinase inhibitors [abstract]. *Blood, 118*, 144a.
71. Leis, J. F., Stepan, D. E., Curtin, P. T., Ford, J. M., Peng, B., Schubach, S., et al. (2004). Central nervous system failure in patients with chronic myelogenous leukemia lymphoid blast crisis and Philadelphia chromosome positive acute lymphoblastic leukemia treated with imatinib (STI-571). *Leukaemia & Lymphoma, 45*, 695–698.
72. Pfeifer, H., Wassmann, B., Hofmann, W. K., Komor, M., Scheuring, U., Bruck, P., et al. (2003). Risk and prognosis of central nervous system leukemia in patients with Philadelphia chromosome-positive acute leukemias treated with imatinib mesylate. *Clinical Cancer Research, 9*, 4674–4681.
73. Armstrong, S. A., Staunton, J. E., Silverman, L. B., Pieters, R., den Boer, M. L., Minden, M. D., et al. (2002). MLL translocations specify a distinct gene expression profile that distinguishes a unique leukemia. *Nature Genetics, 30*, 41–47.
74. DeAngelo, D. J., Stone, R. M., Heaney, M. L., Nimer, S. D., Paquette, R. L., Klisovic, R. B., et al. (2006). Phase 1 clinical results with tandutinib (MLN518), a novel FLT3 antagonist, in patients with acute myelogenous leukemia or high-risk myelodysplastic syndrome: Safety, pharmacokinetics, and pharmacodynamics. *Blood, 108*, 3674–3681.
75. Smith, B. D., Levis, M., Beran, M., Giles, F., Kantarjian, H., Berg, K., et al. (2004). Single-agent CEP-701, a novel FLT3 inhibitor, shows biologic and clinical activity in patients with relapsed or refractory acute myeloid leukemia. *Blood, 103*, 3669–3676.
76. Stone, R. M., DeAngelo, D. J., Klimek, V., Galinsky, I., Estey, E., Nimer, S. D., et al. (2005). Patients with acute myeloid leukemia and an activating mutation in FLT3 respond to a small-molecule FLT3 tyrosine kinase inhibitor, PKC412. *Blood, 105*, 54–60.
77. Weng, A. P., Ferrando, A. A., Lee, W., Morris, J Pt, Silverman, L. B., Sanchez-Irizarry, C., et al. (2004). Activating mutations of NOTCH1 in human T cell acute lymphoblastic leukemia. *Science, 306*, 269–271.
78. DeAngelo, D. J., Stone, R. M., Silverman, L. B., Stock, W., Attar, E. C., Fearen, I., et al. (2006). A phase I clinical trial of the notch inhibitor MK-0752 in patients with T-cell acute lymphoblastic leukemia/lymphoma (T-ALL) and other leukemias [abstract]. *Journal of Clinical Oncology, 24*, 357a.
79. Real, P. J., Tosello, V., Ai, W., Palomero, T., Sulis, M. L., Castillo, M., et al. (2007). Inhibition of NOTCH1 signaling reverses glucocorticoid resistance in T-ALL [abstract]. *Blood, 110*, 52a.
80. Graux, C., Cools, J., Melotte, C., Quentmeier, H., Ferrando, A., Levine, R., et al. (2004). Fusion of NUP214 to ABL1 on amplified episomes in T-cell acute lymphoblastic leukemia. *Nature Genetics, 36*, 1084–1089.
81. Paciucci, P. A., Ohnuma, T., Cuttner, J., Silver, R. T., & Holland, J. F. (1983). Mitoxantrone in acute lymphoblastic leukemia. *Cancer Treatment Reviews, 10 Suppl B*, 65–68.
82. Paciucci, P. A., Keaveney, C., Cuttner, J., & Holland, J. F. (1987). Mitoxantrone, vincristine, and prednisone in adults with relapsed or primarily refractory acute lymphocytic leukemia and terminal deoxynucleotidyl transferase positive blastic phase chronic myelocytic leukemia. *Cancer Research, 47*, 5234–5237.
83. Peterson, B. A., & Bloomfield, C. D. (1978). High-dose methotrexate for the remission induction of refractory adult acute lymphocytic leukemia. *Medical and Pediatric Oncology, 5*, 79–84.
84. Ryan, D. H., Bickers, J. N., Vial, R. H., Hussein, K., Bottomley, R., Hewlett, J. S., et al. (1980). Doxorubicin and ifosfamide combination chemotherapy in previously treated acute leukemia in adults: A Southwest Oncology Group pilot study. *Cancer Treatment Reports, 64*, 869–872.
85. Bassan, R., Cornelli, P. E., Battista, R., Terzi, F., Buelli, M., Rambaldi, A., et al. (1992). Intensive retreatment of adults and children with acute lymphoblastic leukemia. *Hematological Oncology, 10*, 105–110.
86. Bostrom, B., Woods, W. G., Nesbit, M. E., Krivit, W., Kersey, J., Weisdorf, D., et al. (1987). Successful reinduction of patients with acute lymphoblastic leukemia who relapse following bone marrow transplantation. *Journal of Clinical Oncology, 5*, 376–381.
87. Woodruff, R. K., Lister, T. A., Paxton, A. M., Whitehouse, J. M., & Malpas, J. S. (1978). Combination chemotherapy for haematological relapse in adult acute lymphoblastic leukaemia (ALL). *American Journal of Hematology, 4*, 173–177.
88. Yap, B. S., McCredie, K. B., Keating, M. J., Bodey, G. P., & Freireich, E. J. (1981). Asparaginase and methotrexate combination chemotherapy in relapsed acute lymphoblastic leukemia in adults. *Cancer Treatment Reports, 65*(Suppl 1), 83–87.
89. Brochstein, J. A., Kernan, N. A., Groshen, S., Cirrincione, C., Shank, B., Emanuel, D., et al. (1987). Allogeneic bone marrow transplantation after hyperfractionated total-body irradiation and cyclophosphamide in children with acute leukemia. *The New England Journal of Medicine, 317*, 1618–1624.
90. Zwaan, F. E., Hermans, J., Barrett, A. J., & Speck, B. (1984). Bone marrow transplantation for acute lymphoblastic leukaemia: A survey of the European Group for Bone Marrow Transplantation (E.G.B.M.T.). *British Journal Haematology, 58*, 33–42.
91. Sanders, J. E., Thomas, E. D., Buckner, C. D., & Doney, K. (1987). Marrow transplantation for children with acute lymphoblastic leukemia in second remission. *Blood, 70*, 324–326.

92. Barrett, A. J., Horowitz, M. M., Pollock, B. H., Zhang, M. J., Bortin, M. M., Buchanan, G. R., et al. (1994). Bone marrow transplants from HLA-identical siblings as compared with chemotherapy for children with acute lymphoblastic leukemia in a second remission. *The New England Journal of Medicine, 331*, 1253–1258.
93. Uderzo, C., Valsecchi, M. G., Bacigalupo, A., Meloni, G., Messina, C., Polchi, P., et al. (1995). Treatment of childhood acute lymphoblastic leukemia in second remission with allogeneic bone marrow transplantation and chemotherapy: Ten-year experience of the Italian Bone Marrow Transplantation Group and the Italian Pediatric Hematology Oncology Association. *Journal of Clinical Oncology, 13*, 352–358.
94. Weisdorf, D. J., Billett, A. L., Hannan, P., Ritz, J., Sallan, S. E., Steinbuch, M., et al. (1997). Autologous versus unrelated donor allogeneic marrow transplantation for acute lymphoblastic leukemia. *Blood, 90*, 2962–2968.
95. Saarinen-Pihkala, U. M., Gustafsson, G., Ringden, O., Heilmann, C., Glomstein, A., Lonnerholm, G., et al. (2001). No disadvantage in outcome of using matched unrelated donors as compared with matched sibling donors for bone marrow transplantation in children with acute lymphoblastic leukemia in second remission. *Journal of Clinical Oncology, 19*, 3406–3414.

Chapter 18
Allogeneic Stem Cell Transplantation for Acute Lymphoblastic Leukaemia in Adults

David I. Marks

Introduction

The results of all therapies for adults with acute lymphoblastic leukaemia remain disappointing. Five-year survival of the 1,929 intensively treated patients in the UKALL XII/ECOG 2993 study was 39% [1]. Chemotherapy is toxic and prolonged; this study reported a 12% 2-year non-relapse mortality in patients without donors. There is a belief that chemotherapy cannot be pushed much further. Younger (<25–30 years) patients are being treated on more intensive "paediatric" protocols with more asparaginase but there are no mature multicentre data available to evaluate the efficacy of this approach. B cell antibodies are being pursued by a number of groups, nelarabine is being evaluated upfront for T cell disease and the early experience with forodesine looks promising but increasing the doses or intensity of the standard drugs seems unlikely to produce significant survival benefits. There has been better definition of adverse risk factors using cytogenetics [2] in recent times, enabling us to target patients likely to fail chemotherapy with our most aggressive therapies. The 5-year overall survival of patients with t(4;11), low hypodiploidy/near triploidy or >5 abnormalities were 24%, 22%, and 28%, respectively, making these patients valid targets for more aggressive approaches. In addition, a major German study of minimal residual disease (MRD) at nine timepoints in the first year of ALL therapy has found that patients with molecular MRD detectable at week 16 have a very poor outcome (12% vs 66%) [3] making these patients logical candidates for trials of different approaches including upfront allografting.

Rationale and the Graft Versus Leukaemia Effect

Allogeneic stem cell transplantation allows considerably higher doses of chemoradiotherapy to be administered enabling a greater initial leukaemic cell kill. However, careful examination of the evidence reveals an important graft versus leukaemia (GvL) effect. Given that this was the first disease in which a GvL effect was described [4], and given the multiple studies showing a reduced relapse rate in allograft patients it is surprising that many haematologists and even transplanters deny or underrate this effect.

Harnessing the allogeneic GvL effect and using the positive benefits of acute and chronic graft-versus-host disease (GVHD) are essential in curing the high-risk patient or patients with positive

D.I. Marks (✉)
Oncology Day Beds Bristol Children's Hospital, University Hospitals of Bristol,
Upper Maudlin Street, Bristol, UK BS2 8BJ
e-mail: David.Marks@UHBristol.nhs.uk

A.S. Advani and H.M. Lazarus (eds.), *Adult Acute Lymphocytic Leukemia*, Contemporary Hematology,   297
DOI 10.1007/978-1-60761-707-5_18, © Springer Science+Business Media, LLC 2011

MRD prior to transplant. Passweg and colleagues [5] showed 10 years ago that patients with acute, chronic, or both acute and chronic GVHD had a 2.5-fold reduction in relapse risk on multivariate analysis (RR = 0.40).

Other studies have shown that chronic GVHD has more of an effect than acute GVHD. Some forms of T cell depletion (TCD) prevent grade II–IV acute GVHD, but there may still be a significant incidence of chronic GVHD; this may be a strategy worth further investigation.

Further evidence will come from trials of reduced intensity conditioning (RIC) allografting where there is greater reliance on the GvL effect. There are no very large-scale mature data available but the Center for International BMT Research (CIBMTR) has recently analysed the outcomes of 93 patients [6].

Conditioning Regimens

There are no randomised studies comparing conditioning regimens and many large studies have missed opportunities to compare regimens. There are very few data on total body irradiation (TBI)-containing regimens and survival data do not support their use. The City of Hope and Stanford groups have a 20-year experience with etoposide (60 mg/kg) and 13.2 Gy of total body irradiation given in nine fractions and have excellent survival data [7]. Marks and colleagues [8] from the CIBMTR compared this regimen with standard cyclophosphamide and TBI. Cyclophosphamide and 12 Gy of TBI produced markedly inferior survival compared to etoposide containing or higher dose TBI regimens. However, if >13 Gy TBI was given, etoposide/TBI was not superior to cyclophosphamide/TBI. Transplant-related mortality was (perhaps surprisingly) not higher in the etoposide/TBI arm although this is undoubtedly a more toxic regimen. The issue of mucositis will be discussed later in this chapter.

Sibling Allografting in First Remission

There are methodological difficulties establishing the efficacy of allograft in adults with ALL (Table 18.1). A simple comparison of outcome in patients who received an allograft with those who did not would not suffice as the allograft group are on average fitter and had to survive a certain time in remission in order to have an allograft. To overcome these biases, donor versus no-donor analyses were devised. These too are flawed in that they may underestimate the potential benefit of allograft as many patients with matched sibling donors do not proceed to allograft and indeed in many it was never the intention to do so. Nonetheless, they have become widely accepted, and if they do show an advantage, one can be confident that such a difference exists [9].

Sibling allografting has long been established as the therapy of choice in high-risk ALL (Hoelzer criteria [10]). Two French studies compared allografting with chemotherapy and autografting, and there were significant differences in overall survival.

Table 18.1 Studies comparing sibling allografting in CR1 acute lymphoblastic leukaemia with chemotherapy and/or autologous SCT

First Author	Patient no	Donor survival	No donor survival	p Value
Attal [27]	572	46% at 5 years	31%	0.04
Hunault [28][a]	198	75% at 5 years	40%	0.027
Goldstone [1][b]	804	54% at 5 years	44%	0.02

[a] Eligibility for randomisation: age > 35, WBC >30, non-T cell, poor risk cytogenetics, no CR at day 35
[b] Donor versus no donor analysis (chemotherapy only – this arm was superior to autograft)

The results of the recent very large international ALL study have provided clarity [1]. All patients <50 years who were fit for transplant and had a matched sibling donor were eligible to have an allograft. It was a donor versus no donor analysis, which is good at avoiding some known biases towards transplant but which may underestimate the positive effect of allograft. Survival was superior in the donor arm compared with patients without a donor. Subsequently, when chemotherapy was shown to be superior to autografting (in a randomised comparison), a revised comparison was made between patients with donors and chemotherapy-treated patients; the donor arm was still about 10% superior. However, this was not the case in the high-risk group, most of whom where >35 years. The donor arm had 6% better survival at 5 years, but the difference was not significant. There was still excellent protection against relapse (35% vs 67%) but survival was not improved because of a high non-relapse mortality (29% at 1 year and 39% at 2 years). The investigators concluded that if the allogeneic effect could be harnessed more safely in this group, allograft in high-risk patients with ALL in CR1 might be worth pursuing.

The transplant-related mortality (TRM) in low-risk (younger) patients was a disappointing 20% at 2 years; improving this should also be the focus of research efforts.

Unrelated Donor (UD) SCT in First Remission

Encouraging results of sibling allografting and studies showing that UD SCT can produce similar results to sibling allografts for leukaemia have led to many investigating the role of UD SCT in high-risk CR1 ALL (Table 18.2). Marks and colleagues [11] from the CIBMTR recently described 169 adult patients with a median age of 33 years who underwent UD SCT. One hundred and fifty-seven were high risk and 93 had multiple high-risk factors. Overall survival was 40%. Multivariate analysis showed that the following factors affected survival: white cell count at diagnosis, HLA mismatch, >8 weeks to attain CR1 and TCD. This latter finding was a surprise and as there were only 16 patients with TCD (with a variety of techniques) it cannot be regarded as a definite finding.

Patel and colleagues have analysed 55 patients (median age 25 years) who had T-depleted UD SCT for high-risk ALL in CR1 mainly using in vivo alemtuzamab [12] (Patel B et al., submitted). About half of these patients were taken out of UKALL XII to have an "off-protocol" allograft. Survival was an excellent 59% at 3 years, and there was a clear plateau with no events after 2 years. The incidences of grade II–IV, grade III–IV, and chronic GVHD were 25%, 7%, and 22%, respectively. It is difficult to compare the two series but the UK series had a low TRM (19%) and good survival, albeit in a younger population.

Kiehl and colleagues [13] from Germany reported 97 patients, 87 of whom received TCD, who had a TRM of 31% and grades III–IV acute GVHD in only 15%. On a similar note, Dahlke and colleagues [14] compared sibling and UD allografts in 38 and 46 patients in CR1, respectively, and found that survival was the same in the two groups (44% vs 46%, p = NS).

UD SCT clearly has a growing role in this disease. The promising results from (albeit) limited data and the finding that survival is now similar to allografts with sibling donors make it reasonable

Table 18.2 Studies of the outcome of unrelated donor stem cell transplantation for adult patients with acute lymphoblastic leukaemia in CR1

First Author	Patient no	Age	Survival	TRM	Grade 2–4 acute/chronic%
Marks [11]	169	33 years	39%	42%	50/43
Dahlke [14]	38	23 years	44%	NK	36/23
Kiehl [13]	45	29 years	45%	NK	33/NK

NK not known or not specifically stated

Table 18.3 Studies of the outcome of reduced intensity conditioning allogeneic stem cell transplantation for adult ALL

First Author	Patient no	Sibs/UDs%	CR1/CR2/ other%	Regimens	Survival
Mohty [15][a]	97	67/33	29/26/45	Various	21% at 2 years
Martino [29]	27	56/44	15/41/44	Various	31% at 2 years
Massenkeil [30]	9	NK	NK	Flu/Bu/ATG	40% at 3 years
Forman [16]	22	33/67	48/19/33	Flu/Mel	77% at 1 year
Hamaki [31]	33	20/13	19/0/14	Flu/Bu/ATG	30% EFS 1 year
Marks [6]	93	30/63	55/38	various	38%

Reported transplant-related mortality ranged from 4% to 27%
Flu fludarabine, *Bu* busulfan, *ATG* antithymocyte globulin, *Mel* melphalan, *UD* unrelated donor
[a]41% Philadelphia positive. Survival was 52% at 2 years if patient was in CR1

to perform prospective trials of this therapeutic modality. However, patients should be entered in studies so that we learn how to optimise this procedure and the data do not support the use of unrelated donor SCT as standard therapy for standard-risk ALL in CR1.

The Role of RIC Allografting

We have been slow to investigate this transplant modality in adult ALL (Table 18.3). The mistaken notion that the GvL effect was less important in this disease and the view that conditioning regimens had to contain TBI may have led to this attitude. Consequently, it has initially been performed in patients who could not tolerate myeloablative conditioning because of comorbidity or in elderly patients who have little prospect of cure with chemotherapy.

There are no large-scale prospective studies of RIC allografting in this disease. The data we have are relatively small retrospective series of patients with various stem cell sources and heterogeneous disease states.

The largest series from the European Blood and Marrow Transplantation Group (EBMT), reported in 2008 by Mohty and colleagues [15] describes 97 patients, 70 of whom had died at the time of analysis. Two thirds received stem cells from sibling donor and one third from unrelated donors. Survival at 2 years was 21% in the whole group but promisingly exceeded 50% in those with high-risk disease. Patients in CR1 did significantly better with 52% surviving disease free at 2 years. Patients with chronic GVHD had superior OS (RR 0.4, $p<0.01$). There were a variety of RIC regimens used (39% had ATG and 24% had a low-dose TBI containing regimen), but these are not precisely described in the paper.

A smaller series using a uniform protocol (fludarabine and melphalan) was described by the City of Hope group using sibling donors and unrelated donors [16]. Given the variable disease status and risk status of the group, the TRM was low (10%) and survival of 70% at 1 year was promising. Longer follow-up is needed.

Allografting for Relapsed Disease

Selected series have produced some reasonable results for allografting in second complete remission using sibling or unrelated donors. However, the situation in a multicentre setting is less optimistic. Fielding and colleagues [17] described the outcome of 607 adult ALL patients who relapsed and only 7% of these patients survive at 5 years. Forty-two patients had matched sibling allografts and survival at 3 years was 23%. Even more disappointingly 65 patients received stem cells from unrelated donors and only 16% survived at 3 years.

Only two thirds of patients who relapse will achieve CR2 and many will relapse before an appropriate donor is found. I strongly recommend doing a preliminary unrelated donor search in all intensively treated adult ALL patients without sibling donors at diagnosis and referral of the patient to a specialist centre the day the patient is found to have relapsed. More studies need to focus on relapsed ALL but finding donors more rapidly is likely to improve outcome. The Fielding study also shows that allografting (our best antileukaemic therapy) cannot currently be reserved for relapse.

Donor Lymphocyte Infusions

Although there is a pronounced GvL effect for ALL, donor lymphocyte infusion (DLI) has been a relatively ineffective therapy when given for overt relapse of ALL, post allograft. This is likely to be due to the rapid pace of the disease. Kolb and Mackinnon [18] reported the follow-up results of an EBMT study. Only 2 of 22 patients with relapsed ALL responded to DLI without prior chemotherapy. In an American registry study, 2 of 15 patients obtained CR with DLI. The reported 10% response rate may be due to underreporting of unsuccessful cases, and most transplanters do not give DLI as sole therapy for relapse. A recent comprehensive review by Tomblyn and Lazarus describes the data from various small studies [19] and lead the authors to conclude that no firm recommendations can be made on the basis of these (limited) data. However, further studies of DLI after induction chemotherapy or as part of a second transplant strategy are warranted.

A more promising preemptive approach has been followed by German investigators in paediatric patients. In 163 patients who had allografts from a variety of stem cell sources, Bader and colleagues [20] showed that the development of mixed chimerism (defined as a >5% shift in whole blood chimerism) was in the absence of intervention and was associated with universal relapse. Chimerism was monitored very intensively in their study, weekly in the first year. Their intervention was a program of escalating DLI, which resulted in the survival of about a third of such patients. Acute GVHD (of some grade) were seen in 31% of such patients. This approach deserves evaluation in an adult population. Some RIC regimens result in a high incidence of mixed chimerism, and it is standard practice to correct this mixed chimerism with DLI but there are no data available to assess if this approach reduces relapse.

Allografting for Refractory Disease

About 10% of adult patients with ALL are refractory to primary chemotherapy and a very small percentage of these patients can be cured by allogeneic SCT either with a sibling or unrelated donor. Similarly, some patients who relapse fail to respond to reinduction chemotherapy. These patients are often extremely unwell due to prolonged neutropenia and severe infections. The author knows of few such patients who have survived and prefers to attempt to achieve remission with novel agents such as clofarabine, nelarabine, or monoclonal antibodies prior to a curative allograft.

Haploidentical and Cord Blood Transplantation for High-Risk ALL

Patients with ALL who have a low chance of cure with chemotherapy but have no sibling or suitably matched unrelated donor are candidates for allografts with haploidentical or cord blood stem cells. The data are small scale and heterogeneous and come from a small number of centres of excellence.

Aversa described 62 patients with ALL transplanted in remission who had 25% event-free survival [21]. TRM was substantial but there was no chronic GVHD so longer term quality of life was good.

Survival data for patients purely with ALL cannot be gleaned from the reports from Henslee Downey's group in South Carolina, but TRM was seen in 15 of 49 patients and acute and chronic GVHD in about 15%.

The data for cord blood transplant are as limited. Many series do not separate this disease from other diseases. Rocha [22] on behalf of Eurocord reported 98 patients (34% in CR1) who achieved 36% 2-year survival and a 26% incidence of grade 2–4 acute GVHD and 30% incidence of chronic GVHD. The Minneapolis group [23] have some excellent survival data in small numbers of adults with ALL but these data cannot be used to make decisions for individual patients. Further larger-scale studies are required and infection and slow engraftment remain major hurdles.

Other Issues and Supportive Care

Central Nervous System (CNS) Disease

Patients with CNS disease at diagnosis have an inferior outcome to those without CNS disease (29% vs 39% survival, $p=0.03$). However, they can achieve long-term disease-free survival with a sibling allograft. In the Lazarus et al. study [24], 11 of 25 such patients remain alive 21–102 months post allograft. The issue of whether the dose of cranial radiotherapy that is part of TBI is sufficient for control of CNS disease remains uncertain. CNS prophylaxis is a major issue for RIC allografting and additional therapy (such as post transplant intrathecal injections) should be contemplated although there is no evidence to inform practice.

Palifermin

Grade 4 mucositis is a major problem with VP/TBI allografts with cyclosporin and minidose methotrexate prophylaxis. Typical patients have severe symptoms requiring prolonged narcotic analgesia and frank bleeding from the mouth. This may prevent the delivery the four doses of methotrexate, which in turn may affect the chance of acute and chronic GVHD. Some investigators have used mycophenolate mofetil but data showing this to be as effective as methotrexate are lacking. Palifermin (keratinocyte growth factor 1), which has level one evidence after chemoradiotherapy for autologous SCT has been the subject of phase I studies [25].

The Future

Allografting for adults >40 years with ALL is currently too toxic and the TRM is too high. Exploration of RIC in clinical trials will determine whether this is a viable approach and will answer the biologic question of how important conditioning is in obtaining a negative MRD status before the effects of an allogeneic GvL effect. It seems likely that patients with positive MRD prior to transplant and those with resistant disease will not be cured by less intensity conditioning. The next major combined UK and USA trial will examine the role of monoclonal B cell antibodies and will prospectively test RIC allografting in older patients. TBI conditioning may be made less toxic by drugs such as palifermin and velafermin and this may improve outcome (Table 18.4).

Selecting the right patients for allogeneic SCT is also a major issue. Gene profiling may add to our abilities to discriminate using the existing prognostic factors. Further trials are needed to determine

Table 18.4 Likely future developments

Better selection of patients (who will benefit from allograft)
Increased role for reduced intensity allografting, particularly in older patients
Expanded role for alternative donor allografting including cord blood SCT
Recombinant keratinocyte growth factors to mitigate toxicity of TBI

if allografting can overcome the adverse prognostic impact of biologic factors such as a high WCC and adverse cytogenetics. If allografting can do this, the use of allografting will expand if UD allografting can be safely performed on a multicentre basis. Careful matching will be essential if TRM is to be kept low [26]. If it can, then there will be exploration of the use of cord blood as a stem cell source, but again, this is mainly performed in certain specialist centres and there are no data to suggest that it can safely be "rolled out" to large numbers of transplant centres worldwide.

References

1. Goldstone, A. H., Richards, S. M., Lazarus, H. M., Tallman, M. S., Buck, G., Fielding, A. K., et al. (2008). In adults with standard-risk acute lymphoblastic leukemia, the greatest benefit is achieved from a matched sibling allogeneic transplantation in first complete remission, and an autologous transplantation is less effective than conventional consolidation/maintenance chemotherapy in all patients: final results of the International ALL Trial (MRC UKALL XII/ECOG E2993). *Blood, 111*, 1827–1833.
2. Moorman, A. V., Harrison, C. J., Buck, G. A., Richards, S. M., Secker-Walker, L. M., Martineau, M., et al. (2007). Adult Leukaemia Working Party, Medical Research Council/National Cancer Research Institute. Karyotype is an independent prognostic factor in adult acute lymphoblastic leukemia (ALL): Analysis of cytogenetic data from patients treated on the Medical Research Council (MRC) UKALLXII/Eastern Cooperative Oncology Group (ECOG) 2993 trial. *Blood, 109*, 3189–3197.
3. Brüggemann, M., Raff, T., Flohr, T., Gökbuget, N., Nakao, M., Droese, J., et al. (2006). German Multicenter Study Group for Adult Acute Lymphoblastic Leukemia. Clinical significance of minimal residual disease quantification in adult patients with standard-risk acute lymphoblastic leukemia. *Blood, 107*, 1116–23.
4. Thomas, E. D., Buckner, C. D., Clift, R. A., Fefer, A., Johnson, F. L., Neiman, P. E., et al. (1979 Sep 13). Marrow transplantation for acute nonlymphoblastic leukemia in first remission. *The New England Journal of Medicine, 301*(11), 597–599.
5. Passweg, J. R., Cahn, J.-Y., Tiberghien, P., Vowels, M. R., Camitta, B. M., Gale, R. P., et al. (1998). Graft versus leukaemia effect in T-lineage and cALLa + (B-lineage) acute lymphoblastic leukaemia. *Bone Marrow Transplantation, 21*, 153–158.
6. Marks, D. I., Wang, T., Pérez, W. S., et al. (Apr 2010). The outcome of full intensity and reduced intensity conditioning matched sibling or unrelated donor (URD) transplantation in adults with Philadelphia chromosome negative acute lymphoblastic leukemia (PH- ALL) in first and second complete remission (CR1 and CR2). *Blood.* doi:10.1182/blood-2010-01-264077.
7. Snyder, D. S., Chao, N. J., Amylon, M. D., Taguchi, J., Long, G. D., Negrin, R. S., et al. (1993). Fractionated total body irradiation and high-dose etoposide as a preparatory regimen for bone marrow transplantation for 99 patients with acute leukemia in first complete remission. *Blood, 82*, 2920–2928.
8. Marks, D. I., Forman, S. J., Blume, K. G., Perez, W. S., Weisdorf, D. J., Keating, A., et al. (2006). A comparison of cyclophosphamide and total body irradiation with etoposide and total body irradiation as conditioning regimens for patients undergoing sibling allografting for acute lymphoblastic leukemia in first or second complete remission. *Biology of Blood and Marrow Transplantation, 12*, 438–453.
9. Frassoni, F. (2000). Randomised studies in acute myeloid leukaemia: The double truth. *Bone Marrow Transplantation, 25*, 471–473.
10. Hoelzer, D., Thiel, E., Loffler, T., et al. (1988). Prognostic factors in a multicentric study for treatment of acute lymphoblastic leukaemia in adults. *Blood, 71*, 123–131.
11. Marks, D. I., Pérez, W. S., He, W., Zhang, M. J., Bishop, M. R., Bolwell, B. J., et al. (2008). Unrelated donor transplants in adults with Philadelphia-negative acute lymphoblastic leukaemia in first complete remission. *Blood, 112*, 426–434.
12. Patel, B., Kirkland, K. E., Szydlo, R., Pearce, R. M., Clark, R. E., Craddock, C., et al. (2009). Favorable outcomes with alemtuzumab-conditioned unrelated donor stem cell transplantation in adults with high-risk Philadelphia chromosome-negative acute lymphoblastic leukemia in first complete remission. *Haematologica, 94*, 1399–1406.

13. Kiehl, M. G., Kraut, L., Schwerdtfeger, R., et al. (2004). Outcome of allogeneic hematopoietic stem-cell transplantation in adult patients with acute lymphoblastic leukemia: no difference in related compared with unrelated transplant in first complete remission. *Journal of Clinical Oncology, 22,* 2816–2825.
14. Dahlke, J., Kröger, N., Zabelina, T., Ayuk, F., Fehse, N., Wolschke, C., et al. (2006). Comparable results in patients with acute lymphoblastic leukemia after related and unrelated stem cell transplantation. *Bone Marrow Transplantation, 37,* 155–163.
15. Mohty, M., Labopin, M., Rezzi, et al. (2008). Reduced intensity conditioning allogeneic stem cell transplantation for adults with acute lymphoblastic leukaemia: A retrospective study of the European BMT group. *Haematologica, 93,* 303–306.
16. Stein, A., O'Donnell, M., Parker, P., Nademanee, A., Falk, P., Rosenthal, J., et al. (2007). Reduced-intensity stem cell transplantation for high-risk acute lymphoblastic leukemia. *Biology of Blood and Marrow Transplantation, 13,* 134.
17. Fielding, A. K., Richards, S. M., Chopra, R., Lazarus, H. M., Litzow, M., Buck, G., Durrant, I. J., Luger, S. M., Marks, D. I., McMillan, A. K., Tallman, M. S., Rowe, J. M, & Goldstone, A. H. (2006 Oct 10). Outcome of 609 adults after relapse of acute lymphoblastic leukaemia (ALL); an MRC UKALL12/ECOG 2993 study. *Blood* [Epub ahead of print].
18. Kolb, H.-J., & Mackinnon, S. (2004). Adoptive cellular immunotherapy for treatment or prevention of relapse of hematologic malignancy posttransplant, Chapter 65. In K. Atkinson et al. (Eds.), *Clinical bone marrow and blood stem cell transplantation* (3rd ed., pp. 992–1008). Cambridge: Cambridge University Press.
19. Tomblyn, M., Lazarus, HM. (2008 Aug 18). Donor lymphocyte infusions: The long and winding road: How should it be traveled? *Bone Marrow Transplantation* [Epub ahead of print]
20. Bader, P., Kreyenberg, H., Hoelle, W., Dueckers, G., Handgretinger, R., Lang, P., et al. (2004). Increasing mixed chimerism is an important prognostic factor for unfavorable outcome in children with acute lymphoblastic leukemia after allogeneic stem-cell transplantation: possible role for pre-emptive immunotherapy? *Journal of Clinical Oncology, 22,* 1696–1705.
21. Marks, D. I., Aversa, F., & Lazarus, H. (2006). Alternative Donors Transplants For Adult Acute Lymphoblastic Leukaemia: A Comparison of the Three Major Options. *Bone Marrow Transplantation, 38,* 467–475.
22. Rocha, V., Labopin, M., Sanz, G., Arcese, W., Schwerdtfeger, R., Bosi, A., et al. (2004). Transplants of umbilical-cord blood or bone marrow from unrelated donors in adults with acute leukemia. *The New England Journal of Medicine, 351,* 2276–2285.
23. Brunstein, C. G., Barker, J. N., Weisdorf, D. J., DeFor, T. E., Miller, J. S., Blazar, B. R., et al. (2007). Umbilical cord blood transplantation after nonmyeloablative conditioning: impact on transplantation outcomes in 110 adults with hematologic disease. *Blood, 110,* 3064–3370.
24. Lazarus, H. M., Richards, S. M., Chopra, R., Litzow, M. R., Burnett, A. K., Wiernik, P. H., et al. (2006). Medical Research Council (MRC)/National Cancer Research Institute (NCRI) Adult Leukaemia Working Party of the United Kingdom and the Eastern Cooperative Oncology Group. Central nervous system involvement in adult acute lymphoblastic leukemia at diagnosis: results from the international ALL trial MRC UKALL XII/ECOG E2993. *Blood, 108,* 465–472.
25. Spielberger, R., Stiff, P., Bensinger, W., Gentile, T., Weisdorf, D., Kewalramani, T., et al. (2004). Palifermin for oral mucositis after intensive therapy for hematologic cancers. *The New England Journal of Medicine, 351,* 2590–2598.
26. Lee, S. J., Klein, J., Haagenson, M., et al. (2007). High-resolution donor-recipient HLA matching contributes to the success of unrelated donor marrow transplantation. *Blood, 110,* 4576–4583.
27. Attal, M., Blaise, D., Marit, G., Payen, C., Michallet, M., Vernant, J. P., et al. (2005). Consolidation treatment of adult acute lymphoblastic leukemia: a prospective, randomized trial comparing allogeneic versus autologous bone marrow transplantation and testing the impact of recombinant interleukin-2 after autologous bone marrow transplantation BGMT Group. *Blood, 86,* 1619–1628.
28. Hunault, M., Harousseau, J. L., Delain, M., Truchan-Graczyk, M., Cahn, J. Y., Witz, F., et al. (2004). GOELAMS (Groupe Ouest-Est des Leucémies Airguës et Maladies du Sang) Group. Better outcome of adult acute lymphoblastic leukemia after early genoidentical allogeneic bone marrow transplantation (BMT) than after late high-dose therapy and autologous BMT: A GOELAMS trial. *Blood, 104,* 3028–3037.
29. Martino, R., Giralt, S., Caballero, M. D., Mackinnon, S., Corradini, P., Fernández-Avilés, F., et al. (2003). Allogeneic hematopoietic stem cell transplantation with reduced-intensity conditioning in acute lymphoblastic leukemia: a feasibility study. *Haematologica, 88,* 555–560.
30. Massenkeil, G., Nagy, M., Neuburger, S., Tamm, I., Lutz, C., et al. (2005). Survival after reduced-intensity conditioning is not inferior to standard high-dose conditioning before allogeneic haematopoietic cell transplantation in acute leukemias. *Bone Marrow Transplantation, 36,* 683–689.
31. Hamaki, T., Kami, M., Kanda, Y., Yuji, K., Inamoto, Y., Kishi, Y., et al. (2005). Reduced intensity stem-cell transplantation for acute lymphoblastic leukemia: a retrospective study of 33 patients. *Bone Marrow Transplantation, 35,* 549–556.

Chapter 19
Hematopoietic Stem Cell Transplantation in Philadelphia-Positive Acute Lymphoblastic Leukemia

Christy J. Stotler and Edward Copelan

Introduction

The Philadelphia chromosome is present in less than 5% of children with acute lymphoblastic leukemia (ALL), but in approximately 30% of adult cases and in more than 50% of ALL patients over the age of 50 [1]. The Philadelphia chromosome results from the reciprocal translocation which creates a hybrid BCR-ABL gene. A 210 kD BCR-ABL fusion protein (p210) occurs in an overwhelming proportion of patients with chronic myelogenous leukemia (CML) but in less than a third of those with ALL. A shorter 190 kD BCR-ABL fusion protein is present in 50% of adult Ph+ ALL patients and in 80% of childhood Ph+ ALL cases [2].

Historical Perspective

Prior to the use of selective tyrosine kinase inhibitors (TKIs), the presence of the Philadelphia chromosome portended a dismal prognosis in both childhood and adult Philadelphia-positive ALL (Ph+ ALL). While more than 60% of patients with this translocation achieved complete remission (CR), most experienced early relapse (<12 months) and rapid disease progression. Historical data reveal 5-year survival rates with conventional chemotherapy of 10–20% [3, 4]. These poor results stimulated interest in high-dose chemotherapy followed by bone marrow transplantation (BMT). Several small series reported encouraging results with matched sibling donor (MSD) allogeneic transplant in Ph+ ALL patients. Forman et al. [5] reported that of ten patients with Ph+ ALL in first CR or with relapsed or refractory disease, six were alive at a median of 19 months following BMT. A larger study of 38 patients with Ph+ ALL undergoing MSD allogeneic transplant reported a 2-year disease-free survival (DFS) of 46% for patients transplanted in first CR and 28% for patients transplanted after relapse [6]. Registry data from the IBMTR [7] showed a 2-year DFS of 38% for those patients transplanted in first CR and 41% for those transplanted after relapse. The City of Hope reported a 3-year DFS of 65% and an estimated rate of relapse of 12% [8].

C.J. Stotler (✉)
Cleveland Clinic Foundation, Taussig Cancer Institute, Cleveland, OH, USA
e-mail: christy.stotler@yahoo.com

A.S. Advani and H.M. Lazarus (eds.), *Adult Acute Lymphocytic Leukemia*, Contemporary Hematology, DOI 10.1007/978-1-60761-707-5_19, © Springer Science+Business Media, LLC 2011

Allogeneic Stem Cell Transplant

"Donor" Versus "No Donor"

Direct comparison of sibling allogeneic transplantation with chemotherapy is difficult. Lack of a MSD, older age, or comorbidities preclude most adults from allogeneic sibling transplantation. In "genetic randomization," patients with a MSD are assigned to allotransplantation and the remaining patients to chemotherapy or autologous stem cell transplant (ASCT). Ph+ ALL patients have been reported in such studies within subset analyses. LALA 87 [9], a large French multicenter study, compared allogeneic transplantation in ALL in first remission in 116 patients who had a matched donor with those who received either chemotherapy or ASCT (141 patients). Ph+ patients were evaluated within a high-risk ALL category defined as (1) presence of Philadelphia chromosome; (2) undifferentiated or null leukemia (defined by CD10−, CD20− phenotype); (3) common ALL with at least one adverse prognostic factor − (a) age > 35 years, (b) WBC count > 30 × 10⁹/L; or (4) time to achieve remission greater than 4 weeks. For the high-risk patients, there was a significant advantage in the median 5-year DFS for the 41 patients in the transplant arm, 21 months compared to 9 months for the 55 patients in the control arm ($p = 0.01$). The 5-year overall survival (OS) rates were 44% versus 20% respectively. In the following study, LALA-94 [10], 154 patients with Ph+ ALL were treated with an MSD ($n = 56$), matched unrelated donor (MUD) ($n = 14$) or ASCT ($n = 43$). Survival in the MUD group did not differ significantly from survival in the MSD group (RR 0.53, $p = 0.11$) and the 3-year survival in the donor group was 37% versus 12% in the group without a donor (RR in no donor group 1.71, $p = 0.02$). Other studies have shown comparable outcomes in relapse between sibling donors versus well-matched unrelated donor allogeneic transplants. The Medical Research Council UKALL12/ECOG E2993 study of 1,300 ALL patients enrolled 267 Ph+ adults [11]. For patients without a MSD donor, a MUD was sought. Remaining patients were randomized between standard consolidation/maintenance and autograft. The cohort of 267 patients demonstrated a 5-year overall survival (OS) of 22% and leukemia-free survival (LFS) of 16%. Fifty-seven Ph+ ALL patients received a sibling allograft and 30 patients an unrelated allograft. Five-year survival was 42% for patients receiving a matched sibling allograft and 36% for those receiving an unrelated donor graft ($p = 0.6$). MUD transplant recipients had a higher rate of death during remission (57% MUD vs 35% MSD) due to treatment-related mortality, but a low rate of relapse (25% MUD vs 37% MSD), neither of which was found to be statistically significant. Patients with a MSD had a better 5-year OS than the chemotherapy/ autograft arm but no statistically significant differences were noted. Cornelissen [12] described the results of 127 patients with poor-risk ALL who received an HLA-matched unrelated donor transplant. Poor risk was defined by the presence of t(9;22) ($n = 97$), t(4;11) ($n = 25$), or t(1;19) ($n = 5$). Most underwent SCT in CR1 where OS at 2 years was 40%. Two-year survival was 17% for patients in CR ≥ 2, and 5% for patients in relapse. Treatment-related mortality and relapse mortality were 54% and 6%, respectively, for patients in CR1 and 75% and 8% for patients in CR2 or greater. Multivariable analysis revealed that CR1, shorter interval from diagnosis to transplant, DRB1 match, negative CMV serology of patient and donor, and the presence of the Philadelphia chromosome, t(9;22), were independently associated with a better DFS (compared with other poor risk features). Fewer relapses occurred in patients with Ph+ ALL (HR 0.33, $p = 0.05$) compared to patients with t(4;11) or t(1;19) and this effect appeared independent from remission status. The consensus resulting from these reports was that patients with Ph+ ALL and matched sibling or unrelated donors should undergo allogeneic transplant in first remission [13–16].

Umbilical Cord Blood Transplants

There is substantial experience on the use of umbilical cord blood (UCB) as a source of stem cells in the management of pediatric leukemia patients and increasing data on their use in the treatment of adults with ALL [16]. An important benefit of UCB grafts is their permissiveness of HLA mismatches, which is especially important in patients with uncommon HLA haplotypes and racial minorities in whom no well-matched unrelated adult donor may be found. The University of Minnesota [17] reported outcomes of 126 ALL patients (38 with high-risk cytogenetics) using UCB ($n=12$), MSD ($n=85$), unrelated donor (URD) ($n=29$). One-year OS was 75% for the UCB group, 41% in the MSD group, and 33% in the URD group. Relapse rates at 1 year for UCB, MSD, and URD groups were 8%, 21%, and 20%, respectively. Transplant-related mortality at 1 year was 25% for the UCB group, 44% and 53% in the MSD and MUD groups and 86% in the mismatched URD group. While the small number of UCB procedures limits comparison to other stem cell sources, these results suggest that UCB can be an effective alternative graft source in patients without a well-matched sibling or adult unrelated donor. Accumulating data indicate that better HLA matches and higher cell doses dramatically improve engraftment, transplant-related mortality, and survival in UCB transplantation.

Graft Versus Leukemia Effect

Evidence supporting the graft versus leukemia (GVL) effect includes higher relapse rates following autologous and identical twin transplants compared with allogeneic transplants, higher rates of relapse in the absence of graft-vs-host-disease (GVHD) following allogeneic transplant, higher rates of relapse following T-cell depletion and the effectiveness of donor lymphocyte infusions (DLI) [18] in treating relapse in individual patients following allogeneic transplant. Passweg et al. [19] described 1,132 ALL patients from the International Bone Marrow Transplant Registry (IBMTR) who were recipients of an allogeneic transplant in first or second remission. GVHD was associated with a significant reduction in the risk of relapse in ALL of T lineage (RR 0.34, $p=0.005$) and B lineage (RR 0.44, $p=0.002$) in first CR and in ALL of T lineage (RR 0.54, $p=0.05$) and B lineage (RR 0.61, $p=0.01$) transplanted in CR2. Horowitz [20] reported decreased relapse rates in recipients of allogeneic transplants with acute and chronic GVHD (RR 0.33, $p=0.0001$) compared to those without GVHD in a study of 2,254 patients. A decrease in relapse rates in leukemia patients without significant acute or chronic GVHD who were treated with DLI has been reported [21]. In a case report of Ph+ ALL in which residual disease was detected by RT-PCR after transplant, a preemptive infusion of donor lymphocytes prior to hematologic relapse resulted in a negative RT-PCR [22]. DLI might benefit Ph+ patients with molecular relapse following HLA-matched transplant.

Reduced-Intensity Conditioning Regimens

Reduced-intensity conditioning (RIC) regimens have been used increasingly in patients with hematologic malignancies who, because of older age or comorbidities are at high risk of transplant-related mortality, in order to decrease transplant-related morbidity and mortality while exploiting the graft versus tumor effect. This modality, which is immunosuppressive without myeloablative, has been extensively evaluated in patients with myeloid leukemias, while data in ALL are limited. Martino et al. [23] evaluated 27 adults with high-risk ALL (44% of whom were

Ph+) treated with RIC followed by an allogeneic stem cell transplant. A majority of these patients had multiply relapsed or refractory disease and the median age at transplant was 50 years. Thirty percent survived at a median follow-up time of 2.2 years. Most developed acute or chronic GVHD. The 2-year incidence of transplant-related mortality was 23%. Such studies suggest that there may be a role for reduced intensity allogeneic transplant, but larger studies with longer follow-up are needed to discern the role of RIC in Ph+ ALL. Such studies are underway. It is important to note that relapse rates are higher following reduced intensity preparation and that GVHD seems to occur at an incidence similar to that following myeloablative regimens.

Autologous Stem Cell Transplant

Many patients with Ph+ ALL are unable to undergo allogeneic stem cell transplant due to older age, comorbidities, or lack of a suitable donor. Several prospective studies have evaluated the role of ASCT. In the MRC UKALL/ECOG 2993 study [24], autologous transplant was shown to be less effective than conventional consolidation/maintenance chemotherapy due to high rates of relapse. The ASCT arm did not incorporate maintenance chemotherapy. Sirohi et al. [25] reported on 100 patients with ALL undergoing ASCT followed by a maintenance chemotherapy protocol with 6-mercaptopurine, methotrexate, vincristine, and prednisone. An adverse outcome was associated with age > 30 years, greater than 4 weeks to attain remission, and karyotypes t(4,11) and t(9,22). Chemotherapy is generally difficult to administer following ASCT due to marrow suppression. The lack of a GVL effect and residual disease in the graft are likely reasons for the inferior outcomes after ASCT. Results of ALL studies in which purging techniques were used to decrease the risk of relapse have been variable [26–28]. Minimal residual disease can be more effectively addressed with the use of the TKIs in Ph+ ALL.

Myeloablative Preparative Regimens

The most widely utilized regimen of total body irradiation (TBI – 12 Gy/6 fractions) and cyclophosphamide (Cy 120 mg/kg) has been used for more than 30 years and the short and long-term sequelae of this combination have been well established [29]. TBI can kill disease in sanctuary sites such as the central nervous system and the testes, an important advantage in ALL. The use of TBI (13.2 Gy/11 fractions) with etoposide (VP – 60 mg/kg) was first shown to be effective in a phase I/II trial in patients with advanced acute leukemias [30]. Snyder et al. [31] showed that when this combination was used in 34 patients with ALL transplanted in CR1, DFS was 64% at 3 years with a relapse rate of 12%. A report from Stanford University and City of Hope National Medical Center described series of 79 patients with Ph+ ALL with over 20 years of follow-up in which 67 patients (85%) were treated with TBI-VP16 [32]. Sixty-two percent of patients were in CR1 at the time of transplant. Ten-year OS was 54% for patients in CR1 and 29% for patients transplanted beyond CR1. Median time to relapse was 12 months with the latest relapse observed at 27 months suggesting that patients who remained in remission 2 years after transplant were most likely cured. No randomized study has directly compared TBI-Cy and TBI-VP, however, Marks [29] described registry data (CIBMTR) on 298 ALL patients who received Cy-TBI compared with 204 patients who received TBI-VP16. Patients who received ≥ 13 Gy of TBI were also compared to patients who receive doses ≤ 13 Gy. All patients received a MSD allograft. Ph+ ALL patients were analyzed among a subgroup of 71 patients with high-risk cytogenetics. Importantly, the proportion of patients over the age of 30 years and with high-risk cytogenetics was higher in the TBI-VP16 ≥ 13 Gy group.

Relapse and transplant-related mortality (TRM) rates were lower in the group treated with TBI-VP16 regardless of the dose of radiation ($p=0.001$) but for patients who received cyclophosphamide, relapse rates were significantly lower when TBI doses ≥ 13 Gy were used ($p=0.0016$). There appears to be an advantage to substituting etoposide for cyclophosphamide, but when cyclophosphamide is used, doses of TBI ≥ 13 Gy are recommended. TBI does produce late toxicities such as intellectual impairment, growth impairment in children, and an increased risk of secondary malignancies. Registry data from the IBMTR [33] retrospectively compared 451 children who received TBI-Cy with 176 patients who received a chemotherapy-only preparative regimen of busulfan-cyclophosphamide (BuCy) in an attempt to reduce radiation related toxicities. Three-year survival was 55% with TBI-Cy and 40% with BuCy ($p=0.003$ univariate analysis) indicating superior survival with TBI-Cy compared with BuCy conditioning for HLA-identical sibling bone marrow transplants in children with ALL. Although this study was not randomized, most clinicians consider TBI-containing regimens as standard preparation in ALL. The use of targeted busulfan levels or intravenous busulfan might improve results using busulfan regimens.

Tyrosine Kinase Inhibitors (TKIs)

The effectiveness of TKIs has dramatically altered the treatment of patients with Ph + ALL. Imatinib mesylate, the first selective BCR-ABL TKI utilized, was initially approved for the treatment of CML, however, several reports described the feasibility of incorporating imatinib into treatment regimens for Ph+ ALL to increase remission rates. In patients with relapsed or refractory Ph+ ALL, imatinib showed favorable hematologic response rates, but these were generally short-lived [34]. Subsequent studies evaluated the addition of imatinib to the induction or consolidation phase of therapy [35].

Since allogeneic transplantation is most effective and safe in patients in first remission, it was hoped that incorporation of imatinib might permit more patients to undergo transplantation under optimal circumstances and thereby improve results. In a study of 29 Ph+ ALL patients treated with hyper-CVAD and concurrent imatinib 400 600 mg/day who proceeded to allogeneic transplant, the estimated 3-year DFS was 78.1% with a median follow-up of 25 months. The group treated with imatinib had a lower relapse rate when compared with historical controls (4.3% vs 40.7%, $p=0.003$) and allowed a higher rate of allografting when compared to historic controls (86.2% vs 51.5%, $p=0.004$) [36]. The Japan Adult Leukemia Study Group JALSG ALL202 reported on 24 patients with newly diagnosed Ph+ ALL entered onto a phase 2 trial in which imatinib was prescribed concurrently with induction chemotherapy and alternated with chemotherapy during consolidation [37]. Patients were taken to transplant if a HLA-matched donor was found. Twenty-three patients (96%) achieved complete remission after one course of induction chemotherapy plus imatinib with 78% achieving a complete molecular remission. Sixty-three percent of patients (15/24) underwent allotransplantation in CR1 and event-free survival (EFS) and OS were 68% and 89%, respectively, at 1 year. A prospective multicenter trial of 92 Ph+ ALL patients evaluated two separate treatment schedules of imatinib administration in the induction/consolidation chemotherapy setting prior to allogeneic transplant [38]. Forty-seven patients received imatinib alternating with chemotherapy at a dose of 400 mg/day (group 1), while 45 patients received imatinib concurrently with chemotherapy at a dose of 600 mg/day (group 2). Eighty-five percent of patients in group 1 proceeded to allogeneic transplant in CR1 compared with 80% of patients in group 2, with estimated 1 and 2 year probabilities of survival of 72% and 36%, respectively, for patients in group 1 and 61% and 43% for patients in group 2. More patients in group 2 were negative for the BCR-ABL transcript by RT-PCR compared to group 1 (52% vs 19%, $p=0.01$) but group 2 patients also exhibited more grade III–IV cytopenias and toxicities requiring treatment disruptions (87% vs 53%). Thus, while both schedules of imatinib facilitate transplantation in first complete remission, the concurrent administration of chemotherapy and imatinib appeared to exert an improved antileukemic effect. Imatinib is useful in getting more patients to allotransplantation.

Even after allotransplant in CR1, a substantial proportion of patients with Ph+ ALL will relapse, and following allotransplantation in patients not in CR1, relapse is more frequent. The detection of minimal residual disease (MRD) following transplant is associated with increased risk of relapse. Several studies have evaluated the role of imatinib following transplant used prophylactically to prevent relapse or to eliminate MRD. Carpenter et al. [39] treated 22 patients, 15 with Ph+ ALL and seven with high-risk CML with imatinib 400 mg daily from engraftment following transplantation for 1 year. Imatinib was tolerated in 17/19 adults. Fifteen patients were alive without detectable BCR-ABL at a median of almost 6 months beyond the discontinuation of imatinib at 1 year post-transplant. Detectable MRD following transplant is associated with a greater than 90% risk of relapse in Ph+ ALL [40]. Wassman et al. [41] evaluated the role of imatinib in MRD post-transplant in 27 Ph+ ALL patients who had molecular evidence of recurrent disease. Fifty-two percent achieved a molecular remission at a median of 1.5 months from initiation of treatment. Of 16 patients entered onto study because of molecular relapse, eight became PCR negative and the other eight went on to hematologic relapse. DFS at 1 and 2 years in patients who achieved an early complete molecular remission was 91% and 54% compared with 8% at 1 year for those who continued to have molecular evidence of disease. A shorter time to complete molecular remission predicted for a prolonged DFS. Acquired resistance to imatinib may result from point mutations in BCR-ABL that result in the inactivation of imatinib. Dasatinib and Nilotinib are other TKIs that are FDA approved at this time for Ph+ disease, but their particular role in the peri-transplant period has yet to be fully studied. [35].

Since the inclusion of TKIs into the treatment regime of Ph+ ALL have improved achievement and depth of first CR, it is reasonable to ask whether allogeneic transplant in first CR is still imperative [15, 35]. A phase II Japanese study treated 80 Ph+ ALL patients with combination induction chemotherapy and imatinib 49 of whom went on to allogeneic stem cell transplant. The probability for OS at 1 year was 73% for those who underwent allogeneic transplant and 84% for those who did not, a difference which was not statistically significant ($p=0.94$) [42]. The UKALLXII/ECOG 2993 study evaluated the 267 patients with Ph+ ALL treated in the pre-imatinib era and compared them with 153 patients treated in the post-imatinib era (after 2003) when the study was amended to add imatinib 600 mg/day following induction and after BMT for 2 years or until relapse. Of 153 patients treated with imatinib, 128 were eligible for BMT, and 57 (58%) underwent transplant. Overall survival of the imatinib-treated group was 23% at 3 years similar to the overall survival of 26% from the pre-imatinib era. It is unclear that imatinib improves sustained LFS in Ph+ ALL. Imatinib given with induction therapy does improve the CR rate and increases the number of patients able to undergo transplant. There is insufficient evidence to assess its impact on survival rates following transplantation. Allogeneic transplantation in first CR remains the standard of care for patients with Ph+ ALL patients [43].

Conclusion

Allogeneic stem cell transplant provides the best curative option for patients with Ph+ ALL, and is recommended for patients who achieve a complete remission. In counseling patients prior to transplant for whom a MSD is not available, a well-matched URD or UCB donor is generally recommended with the understanding that the risk of transplant-related morbidity and mortality may be higher. TKIs should be incorporated into first-line therapy. Imatinib has improved the rate, quality, and duration of first remission permitting more patients with Ph+ ALL to undergo allogeneic transplant in first remission. Ongoing studies will define the role of these agents in the post-transplant setting. Further studies are needed to determine whether some patients with Ph+ ALL might not require transplantation in first complete remission. The effectiveness of transplantation will be improved by incorporation of immune therapies (e.g., monoclonal antibodies) into preparative regimens, better methods to prevent and treat GVHD, and new sources of hematopoietic stem cells, such as cells derived from embryonal stem cells.

References

1. Radich, J. P. (2001). Philadelphia positive acute lymphocytic leukemia. *Hematology/Oncology Clinics of North America, 15*, 21–36.
2. Faderl, S., Kantarjian, H. M., Talpaz, M., et al. (1998). Clinical significance of cytogenetic abnormalities in adult acute lymphoblastic leukemia. *Blood, 91*, 3995–4019.
3. Faderl, S., Kantarjian, H. M., Thomas, D. A., et al. (2000). Outcome of Philadelphia chromosome positive adult acute lymphoblastic leukemia. *Leukaemia & Lymphoma, 36*, 263–273.
4. Larson, R. A., Dodge, R. K., Burns, C. P., et al. (1995). A five-drug remission induction regimen with intensive consolidation for adults with acute lymphoblastic leukemia: cancer and leukemia group B study 8811. *Blood, 85*, 2025–2037.
5. Forman, S. J., O'Donnell, M. R., Nadamanee, A. P., et al. (1987). Bone marrow transplant for patients with Philadelphia chromosome-positive acute lymphoblastic leukemia. *Blood, 70*, 587–588.
6. Chao, N. J., Blume, K. G., Forman, S. J., et al. (1995). Long-term follow-up of allogeneic marrow recipients for Philadelphia chromosome-positive acute lymphoblastic leukemia. *Blood, 85*, 3353–3354.
7. Barrett, A. J., Horowitz, M. M., Ash, R. C., et al. (1992). Bone marrow transplantation for Philadelphia chromosome-positive acute lymphoblastic leukemia. *Blood, 79*, 3067–3070.
8. Snyder, D. S., Nademanee, A. P., O'Donnell, M. R., et al. (1999). Long-term follow-up of 23 patients with Philadelphia chromosome-positive acute lymphoblastic leukemia treated with allogeneic bone marrow transplant in first complete remission. *Leukemia, 13*, 2053–2058.
9. Sebban, C., Lepage, E., Vernant, J. P., et al. (1994). Allogeneic bone marrow transplantation in adult acute lymphoblastic leukemia in first complete remission: A comparative study. *Journal of Clinical Oncology, 12*, 2580–2587.
10. Dombret, H., Gabert, J., Boiron, J. M., et al. (2002). Outcome of treatment in adults with Philadelphia chromosome-positive acute lymphoblastic leukemia – results of a prospective multicenter LALA-94 trial. *Blood, 100*, 2357–2366.
11. Goldstone, A. H., Chopra, R., Buck, G., et al. (2003). The outcome of 67 Philadelphia positive adults in the international UKALL12/ECOG E 2993 Study. Final analysis and the role of allogeneic transplant in those under 50 years [abstract]. *Blood, 104*, 268a.
12. Cornelissen, J. J., Carston, M., Kollman, C., et al. (2001). Unrelated marrow transplantation for adult patients with poor-risk acute lymphoblastic leukemia: strong graft-versus-leukemia effect and risk factors determining outcome. *Blood, 97*, 1572–1577.
13. Stein, A., & Forman, S. J. (2008). Allogeneic transplantation in ALL. *Bone Marrow Transplantation, 41*, 439–446.
14. Avivi, I., & Goldstone, A. H. (2003). Bone marrow transplant in Ph + ALL patients. *Bone Marrow Transplantation, 31*, 623–632.
15. Rowe, J. M., & Goldstone, A. H. (2007). How I treat acute lymphocytic leukemia in adults? *Blood, 110*, 2268–2275.
16. Bachanova, V., & Weisdorf, D. (2008). Unrelated donor allogeneic transplantation for adult acute lymphoblastic leukemia: a review. *Bone Marrow Transplantation, 41*, 455–464.
17. Kumar, P., Defor, T. E., Brunstein, C., et al. (2005). Allogeneic hematopoietic stem cell transplantation (HSCT) in the treatment of acute lymphocytic leukemia (ALL) in 126 adults: Impact of donor source on leukemia free survival [abstract]. *Blood, 106*, 2064.
18. Tomblyn, M., & Lazarus, H. M. (2008). Donor lymphocyte infusions: The long and winding road: How should it be traveled? *Bone Marrow Transplantation, 42*, 569–579.
19. Passweg, J. R., Tiberghien, P., Cahn, J. Y., et al. (1998). Graft-versus-leukemia effects in T lineage and B lineage acute lymphoblastic leukemia. *Bone Marrow Transplantation, 21*, 153–158.
20. Horowitz, M. M., Gale, R. P., Sondel, P. M., et al. (1990). Graft-versus-leukemia reactions after bone marrow transplantation. *Blood, 75*, 555–562.

21. Schaap, N., Schattenberg, A., Bar, B., et al. (2001). Induction of graft-versus-leukemia to prevent relapse after partially lymphocyte-depleted allogeneic bone marrow transplantation by pre-emptive donor leukocyte infusion. *Leukemia, 15*, 1339–1346.

22. Yazaki, M., Andoh, M., Ito, T., et al. (1997). Successful prevention of hematological relapse for a patient with Philadelphia chromosome-positive acute lymphoblastic leukemia after allogeneic bone marrow transplantation by donor leukocyte infusion. *Bone Marrow Transplantation, 19*, 393–394.

23. Martino, R., Giralt, S., Cabarello, M. D., et al. (2003). Allogeneic hematopoietic stem cell transplant with reduced intensity conditioning in acute lymphoblastic leukemia: A feasibility study. *Haematologica, 88*, 555–560.

24. Goldstone, A. H., Richards, S. M., Lazarus, H. M., Tallman, M. S., et al. (2008). In adults with standard-risk acute lymphoblastic leukemia (ALL) the greatest benefit is achieved from an allogeneic transplant in first complete remission (CR) and an autologous transplant is less effective than conventional consolidation/maintenance chemotherapy: Final results of the international ALL trial (MRC UKALL XII/ECOG E2993). *Blood, 111*, 1827–1833.

25. Sirohi, B., Powles, R., Treleaven, J., et al. (2008). The role of maintenance chemotherapy after autotransplantation for acute lymphoblastic leukemia in first remission: Single-center experience of 100 patients. *Bone Marrow Transplantation, 42*, 105–112.

26. Simonsson, B., Burnett, A. K., Prentice, H. G., et al. (1989). Autologous bone marrow transplantation with monoclonal antibody purged marrow for high risk acute lymphoblastic leukemia. *Leukemia, 9*, 631–636.

27. Gilmore, M. J., Hamon, M. D., Prentice, H. G., et al. (1991). Failure of purged autologous bone marrow transplantation in high risk acute lymphoblastic leukaemia in first complete remission. *Bone Marrow Transplantation, 8*, 19–26.

28. Soiffer, R. J., Roy, D. C., Gonin, R., et al. (1993). Monoclonal antibody-purged autologous bone marrow transplantation in adults with acute lymphoblastic leukemia at high risk of relapse. *Bone Marrow Transplantation, 3*, 243–251.

29. Marks, D. I., Forman, S. J., Blume, K. G., et al. (2006). A comparison of cyclophosphamide and total body irradiation with etoposide and total body irradiation as conditioning regimens for patients undergoing sibling allografting for acute lymphoblastic leukemia in first or second complete remission. *Biology of Blood and Marrow Transplantation, 12*, 293–300.

30. Blume, K. G., Forman, S. J., O'Donnell, M. R., et al. (1987). Total body irradiation and high-dose etoposide: A new preparatory regimen for bone marrow transplantation in patients with advanced hematologic malignancies. *Blood, 69*, 1015–1020.

31. Snyder, D. S., Chao, N. J., Amylon, M. D., et al. (1993). Fractionated total body irradiation and high-dose etoposide as a preparatory regimen for bone marrow transplantation for 99 patients with acute leukemia in first complete remission. *Blood, 82*, 2920–2928.

32. Laport, G. G., Alvarnas, J. C., Palmer, J. M., et al. (2008). Long-term remission of Philadelphia chromosome positive acute lymphoblastic leukemia after allogeneic hematopoietic cell transplantation from matched sibling donors: A 20-year experience with the fractionated total body irradiation etoposide regimen. *Blood, 112*, 903–909.

33. Davies, S. M., Ramsay, N. K., Klein, J. P., et al. (2000). Comparison of preparative regimens in transplants for children with acute lymphoblastic leukemia. *Journal of Clinical Oncology, 18*, 340–347.

34. Ottmann, O. G., Druker, B. J., Sawyers, C. L., et al. (2002). A phase 2 study of imatinib in patients with relapsed or refractory Philadelphia chromosome-positive acute lymphoid leukemias. *Blood, 100*, 1965–1971.

35. Abou Mourad, Y. R., Fernandez, H. F., & Kharfan-Dabaja, M. A. (2008). Allogeneic hematopoietic cell transplantation for adult Philadelphia-positive acute lymphoblastic leukemia in the era of tyrosine kinase inhibitors. *Biology of Blood and Marrow Transplantation, 14*, 949–958.

36. Lee, S., Kim, Y. J., Min, C. K., et al. (2005). The effect of first-line imatinib interim therapy on the outcome of allogeneic stem cell transplantation in adults with newly diagnosed Philadelphia chromosome-positive acute lymphoblastic leukemia. *Blood, 105*, 3449–3457.

37. Towatari, M., Yanada, M., Usui, N., et al. (2004). Combination of intensive chemotherapy and imatinib can rapidly induce high-quality complete remission for a majority of patients with newly diagnosed BCR-ABL-positive acute lymphoblastic leukemia. *Blood, 104*, 3507–3512.

38. Wassman, B., Pfeifer, H., Goekbuget, N., et al. (2006). Alternating versus concurrent schedules of imatinib and chemotherapy as frontline therapy for Philadelphia-positive acute lymphoblastic leukemia (Ph + ALL). *Blood, 108*, 1469–1477.

39. Carpenter, P. A., Snyder, D. S., Flowers, M. E., et al. (2007). Prophylactic administration of imatinib after hematopoietic cell transplantation for high-risk Philadelphia chromosome-positive leukemia. *Blood, 109*, 2791–2793.

40. Radich, J., Gehly, G., Lee, A., et al. (1997). Detection of BCR-ABL transcripts in Philadelphia chromosome-positive acute lymphoblastic leukemia after marrow transplantation. *Blood, 89*, 2602–2609.

41. Wassman, B., Pheifer, H., Stadler, M., et al. (2005). Early molecular response to post-transplantation imatinib determines outcome in MRD + Philadelphia-positive acute lymphoblastic leukemia (Ph + ALL). *Blood, 106,* 458–463.
42. Yanada, M., Takeuchi, J., Sugiura, I., et al. (2006). High complete remission rate and promising outcome by combination of imatinib and chemotherapy for newly diagnosed BCR-ABL-positive acute lymphoblastic leukemia: a phase II study by the Japan adult leukemia study group. *Journal of Clinical Oncology, 24,* 460–466.
43. Fielding, A. K., Richards, S. M., Lazarus, H. M., et al. (2007). Does imatinib change the outcome in Philadelphia chromosome positive acute lymphoblastic leukaemia in adults? Data from the UKALLXII/ECOG 2993 study [abstract]. *Blood, 110,* 10.

Chapter 20
Special Challenges: Genetic Polymorphisms and Therapy

Maja Krajinovic

Pharmacogenetics contributes to understanding the variability in treatment responses and identifying genetic polymorphisms that may predict patient response prior to drug administration [1]. The identification of genetic polymorphisms may lead to different treatment schedules, allowing for a reduction in drug side effects while improving or maintaining the efficacy of treatment. This chapter will summarize the pharmacogenetic studies of acute lymphocytic leukemia (ALL) including polymorphisms in genes involved in drug metabolism, as well as genes involved with acquisition of the disease and risk of relapse. ALL has a much higher incidence in children than adults [2], thus the majority of pharmacogenetic studies have been carried out in childhood ALL patients. ALL is also the most common cancer in children, comprising 25–30% of all childhood malignancies. The treatment of this disease has greatly improved in the past four decades due to the introduction of effective combination risk-adapted therapies resulting in long-term disease-free survival in approximately 80% of childhood ALL patients [3]. However, resistance to therapy is still a major obstacle to successful treatment, rendering ALL the leading cause of cancer-related deaths in children. Intensive chemotherapy treatment also has significant short-term and long-term toxicities [4], indicating the need to identify the factors that contribute to this variability.

Thiopurines

Thiopurines (including 6-mercaptopurine, 6-MP) are an integral component of ALL treatment. The methylation pathway of 6-MP (Fig. 20.1) in ALL has been studied by several research groups and differences in this pathway have been shown to influence the response to treatment. Excessive cellular accumulation of the thioguanine nucleotide (TGN) due to low thiopurine methyltransferase (TPMT) activity leads to 6-MP intolerance manifested as severe hematopoietic toxicity [4]. Several polymorphisms in the TPMT gene have been identified (described in Table 20.1). They are defined by DNA base substitutions leading to amino acid replacements and a reduction in enzyme activity. The most frequent variants are TPMT *2 (defined by G to C substitution at position 238 of the gene), TPMT *3A (defined by G640A and A719G nucleotide transitions), and TPMT *3C (defined by G719A) [4, 5]. In Caucasians, low-activity TPMT variants are observed with a frequency of 4–7%, with the *3A variant being the most prevalent. Variant TPMT alleles are found in 5–7% of the African population with the most prevalent variant being the *3C allele. Asians have the lowest

M. Krajinovic (✉)
Cancer Research Center Charles Bruneau; Research Center CHU Sainte-Justine,
Departments of Paediatrics and Pharmacology, University of Montreal, 3175 Côte Ste-Catherine,
Montréal (Québec), H3T 1C5, Canada
e-mail: maja.krajinovic@umontreal.ca

A.S. Advani and H.M. Lazarus (eds.), *Adult Acute Lymphocytic Leukemia*, Contemporary Hematology,
DOI 10.1007/978-1-60761-707-5_20, © Springer Science+Business Media, LLC 2011

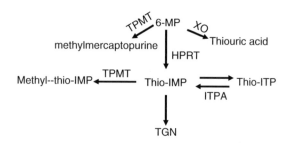

Fig. 20.1 Schematic representation of the metabolism of 6-mercaptopurine. *6MP* 6-mercaptopurine, *TPMT* thiopurine *S*-methyltransferase, *XO* xanthine oxidase, *HPRT* hypoxanthine phosphoribosyltransferase, *TGN* thioguanine nucleotide, *ITPA* inosine triphosphate pyrophosphatase, *IDP* inosine diphosphate, *IMP* inosine monophosphate, *ITP* inosine triphosphate

frequency of TPMT variants (1–2%), mostly represented by the *3A allele in Southwest Asians and by the *3C allele in Eastern Asians [6]. Approximately 10% of the population is heterozygous for nonfunctional variants, resulting in intermediate enzyme activity; whereas 1 in 300 people inherit two nonfunctional alleles, resulting in very low or no enzyme activity [4].

When treated with conventional doses of 6-MP, patients with very low or no TPMT enzyme activity develop severe myelosuppression. Up to half of heterozygous individuals (those with intermediate TPMT enzyme activity) develop milder forms of hematological toxicity [7]. Numerous studies demonstrating a clear correlation between TPMT genotypes and 6-MP intolerance prompted the Food and Drug Administration (FDA) to recommend TPMT testing in patients with clinical evidence of myelosuppression [8]. Reduction to 10% of standard 6-MP doses is recommended for individuals that are homozygous for variant TPMT alleles. Heterozygous individuals might also benefit from dose reduction [7]. In certain institutions, TPMT genotypes are routinely determined before 6-MP administration [7].

In addition to influencing hematologic toxicity after treatment with 6-MP, TPMT variants might also influence long-term morbidity, such as the development of secondary malignancies. A higher frequency of brain tumors following radiation therapy and a higher frequency of therapy-related acute myeloid leukemia was observed among patients with variant TPMT alleles [7]. Patients homozygous for TPMT alleles conferring no reduction in enzyme activity are less likely to have increased treatment-related toxicity. However, this subgroup of patients may have a suboptimal response to treatment, as demonstrated by the more frequent incidence of minimal residual disease in these patients [9].

Other enzymes involved in 6-MP metabolism may also influence 6-MP response. These corresponding genes may be interesting candidates for 6-MP pharmacogenetics. Xanthine oxidase (XO) is an alternative pathway to TPMT for 6-MP inactivation (Fig. 20.1). Several polymorphisms have been recently described in the XO gene in the Japanese population [10]. However, no association with 6-MP related toxicity was found in ALL patients [11]. A more detailed analysis of XO polymorphisms is needed. Inosine triphosphate pyrophosphatase (ITPA) catalyzes the conversion of inosine triphosphate (ITP) into inosine monophosphate, thereby preventing the accumulation of ITP in normal cells (Fig. 20.1). In ITPA-deficient patients treated with thiopurines, accumulation of ITP can occur, resulting in drug-related toxicity [12]. Two polymorphisms are associated with ITPA deficiency: C94A substitution leading to amino acid replacement (Pro32 to Thr) and an A to C substitution at the position 21 of the second intron. These polymorphisms occur in 7% and 13% of Caucasians, respectively [13]. The C94A polymorphism is found in Africans at a similar frequency as in Caucasians, whereas it occurs in 14–19% of the Asian population [14]. In childhood ALL, a significant association exists between intronic A to C polymorphism and thrombocytopenia [15], and between the C94A variant and febrile neutropenia [16] (Table 20.1).

Table 20.1 Summary of studies demonstrating an association between therapeutic response in ALL patients and polymorphisms in genes controlling drug pharmacokinetics and pharmacodynamics

Gene	Polymorphism	Impact	Function	Association	Population	Drug	References
TPMT	*2 G238C	Ala80Pro	Reduced	Toxicity (myelosuppression, secondary malignancies) MRD	Childhood	Thiopurines	[4–7, 9]
	*3A (G460A; A719G)	Ala154Thr; Tyr240Cys					
	*3B (G460A)	Ala154Thr					
	*3C (A719G)	Tyr240Cys					
IPTA	C94A	Pro32Thr	Reduced	Febrile neutropenia	Childhood	Thiopurines	[16]
	A IVS2+21 C	Intron		Thrombocytopenia			[15]
DHFR	C-1610G/T	Promoter transcription	Increased	EFS, DFS	Childhood	MTX	[21]
	A-317G						
MTHFR	C677T	Ala222Val	Reduced	EFS, DFS	Childhood	MTX	[32, 33]
				OS	Adult		[34]
				Toxicity (bone marrow and hepatic)	Adult		[34, 37]
TS	2R-97 3R	5'UTR transcription	Increased	EFS, DFS, CNS relapse, osteonecrosis	Childhood	MTX	[46–49]
CCND1	A870G	Exon/intron junction	Alternative splicing	EFS, DFS	Childhood	MTX	[54, 55]
RFC1	G80A	His27Arg	Unknown	EFS, DFS (gastrointestinal, hepatic)	Childhood	MTX	[59–62]
MDR1	C3435T	Synonymous	Reduced	ALL outcome, infectious complications	Childhood	Glucocorticoids, anthracycline, vincristine, etoposide, cyclophosphamide	[75–77]
MRP2	C-24T	5'UTR transcription	Reduced	MTX levels	Childhood	MTX	[79]
GR	C IVS2 +646 G, Bcl I	Intron	Altered	OS	Childhood	CS	[91]
CRHR1	G IVS2 +8507 T	Intron	Unknown	CS-induced hypertension	Childhood	CS	[97]
	A IVS12 +111 G	Intron	Unknown	CS-induced hypertension osteonecrosis	Childhood	CS	[97, 98]
IL-10	A-1082G	Promoter	Increased	Prednisone response	Childhood	CS	[100]

TPMT thiopurine methyltransferase, *IPTA* inosine triphosphate pyrophosphatase, *DHFR* dihydrofolate reductase, *MTHFR* methylene tetrahydrofolate reductase, *TS* thymidylate synthase, *CCND1* cyclin D, *RFC1* reduced folate carrier, *MDR1* multidrug-resistance protein, *MRP2* multidrug-resistance-associated protein 2, *GR* glucocorticoid receptor, *CRHR1* corticotrophin releasing factor receptor, *TNF* tumor necrosis factor, *IL* interleukin, *MRD* minimal residual disease, *EFS* event-free survival, *DFS* disease-free survival, *OS* overall survival, *6-MP* mercaptopurine, *MTX* methotrexate, *CS* corticosteroids. More details on these polymorphisms can be also found in [131, 132]

Methotrexate

Methotrexate (MTX), a folate antagonist, competitively inhibits dihydrofolate reductase (DHFR) [17] (Fig. 20.2). Altered levels of DHFR are found at diagnosis in childhood ALL, particularly in patients with a shorter event-free survival (EFS) [18–20]. Changes in the level of DHFR expression and consequently in the sensitivity to MTX can also be due to genetic polymorphisms. Recently, a comprehensive study of promoter polymorphisms in the DHFR gene was performed [21], identifying 15 variations that were in linkage disequilibrium. Three polymorphisms (C-1610G/T; C-680A; A-317G) were identified as sufficient to define all observed haplotypes. These polymorphisms were found in Caucasians with a frequency of 35%, 11%, 29%, and 42%, respectively. Lower EFS in childhood ALL patients was associated with homozygosity for the alleles A-317 and C-1610 (Table 20.1). Both alleles are associated with higher DHFR expression, likely explaining the worse prognosis in this subset of patients [21]. An additional polymorphism, a C829T substitution in the 3'-untranslated region of the DHFR gene transcript, has been described in the Japanese population with a frequency of 24% [22]. This polymorphism is located near the binding site for microRNA [23]. Moreover, in vitro, this polymorphism affects DHFR expression by interfering with the binding of microRNA, resulting in DHFR overexpression and MTX resistance [23]. Although this polymorphism has significant potential to influence the outcome of diseases treated with MTX, no data analyzing the effects of this polymorphism on clinical outcome have been described. One potential reason for this might be the fact this substitution was originally investigated in the DHFR transcript and the DNA sequence at this particular locus renders the design of appropriate genotyping assay difficult (personal observation).

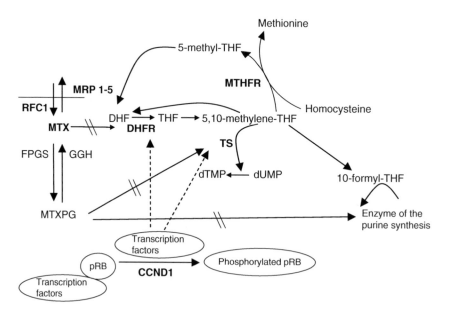

Fig. 20.2 The effect of methotrexate on the folate cycle. Enzymes whose corresponding genetic polymorphisms are described in the text are in bold font. *DHF* dihydrofolate, *THF* tetrahydrofolate, *DHFR* dihydrofolate reductase, *dUMP* deoxyuridine monophosphate, *dTMP* deoxythymidine monophosphate, *TS* thymidylate synthase, *FPGS* folylpolyglutamate synthase, *GGH* gamma-glutamyl hydrolase, *MTX* methotrexate, *MTXPG* methotrexate polyglutamate, *MTHFR* methylene tetrahydrofolate reductase, *RFC1* reduced folate carrier, *MRP* multidrug-resistance-associated proteins, *CCND1* cyclin D1, *pRB* retinoblastoma protein (Modified and reproduced from [131]. With permission of Lippincott Williams & Wilkins)

Methylene Tetrahydrofolate Reductase

The 5,10-methylene tetrahydrofolate reductase (MTHFR) gene plays a key role in folate metabolism by channeling one-carbon units between nucleotide synthesis and methylation reactions. MTHFR catalyzes the conversion of 5,10-MTHF into 5-MTHF, a major circulating form of folate that provides a methyl group for homocysteine methylation. 5,10-MTHF and its derivatives are essential cofactors for thymidylate and de novo purine synthesis (Fig. 20.2) [24]. Reduced 5-MTHF levels may decrease homocysteine methylation to methionine, resulting in hyperhomocysteinemia and DNA hypomethylation; whereas, reduced levels of 5,10-MTHF, required for thymidylate synthesis, could lead to uracil misincorporation into DNA and increase the frequency of chromosome damage [25].

Reduced levels of 5,10-MTHF facilitate the action of certain chemotherapeutics, including that of methotrexate (MTX). In contrast, an increase in 5,10-MTHF can antagonize the action of MTX and contribute to MTX resistance (Fig. 20.2) [26]. Two common polymorphisms, a C677 to T transition causing an alanine to valine substitution at codon 222 (Ala222Val) and an A1298 to C transversion causing a glutamic acid to alanine replacement at codon 429 (Glu429Ala), have been described in the MTHFR gene [27, 28]. Both variants have an impact on enzyme function. T677 affects the catalytic domain, and C1298 affects the regulatory MTHFR domain. Reduced enzymatic activity has been observed in TT677 or CC1298 homozygotes, and to a lesser extent in heterozygous individuals [27, 28]. The frequency of the MTHFR 677T allele varies substantially in different populations. The T677 allele is found with a frequency of 34% in Caucasians, 42% in Eastern Asians, and 8% in Africans. Frequencies of the C1298 allele in Caucasians, Japanese, and Africans are 34%, 21%, and 9%, respectively [29]. Both MTHFR polymorphisms are in linkage disequilibrium [30].

The role of MTHFR variants in a number of disorders, involving disturbances in folate metabolism, such as neural tube defects (NTD), vascular disease, and cancer susceptibility, is well documented [24]. Sohn et al. [31] demonstrated that cells transfected with the T677 MTHFR allele had an altered intracellular folate distribution, increased thymidylate synthase activity, and decreased chemosensitivity to MTX. Two studies have demonstrated an increased risk of relapse for childhood ALL patients having at least one T677 MTHFR allele [32, 33] (Table 20.1). A similar association was demonstrated with the T677 variant allele and a decreased overall survival in adult ALL patients receiving MTX-based maintenance treatment [34]. Childhood ALL patients with the T677 allele rarely develop MTX-related toxicity at least in some studies [33, 35, 36]. In contrast, adult ALL patients with the T677 allele have an increased risk of toxicity. Individuals homozygous for the T677 allele experience a higher frequency of MTX intolerance, requiring dose modification and temporary MTX withdrawal during the maintenance phase of treatment (Table 20.1) [34, 37]. Toxicity affecting both liver and bone marrow function was seen more often in these individuals. The reason for this difference in toxicity between children and adults with ALL is unclear. Potential explanations may include differences in MTX dose and administration schedule, concurrent medications, folate status, diet, and a different mechanism of toxicity (i.e., driven by 5-MTHF vs 5,10 MTHF levels).

Thymidylate Synthase

Thymidylate synthase (TS) is a key enzyme in the nucleotide biosynthetic pathway that catalyzes conversion of deoxyuridylate to deoxythymidylate (Fig. 20.2). Several enzymes of purine and pyrimidine synthesis, including TS, are inhibited by MTX polyglutamates [17]. A repeat polymorphism was identified in the enhancer element of the 5′UTR region [38]. This polymorphism contains variable numbers of a 28-bp repeat element with the double (2R) and triple repeat (3R) alleles being the most frequent. The 3R allele is found with a frequency of 50–60%, 60%, and 80% in Caucasians, Southwest Asians, and Eastern Asians, respectively [39]. The repeat element appears to function as an enhancer element. In vitro studies have demonstrated increased TS expression associated with the 3R allele compared to that of the 2R variant [40, 41]. These findings have been confirmed in patients homozygous for the 3R allele [40–43].

A TS repeat genotype correlates with the clinical efficacy of MTX [44, 45]. Several studies evaluating TS genotype and outcome have been conducted in childhood ALL patients. Individuals homozygous for the 3R allele have a higher risk of relapse (at any site) [46, 47]. Another study demonstrated that low-risk patients with the TS 3R3R genotype had a predisposition for central nervous system (CNS) relapse, whereas high-risk patients with a combined TS 3R3R and glutathione-*S*-transferase non-null genotype had an increased risk of hematologic relapse (Table 20.1) [48]. Higher TS expression associated with a 3R allele would provide cells with enough nucleotides required for DNA synthesis, preventing initiation of a DNA damage response pathway. From a clinical perspective, patients with higher TS levels might need higher doses of methotrexate to effectively inhibit TS. The data on drug-related toxicity favors such a hypothesis. A higher incidence of osteonecrosis of the hip has been demonstrated in ALL patients with the 2R2R genotype (low TS activity) [49].

Cyclin D1 (CCND1)

CCND1 is a key protein that regulates the G1 phase of the cell cycle. CCND1 has an important role in the phosphorylation and the functional inactivation of the retinoblastoma protein (pRB) (Fig. 20.2). The phosphorylation state of pRB can be affected by the increased expression of CCND1, thus resulting in higher E2F levels and increased transcription of MTX targets like DHFR and TS. This, in turn, can reduce the sensitivity of leukemia cells to MTX [50–52]. CCND1 A870G polymorphisms modify mRNA splicing [53]. The variant A870 allele results in a CCND1 with a longer half-life, potentially affecting transition through the G1/S checkpoint and mimicking CCND1 overexpression. This allele is present at a frequency of 50% in Caucasians, 39–54% in Asians, and 20% in Africans, based on the HapMap data available at SNP data base (rs603965) at NCBI http://www.ncbi.nlm.nih.gov/SNP. Two studies have demonstrated an increased risk of relapse or treatment failure in childhood ALL patients with the AA genotype (Table 20.1) [54, 55]. Since CCND1 can upregulate DHFR and TS, the combined effect of genetic polymorphisms in these three genes is more pronounced and leads to a further reduction in EFS in childhood ALL patients [21].

Reduced Folate Carrier

Reduced folate carrier (RFC1) is a major MTX transporter, whose expression/function may also affect MTX sensitivity [17] (Fig. 20.2). Impaired RFC1 function has been recognized as a frequent mechanism of antifolate resistance [17]. A G80A polymorphism, leading to His27Arg replacement in the first transmembrane domain of the RFC1 protein, is considered to play a key role in folate–antifolate binding [56, 57]. The G allele is present in 45–55% of Caucasians, 30% of Africans, and 50% of Asians [58]. This polymorphism is associated with an increased risk of relapse in children with ALL and a higher risk of gastrointestinal toxicity during consolidation and maintenance treatment [59–62]. The mechanism for these associations is still unknown since in vitro, MTX uptake is similar for the A and G alleles [63]. The effect of another functional variant in linkage disequilibrium with the G80A substitution might explain this difference in outcomes [60]. It is also possible that the G80A allele affects folate homeostasis and not MTX transport [17]. The association of the G80A allele with conditions characterized by folate deficiencies, such as NTD and chromosome nondisjunction, favors this latter hypothesis [64, 65].

Multidrug-Resistance Protein and Multidrug-Resistance-Associated Proteins

Multidrug-resistance (MDR) proteins are membrane-bound proteins that transport drugs out of the cell and determine drug absorption, distribution, and excretion [66]. MDR proteins are members of the ATP-binding cassette (ABC) family of transporters (Fig. 20.2). They use ATP as an energy source, have highly conserved ATP-binding domain(s) in their protein structure, and are expressed in a variety of tissues including intestine, liver, kidney, brain, and hematopoietic cells.

P-glycoprotein (P-gp) is controlled by the MDR1 gene, and several multidrug-resistance-associated proteins (MRP) are controlled by MRP genes. These proteins are involved in the efflux of many chemotherapeutic agents used in leukemia treatment (i.e., MTX, 6-MP, corticosteroids (CS), anthracycline, vincristine, etoposide, and cyclophosphamide) [17, 67]. Activity and expression of P-gp and MRPs may affect bioavailability of these drugs. An increase in MRP1 and MRP3 expression is associated with a poor prognosis in adult ALL [68, 69]. Increased MDR1 expression is associated with an inferior outcome in both childhood and adult ALL patients [70, 71].

Pharmacogenetic studies have analyzed the MDR1 gene, with emphasis on the C3435T substitution (Table 20.1). The T allele is present in 55% of Caucasians, 42% of Eastern Asians, and 21% of Africans [72], and is associated with reduced P-gp function [73, 74]. Clinically, the T allele is associated with a better prognosis and lower rate of CNS relapse in childhood ALL patients [75, 76]. However, there is also an increased risk of infectious complications in this subgroup of patients [77]. No association of the T allele with prognosis has been demonstrated in adult ALL patients [78]. One study analyzed the C24T polymorphism of the MRP2 gene in leukemia patients [79]. The frequency of this allele is 15–17% in both Caucasians and Eastern Asians [80, 81]. This polymorphism is located in the regulatory region of the gene and has been associated with lower mRNA levels of MRP2 [82]. MTX levels following high-dose MTX were higher in childhood ALL patients with this variant allele, and intensification of leucovorin rescue was needed [79] (Table 20.1).

Corticosteroids

CS are an integral part of the therapeutic armamentarium in ALL. However, resistance and toxicity are associated with the use of these drugs [83]. The percentage of children resistant to CS increases from 20% to 30% at diagnosis to 70% at relapse [84]. CS are also associated with toxicity [85]. In 20% of children treated for ALL, a significant decrease in bone mineral density is reported, resulting in osteoporosis and avascular bone necrosis [86]. Clinical observations demonstrate variations in patients' sensitivity to CS therapy with respect to both efficacy and toxicity [85–88].

Genes of CS Action Pathways

Polymorphisms of the glucocorticoid receptor are known to influence the response to endogenous steroids and to correlate with changes in metabolism, cardiovascular control, and stress response [89, 90]. These polymorphisms have been studied in childhood ALL patients [91, 92]. Reduced overall survival was reported for individuals with the GG genotype (a C to G substitution at the position 646 of intron 2, Table 20.1) [91]. The G allele occurs with a frequency of 30–35% in Caucasians, 32% in Asians, and 20% in Africans [93, 94].

Corticotropin-releasing hormone receptor (CRHR1) plays a pivotal role in steroid biology by regulating endogenous cortisol levels [95]. Variation in its activity may also affect the response to exogenous steroids. Polymorphism of this gene influences the asthmatic response to CS in both adult and pediatric patients [96]. This same variant (G to T substitution in intron 2, rs242941 together with A to T replacement in intron 12 [rs1876828]) is associated with corticosteroid-induced hypertension and a lower bone density in childhood ALL patients [97, 98] (Table 20.1).

Interleukin 10 (IL-10) also influences transcriptional activity of the glucocorticoid receptor. The binding capacity for dexamethasone can be upregulated by high IL-10 production [99, 100]. A polymorphism in the regulatory region of the IL-10 gene (A-1082G) has been described. The G allele is associated with increased expression of IL-10, and childhood ALL patients with the GG genotype have an improved response to prednisone (Table 20.1) [100].

Genes Coding for Xenobiotic Metabolizing Enzymes

Xenobiotic metabolizing enzymes are involved in the biotransformation of a wide range of carcinogens and drugs, including those used in the treatment of ALL. Several glutathione-S-transferase (GSTs) subfamilies exist, and multiple polymorphisms are present in the respective genes. Genotypes with lower GST activity may confer a therapeutic advantage to patients undergoing chemotherapy treatment. The GSTM1 and GSTT1 null genotypes result from homozygous gene deletions. Individuals with these genotypes lack the respective GST activities. In the GSTP1 gene, two single-nucleotide polymorphisms (SNPs) leading to amino acid substitutions have been described [101]. A lower incidence of relapse is found in pediatric ALL patients with the null genotype of GSTT1 and the GSTM1 genes [48, 102, 103], and an improved prednisone response has been demonstrated in GSTT1 null individuals [102, 104] (Table 20.2). Etoposide clearance is increased in carriers of the low-activity GSTP1 allele (Val allele of Ile105Val polymorphism) [105].

Genotypes with lower GST activity also have the potential to increase the risk of cancer in an individual because GST is involved in the metabolism of carcinogens. An increased susceptibility to adult ALL has been associated with the GSTT1 null genotype [106]. However, no data exists in adult ALL patients regarding the modulation of treatment response by GST polymorphisms.

Cytochrome P4501A1 (CYP1A1) is another xenobiotic metabolizing enzyme. CYP1A1*2A has a T6235C polymorphism located in the 3' UTR of the gene and is associated with increased enzyme inducibility. This variant is associated with a decreased EFS in childhood ALL (Table 20.2) [107]. Corticosteroids can affect the induction and catalytic activity of CYP1A1 by acting through CYP1A1 glucocorticoid-responsive elements [108, 109].

Disease-Associated Genes

One of the adverse effects of CS therapy is hypertension. A comprehensive analysis of a large number of candidate genes possibly involved in CS-induced hypertension has been performed [97]. This analysis identified genes related to the development of hypertension, metabolic syndrome, and atherosclerosis (Table 20.2). Genes identified include the leptin receptor (LEPR, Gln223Arg), [110] the sodium chloride transporter (SLC12A3, G2744A, Arg913Gln) [111], and apolipoprotein B (APOB, XbaI polymorphism) [112]. Contactin-associated protein-like-2 (CNTNAP2, C to T substitution in exon 11, rs2286128) was also identified as an important predictor of hypertension. Although its role in the development of hypertension is not clear, CNTNAP2 is expressed in the pituitary gland and kidney and may modulate glucocorticoid effects on blood pressure via interaction with the potassium and sodium ion channels [97]. This variant allele is not present in Caucasians but is present in Africans and Asians with frequencies of 5% and 9%, respectively.

Table 20.2 Summary of studies demonstrating an association between therapeutic response in ALL and polymorphisms in xenobiotic metabolizing and disease-related genes

Gene	Polymorphism	Impact	Function	Association	Population	Drug	Ref
GSTT1	Null genotype	Deletion	Reduced	Risk of relapse, prednisone response	Childhood	Alkylating agents, anthracyclines, CS,	[102–104]
GSTM1	Null genotype	Deletion	Reduced	Risk of relapse	Childhood		[48]
GSTP1	A1578G	Ile105Val	Reduced	Lower etoposide clearance	Childhood	etoposide	[105]
CYP1A1	*2A (T6235C)	3′ UTR	Increased	EFS,DFS	Childhood		[107]
SLC12A3	G 2744A	Arg913Gln		CS-induced hypertension	Childhood		[97]
APOB	C7673T,XbaI	Synonymous					
LEPR	C870T	Arg223Gln					
CNTNAP2	C2226T	Synonymous					
PAI-1	G118A	A1a15Thr		Osteonecrosis	Childhood		[115]
UGT1A1	*28 [TA(6)-41 TA(7)]	Promoter transcription	Reduced	Hyperbilirubinemia	Adult	Nilotinib	[120]
NOD2/CARD15	C2104T	Arg702Trp		OS, DFS	Adult	Transplantation	[121]
	G2722C	Gly908Arg					
	insC3019	Frameshift 1007					

GSTT1, GSTM1, GSTP1, glutathione-S-transferase T1, M1, P1; *CYP1A1*, cytochrome P-450 1A1; *SLC12A3*, sodium chloride transporter; *APOB*, apolipoprotein B; *LEPR*, leptin receptor; *CNTNAP2*, contactin-associated protein-like-2; *PAI-1*, serpine 1; UGT1A1 uridine diphosphate glucuronosyltransferase 1, isoform A1; *NOD2/CARD15*, nucleotide-binding oligomerization domain 2/caspase recruitment domain 15

High levels of serpine 1 (PAI-1), induced by corticosteroid treatment, or through polymorphisms in PAI-1, lead to suppression of fibrinolysis through inhibition of tissue plasminogen activator and promotion of thrombosis, ultimately resulting in hypoxic bone death or osteonecrosis [113, 114]. An association between the PAI-1 G118A polymorphism (rs6092) and osteonecrosis has been demonstrated in childhood ALL patients (Table 20.2) [115]. Allele frequencies of this gene differ significantly between populations. The combined GA and AA genotypes were present in 30.9% of Caucasians, 12.5% of African-Americans, and 20% of Hispanics [115]. These genotypes are in linkage disequilibrium with a 4G/5G repeat promoter insertion/deletion polymorphism [116]. The 4G allele has been associated with an increased risk of osteonecrosis among renal transplant recipients who received glucocorticoids [117].

Other Genes Modulating the Therapeutic Response in Acute Lymphoblastic Leukemia

The A1 isoform of uridine diphosphate glucuronosyltransferase 1 (UGT1A1) catalyzes glucuronidation of hepatic bilirubin in humans. An $A(TA)_7TAA$ polymorphism in a TATAA element in the promoter region reduces UGT1A1 expression and contributes to the benign elevation of bilirubin, as compared to the common $A(TA)_6TAA$ allele [118]. The $(TA)_7$ allele occurs at frequencies up to 42% in some African and South Asian populations, and is seen in Asian and European populations at lower rates (1–15%).

Nilotinib is an inhibitor of the BCR-ABL kinase [119]. In a Phase 1 trial of Nilotinib for patients with imatinib-resistant or imatinib-intolerant chronic myeloid leukemia or refractory Philadelphia chromosome positive ALL, homozygosity for the (TA)7 allele was associated with an increased risk of hyperbilirubinemia (Table 20.2) [120]. Although Nilotinib is not metabolized by UGT1A1, it can inhibit UGT1A1 activity leading to hyperbilirubinemia in susceptible (TA)7 homozygous individuals.

Hematopoietic Stem Cell Transplantation

Hematopoietic stem cell transplantation (HSCT) is an important option in the management of acute leukemia, but the risk of disease relapse and death remains high. It has been recently demonstrated that the presence of nucleotide-binding oligomerization domain 2 (NOD2)/caspase recruitment domain 15 (CARD15) polymorphisms have a significant impact on the outcome in patients receiving HSCT for ALL [121]. The NOD2/CARD15 gene encodes the NOD2 protein, which is involved in the formation of a protein complex termed the inflammasome. The inflammasome has widespread effects on innate immunity, cytokine secretion, cell survival, and apoptosis [122]. Three SNPs within the NOD2/CARD15 gene have been associated with functional immune defects and with the occurrence of inflammatory bowel disorders [123]. Two of these, C2104T in exon 4 and G2722C in exon 8 (labeled SNP8 and SNP12), cause amino acid substitutions (Arg702Trp and Gly908Arg, respectively). The insertion of a C at the position 3019 in exon 11 (labeled SNP13) causes a frameshift mutation and truncation of the protein. These three mutations could potentially alter activation of NFκB [124].

In adult ALL patients receiving transplants from unrelated donors, the presence of any of three NOD2/CARD15 polymorphisms in donor/recipient pairs was associated with worse overall survival and disease-free survival (Table 20.2) [121]. The effect of NOD2/CARD15 polymorphisms (and possibly other variants as well) is largely dependent on transplant regimen, donor source, underlying disease, and ethnicity [125]. Several other studies analyzing heterogeneous patient populations in terms of diagnosis and transplant regimen reported an association between NOD2/CARD15 polymorphisms and different outcomes [126–129]. The SNPs 8, 12, and 13 of NOD2/CARD15 gene are relatively rare, appearing only in individuals of European descendent with a frequency of 5–7%, 1–2%, and 2.5–5%, respectively, as defined by HapMap data and literature reports [130].

Conclusion

Our understanding of the role of genetic variants in the therapeutic response of ALL has only begun to unravel. Certain studies are still inconclusive and require further validation. Most studies have addressed only one enzyme or one polymorphism at a time and are insufficient to explain the complex web of influences that surrounds the host-related genetic factors of therapeutic response. There is no doubt that several factors will have to be considered simultaneously to accurately predict disease outcome. Towards this goal, future studies will have to simultaneously address all mediators of resistance to one drug and, beyond that, to consider the whole spectrum of genetic polymorphisms that are relevant to multi-agent leukemia treatment protocols. Achievement of this goal will allow individualized treatment according to a patient's genetic profile. This will both increase drug efficacy and reduce long-term side effects.

References

1. Goldstein, D. B., Tate, S. K., & Sisodiya, S. M. (2003). Pharmacogenetics goes genomic. *Nature Reviews Genetics, 4*, 937–947.
2. Bleyer, W. A. (1990). The impact of childhood cancer on the United States and the world. *CA: A Cancer Journal for Clinicians, 40*, 355–367.
3. Pui, C. H. (2000). Acute lymphoblastic leukemia in children. *Current Opinion in Oncology, 12*, 3–12.
4. Cheok, M. H., & Evans, W. E. (2006). Acute lymphoblastic leukaemia: a model for the pharmacogenomics of cancer therapy. *Nature Reviews Cancer, 6*, 117–129.
5. Cheok, M. H., Lugthart, S., & Evans, W. E. (2006). Pharmacogenomics of acute leukemia. *Annual Review of Pharmacology and Toxicology, 46*, 317–353.
6. McLeod, H. L., Krynetski, E. Y., Relling, M. V., & Evans, W. E. (2000). Genetic polymorphism of thiopurine methyltransferase and its clinical relevance for childhood acute lymphoblastic leukemia. *Leukemia, 14*, 567–572.
7. Evans, W. E., & Relling, M. V. (2004). Moving towards individualized medicine with pharmacogenomics. *Nature, 429*, 464–468.
8. Maitland, M. L., Vasisht, K., & Ratain, M. J. (2006). TPMT, UGT1A1 and DPYD: genotyping to ensure safer cancer therapy? *Trends in Pharmacological Sciences, 27*, 432–437.
9. Stanulla, M., Schaeffeler, E., Flohr, T., et al. (2005). Thiopurine methyltransferase (TPMT) genotype and early treatment response to mercaptopurine in childhood acute lymphoblastic leukemia. *Journal of the American Medical Association, 293*, 1485–1489.
10. Kudo, M., Moteki, T., Sasaki, T., et al. (2008). Functional characterization of human xanthine oxidase allelic variants. *Pharmacogenetics and Genomics, 18*, 243–251.
11. Hawwa, A. F., Millership, J. S., Collier, P. S., et al. (2008). Pharmacogenomic studies of the anticancer and immunosuppressive thiopurines mercaptopurine and azathioprine. *British Journal of Clinical Pharmacology, 66*, 517–528.
12. Marinaki, A. M., Ansari, A., Duley, J. A., et al. (2004). Adverse drug reactions to azathioprine therapy are associated with polymorphism in the gene encoding inosine triphosphate pyrophosphatase (ITPase). *Pharmacogenetics, 14*, 181–187.
13. von Ahsen, N., Oellerich, M., & Armstrong, V. W. (2008). Characterization of the inosine triphosphatase (ITPA) gene: haplotype structure, haplotype-phenotype correlation and promoter function. *Therapeutic Drug Monitoring, 30*, 16–22.

14. Marsh, S., King, C. R., Ahluwalia, R., & McLeod, H. L. (2004). Distribution of ITPA P32T alleles in multiple world populations. *Journal of Human Genetics, 49*, 579–581.

15. Hawwa, A. F., Collier, P. S., Millership, J. S., et al. (2008). Population pharmacokinetic and pharmacogenetic analysis of 6-mercaptopurine in paediatric patients with acute lymphoblastic leukaemia. *British Journal of Clinical Pharmacology, 66*(6), 826–837.

16. Stocco, G., Cheok, M., Crews, K., et al. (2009). Genetic polymorphism of inosine triphosphate pyrophosphatase is a determinant of mercaptopurine metabolism and toxicity during treatment for acute lymphoblastic leukemia. *Clinical Pharmacology and Therapeutics, 85*(2), 164–172.

17. Assaraf, Y. G. (2007). Molecular basis of antifolate resistance. *Cancer and Metastasis Reviews, 26*, 153–181.

18. Matherly, L. H., Taub, J. W., Ravindranath, Y., et al. (1995). Elevated dihydrofolate reductase and impaired methotrexate transport as elements in methotrexate resistance in childhood acute lymphoblastic leukemia. *Blood, 85*, 500–509.

19. Matherly, L. H., Taub, J. W., Wong, S. C., et al. (1997). Increased frequency of expression of elevated dihydrofolate reductase in T-cell versus B-precursor acute lymphoblastic leukemia in children. *Blood, 90*, 578–589.

20. Rots, M. G., Willey, J. C., Jansen, G., et al. (2000). mRNA expression levels of methotrexate resistance-related proteins in childhood leukemia as determined by a standardized competitive template-based RT-PCR method. *Leukemia, 14*, 2166–2175.

21. Dulucq, S., St-Onge, G., Gagne, V., et al. (2008). DNA variants in the dihydrofolate reductase gene and outcome in childhood ALL. *Blood, 111*, 3692–3700.

22. Goto, Y., Yue, L., Yokoi, A., et al. (2001). A novel single-nucleotide polymorphism in the 3′-untranslated region of the human dihydrofolate reductase gene with enhanced expression. *Clinical Cancer Research, 7*, 1952–1956.

23. Mishra, P. J., Humeniuk, R., Mishra, P. J., Longo-Sorbello, G. S., Banerjee, D., & Bertino, J. R. (2007). A miR-24 microRNA binding-site polymorphism in dihydrofolate reductase gene leads to methotrexate resistance. *Proceedings of the National Academy of Sciences of the United States of America, 104*, 13513–13518.

24. Schwahn, B., & Rozen, R. (2001). Polymorphisms in the methylenetetrahydrofolate reductase gene: clinical consequences. *American Journal of Pharmacogenomics, 1*, 189–201.

25. Blount, B. C., Mack, M. M., Wehr, C. M., et al. (1997). Folate deficiency causes uracil misincorporation into human DNA and chromosome breakage: implications for cancer and neuronal damage. *Proceedings of the National Academy of Sciences of the United States of America, 94*, 3290–3295.

26. Krajinovic, M., & Moghrabi, A. (2004). Pharmacogenetics of methotrexate. *Pharmacogenomics, 5*, 819–834.

27. Frosst, P., Blom, H. J., Milos, R., et al. (1995). A candidate genetic risk factor for vascular disease: a common mutation in methylenetetrahydrofolate reductase. *Nature Genetics, 10*, 111–113.

28. van der Put, N. M., Gabreels, F., Stevens, E. M., et al. (1998). A second common mutation in the methylenetetrahydrofolate reductase gene: an additional risk factor for neural-tube defects? *American Journal of Human Genetics, 62*, 1044–1051.

29. Rosenberg, N., Murata, M., Ikeda, Y., et al. (2002). The frequent 5, 10-methylenetetrahydrofolate reductase C677T polymorphism is associated with a common haplotype in whites, Japanese, and Africans. *American Journal of Human Genetics, 70*, 758–762.

30. Ogino, S., & Wilson, R. B. (2003). Genotype and haplotype distributions of MTHFR677C>T and 1298A>C single nucleotide polymorphisms: a meta-analysis. *Journal of Human Genetics, 48*, 1–7.

31. Sohn, K. J., Croxford, R., Yates, Z., Lucock, M., & Kim, Y. I. (2004). Effect of the methylenetetrahydrofolate reductase C677T polymorphism on chemosensitivity of colon and breast cancer cells to 5-fluorouracil and methotrexate. *Journal of the National Cancer Institute, 96*, 134–144.

32. Krajinovic, M., Lemieux-Blanchard, E., Chiasson, S., Primeau, M., Costea, I., & Moghrabi, A. (2004). Role of polymorphisms in MTHFR and MTHFD1 genes in the outcome of childhood acute lymphoblastic leukemia. *The Pharmacogenomics Journal, 4*, 66–72.

33. Aplenc, R., Thompson, J., Han, P., et al. (2005). Methylenetetrahydrofolate reductase polymorphisms and therapy response in pediatric acute lymphoblastic leukemia. *Cancer Research, 65*, 2482–2487.

34. Chiusolo, P., Reddiconto, G., Farina, G., et al. (2007). MTHFR polymorphisms' influence on outcome and toxicity in acute lymphoblastic leukemia patients. *Leukemia Research, 31*, 1669–1674.

35. Costea, I., Moghrabi, A., Laverdiere, C., Graziani, A., & Krajinovic, M. (2006). Folate cycle gene variants and chemotherapy toxicity in pediatric patients with acute lymphoblastic leukemia. *Haematologica, 91*, 1113–1116.

36. Kishi, S., Griener, J., Cheng, C., et al. (2003). Homocysteine, pharmacogenetics, and neurotoxicity in children with leukemia. *Journal of Clinical Oncology, 21*, 3084–3091.

37. Chiusolo, P., Reddiconto, G., Casorelli, I., et al. (2002). Preponderance of methylenetetrahydrofolate reductase C677T homozygosity among leukemia patients intolerant to methotrexate. *Annals of Oncology, 13*, 1915–1918.

38. Horie, N., Aiba, H., Oguro, K., Hojo, H., & Takeishi, K. (1995). Functional analysis and DNA polymorphism of the tandemly repeated sequences in the 5′-terminal regulatory region of the human gene for thymidylate synthase. *Cell Structure and Function, 20*, 191–197.

39. Marsh, S., Collie-Duguid, E. S., Li, T., Liu, X., & McLeod, H. L. (1999). Ethnic variation in the thymidylate synthase enhancer region polymorphism among Caucasian and Asian populations. *Genomics, 58*, 310–312.

40. Kawakami, K., & Watanabe, G. (2003). Identification and functional analysis of single nucleotide polymorphism in the tandem repeat sequence of thymidylate synthase gene. *Cancer Research, 63*, 6004–6007.

41. Mandola, M. V., Stoehlmacher, J., Muller-Weeks, S., et al. (2003). A novel single nucleotide polymorphism within the 5′ tandem repeat polymorphism of the thymidylate synthase gene abolishes USF-1 binding and alters transcriptional activity. *Cancer Research, 63*, 2898–2904.

42. Kawakami, K., Omura, K., Kanehira, E., & Watanabe, Y. (1999). Polymorphic tandem repeats in the thymidylate synthase gene is associated with its protein expression in human gastrointestinal cancers. *Anticancer Research, 19*, 3249–3252.

43. Pullarkat, S. T., Stoehlmacher, J., Ghaderi, V., et al. (2001). Thymidylate synthase gene polymorphism determines response and toxicity of 5-FU chemotherapy. *The Pharmacogenomics Journal, 1*, 65–70.

44. Robien, K., Bigler, J., Yasui, Y., et al. (2006). Methylenetetrahydrofolate reductase and thymidylate synthase genotypes and risk of acute graft-versus-host disease following hematopoietic cell transplantation for chronic myelogenous leukemia. *Biology of Blood and Marrow Transplantation, 12*, 973–980.

45. Robien, K., Schubert, M. M., Chay, T., et al. (2006). Methylenetetrahydrofolate reductase and thymidylate synthase genotypes modify oral mucositis severity following hematopoietic stem cell transplantation. *Bone Marrow Transplantation, 37*, 799–800.

46. Krajinovic, M., Costea, I., & Chiasson, S. (2002). Polymorphism of the thymidylate synthase gene and outcome of acute lymphoblastic leukaemia. *Lancet, 359*, 1033–1034.

47. Krajinovic, M., Costea, I., Primeau, M., Dulucq, S., & Moghrabi, A. (2005). Combining several polymorphisms of thymidylate synthase gene for pharmacogenetic analysis. *The Pharmacogenomics Journal, 5*, 374–380.

48. Rocha, J. C., Cheng, C., Liu, W., et al. (2005). Pharmacogenetics of outcome in children with acute lymphoblastic leukemia. *Blood, 105*, 4752–4758.

49. Relling, M. V., Yang, W., Das, S., et al. (2004). Pharmacogenetic risk factors for osteonecrosis of the hip among children with leukemia. *Journal of Clinical Oncology, 22*, 3930–3936.

50. Hochhauser, D. (1997). Modulation of chemosensitivity through altered expression of cell cycle regulatory genes in cancer. *Anti-Cancer Drugs, 8*, 903–910.

51. Hochhauser, D., Schnieders, B., Ercikan-Abali, E., et al. (1996). Effect of cyclin D1 overexpression on drug sensitivity in a human fibrosarcoma cell line. *Journal of the National Cancer Institute, 88*, 1269–1275.

52. Li, W., Fan, J., Hochhauser, D., et al. (1995). Lack of functional retinoblastoma protein mediates increased resistance to antimetabolites in human sarcoma cell lines. *Proceedings of the National Academy of Sciences of the United States of America, 92*, 10436–10440.

53. Betticher, D. C., Thatcher, N., Altermatt, H. J., Hoban, P., Ryder, W. D., & Heighway, J. (1995). Alternate splicing produces a novel cyclin D1 transcript. *Oncogene, 11*, 1005–1011.

54. Costea, I., Moghrabi, A., & Krajinovic, M. (2003). The influence of cyclin D1 (CCND1) 870A>G polymorphism and CCND1-thymidylate synthase (TS) gene-gene interaction on the outcome of childhood acute lymphoblastic leukaemia. *Pharmacogenetics, 13*, 577–580.

55. Hou, X., Wang, S., Zhou, Y., et al. (2005). Cyclin D1 gene polymorphism and susceptibility to childhood acute lymphoblastic leukemia in a Chinese population. *International Journal of Hematology, 82*, 206–209.

56. Drori, S., Jansen, G., Mauritz, R., Peters, G. J., & Assaraf, Y. G. (2000). Clustering of mutations in the first transmembrane domain of the human reduced folate carrier in GW1843U89-resistant leukemia cells with impaired antifolate transport and augmented folate uptake. *The Journal of Biological Chemistry, 275*, 30855–30863.

57. Chango, A., Emery-Fillon, N., de Courcy, G. P., et al. (2000). A polymorphism (80G->A) in the reduced folate carrier gene and its associations with folate status and homocysteinemia. *Molecular Genetics and Metabolism, 70*, 310–315.

58. Shi, M., Caprau, D., Romitti, P., Christensen, K., & Murray, J. C. (2003). Genotype frequencies and linkage disequilibrium in the CEPH human diversity panel for variants in folate pathway genes MTHFR, MTHFD, MTRR, RFC1, and GCP2. *Birth Defects Research, 67*, 545–549.

59. Imanishi, H., Okamura, N., Yagi, M., et al. (2007). Genetic polymorphisms associated with adverse events and elimination of methotrexate in childhood acute lymphoblastic leukemia and malignant lymphoma. *Journal of Human Genetics, 52*, 166–171.

60. Kishi, S., Cheng, C., French, D., et al. (2007). Ancestry and pharmacogenetics of antileukemic drug toxicity. *Blood, 109*, 4151–4157.

61. Laverdiere, C., Chiasson, S., Costea, I., Moghrabi, A., & Krajinovic, M. (2002). Polymorphism G80A in the reduced folate carrier gene and its relationship to methotrexate plasma levels and outcome of childhood acute lymphoblastic leukemia. *Blood, 100*, 3832–3834.

62. Shimasaki, N., Mori, T., Samejima, H., et al. (2006). Effects of methylenetetrahydrofolate reductase and reduced folate carrier 1 polymorphisms on high-dose methotrexate-induced toxicities in children with acute lymphoblastic leukemia or lymphoma. *Journal of Pediatric Hematology/Oncology, 28*, 64–68.

63. Whetstine, J. R., Gifford, A. J., Witt, T., et al. (2001). Single nucleotide polymorphisms in the human reduced folate carrier: characterization of a high-frequency G/A variant at position 80 and transport properties of the His(27) and Arg(27) carriers. *Clinical Cancer Research, 7*, 3416–3422.

64. Wang, L., Chen, W., Wang, J., et al. (2006). Reduced folate carrier gene G80A polymorphism is associated with an increased risk of gastroesophageal cancers in a Chinese population. *European Journal of Cancer, 42*, 3206–3211.

65. Scala, I., Granese, B., Sellitto, M., et al. (2006). Analysis of seven maternal polymorphisms of genes involved in homocysteine/folate metabolism and risk of Down syndrome offspring. *Genetics in Medicine, 8*, 409–416.

66. Gradhand, U., & Kim, R. B. (2008). Pharmacogenomics of MRP transporters (ABCC1-5) and BCRP (ABCG2). *Drug Metabolism Reviews, 40*, 317–354.

67. Bradshaw, D. M., & Arceci, R. J. (1998). Clinical relevance of transmembrane drug efflux as a mechanism of multidrug resistance. *Journal of Clinical Oncology, 16*, 3674–3690.

68. Steinbach, D., & Legrand, O. (2007). ABC transporters and drug resistance in leukemia: was P-gp nothing but the first head of the Hydra? *Leukemia, 21*, 1172–1176.

69. Plasschaert, S. L., de Bont, E. S., Boezen, M., et al. (2005). Expression of multidrug resistance-associated proteins predicts prognosis in childhood and adult acute lymphoblastic leukemia. *Clinical Cancer Research, 11*, 8661–8668.

70. Kourti, M., Vavatsi, N., Gombakis, N., et al. (2007). Expression of multidrug resistance 1 (MDR1), multidrug resistance-related protein 1 (MRP1), lung resistance protein (LRP), and breast cancer resistance protein (BCRP) genes and clinical outcome in childhood acute lymphoblastic leukemia. *International Journal of Hematology, 86*, 166–173.

71. Vitale, A., Guarini, A., Ariola, C., et al. (2006). Adult T-cell acute lymphoblastic leukemia: biologic profile at presentation and correlation with response to induction treatment in patients enrolled in the GIMEMA LAL 0496 protocol. *Blood, 107*, 473–479.

72. Tang, K., Wong, L. P., Lee, E. J., Chong, S. S., & Lee, C. G. (2004). Genomic evidence for recent positive selection at the human MDR1 gene locus. *Human Molecular Genetics, 13*, 783–797.

73. Hoffmeyer, S., Burk, O., von Richter, O., et al. (2000). Functional polymorphisms of the human multidrug-resistance gene: multiple sequence variations and correlation of one allele with P-glycoprotein expression and activity in vivo. *Proceedings of the National Academy of Sciences of the United States of America, 97*, 3473–3478.

74. Kimchi-Sarfaty, C., Oh, J. M., Kim, I. W., et al. (2007). A "silent" polymorphism in the MDR1 gene changes substrate specificity. *Science, 315*, 525–528.

75. Stanulla, M., Schaffeler, E., Arens, S., et al. (2005). GSTP1 and MDR1 genotypes and central nervous system relapse in childhood acute lymphoblastic leukemia. *International Journal of Hematology, 81*, 39–44.

76. Jamroziak, K., Mlynarski, W., Balcerczak, E., et al. (2004). Functional C3435T polymorphism of MDR1 gene: an impact on genetic susceptibility and clinical outcome of childhood acute lymphoblastic leukemia. *European Journal of Hematology, 72*, 314–321.

77. Erdelyi, D. J., Kamory, E., Zalka, A., et al. (2006). The role of ABC-transporter gene polymorphisms in chemotherapy induced immunosuppression, a retrospective study in childhood acute lymphoblastic leukaemia. *Cellular Immunology, 244*, 121–124.

78. Jamroziak, K., Balcerczak, E., Cebula, B., et al. (2005). Multi-drug transporter MDR1 gene polymorphism and prognosis in adult acute lymphoblastic leukemia. *Pharmacological Reports, 57*, 882–888.

79. Rau, T., Erney, B., Gores, R., Eschenhagen, T., Beck, J., & Langer, T. (2006). High-dose methotrexate in pediatric acute lymphoblastic leukemia: impact of ABCC2 polymorphisms on plasma concentrations. *Clinical Pharmacology and Therapeutics, 80*, 468–476.

80. Sai, K., Saito, Y., Itoda, M., et al. (2008). Genetic variations and haplotypes of ABCC2 encoding MRP2 in a Japanese population. *Drug Metabolism and Pharmacokinetics, 23*, 139–147.

81. Daly, A. K., Aithal, G. P., Leathart, J. B., Swainsbury, R. A., Dang, T. S., & Day, C. P. (2007). Genetic susceptibility to diclofenac-induced hepatotoxicity: contribution of UGT2B7, CYP2C8, and ABCC2 genotypes. *Gastroenterology, 132*, 272–281.

82. Haenisch, S., Zimmermann, U., Dazert, E., et al. (2007). Influence of polymorphisms of ABCB1 and ABCC2 on mRNA and protein expression in normal and cancerous kidney cortex. *The Pharmacogenomics Journal, 7*, 56–65.

83. Tissing, W. J., Meijerink, J. P., den Boer, M. L., & Pieters, R. (2003). Molecular determinants of glucocorticoid sensitivity and resistance in acute lymphoblastic leukemia. *Leukemia, 17*, 17–25.

84. Bailey, S., Hall, A. G., Pearson, A. D., Reid, M. M., & Redfern, C. P. (1999). Glucocorticoid resistance and the AP-1 transcription factor in leukaemia. *Advances in Experimental Medicine and Biology, 457*, 615–619.

85. Gaynon, P. S., & Carrel, A. L. (1999). Glucocorticosteroid therapy in childhood acute lymphoblastic leukemia. *Advances in Experimental Medicine and Biology, 457*, 593–605.

86. Bianchi, M. L. (2002). Glucocorticoids and bone: some general remarks and some special observations in pediatric patients. *Calcified Tissue International, 70*, 384–390.

87. Ito, C., Evans, W. E., McNinch, L., et al. (1996). Comparative cytotoxicity of dexamethasone and prednisolone in childhood acute lymphoblastic leukemia. *Journal of Clinical Oncology, 14*, 2370–2376.

Chapter 5
Cytogenetics

Anthony V. Moorman and Christine J. Harrison

Introduction

Acquired chromosomal abnormalities in the leukemic blasts of patients with acute lymphoblastic leukemia (ALL) are hallmarks of the disease. The discovery and characterization of these genetic lesions have increased our understanding of the biology of ALL, have shaped our current classification system, and are now used to direct therapy. Moreover, deciphering the underlying molecular consequences of chromosomal translocations has led to the development of therapies that target specific molecular lesions. Since acquired clonal chromosomal abnormalities were first identified in the early 1960s, the number and spectrum of these aberrations have increased dramatically. To date, more than 150 recurrent balanced aberrations have been reported in ALL, including more than 80 gene fusions [1].

Cytogenetic investigations form a vital part of the standard diagnostic work-up of adults with ALL. Certain chromosomal abnormalities are considered to be pathognomic of particular disease subtypes and point to treatment with specific protocols or drugs. Hence, an increasing number and type of healthcare professionals encounter and are required to understand and interpret cytogenetic reports and terminology. This chapter provides an overview of the main cytogenetic and genetic techniques, their associated terminology, and a description of the principal genetic abnormalities so far identified in adult ALL in relation to their clinical significance.

Cytogenetic Techniques and Nomenclature

A range of genetic techniques can be employed to detect chromosomal and genetic abnormalities in patients with ALL. Table 5.1 provides an overview of the principal cytogenetic techniques and contrasts them with the main analogous molecular methods. Although these procedures are principally performed at diagnosis, they can also be used at subsequent time points to confirm remission or relapse.

A.V. Moorman (✉)
Leukaemia Research Cytogenetics Group, Northern Institute for Cancer Research,
Newcastle University, Newcastle-upon-Tyne, UK
e-mail: anthony.moorman@newcastle.ac.uk

A.S. Advani and H.M. Lazarus (eds.), *Adult Acute Lymphocytic Leukemia*, Contemporary Hematology,
DOI 10.1007/978-1-60761-707-5_5, © Springer Science+Business Media, LLC 2011

Table 5.1 Overview of the principal cytogenetic and molecular-genetic techniques used in the diagnosis and classification of adult ALL

Technique	Scope of Test	Target / Unit of analysis	Detection Limit	Detectable Abnormalities
G banded Cytogenetics	Whole genome	Chromosomes*	10^{-1} to 10^{-2}	Translocations, Deletions,
Locus specific FISH	Specific Target(s)	Genes / DNA sequences	10^{-2}	Amplifications, Aneuploidy
Multiplex FISH	Whole genome	Chromosomes*	10^{-1} to 10^{-2}	
Chromosome Painting	Specific Target(s)	Chromosomes*	10^{-1} to 10^{-2}	
RT-PCR	Specific Target(s)	Fusion transcripts	10^{-5}	Translocations
Quantitative PCR	Specific Target(s)	Gene copy number	10^{-5}	Deletions and Amplifications

*By definition these techniques require metaphases

Abbreviations: FISH - Fluorescence in situ Hybridisation; PCR - Polymerase Chain Reaction; RT - Reverse Transcriptase

Conventional Cytogenetic Analysis

Conventional cytogenetic analysis is the examination of chromosomes by bright-field microscopy during the metaphase stage of cell division, when they are condensed into discrete bodies within the nucleus. When a sample of bone marrow or peripheral blood is processed for cytogenetics, the addition of a spindle poison (e.g., colcemid) to the culture arrests cells at this stage of mitosis, thereby increasing the number of metaphases available for analysis. The chromosomes are then enzymatically treated and Giemsa stained to create a black and white banding pattern resembling a bar-code (G-banding) which is used to identify individual chromosomes (see Fig. 5.1). The total number of bands visible across the whole cell is proportional to the length of the chromosomes, which, in turn, depends on the level of chromosome condensation and the precise time during cell division at which the cell was arrested. In leukemic cells, usually only 240–330 bands are visible. Chromosomal analysis determines changes in chromosome number and the presence of structural abnormalities (see Fig. 5.2).

The major advantage of cytogenetics (see Table 5.1) is that it represents a whole genome analysis that identifies the majority of clinically relevant aberrations identified to date. Its major limitation is that it relies on the presence of metaphases which are representative of the leukemic clone. Thus a proportion of samples will fail or be classified as having a normal karyotype. In the absence of a clonal abnormality, samples are usually considered to have failed if fewer than 20 metaphases were available for analysis; otherwise they would be classified as having a normal karyotype. The rapid transport of bone marrow, in the correct medium to the cytogenetic laboratory, has been shown to maximize the chromosomal abnormality detection rate [3, 4].

Cytogenetic Terminology

The normal human chromosome complement of 46 chromosomes comprises 22 pairs of autosomes (numbered 1–22) and two sex chromosomes (XX in females and XY in males). Autosomes are numbered according to their size and the position of their centromere (see Fig. 5.1). Chromosomes are usually depicted "standing up" with the short (p) arm above and the long (q) arm below the centromere. Each chromosome arm is further divided into regions, bands, and subbands (see Fig. 5.1b), all of which are numbered outward from the centromere. Thus, the banding pattern produced by the

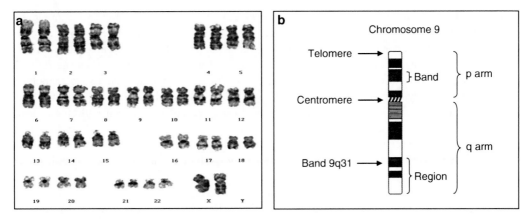

Fig. 5.1 (**a**) Karyogram of a G-banded metaphase from a normal female. (**b**) Ideogram of chromosome 9 illustrating the main components of a chromosome

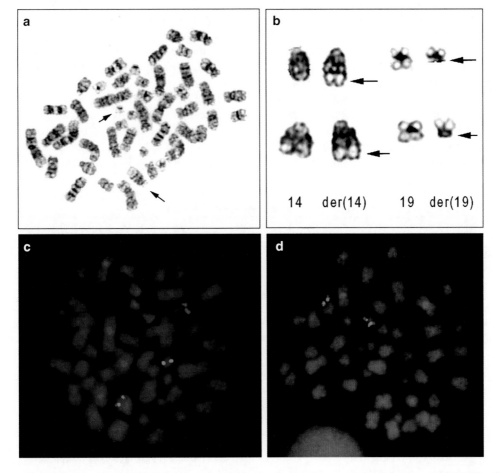

Fig. 5.2 (**a**) G-banded metaphase chromosomes from a young adult female with ALL and a t(14;19)(q32;q13). (**b**) Partial G-banded karyograms confirming the translocation breakpoints – 14q32 and 19q13. (**c**) Involvement of the *IGH@* locus was confirmed using the LSI© IGH Dual Color Break Apart Rearrangement Probe (Abbot Diagnostics), which showed a split signal pattern (1R-1G-1F). The 5′ *IGH@* green probe was translocated to the derived chromosome 19 while the 3′ *IGH@* red probe remaining on the derived chromosome 14. (**d**) Involvement of the *BCL3* gene (located at 19q13) was excluded using home-grown FISH probes, which flanked the gene and did not separate. Both probes were translocated to the derived chromosome 14; therefore, it was concluded that the breakpoint lay centromeric of the *BCL3* gene. This figure was original published in [2] (Copyright © 2004 Wiley-Liss, Inc.)

staining process provides a unique location for any breakpoint within the genome. For example, the region highlighted in Fig. 5.1b is 9q31, i.e., the long arm (q) of chromosome 9, region 3, band 1.

The spectrum of numerical and structural chromosomal abnormalities reported in leukemia is vast. The main types of aberrations seen in adult ALL are listed in Table 5.2, along with the possible molecular consequences of each type. Numerical chromosomal abnormalities give rise to aneuploidy and range from ploidy changes to the gain (trisomy) or loss (monosomy) of single chromosomes. Normal human cells are diploid (2n, 46 chromosomes). Loss or gain of an entire chromosome set leads to haploidy (n, 23 chromosomes), triploidy (3n, 69 chromosomes), or tetraploidy (4n, 92 chromosomes. Clones with fewer or more than 46 chromosomes are termed hypodiploid or hyperdiploid, respectively. Within the context of ALL, the following ploidy subgroups are recognized: near-haploidy (23–29 chromosomes), low hypodiploidy (30–39 chromosomes), hypodiploidy (40–45 chromosomes), low hyperdiploidy (47–50 chromosomes), high hyperdiploidy (51–65 chromosomes), near-triploidy (60–78 chromosomes), and near-tetraploidy (79–100 chromosomes). The overlap between the upper limit of high hyperdiploidy and the lower limit of near-triploidy will be discussed below in relation to these specific subgroups. Structural abnormalities arise from one or more double-stranded DNA breaks. The resulting acentric chromosome fragments (i.e., sections without a centromere) are lost, duplicated, amplified, inverted, or translocated to another chromosome (see Table 5.2).

The International System for Human Cytogenetic Nomenclature (ISCN 2009) [5] provides a standard system to describe the results of conventional cytogenetic analysis as a text string known as the karyotype. The different elements of a karyotype are separated using commas. The first two elements of any karyotype are the number of chromosomes (modal number) and the sex chromosomes. The number of cells with that particular chromosome makeup is stated at the end within square brackets. For example, a normal male karyotype seen in ten cells is written as 46,XY[10]. The chromosomal abnormalities are then listed in numerical order of the affected chromosome again delineated by commas. For example, the karyotype 47,XY,del(6)(q21),+8,t(9;22)(q34;q11) [10] represents an abnormal male cell line seen in ten cells with three abnormalities: (1) a deletion

Table 5.2 Summary of the main types of chromosomal abnormality in adult ALL

Chromosomal abnormality	Example(s)	Description	Possible molecular consequence
Deletion	del(6)(q21), del(6) (q21q25)	Loss of material distal to the breakpoint or between two breakpoints	Loss of a tumor suppressor gene; unmasking of a mutation present in the other allele; under-expression of genes in region (haplo-insufficiency)
Dicentric chromosome	dic(9;20)(p13;q11)	Loss of material distal to the two breakpoints and subsequent fusion of the two chromosomes	Chimeric gene fusion; loss of a tumor suppressor gene; under-expression of genes in the region (haplo-insufficiency)
Inversion	inv(7)(p13q35)	Inversion of chromosome segment between the two breakpoints	Chimeric gene fusion; juxtaposition of oncogene to foreign regulatory elements
Monosomy	−7	Loss of a whole chromosome	Loss of a tumor suppressor gene; unmasking of a mutation present in the other allele; under-expression of genes in region (haplo-insufficiency)
Translocation	t(4;11)(q21;q23)	Exchange of material distal to the breakpoints between two (or more) chromosomes	Chimeric gene fusion; juxtaposition of oncogene to foreign regulatory elements
Trisomy	+8	Gain of a whole chromosome	Over expression of genes on the affected chromosome

Table 21.1 Subtypes of late sequelae of treatment of acute lymphoblastic leukemia and blood and marrow transplantation

- Neurocognitive
- Endocrine
  - ○ Height and weight
  - ○ Thyroid
  - ○ Fertility and sterility
  - ○ Bone
- Cardiac
- Respiratory
- Hepatic
- Genitourinary
- Ophthalmologic
- Dental
- Second malignancies
- Psychosocial

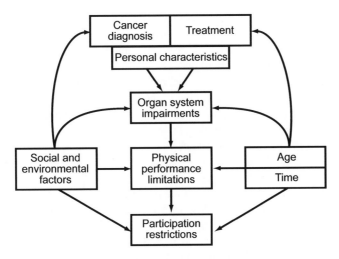

Fig. 21.2 Conceptual model of disability among cancer survivors (From [5])

malignancies developed. Over half of these second malignancies were in the central nervous system with the others affecting multiple organs.

Outcomes of survivors were compared to a sibling cohort of nearly 4,000 individuals. Survivors of ALL reported more chronic medical conditions than siblings with an odds ratio of 2.8 (95% CI, 2.4–3.2). Severe chronic medical conditions, including death, were 21% (95% CI 18–24%) for patients who had received RT and 13% (95% CI 8–18%) for those who had not received RT. Survivors of ALL reported more adverse general and mental health outcomes and had more activity limitation and functional impairment compared to their siblings. Rates of marriage, employment, attainment of health insurance, and college graduation were lower than sibling cohorts. Thus, survivors of ALL treatment in childhood experience excessive mortality and morbidity compared to their siblings, and this is particularly severe in recipients of RT [9]. A recent review has also indicated that females are at higher risk than males for many long-term sequelae including cognitive dysfunction after cranial RT, cardiotoxicity, obesity, radiation-associated early onset of puberty, primary hypothyroidism, breast cancer, and possibly osteonecrosis [10]. Subsequent sections of this chapter will detail the adverse consequences of therapy in various organ systems.

Neurologic

Of the multiple complications that can occur following successful therapy of ALL, neurocognitive deficits are perhaps the most distressing to both survivors and parents. These complications most commonly manifest as difficulties in school and include declines in memory, visual and motor integration, executive function, math achievement, nonverbal intelligence, processing speed, and attention. Guidelines for the identification of these deficits and how to advocate for patients and intervene in their care have been published [11]. Although these effects have been most pronounced in children with ALL receiving whole brain RT and intrathecal chemotherapy, they have also been noted in patients who have not received whole brain RT. Two meta-analyses of the neuropsychological outcomes of RT have documented these changes [12, 13]. However, a recent meta-analysis published this year assessing neuropsychological sequelae of chemotherapy-only treatment for ALL without RT indicated that intellectual functioning is also impaired in these patients. This latter analysis suggested that selected verbal skills may not be as significantly affected. However, overall, ALL survivors exhibit difficulty achieving academic progress in both reading and math [14]. Chemotherapeutic agents most commonly associated with neurocognitive decline include methotrexate, corticosteroids, and high-dose cytarabine [15–19]. Risk factors for these sequelae include younger age (especially under the age of 3 years), female gender, and increasing time from the date of treatment [20–23].

In addition to the neurocognitive difficulties noted above, other difficulties can include hyperactivity, which can manifest as deficits in attention, apathy, or poor behavior [24]. Academic performance can be inconsistent, and students may make careless errors and not complete their assignments on time. These individuals may need extra time to complete their work. Difficulties with organizational skills and planning may aggravate these problems [25]. These difficulties may be less evident in children in the primary grades where rote learning is emphasized but can become more evident as children enter high school where academic success depends more on reasoning and organizational skills [11].

Attempts have been made to screen asymptomatic ALL survivors with electroencephalograms, visual evoked potentials, cerebral blood flow measurements, and positron emission tomography. These studies have not been found to be predictive of neurophysiologic disturbances [26, 27]. A study of 35 asymptomatic survivors of ALL who had received prophylactic cranial RT was conducted. MRI and MR angiogram results were compared to a group of 24 patients who were cured of other childhood malignancies without the use of cranial RT. In 26% of the ALL patients, abnormalities were found including a meningioma, a paranasal sinus rhabdomyosarcoma, and an anaplastic astrocytoma. One control patient had a cerebellar infarct [28].

Given the similarities of some of these neurocognitive deficits to patients with attention-deficit hyperactivity disorder, trials of the psychostimulant methylphenidate have been conducted. Treatment with this medication can reduce some social and attentional deficits amongst these patients and is well tolerated [29,30]. However, further study of the long-term effects of use of stimulants like methylphenidate is still required [31].

Endocrine

Height and Weight

The hypothalamic-pituitary axis plays a key role in the central control of endocrine function. It is sensitive to the impact of cancer therapy and is particularly impacted by RT [32]. Growth hormone (GH) secretion seems to be most sensitive to RT [33]. Decreased growth and short stature clearly occurs following treatment of ALL, with 10–15% of survivors having final heights below the 5th percentile [34, 35]. Cranial RT has a greater impact on children, particularly under the age of 5, and on females. However, the precise mechanisms by which cranial RT induces growth retardation are not clear since GH production has not been found to correlate well with growth patterns [36, 37]. A recent report from the CCSS confirms that survivors of childhood ALL are at a higher risk of having short stature in adulthood, and the risk is highest for those who received cranial and cranio-spinal radiotherapy at a young age [38]. A study from the Dana-Farber Cancer Institute indicated that children under the age of 13 had a statistically significant decrease in their height and an increase in their body mass index (BMI), and this occurred regardless of whether or not they received cranial RT. Increased intensity of chemotherapy and young age at diagnosis were major risk factors for these changes. The authors speculated that patients may be more obese because of normal weight gain in the face of relative height loss [39].

Several studies have demonstrated an increased prevalence of obesity in survivors of childhood ALL. One analysis compared 1,765 adult survivors of childhood ALL to 2,565 adult siblings of childhood cancer survivors. In this study, doses of cranial RT ≥ 20 Gy were associated with an increased prevalence of obesity that was not seen in patients who received chemotherapy alone or cranial irradiation doses of 10–19 Gy [40]. Another report from the CCSS found that cranial RT administered during the treatment of childhood ALL was associated with a greater risk of an increased BMI, particularly among women who received cranial RT during the first decade of life [41]. Higher BMI may also be associated with a polymorphism in the leptin receptor, which leads to higher serum levels of leptin. Ross et al. found that female ALL survivors with a BMI ≥ 25 kg/m^2 were more likely to be homozygous for an arginine residue in the leptin receptor than those with a BMI <25 kg/m^2. This difference was not observed in males [42].

A recent study from St. Jude's has suggested that the overall percentage of ALL survivors who are overweight or obese approximates the rates in the general population of the United States. Young age and obesity at diagnosis were the best predictors of obesity at adult height [43]. The reason for the disparate results in this latter study is not known.

Thyroid

Thyroid disorders that occur following ALL treatment are thought to arise either via disruption of the hypothalamic–pituitary–thyroid axis or as a result of direct damage to the thyroid gland itself. The most common nonmalignant late effect is hypothyroidism [44]. Neoplastic tumors of the thyroid gland, both benign and malignant, are more frequent following RT involving the neck, but may occur even when the thyroid gland is outside the radiation field because of the intrinsic sensitivity of the thyroid gland in children [45]. Hyperthyroidism is the least common disorder, but can occur following neck irradiation [44].

Fertility and Sterility

Problems with fertility and sterility can also occur following ALL treatment [46]. The ovaries are relatively resistant to chemotherapy-induced damage during childhood and adolescence but are sensitive to RT. In the CCSS, a loss of ovarian function was found in 6.3% of 3,390 women during or immediately following completion of therapy. However, 70% of women who had received 2 Gy or more of ovarian RT had acute ovarian failure. Doses of <1 Gy induced ovarian failure mainly in women who were also treated with alkylating agents or who were older [47]. Females with preserved ovarian function are still at risk to develop premature menopause (before age 40) and/or have reduced ovarian reserve. In a CCSS cohort, a relative risk (RR) of nonsurgical premature menopause of 13.2 [95% confidence intervals (CI) 3.3–53.5] was found [48].

Attempts to preserve fertility in females undergoing cancer therapy during their childhood years can include laparoscopic oophoropexy. However, this technique is not always successful [49, 50]. The use of cryopreservation of unfertilized oocytes is also not frequently successful and has rarely been applied [51, 52]. Protection of the ovaries by suppression with gonadotropin-releasing hormone analogs has been attempted with varying success.

Fortunately, outcomes of pregnancy following childhood malignancies are generally favorable. In the CCSS, 4,029 live births were reported from 1953 women. There was no association between an adverse pregnancy outcome and use of chemotherapy. Previous pelvic RT was associated with lower birth weight [53].

In the testis, the germinal epithelium is exquisitely sensitive to radiation. Doses above 200 cGy nearly always result in at least, transient oligospermia or azoospermia [54]. Thus, males who receive RT to the testes for a testicular relapse or total body irradiation as part of a transplant are frequently rendered infertile. Even scatter radiation from radiation fields to the pelvis, spine, or inguinal area can inhibit sperm production [54–56]. Alkylating agents such as cyclophosphamide, ifosphamide, and cisplatin can cause significant damage to spermatogenesis. Combinations of these agents can have a high incidence of inducing infertility [54]. RT to the hypothalamic–pituitary axis, resulting in gonadotropin deficiency, can also indirectly affect spermatogenesis.

Preservation of fertility via semen cryopreservation is straightforward and effective in males. However, in children, this technique can only be utilized in adolescence. Cryopreservation of testicular tissue has not been successfully implemented to date.

Proven fertility, i.e., fathered a pregnancy, was evaluated by self-report in a series of 213 men treated for ALL before age 18. Controls were male siblings. Overall, the fertility of the males with ALL was not different from that of controls except in men treated before age 10 with 2.4 Gy of cranial RT, where their fertility was only 9% that of controls. High-dose cranial RT at older ages was not associated with decreased fertility [57]. A similar study in women treated with cranial RT for childhood ALL found that among 182 females and 170 sibling controls, decreased fertility was noted in the female ALL patients who were treated with cranial RT around the time of menarche [58].

Treatment of childhood ALL does not delay the onset of menarche in females. In patients treated with chemotherapy alone, menarche occurs at a similar rate compared to siblings. Of interest, patients who receive cranial RT may actually have an earlier onset of menarche. Exposure to alkylating agents does not delay onset of menarche [59].

Bone

The impact of ALL and its treatment on subsequent bone density is uncertain. Many studies in the literature have assessed this and come to conflicting results [60, 61]. Mandel et al. found that most childhood ALL survivors recover normal bone mineral density. It did appear that patients who received a total methotrexate dose >40,000 mg/m^2 or a total corticosteroid dose of >9,000 mg/m^2 may not recover normal bone mineral density and should undergo bone density screening [60]. A recent study suggested that polymorphisms in the corticotrophin-releasing hormone receptor-1 (CRHR1) gene are associated with decreased bone mineral density in long-term survivors of ALL [62].

Osteonecrosis is another complication of ALL treatment, and is associated with corticosteroid use. In 2000, the Children's Cancer Group (CCG) reported a 9.3% incidence of osteonecrosis in 1,409 children between the ages of 1 and 20 years receiving therapy for high-risk ALL. The incidence was highest for children over the age of 10, especially females 10–15 years of age and males

16–20 years of age. Caucasians had a higher incidence than other ethnic groups. The diagnosis of osteonecrosis was made within 3 years of starting ALL therapy in almost all patients and seemed to occur more frequently in patients who received higher cumulative doses of corticosteroids [63]. A study from the Italian Pediatric Oncology Group (AIEOP) demonstrated a lower incidence of osteonecrosis (1.1%). However, similar to the CCG study, there was an increased risk in females and older children [64]. A prospective study of 24 patients with ALL who underwent MRI scanning of the lower extremities at the beginning of, during, and at the cessation of chemotherapy found that 9 of 24 patients developed osteonecrosis radiographically, but 6 of these 9 patients were asymptomatic. The MRI lesions subsequently regressed in 6 patients and returned to normal in 3 [65]. A study with a similar design from the Nordic ALL Group found osteonecrosis in 23 (24%) of 97 patients, but only 7 of the patients were symptomatic. Shorter duration of dexamethasone exposure was associated with a decreased incidence of osteonecrosis, and a high BMI was associated with an increased risk of osteonecrosis [66]. The CCSS recently reported that amongst 9,621 patients with all types of childhood cancer, there were 52 individuals who reported osteonecrosis in 78 joints. The risk was higher in survivors of stem cell transplants and in non-transplant patients with ALL and bone sarcoma. Older age, earlier treatment era, exposure to dexamethasone, and the use of RT were independently associated with an increased incidence of osteonecrosis [67]. Other studies have suggested an increased incidence of osteonecrosis in children treated with dexamethasone as opposed to prednisone. However, not all trials have supported this finding [68, 69].

Cardiac

The heart is an important target of toxicity following ALL treatment. One of the major risk factors is exposure to anthracycline chemotherapy. A seminal study in the *New England Journal of Medicine* in 1991 demonstrated that in up to 65% of survivors, exposure to doxorubicin impairs myocardial growth in a dose-related fashion. This leads to a progressive increase in left ventricular afterload, which is sometimes accompanied by reduced contractility [70]. In a follow-up study, female sex and higher cumulative doses of doxorubicin were associated with an increased risk of cardiac abnormalities. These abnormalities can result in late-onset congestive heart failure, symptomatic arrhythmias, and even sudden death [71]. Lower doses of anthracycline can decrease the risk of this complication, but there is no "safe" anthracycline dose that has been identified [72]. The risk of cardiac dysfunction continues following completion of therapy [73]. Cardioprotectants, such as dexrazoxane, have been evaluated in children treated with anthracyclines. Although short-term benefits have been observed, the long-term benefits are unclear [74, 75].

A study comparing 23 young adult ALL survivors with 12 healthy controls assessed the response to exercise echocardiography and found significant differences in systolic function at maximal exercise, despite an absence of reported symptoms from the patients. Ten out of the 23 ALL patients reduced their ejection fraction at stress compared with at rest, whereas this was not found in any of the controls [76]. Based on these findings, it is recommended that survivors of ALL treatment undergo periodic echocardiography.

The increased incidence of obesity in survivors may also be a risk factor for coronary artery disease. The metabolic syndrome, which is a constellation of disorders related to insulin resistance can result in central obesity, elevated plasma glucose, dyslipidemia, hypertension, and a prothrombotic and proinflammatory state and contribute to adverse cardiovascular and diabetic risks [77]. Use of methotrexate therapy in the treatment of ALL can also result in hyperhomocysteinemia, which is a known risk factor for the development of cardiovascular disease. Thus, these factors can put survivors of ALL at increased risk of cardiovascular disease. Patients should be carefully assessed and should be educated regarding lifestyle modifications in an effort to reduce their risk of cardiovascular disease [78].

Respiratory

Relatively few studies have assessed the impact of ALL and its treatment on subsequent respiratory function. In a small trial from the 1980s, 38 patients with a history of leukemia had spirometry and lung volumes measured. Of the 26 patients with complete data available, 17 (65%) had one or more pulmonary function parameters that were abnormal. Few patients had symptoms of respiratory disease [79]. The CCSS assessed pulmonary complications from a cohort of 12,390 childhood cancer survivors and 3,546 randomly selected siblings and looked at the rate of first occurrence of 15 selected pulmonary conditions either during therapy, from the end of therapy to 5 years post-diagnosis, and beyond 5 years post-diagnosis. Pulmonary complications were assessed in relation to exposure to RT to the chest and to chemotherapeutic agents including bleomycin and selected alkylating agents. Compared with siblings, cancer survivors had statistically significantly increased risks of lung fibrosis, recurrent pneumonia, chronic cough, pleurisy, use of supplemental oxygen, abnormal chest wall, dyspnea on exertion, recurrent sinus infections, and tonsillitis for all three periods studied. During the period >5 years post-diagnosis, there was an association between the presence of lung fibrosis and chest radiation (RR 4.3, 95% CI 2.9–6.6). During this same period, an association was seen for supplemental oxygen use and chest radiation (RR 1.8, 95% CI 1.5–2.2), BCNU (RR 1.4, 95% CI 1.0–2.0), bleomycin (RR 1.7, 95% CI 1.2–2.3), busulfan (RR 3.2, 95% CI 1.5–7.0), CCNU (RR 2.1, 95% CI 1.4–2.9), and cyclophosphamide (RR 1.5, 95% CI 1.3–1.9) (relative risks all statistically significant). For recurrent pneumonia, chest RT and cyclophosphamide were significant associations. For chronic cough, chest RT, bleomycin, and cyclophosphamide were significant associations. Chest RT was associated with a 3.5% cumulative incidence of lung fibrosis at 20 years after diagnosis [80]. In a survey of adult survivors of childhood ALL, there was a significantly lower risk of being a smoker compared to sibling controls [81].

Hepatic

A small study from Japan assessed liver function in 27 children with ALL after cessation of therapy. Most of the patients were transfused during their therapy. The ALT level was more than three times normal during maintenance therapy but normalized in all patients within 3 months after the completion of maintenance therapy. Bilirubin, albumin, and prothrombin times were within normal limits. The bile acid profile was low in all but two patients, whereas it was normal in all controls. The authors suggested that long-term follow-up of survivors of ALL treated with hepatotoxic chemotherapy needs to be done to look for late hepatic damage [82]. Chemotherapy drugs can contribute to hepatotoxicity. A small study reported 6 children treated with 6-thioguanine who developed splenomegaly, hepatomegaly, and an elevated AST. In some of these patients, ultrasonography demonstrated an altered liver parenchymal texture and biopsy demonstrated occlusive venopathy and nodular regenerative hyperplasia [83]. Viral hepatitis can also occur in ALL patients. However, the incidence of these infections is low in the modern era, due to the screening of blood products.

Genitourinary

The genitourinary side effects of ALL and its treatment are infrequently reported. Two adolescent girls with high-risk ALL who developed progressive renal dysfunction have been reported. Renal biopsies showed focal segmental glomerulosclerosis. One patient progressed to chronic renal failure and required prolonged dialysis, whereas the other had persistent proteinuria but preserved renal function and was treated with high-dose steroids at the time of the report [84]. Other toxicities can include glomerular dysfunction, renal arterial sclerosis, tubular dysfunction, nephrotic syndrome, bladder fibrosis, cystitis, ureteral fibrosis, or urethral stricture [85].

Ophthalmologic

A prospective study of 82 survivors of ALL assessed for ocular sequelae of the disease and its treatment. The mean interval from the end of treatment to their ophthalmologic examination was 32 months. Only one patient had symptomatic visual changes. In 52% of the patients, posterior subcapsular cataracts were noted, whereas none of these types of cataracts was seen in 15 survivors of acute myeloid leukemia. Despite the presence of these cataracts, the median visual acuity was 20/20 [86].

Dental

The oral cavity can be a source of significant morbidity following ALL treatment although few studies in the literature have documented this. Sixty-eight children diagnosed with ALL prior to age 5 who were treated either with chemotherapy alone, chemotherapy plus 1.8 Gy cranial RT, or chemotherapy plus 2.4 Gy were assessed clinically for their overall dental health. All patients had been in remission for at least 5 years. No significant difference in the development of dental caries was noted between the three groups, nor was there a difference compared with the normal population. Patients who had received 2.4 Gy of radiation therapy had significantly higher plaque and periodontal index scores compared to patients in the other treatment modalities [87]. Dental abnormalities were also assessed in 423 ALL survivors at St. Jude's Hospital. Abnormalities included root stunting in 24%, microdontia in 19%, hypodontia in 9%, taurodontia in 6%, and over-retention of primary dentition in 4%. Patients under 8 years of age at diagnosis or patients who had received cranial RT had more dental abnormalities than older children and those who did not receive cranial RT (42% vs. 32%). Dental evaluation at diagnosis and frequent follow-up is recommended [88]. An important consideration in the treatment of pediatric patients is how to manage orthodontic needs during treatment. A review in 2004 addressed this issue and concluded that ideally, orthodontic treatments should be delayed until 2 years after completion of cancer therapy, but that orthodontic therapy during cancer treatment does not produce harmful side effects [89].

Second Malignancies

With the long-term survival and cure of children and adolescents with ALL came the recognition of the development of secondary malignancies. These have been evaluated in multiple large cohorts of patients from different cooperative groups. The BFM demonstrated that the risk was highest in patients who had received cranial RT. Among the 52 patients with secondary neoplasms, nearly half ($n=23$) had hematologic malignancies including lymphoma (Hodgkin's and non-Hodgkin's), acute myeloid leukemia (AML), and chronic myeloid leukemia. Thirteen patients had CNS tumors, and 16 had a variety of other malignancies. The cumulative risk of secondary neoplasm at 15 years was 3.3% with a risk of 3.5% in patients who had received cranial RT, but only 1.2% in patients not receiving any RT [90].

CCG reported in a cohort of 8,831 children with ALL that relapse of ALL, female gender, and RT of the craniospinal axis were independently associated with an increased risk of second neoplasms. The cumulative incidence at 15 years was approximately 2%. The actuarial survival at

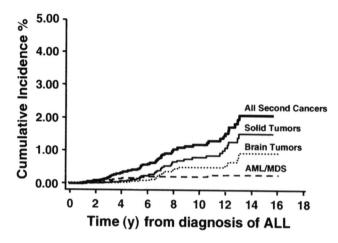

Fig. 21.3 Cumulative incidence of all second neoplasms, AML/MDS, all solid tumors, and brain tumors in 8,831 children with ALL (From [91])

10 years from diagnosis of a second neoplasm was 39%. The most common second malignancies were AML or myelodysplastic syndrome (MDS), lymphoma (non-Hodgkin's or Hodgkin's disease), and solid tumors including brain tumors, soft tissue sarcoma, thyroid cancer, and parotid gland tumors (Fig. 21.3) [91]. The experience from the Polish Pediatric Leukemia/Lymphoma Group in 3,252 patients showed a cumulative incidence of approximately 1% at 15 years with a similar distribution of malignancies [92]. At St. Jude's Hospital, amongst 2,169 patients, 123 patients in first complete remission developed a second neoplasm, including 46 myeloid malignancies, 3 Hodgkin's lymphoma, 14 basal cell carcinomas, 16 other carcinomas, 6 sarcomas, 16 meningiomas, and 22 other types of brain tumors. The cumulative incidence at 30 years was 2.2% [93]. Other smaller series have found similar incidences.

Two correlative laboratory studies have documented that survivors of pediatric ALL have increased mutant frequencies at the hypoxanthine phosphoribosyl transferase (HPRT) locus. In one study, a significant increase in mutant frequencies occurred through different phases of treatment and following completion of treatment. These mutation frequencies were independent of the risk group for the patients' disease. These studies suggest that chemotherapy can cause persistent genotoxicity in vivo in some pediatric ALL patients. The clinical significance of these observations is as yet unknown [94, 95].

Psychosocial

Understandably, a diagnosis of ALL and the burden and stress of treatment can put significant psychological strain on both a patient's family and the patients themselves. Despite this trauma, many survivors appear less likely to practice risky behaviors such as drug use or cigarette smoking [96,97]. In aggregate, however, survivors of childhood cancer are more likely to have chronic somatic symptoms including chronic pain and fatigue and mental health disorders than the general population. In the CCSS cohort, 17% of nearly 10,000 young adult survivors of childhood cancer had depression, somatic, or anxiety symptoms, and 10% reported moderate to extreme pain as a result of their cancer [98]. Posttraumatic stress disorder where survivors experience aspects of their prior cancer experience and its associated emotions is reported in 1 out of 5 young adult survivors. They may avoid people or places that remind them of their previous malignancy [99, 100].

Long-term survivors of childhood cancer also have higher utilizations of special education services, and their educational achievement is lower than that of their siblings [101, 102]. Adult survivors of childhood ALL on CCSG protocols report more tension, depression, anger, and confusion, and this was highest among females, minority patients, and unemployed survivors [103]. Global self-worth scores were also significantly lower in ALL survivors compared to sibling controls, although 81% of survivors were able to mount a positive self-concept [104]. Fatigue and sleep disturbances are also seen more frequently in cancer survivors as demonstrated in the CCSS [105]. Most survivors become socially independent and leave home at ages similar to the general population, but rates of marriage do tend to be slightly lower [106]. The CCSS has also demonstrated that adult survivors of childhood ALL tend to be more physically inactive and not meet Centers for Disease Control recommendations for physical activity. The authors concluded that their level of inactivity could increase their risk of cardiovascular disease, osteoporosis, and all cause mortality [107]. Books have been written to provide survivors and their families with information that addresses the particular challenges related to the experience of cancer and subsequent survival [108].

One of the few studies to address quality of life of adult leukemia survivors was reported in 1997. Two hundred and six survivors with AML (77%) or ALL (23%) treated on any of 13 CALGB trials from 1971 to 1988 were evaluated. Patients were interviewed by telephone at least 1 year after completion of their treatment. While most survivors adapted well, 14% were 1.5 standard deviations above normal on the global severity index of the brief symptom inventory. The predictors of increased psychological stress included lower education, younger age, anticipatory distress during chemotherapy treatment, and the combination of more medical problems after treatment and poor family functioning. Patients at higher risk should be monitored for depressive symptoms in later years [109].

Blood and Marrow Transplantation

Blood and marrow transplantation (BMT) poses many challenges similar to those experienced by long-term survivors of ALL chemotherapy and/or RT but also poses some unique challenges in its own right. Patients with ALL or AML often undergo BMT in addition to chemotherapy because their risk of relapse is felt to be inordinately high or because they have relapsed and BMT is now their only long-term curative option. A study from the Late Effects Working Committee of the Center for International Blood and Marrow Transplant Research (CIBMTR) assessed the outcome of 6,691 patients who were free of their original disease 2 years following allogeneic BMT. The probability of living an additional 5 years was 89%. For patients with aplastic anemia, the risk of death by the sixth year after transplantation was not significantly different from the normal population but mortality remains significantly higher than normal throughout the study for patients transplanted for malignancy. Recurrent leukemia was the chief cause of death for patients transplanted for leukemia, whereas chronic graft vs. host disease (GVHD) was the chief cause for those transplanted for aplastic anemia [110].

A single center study assessed the outcome of adult acute leukemia patients who were alive and well 2 years following autologous BMT. Approximately half of the 87 patients studied had AML and half had ALL. Nine patients relapsed 2–4 years after transplantation. Four of the nine patients were still alive at the time of the report. Two other patients died of complications related to the transplant and one of ischemic heart disease. Seventy-nine patients remained alive and in remission after transplant [111].

In children, a study of 13 patients who had undergone allogeneic BMT for treatment of their ALL and had long-term follow-up were reported. In 8 of the cases, TBI was part of the conditioning regimen. Pubertal development was normal in 3 children and delayed in 1 of the 4 where it was evaluable. Thyroid function and left ventricular function were normal in all cases. Three patients had mild abnormalities of pulmonary function, and 2 patients had cataracts develop 7 and 10 years after TBI. Most patients had normal memory [112]. Long-term follow-up has also been described in children under the age of 3 who underwent BMT for AML or ALL. In these children, GH deficiency was noted in 60%, hypothyroidism in 35%, osteochondromas in 24%, decreased bone marrow density in 24%, and dyslipidemias in 59%. Of the 17 patients evaluated, 2 developed a second malignancy. Neuropsychological testing revealed average IQ, but attention deficits were noted in many patients [113]. Studies thus far have not demonstrated an adverse impact of BMT on quality of life. The quality of life in 22 young adults who had received a BMT an average of 14 years previously during childhood at Leiden University Medical Center was described. Quality of life as assessed by the functional assessment of cancer therapy, bone marrow transplant scale (FACT-BMT), showed quality of life measures within the normal range of functioning and, compared to a reference sample of patients who had received BMT as an adult, the patients in this study scored significantly higher; it did not appear that BMT had negatively impacted on their quality of life [114].

In adults, the Toronto group reported the incidence of second malignancies post-allogeneic BMT in a cohort of 557 patients and found a cumulative estimated incidence rate of secondary malignancy of 4.2% at 10 years posttransplant. The observed vs. expected ratio compared to the general population was 5:13. Older age was the only significant predictor for development of a secondary malignancy. Non-melanomatous skin cancers and squamous cell cancers of the buccal cavity were the most common malignancy [115].

The European Group for Blood and Marrow Transplantation assessed 1,036 consecutive patients who had undergone transplantation for a variety of diseases and had survived for more than 5 years. In 53 patients, a malignant neoplasm was seen, giving an actuarial incidence of 3.5% at 10 years and 12.8% at 15 years. The most frequent malignant diseases were neoplasms of the skin in 14 patients, oral cavity in 7, uterus including the cervix in 5, thyroid gland in 5, breast in 4 patients, and glial tissue in 3. Older age and treatment of chronic graft vs. host disease with cyclosporin were significant risk factors [116].

The largest series assessing secondary solid tumors after transplantation has come from the CIBMTR and Fred Hutchinson Cancer Research Center where 19,229 patients were assessed who had received allogeneic BMT. The observed vs. expected ratio of cases compared to the general population was 8.3 with a cumulative incidence of 2.2% at 10 years and 6.7% at 15 years. In this series, younger patients had a higher risk of secondary malignancy, and a higher dose of TBI was associated with a higher risk of solid cancers. Chronic GVHD and male sex were strongly linked with an excess risk of squamous cell carcinomas of the buccal cavity and skin [117].

A large number of nonmalignant late effects after allogeneic BMT have been described and include ocular, pulmonary, hepatic, joint, dental, and endocrine effects. Many of these mirror those seen following treatment for ALL as described above. These are summarized in an excellent review by Socie et al. [118]. Among these late effects are cardiovascular events including cerebrovascular, coronary artery, peripheral arterial events, and late congestive failure [119]. These events have been identified a median of 3 years posttransplant in 60 of nearly 3,000 patients assessed at the City of Hope National Medical Center [120].

Health and functional status of adult recipients of allogenic BMT who are 1 year out from BMT has been assessed in 105 adult patients. At the time of screening, 52% had returned to work. Their general health status was normal in 67%. In 47% of patients, sexual activity had returned. Female patients and older patients were more likely to have not returned to work. Sexual inactivity was associated with younger age and chronic GVHD. Risk factors for altered pulmonary function tests were previous smoking habits, irradiation, and chronic GVHD [121].

On the psychological level, despite the trauma of BMT, many survivors report normal psychologic health and more score higher on measures of psychological and interpersonal growth compared to age and sex-matched controls [122].

Follow-up Care

Several groups have established guidelines for follow-up care of survivors of ALL and survivors of BMT [123,124]. The pediatric ALL follow-up guidelines can also be accessed at the following website: www.survivorshipguidelines.org. A table with resources for childhood cancer survivors, their parents, and caregivers has been published (Table 21.2) [11]. These guidelines provide comprehensive recommendations for management of this challenging population of patients that span the spectrum of conditions managed by general pediatricians and internists.

Table 21.2 North American resources for pediatric cancer survivors and their caregivers related to neurocognitive late effects (Taken from Table 21.1 of [11])

Service or disability organization	Service provided
National Childhood Cancer Foundation 440 Huntington Dr Arcadia, CA 91066-60612 (800) 458-6223 http://www.curesearch.org	Provides information and resources for pediatric cancer survivors
American Cancer Society 1599 Clifton RD NE Atlanda, GA 30329-4215 (800) ACS-2345 http://www.cancer.org	Programs include equipment and supplies, support groups, educational literature, and summer camps for childhood cancer survivors
Canadian Cancer Society 565 W 10th Ave Vancouver, BC V5Z 4J4 Canada http://www.bc.cancer.ca	Programs include those provided by the American Cancer Society
Association of Cancer Online Resources http://www.acor.org	Online information and electronic support groups for pediatric cancer survivors and their caregivers
Candle lighters Childhood Cancer Foundation 3910 Warner St Kensington, MD 20895 (800) 366-CCCF http://www.candlelighters.org	Provides resource guides quarterly, newsletters, referrals and information and publish book for pediatric cancer survivors including *Educating the Child with Cancer: A Guide for Parents and Teachers* [125]
Childhood Cancer Foundation Candle lighters Canada 1300 Yonge St, Ste 405 Toronto, ON M4T 1X3,Canda (800) 363-1062 http://www.Candlelighters.ca	Provides resource guides, newsletters, and information
Childhood Cancer Ombudsman Program 27 Witch Duck Ln Heathsville, VA 22473 gpmonaco@rivnet.net	Provides help for pediatric cancer survivors experiencing problems gaining access to appropriate education, medical care, health care cost coverage and employment
Federation for Children with special needs 1135 Tremont St, Ste 420 Boston, MA 02120 (617) 236-7210 http://www.fcsn.org	Federally funded organization providing information on special education rights and laws, conferences, referrals for services, parent training workshops, publications, and advocacy information
Lance Armstrong Foundations PO BOX 161150 Austin, TX 78716 (866) 235-7205 http://www.livestrong.org	A nonprofit organizations that offers extensive educational advocacy, and public health resources
National Cancer For Learning Disabilities 381 Park Ave S, Ste 1401 New York, NY 10016 (888) 575-7373 http://www.ncld.org	Offer extensive resources, referral services, and educational programs related to learning disabilities
US Department of Justice ADA information Line, Civil Rights Division PO Box 66738 Washington, DC 20035 (800) 514-0301 http://www.usdoj.gov/crt/ada/ adahom1.htm	Answers questions about the Americans with Disabilities Act (ADA), explains how to file a complaint, and provides dispute resolution information

Conclusion

In this review, I have attempted to comprehensively describe the psychosocial and physical challenges faced by survivors of ALL and BMT. While survivors of ALL treatment and BMT are heroes in their own right, these patients face numerous physical and psychological challenges that require the resources of multiple healthcare professionals to help them navigate the numerous potential complications they can experience. These complications encompass nearly every organ system and challenge physicians and psychologists to take a broad and comprehensive overview to their care.

References

1. Farber, S., & Diamond, L. K. (1948). Temporary remissions in acute leukemia in children produced by folic acid antagonist, 4-aminopteroyl-glutamic acid. *The New England Journal of Medicine, 238*(23), 787–793.
2. Ravindranath, Y. (1999). Forty-five-year follow-up of a childhood leukemia survivor: Serendipity or karma? [See comment]. *Medical and Pediatric Oncology, 33*(4), 409–410.
3. Pui, C. H., & Evans, W. E. (2006). Treatment of acute lymphoblastic leukemia. *The New England Journal of Medicine, 354*(2), 166–178.
4. Langebrake, C., Reinhardt, D., & Ritter, J. (2002). Minimising the long-term adverse effects of childhood leukaemia therapy. *Drug Safety, 25*(15), 1057–1077.
5. Ness, K. K., & Gurney, J. G. (2007). Adverse late effects of childhood cancer and its treatment on health and performance. *Annual Review of Public Health, 28*, 279–302.
6. Pastore, G., Viscomi, S., Gerov, G. L., Terracini, B., Madon, E., & Magnani, C. (2003). Population-based survival after childhood lymphoblastic leukaemia in time periods corresponding to specific clinical trials from 1979 to 1998 – A report from the Childhood Cancer Registry of Piedmont (Italy). *European Journal of Cancer, 39*(7), 952–960.
7. Pui, C. H., Cheng, C., Leung, W., et al. (2003). Extended follow-up of long-term survivors of childhood acute lymphoblastic leukemia. *The New England Journal of Medicine, 349*(7), 640–649.
8. Robison, L. L., Mertens, A. C., Boice, J. D., et al. (2002). Study design and cohort characteristics of the Childhood Cancer Survivor Study: A multi-institutional collaborative project. *Medical and Pediatric Oncology, 38*(4), 229–239.
9. Mody, R., Li, S., Dover, D. C., et al. (2008). Twenty-five-year follow-up among survivors of childhood acute lymphoblastic leukemia: A report from the Childhood Cancer Survivor Study. *Blood, 111*(12), 5515–5523.
10. Armstrong, G., Sklar, C., Hudson, M., et al. (2007). Long-term health status among survivors of childhood cancer: Does sex matter? *Journal of Clinical Oncology, 25*(28), 4477–4489.
11. Nathan, P. C., Patel, S. K., Dilley, K., et al. (2007). Guidelines for identification of, advocacy for, and intervention in neurocognitive problems in survivors of childhood cancer: A report from the Children's Oncology Group. *Archives of Pediatrics & Adolescent Medicine, 161*(8), 798–806.
12. Cousens, P., Waters, B., Said, J., & Stevens, M. (1988). Cognitive effects of cranial irradiation in leukaemia: A survey and meta-analysis. *Journal of Child Psychology and Psychiatry, and Allied Disciplines, 29*(6), 839–852.
13. Campbell, L. K., Scaduto, M., Sharp, W., et al. (2007). A meta-analysis of the neurocognitive sequelae of treatment for childhood acute lymphocytic leukemia. *Pediatric Blood & Cancer, 49*(1), 65–73.
14. Peterson, C. C., Johnson, C. E., Ramirez, L. Y., et al. (2008). A meta-analysis of the neuropsychological sequelae of chemotherapy-only treatment for pediatric acute lymphoblastic leukemia. *Pediatric Blood & Cancer, 51*(1), 99–104.
15. Brown, R. T., Madan-Swain, A., Walco, G. A., et al. (1998). Cognitive and academic late effects among children previously treated for acute lymphocytic leukemia receiving chemotherapy as CNS prophylaxis. *Journal of Pediatric Psychology, 23*(5), 333–340.
16. Espy, K. A., Moore, I. M., Kaufmann, P. M., Kramer, J. H., Matthay, K., & Hutter, J. J. (2001). Chemotherapeutic CNS prophylaxis and neuropsychologic change in children with acute lymphoblastic leukemia: A prospective study. *Journal of Pediatric Psychology, 26*(1), 1–9.
17. Moleski, M. (2000). Neuropsychological, neuroanatomical, and neurophysiological consequences of CNS chemotherapy for acute lymphoblastic leukemia. *Archives of Clinical Neuropsychology, 15*(7), 603–630.
18. Nand, S., Messmore, H. L., Jr., Patel, R., Fisher, S. G., & Fisher, R. I. (1986). Neurotoxicity associated with systemic high-dose cytosine arabinoside. *Journal of Clinical Oncology, 4*(4), 571–575.
19. Waber, D. P., Carpentieri, S. C., Klar, N., et al. (2000). Cognitive sequelae in children treated for acute lymphoblastic leukemia with dexamethasone or prednisone. *Journal of Pediatric Hematology/Oncology, 22*(3), 206–213.

20. Christie, D., Leiper, A. D., Chessells, J. M., & Vargha-Khadem, F. (1995). Intellectual performance after presymptomatic cranial radiotherapy for leukaemia: Effects of age and sex. *Archives of Disease in Childhood, 73*(2), 136–140.
21. Kaleita, T. A., Reaman, G. H., MacLean, W. E., Sather, H. N., & Whitt, J. K. (1999). Neurodevelopmental outcome of infants with acute lymphoblastic leukemia: A Children's Cancer Group report. *Cancer, 85*(8), 1859–1865.
22. Packer, R. J., Sutton, L. N., Atkins, T. E., et al. (1989). A prospective study of cognitive function in children receiving whole-brain radiotherapy and chemotherapy: 2-year results. *Journal of Neurosurgery, 70*(5), 707–713.
23. Waber, D. P., Tarbell, N. J., Kahn, C. M., Gelber, R. D., & Sallan, S. E. (1992). The relationship of sex and treatment modality to neuropsychologic outcome in childhood acute lymphoblastic leukemia. *Journal of Clinical Oncology, 10*(5), 810–817.
24. Armstrong, F. D., & Briery, B. G. (2004). Childhood cancer and the school. In R. T. Brown (Ed.), *Handbook of pediatric psychology in school settings* (pp. 263–281). Mahway: Lawrence Erlbaum Associates, Inc.
25. Mulhern, R. K., & Palmer, S. L. (2003). Neurocognitive late effects in pediatric cancer. *Current Problems in Cancer, 27*(4), 177–197.
26. Kahkonen, M., Harila-Saari, A., Metsahonkala, L., et al. (1999). Cerebral blood flow and glucose metabolism in long-term survivors of childhood acute lymphoblastic leukaemia. *European Journal of Cancer, 35*(7), 1102–1108.
27. Ueberall, M. A., Skirl, G., Strassburg, H. M., et al. (1997). Neurophysiological findings in long-term survivors of acute lymphoblastic leukaemia in childhood treated with the BFM protocol 81 SR-A/B. *European Journal of Pediatrics, 156*(9), 727–733.
28. Laitt, R. D., Chambers, E. J., Goddard, P. R., Wakeley, C. J., Duncan, A. W., & Foreman, N. K. (1995). Magnetic resonance imaging and magnetic resonance angiography in long term survivors of acute lymphoblastic leukemia treated with cranial irradiation. *Cancer, 76*(10), 1846–1852.
29. Conklin, H. M., Khan, R. B., Reddick, W. E., et al. (2007). Acute neurocognitive response to methylphenidate among survivors of childhood cancer: A randomized, double-blind, cross-over trial. *Journal of Pediatric Psychology, 32*(9), 1127–1139.
30. Mulhern, R. K., Khan, R. B., Kaplan, S., et al. (2004). Short-term efficacy of methylphenidate: A randomized, double-blind, placebo-controlled trial among survivors of childhood cancer. *Journal of Clinical Oncology, 22*(23), 4795–4803.
31. Daly, B. P., & Brown, R. T. (2007). Scholarly literature review: Management of neurocognitive late effects with stimulant medication. *Journal of Pediatric Psychology, 32*(9), 1111–1126.
32. Littley, M. D., Shalet, S. M., Beardwell, C. G., Robinson, E. L., & Sutton, M. L. (1989). Radiation-induced hypopituitarism is dose-dependent. *Clinical Endocrinology, 31*(3), 363–373.
33. Littley, M. D., Shalet, S. M., Beardwell, C. G., Ahmed, S. R., Applegate, G., & Sutton, M. L. (1989). Hypopituitarism following external radiotherapy for pituitary tumours in adults. *The Quarterly Journal of Medicine, 70*(262), 145–160.
34. Robison, L. L., Nesbit, M. E., Jr., Sather, H. N., Meadows, A. T., Ortega, J. A., & Hammond, G. D. (1985). Height of children successfully treated for acute lymphoblastic leukemia: A report from the Late Effects Study Committee of Childrens Cancer Study Group. *Medical and Pediatric Oncology, 13*(1), 14–21.
35. Sklar, C., Mertens, A., Walter, A., et al. (1993). Final height after treatment for childhood acute lymphoblastic leukemia: Comparison of no cranial irradiation with 1800 and 2400 centigrays of cranial irradiation. *The Journal of Pediatrics, 123*(1), 59–64.
36. Blatt, J., Bercu, B. B., Gillin, J. C., Mendelson, W. B., & Poplack, D. G. (1984). Reduced pulsatile growth hormone secretion in children after therapy for acute lymphoblastic leukemia. *The Journal of Pediatrics, 104*(2), 182–186.
37. Shalet, S. M., Price, D. A., Beardwell, C. G., Jones, P. H., & Pearson, D. (1979). Normal growth despite abnormalities of growth hormone secretion in children treated for acute leukemia. *The Journal of Pediatrics, 94*(5), 719–722.
38. Chow, E. J., Friedman, D. L., Yasui, Y., et al. (2007). Decreased adult height in survivors of childhood acute lymphoblastic leukemia: A report from the Childhood Cancer Survivor Study. *The Journal of Pediatrics, 150*(4), 370–375. 5 e1.
39. Dalton, V. K., Rue, M., Silverman, L. B., et al. (2003). Height and weight in children treated for acute lymphoblastic leukemia: Relationship to CNS treatment. *Journal of Clinical Oncology, 21*(15), 2953–2960.
40. Oeffinger, K. C., Mertens, A. C., Sklar, C. A., et al. (2003). Obesity in adult survivors of childhood acute lymphoblastic leukemia: A report from the Childhood Cancer Survivor Study. *Journal of Clinical Oncology, 21*(7), 1359–1365.
41. Garmey, E. G., Liu, Q., Sklar, C. A., et al. (2008). Longitudinal changes in obesity and body mass index among adult survivors of childhood acute lymphoblastic leukemia: A report from the Childhood Cancer Survivor Study. *Journal of Clinical Oncology, 26*(28), 4639–4645.

42. Ross, J. A., Oeffinger, K. C., Davies, S. M., et al. (2004). Genetic variation in the leptin receptor gene and obesity in survivors of childhood acute lymphoblastic leukemia: A report from the Childhood Cancer Survivor Study. *Journal of Clinical Oncology, 22*(17), 3558–3562.
43. Razzouk, B. I., Rose, S. R., Hongeng, S., et al. (2007). Obesity in survivors of childhood acute lymphoblastic leukemia and lymphoma. *Journal of Clinical Oncology, 25*(10), 1183–1189.
44. Brougham, M. F., Kelnar, C. J., & Wallace, W. H. (2002). The late endocrine effects of childhood cancer treatment. *Pediatric Rehabilitation, 5*(4), 191–201.
45. Inskip, P. D. (2001). Thyroid cancer after radiotherapy for childhood cancer. *Medical and Pediatric Oncology, 36*(5), 568–573.
46. Oeffinger, K. C., Nathan, P. C., & Kremer, L. C. (2008). Challenges after curative treatment for childhood cancer and long-term follow up of survivors. *Pediatric Clinics of North America, 55*(1), 251–273. xiii.
47. Chemaitilly, W., Mertens, A. C., Mitby, P., et al. (2006). Acute ovarian failure in the childhood cancer survivor study. *The Journal of Clinical Endocrinology and Metabolism, 91*(5), 1723–1728.
48. Sklar, C. A., Mertens, A. C., Mitby, P., et al. (2006). Premature menopause in survivors of childhood cancer: A report from the childhood cancer survivor study. *Journal of the National Cancer Institute, 98*(13), 890–896.
49. Bisharah, M., & Tulandi, T. (2003). Laparoscopic preservation of ovarian function: An underused procedure. *American Journal of Obstetrics and Gynecology, 188*(2), 367–370.
50. Williams, R. S., Littell, R. D., & Mendenhall, N. P. (1999). Laparoscopic oophoropexy and ovarian function in the treatment of Hodgkin disease. *Cancer, 86*(10), 2138–2142.
51. Blumenfeld, Z., Dann, E., Avivi, I., Epelbaum, R., & Rowe, J. M. (2002). Fertility after treatment for Hodgkin's disease. *Annals of Oncology, 13*(Suppl 1), 138–147.
52. Oktay, K., Cil, A. P., & Bang, H. (2006). Efficiency of oocyte cryopreservation: A meta-analysis. *Fertility and Sterility, 86*(1), 70–80.
53. Green, D. M., Whitton, J. A., Stovall, M., et al. (2002). Pregnancy outcome of female survivors of childhood cancer: A report from the Childhood Cancer Survivor Study. *American Journal of Obstetrics and Gynecology, 187*(4), 1070–1080.
54. Howell, S. J., & Shalet, S. M. (2005). Spermatogenesis after cancer treatment: Damage and recovery. *Journal of the National Cancer Institute Monographs, 34*, 12–17.
55. Rovo, A., Tichelli, A., Passweg, J. R., et al. (2006). Spermatogenesis in long-term survivors after allogeneic hematopoietic stem cell transplantation is associated with age, time interval since transplantation, and apparently absence of chronic GvHD. *Blood, 108*(3), 1100–1105.
56. Sklar, C. A., Robison, L. L., Nesbit, M. E., et al. (1990). Effects of radiation on testicular function in long-term survivors of childhood acute lymphoblastic leukemia: A report from the Children Cancer Study Group. *Journal of Clinical Oncology, 8*(12), 1981–1987.
57. Byrne, J., Fears, T. R., Mills, J. L., et al. (2004). Fertility of long-term male survivors of acute lymphoblastic leukemia diagnosed during childhood. *Pediatric Blood & Cancer, 42*(4), 364–372.
58. Byrne, J., Fears, T. R., Mills, J. L., et al. (2004). Fertility in women treated with cranial radiotherapy for childhood acute lymphoblastic leukemia. *Pediatric Blood & Cancer, 42*(7), 589–597.
59. Chow, E. J., Friedman, D. L., Yasui, Y., et al. (2008). Timing of menarche among survivors of childhood acute lymphoblastic leukemia: A report from the Childhood Cancer Survivor Study. *Pediatric Blood & Cancer, 50*(4), 854–858.
60. Mandel, K., Atkinson, S., Barr, R. D., & Pencharz, P. (2004). Skeletal morbidity in childhood acute lymphoblastic leukemia. *Journal of Clinical Oncology, 22*(7), 1215–1221.
61. Nysom, K., Holm, K., Michaelsen, K. F., Hertz, H., Muller, J., & Molgaard, C. (1998). Bone mass after treatment for acute lymphoblastic leukemia in childhood. *Journal of Clinical Oncology, 16*(12), 3752–3760.
62. Jones, T. S., Kaste, S. C., Liu, W., et al. (2008). CRHR1 polymorphisms predict bone density in survivors of acute lymphoblastic leukemia. *Journal of Clinical Oncology, 26*(18), 3031–3037.
63. Mattano, L. A., Sather, H. N., Trigg, M. E., et al. (2000). Osteonecrosis as a complication of treating acute lymphoblastic leukemia in children: A report from the Children's Cancer Group. *Journal of Clinical Oncology, 18*(18), 3262–3272.
64. Arico, M., Boccalatte, M. F., Silvestri, D., et al. (2003). Osteonecrosis: An emerging complication of intensive chemotherapy for childhood acute lymphoblastic leukemia. *Haematologica, 88*(7), 747–753.
65. Ojala, A. E., Paakko, E., Lanning, F. P., & Lanning, M. (1999). Osteonecrosis during the treatment of childhood acute lymphoblastic leukemia: A prospective MRI study. *Medical and Pediatric Oncology, 32*(1), 11–17.
66. Niinimaki, R. A., Harila-Saari, A. H., Jartti, A. E., et al. (2007). High body mass index increases the risk for osteonecrosis in children with acute lymphoblastic leukemia. *Journal of Clinical Oncology, 25*(12), 1498–1504.
67. Kadan-Lottick, N. S., Dinu, I., Wasilewski-Masker, K., et al. (2008). Osteonecrosis in adult survivors of childhood cancer: A report from the childhood cancer survivor study. *Journal of Clinical Oncology, 26*(18), 3038–3045.

68. Mattano, L. A., Nachman, J. B., Devidas, M., et al. (2008). Increased incidence of osteonecrosis (ON) with a dexamethasone (DEX) induction for high risk acute lymphoblastic leukemia (HR-ALL): A report from the Children's Oncology Group (COG) (Abstract 898). *Blood, 112*, 333.

69. Moricke, A., Zimmermann, M., Schrauder, A., et al. (2008). No influence on the incidence of osteonecroses when dexamethasone replaces prednisone during induction treatment for childhood ALL: Results of trial ALL-BFM 2000 (Abstract 899). *Blood, 112*, 334.

70. Lipshultz, S. E., Colan, S. D., Gelber, R. D., Perez-Atayde, A. R., Sallan, S. E., & Sanders, S. P. (1991). Late cardiac effects of doxorubicin therapy for acute lymphoblastic leukemia in childhood. *The New England Journal of Medicine, 324*(12), 808–815.

71. Lipshultz, S. E., Lipsitz, S. R., Mone, S. M., et al. (1995). Female sex and drug dose as risk factors for late cardiotoxic effects of doxorubicin therapy for childhood cancer. *The New England Journal of Medicine, 332*(26), 1738–1743.

72. Sorensen, K., Levitt, G., Bull, C., Chessells, J., & Sullivan, I. (1997). Anthracycline dose in childhood acute lymphoblastic leukemia: Issues of early survival versus late cardiotoxicity. *Journal of Clinical Oncology, 15*(1), 61–68.

73. Lipshultz, S. E., Lipsitz, S. R., Sallan, S. E., et al. (2005). Chronic progressive cardiac dysfunction years after doxorubicin therapy for childhood acute lymphoblastic leukemia. *Journal of Clinical Oncology, 23*(12), 2629–2636.

74. Bryant, J., Picot, J., Baxter, L., Levitt, G., Sullivan, I., & Clegg, A. (2007). Clinical and cost-effectiveness of cardioprotection against the toxic effects of anthracyclines given to children with cancer: A systematic review. *British Journal of Cancer, 96*(2), 226–230.

75. Lipshultz, S. E., Rifai, N., Dalton, V. M., et al. (2004). The effect of dexrazoxane on myocardial injury in doxorubicin-treated children with acute lymphoblastic leukemia. *The New England Journal of Medicine, 351*(2), 145–153.

76. Jarfelt, M., Kujacic, V., Holmgren, D., Bjarnason, R., & Lannering, B. (2007). Exercise echocardiography reveals subclinical cardiac dysfunction in young adult survivors of childhood acute lymphoblastic leukemia. *Pediatric Blood & Cancer, 49*(6), 835–840.

77. Gurney, J. G., Ness, K. K., Sibley, S. D., et al. (2006). Metabolic syndrome and growth hormone deficiency in adult survivors of childhood acute lymphoblastic leukemia. *Cancer, 107*(6), 1303–1312.

78. Oeffinger, K. C. (2008). Are survivors of acute lymphoblastic leukemia (ALL) at increased risk of cardiovascular disease? *Pediatric Blood & Cancer, 50*(Suppl. 2), 462–467. discussion 8.

79. Shaw, N. J., Tweeddale, P. M., & Eden, O. B. (1989). Pulmonary function in childhood leukaemia survivors. *Medical and Pediatric Oncology, 17*(2), 149–154.

80. Mertens, A. C., Yasui, Y., Liu, Y., et al. (2002). Pulmonary complications in survivors of childhood and adolescent cancer a report from the Childhood Cancer Survivor Study. *Cancer, 95*(11), 2431–2441.

81. Tao, M. L., Guo, M. D., Weiss, R., et al. (1998). Smoking in adult survivors of childhood acute lymphoblastic leukemia. *Journal of the National Cancer Institute, 90*(3), 219–225.

82. Bessho, F., Kinumaki, H., Yokota, S., Hayashi, Y., Kobayashi, M., & Kamoshita, S. (1994). Liver function studies in children with acute lymphocytic leukemia after cessation of therapy. *Medical and Pediatric Oncology, 23*(2), 111–115.

83. De Bruyne, R., Portmann, B., Samyn, M., et al. (2006). Chronic liver disease related to 6-thioguanine in children with acute lymphoblastic leukaemia. *Journal of Hepatology, 44*(2), 407–410.

84. Sathiapalan, R. K., Velez, M. C., McWhorter, M. E., et al. (1998). Focal segmental glomerulosclerosis in children with acute lymphocytic leukemia: Case reports and review of literature. *Journal of Pediatric Hematology/Oncology, 20*(5), 482–485.

85. Alvarez, J. A., Scully, R. E., Miller, T. L., et al. (2007). Long-term effects of treatments for childhood cancers. *Current Opinion in Pediatrics, 19*(1), 23–31.

86. Hoover, D. L., Smith, L. E., Turner, S. J., Gelber, R. D., & Sallan, S. E. (1988). Ophthalmic evaluation of survivors of acute lymphoblastic leukemia. *Ophthalmology, 95*(2), 151–155.

87. Sonis, A. L., Waber, D. P., Sallan, S., & Tarbell, N. J. (1995). The oral health of long-term survivors of acute lymphoblastic leukaemia: A comparison of three treatment modalities. *European Journal of Cancer, 31B*(4), 250–252.

88. Kaste, S. C., Hopkins, K. P., Jones, D., Crom, D., Greenwald, C. A., & Santana, V. M. (1997). Dental abnormalities in children treated for acute lymphoblastic leukemia. *Leukemia, 11*(6), 792–796.

89. Dahllöf, G., & Huggare, J. (2004). Orthodontic considerations in the pediatric cancer patient: A review. *Seminars in Orthodontics, 10*(4), 266–276.

90. Loning, L., Zimmermann, M., Reiter, A., et al. (2000). Secondary neoplasms subsequent to Berlin-Frankfurt-Munster therapy of acute lymphoblastic leukemia in childhood: Significantly lower risk without cranial radiotherapy. *Blood, 95*(9), 2770–2775.

91. Bhatia, S., Sather, H. N., Pabustan, O. B., Trigg, M. E., Gaynon, P. S., & Robison, L. L. (2002). Low incidence of second neoplasms among children diagnosed with acute lymphoblastic leukemia after 1983. *Blood, 99*(12), 4257–4264.

92. Kowalczyk, J., Nurzynska-Flak, J., Armata, J., et al. (2004). Incidence and clinical characteristics of second malignant neoplasms in children: A multicenter study of a polish pediatric leukemia/lymphoma group. *Medical Science Monitor, 10*(3), CR117–CR122.

93. Hijiya, N., Hudson, M. M., Lensing, S., et al. (2007). Cumulative incidence of secondary neoplasms as a first event after childhood acute lymphoblastic leukemia. *JAMA, 297*(11), 1207–1215.

94. Koishi, S., Kubota, M., Sawada, M., et al. (1998). Biomarkers in long survivors of pediatric acute lymphoblastic leukemia patients: Late effects of cancer chemotherapy. *Mutation Research, 422*(2), 213–222.

95. Rice, S. C., Vacek, P., Homans, A. H., et al. (2004). Genotoxicity of therapeutic intervention in children with acute lymphocytic leukemia. *Cancer Research, 64*(13), 4464–4471.

96. Clarke, S. A., & Eiser, C. (2007). Health behaviours in childhood cancer survivors: A systematic review. *European Journal of Cancer, 43*(9), 1373–1384.

97. Larcombe, I., Mott, M., & Hunt, L. (2002). Lifestyle behaviours of young adult survivors of childhood cancer. *British Journal of Cancer, 87*(11), 1204–1209.

98. Hudson, M. M., Mertens, A. C., Yasui, Y., et al. (2003). Health status of adult long-term survivors of childhood cancer: A report from the Childhood Cancer Survivor Study. *JAMA, 290*(12), 1583–1592.

99. Rourke, M. T., Hobbie, W. L., Schwartz, L., & Kazak, A. E. (2007). Posttraumatic stress disorder (PTSD) in young adult survivors of childhood cancer. *Pediatric Blood & Cancer, 49*(2), 177–182.

100. Schwartz, L., & Drotar, D. (2006). Posttraumatic stress and related impairment in survivors of childhood cancer in early adulthood compared to healthy peers. *Journal of Pediatric Psychology, 31*(4), 356–366.

101. Kingma, A., Rammeloo, L. A., van der Does-van den Berg, A., Rekers-Mombarg, L., & Postma, A. (2000). Academic career after treatment for acute lymphoblastic leukaemia. *Archives of Disease in Childhood, 82*(5), 353–357.

102. Mitby, P. A., Robison, L. L., Whitton, J. A., et al. (2003). Utilization of special education services and educational attainment among long-term survivors of childhood cancer: A report from the Childhood Cancer Survivor Study. *Cancer, 97*(4), 1115–1126.

103. Zeltzer, L. K., Chen, E., Weiss, R., et al. (1997). Comparison of psychologic outcome in adult survivors of childhood acute lymphoblastic leukemia versus sibling controls: A cooperative Children's Cancer Group and National Institutes of Health study. *Journal of Clinical Oncology, 15*(2), 547–556.

104. Seitzman, R. L., Glover, D. A., Meadows, A. T., et al. (2004). Self-concept in adult survivors of childhood acute lymphoblastic leukemia: A cooperative Children's Cancer Group and National Institutes of Health study. *Pediatric Blood & Cancer, 42*(3), 230–240.

105. Mulrooney, D. A., Ness, K. K., Neglia, J. P., et al. (2008). Fatigue and sleep disturbance in adult survivors of childhood cancer: A report from the childhood cancer survivor study (CCSS). *Sleep, 31*(2), 271–281.

106. Rauck, A. M., Green, D. M., Yasui, Y., Mertens, A., & Robison, L. L. (1999). Marriage in the survivors of childhood cancer: A preliminary description from the Childhood Cancer Survivor Study. *Medical and Pediatric Oncology, 33*(1), 60–63.

107. Florin, T. A., Fryer, G. E., Miyoshi, T., et al. (2007). Physical inactivity in adult survivors of childhood acute lymphoblastic leukemia: A report from the childhood cancer survivor study. *Cancer Epidemiology Biomarkers and Prevention, 16*(7), 1356–1363.

108. Keene, N., Hobbie, W., & Ruccione, K. (2007). *Childhood cancer survivors: A practical guide to your future.* Sebastopol: O'Reilly & Associates.

109. Greenberg, D. B., Kornblith, A. B., Herndon, J. E., et al. (1997). Quality of life for adult leukemia survivors treated on clinical trials of Cancer and Leukemia Group B during the period 1971-1988: Predictors for later psychologic distress. *Cancer, 80*(10), 1936–1944.

110. Socie, G., Stone, J. V., Wingard, J. R., et al. (1999). Long-term survival and late deaths after allogeneic bone marrow transplantation. Late Effects Working Committee of the International Bone Marrow Transplant Registry. *The New England Journal of Medicine, 341*(1), 14–21.

111. Singhal, S., Powles, R., Treleaven, J., Kulkarni, S., Horton, C., & Mehta, J. (1999). Long-term outcome of adult acute leukemia patients who are alive and well 2 years after autologous blood or marrow transplantation. *Bone Marrow Transplantation, 23*(9), 875–879.

112. Thuret, I., Michel, G., Carla, H., et al. (1995). Long-term side-effects in children receiving allogeneic bone marrow transplantation in first complete remission of acute leukaemia. *Bone Marrow Transplantation, 15*(3), 337–341.

113. Perkins, J. L., Kunin-Batson, A. S., Youngren, N. M., et al. (2007). Long-term follow-up of children who underwent hematopoeitic cell transplant (HCT) for AML or ALL at less than 3 years of age. *Pediatric Blood & Cancer, 49*(7), 958–963.

114. Helder, D. I., Bakker, B., de Heer, P., et al. (2004). Quality of life in adults following bone marrow transplantation during childhood. *Bone Marrow Transplantation, 33*(3), 329–336.
115. Hasegawa, W., Pond, G. R., Rifkind, J. T., et al. (2005). Long-term follow-up of secondary malignancies in adults after allogeneic bone marrow transplantation. *Bone Marrow Transplantation, 35*(1), 51–55.
116. Kolb, H. J., Socie, G., Duell, T., et al. (1999). Malignant neoplasms in long-term survivors of bone marrow transplantation Late Effects Working Party of the European Cooperative Group for Blood and Marrow Transplantation and the European Late Effect Project Group. *Annals of Internal Medicine, 131*(10), 738–744.
117. Curtis, R. E., Rowlings, P. A., Deeg, H. J., et al. (1997). Solid cancers after bone marrow transplantation. *The New England Journal of Medicine, 336*(13), 897–904.
118. Socie, G., Salooja, N., Cohen, A., et al. (2003). Nonmalignant late effects after allogeneic stem cell transplantation. *Blood, 101*(9), 3373–3385.
119. Tichelli, A., Passweg, J., Wojcik, D., et al. (2008). Late cardiovascular events after allogeneic hematopoietic stem cell transplantation: A retrospective multicenter study of the Late Effects Working Party of the European Group for Blood and Marrow Transplantation. *Haematologica, 93*(8), 1203–1210.
120. Armenian, S. H., Sun, C. L., Francisco, L., et al. (2008). Late congestive heart failure after hematopoietic cell transplantation. *Journal of Clinical Oncology, 26*(34), 5537–5543.
121. Socie, G., Mary, J. Y., Esperou, H., et al. (2001). Health and functional status of adult recipients 1 year after allogeneic haematopoietic stem cell transplantation. *British Journal Haematology, 113*(1), 194–201.
122. Andrykowski, M. A., Bishop, M. M., Hahn, E. A., et al. (2005). Long-term health-related quality of life, growth, and spiritual well-being after hematopoietic stem-cell transplantation. *Journal of Clinical Oncology, 23*(3), 599–608.
123. Landier, W., Bhatia, S., Eshelman, D. A., et al. (2004). Development of risk-based guidelines for pediatric cancer survivors: The Children's Oncology Group Long-Term Follow-Up Guidelines from the Children's Oncology Group Late Effects Committee and Nursing Discipline. *Journal of Clinical Oncology, 22*(24), 4979–4990.
124. Rizzo, J. D., Wingard, J. R., Tichelli, A., et al. (2006). Recommended screening and preventive practices for long-term survivors after hematopoietic cell transplantation: Joint recommendations of the European Group for Blood and Marrow Transplantation, the Center for International Blood and Marrow Transplant Research, and the American Society of Blood and Marrow Transplantation. *Biology of Blood and Marrow Transplantation, 12*(2), 138–151.
125. Keene N. (2003). Educating the Child with Cancer: A Guide for Parents and Teachers. Kensington, MD: Candlelighters Childhood Cancer Foundation.

Chapter 22
Immunotherapy for Acute Lymphocytic Leukemia

Jacalyn Rosenblatt and David Avigan

Introduction

While a majority of patients with acute lymphocytic leukemia (ALL) demonstrate response following treatment with standard chemotherapy, subsequent progression due to the emergence of resistant disease is often encountered. The failure to eradicate disease is most commonly observed in adult patients particularly with high-risk features such as adverse cytogenetics. In contrast, immunotherapy may be successful in targeting chemotherapy-resistant clones. The role of immune-based therapy in the treatment of ALL is highlighted by the observation that allogeneic hematopoietic stem cell transplantation is uniquely curative for a subset of patients in this setting [1]. The efficacy of transplant is derived from the dose intensity of the transplant conditioning regimen as well as the antitumor effect mediated by donor-derived immune effector cells. Improved outcomes as compared to standard chemotherapy have been observed in patients in first complete remission (CR) who exhibit negative prognostic factors as well as those with relapsed or refractory disease.

Allogeneic Transplantation as Cellular Immunotherapy

Standard allogeneic transplantation involves the use of high dose chemotherapy alone or in conjunction with myeloablative radiation therapy followed by the infusion of hematopoietic stem cells derived from a HLA matched sibling or alternative donor. The importance of the ablative regimen in determining outcome is supported by the lower risk of relapse observed in patients treated with total body irradiation as compared to busulfan-based regimens [2, 3]. In addition, regimens involving greater than 13 cGy or the use of etoposide as compared to cyclophosphamide have also been shown to be associated with lower relapse rate [4, 5]. However, dose intensity alone is insufficient to achieve long-term disease control in patients with high risk or recurrent ALL. A vital component of allogeneic transplantation responsible for the prevention of disease relapse is the anti-leukemia effect mediated by alloreactive lymphocytes.

Evidence of the unique efficacy of allogeneic transplant has been observed in patients undergoing transplantation in first complete remission. Patients with ALL with high-risk features such as the presence of chromosomal abnormalities including translocation of (9;22), (4;11), and (8;14) rarely

D. Avigan (✉)
Beth Israel Deaconess Medical Center, Harvard Medical School, Kirstein RM 135, 330 Brookline Ave,
Boston, MA 02215, USA
e-mail: davigan@bidmc.harvard.edu

A.S. Advani and H.M. Lazarus (eds.), *Adult Acute Lymphocytic Leukemia*, Contemporary Hematology,
DOI 10.1007/978-1-60761-707-5_22, © Springer Science+Business Media, LLC 2011

experience durable remissions following standard chemotherapy [6, 7]. In contrast, allogeneic transplantation has been associated with improved disease-free survival [3, 8]. In one study, high-risk ALL was defined by the presence of abnormal cytogenetics, elevated WBC, age older than 30, extramedullary disease, or prolonged time to achieve CR. With a median follow up of 5 years, an event-free survival of 64% was observed following allogeneic transplantation [8]. In another study, patients with ALL were assigned to receive an allogeneic as compared to autologous transplant based on the presence of an HLA-matched donor. In the subset exhibiting high-risk features, the 5-year disease free survival was 45% and 23% for the 100 patients who had a sibling donor and the 159 patients who did not, respectively [9].

The efficacy of allogeneic as compared to autologous transplant for high risk ALL was confirmed in a meta-analysis of 10 trials (1,274 patients) comparing outcomes in which patients with an available sibling donor underwent allogeneic transplantation [10]. In a retrospective analysis of 712 patients, allogeneic transplant from unrelated donor in CR1 or CR2 was associated with lower risk of relapse as compared to autologous transplant (49% vs. 14%). However, because of significant treatment related mortality, the 5 year survival was equivalent after CR1. In contrast, allogeneic transplantation was associated with improved survival (50% vs. 14%) in patients with more advanced disease (CR2) [11].These findings highlight the importance of the donor graft in preventing disease relapse.

In a prospective joint study between the Medical Research Council (MRC) of the United Kingdom and ECOG, nearly 2,000 patients with ALL were treated with induction therapy followed by transplantation or standard chemotherapy. Those with a sibling donor were offered an allogeneic transplant while the remaining patients were randomized to receive an autologous transplant or standard chemotherapy including maintenance therapy [12]. Risk of relapse was significantly higher for Philadelphia chromosome (Ph) negative patients not undergoing allogeneic transplant while the benefit with respect to survival was reserved for those patients younger than age 35 due to higher levels of transplant associated toxicity in older patients. Of note, autologous transplantation did not offer any benefit as compared to standard chemotherapy suggesting that improved disease control following allogeneic transplantation was not due to dose intensity.

Patients with Ph+ALL are considered to have intrinsically chemotherapy resistant disease. In one study, 103 patients with Ph+ALL achieved complete remission to initial therapy and were randomized to receive an autologous or allogeneic transplant based on the availability of an appropriate HLA matched donor. Those patients randomized to the allogeneic transplant arm demonstrated a better 3 year overall survival (37% vs. 12%) and decreased relapse rate (50% vs. 90%) as compared to those patients without an HLA-matched donor. On multivariate analysis, the presence of a donor and persistence of molecular evidence of BRC-ABL prior to transplant remained highly significant in predicting outcome [18]. These data suggest that while relapse remains a major concern after allogeneic transplantation, the presence of alloreactive cells following intensive therapy is potentially crucial to eliminate chemotherapy resistant disease in this setting. In several studies, disease-free survival was similar following allogeneic transplant from a sibling and unrelated donor [19, 20].

As suggested above, prevention of disease relapse is thought to be mediated, in part, by alloreactive lymphocytes that target patient-derived leukemia cells [13, 14]. The importance of the graft versus leukemia effect is supported by the association of graft versus host disease with a lower incidence of disease relapse. In one study of 192 patients with ALL who were predominantly transplanted in second complete remission, the actuarial risk of relapse was 40% for patients with grade II or higher graft versus host disease (GVHD) as compared to 80% in patients without evidence of GVHD [15]. A subsequent study of 1,132 patients with ALL also demonstrated that the presence of acute or chronic GVHD was associated with decreased risk of relapse [16]. Similarly, T cell depletion of the hematopoietic graft has been associated with decreased toxicity but a high risk of relapse [17].

Reduced Intensity Conditioning

Allogeneic transplantation following reduced intensity conditioning has been explored in an effort to minimize transplant associated toxicity while relying on the potency of the graft versus disease effect. Limited data is available regarding its efficacy in ALL. In a study of 22 patients with ALL many of which resistant disease long-term survival was only observed in patients transplanted in CR [21]. In another study of 27 patients with high risk ALL who underwent transplant with reduced intensity conditioning, the 2 year overall survival was 31% suggesting that this treatment approach was effective for a subset of patients with ALL not curable with chemotherapy [22]. One study reported on the results of 43 patients with ALL in CR2 undergoing reduced intensity conditioning with busulfan, cyclophosphamide, and fludarabine [23]. The overall survival at 3 years was 31% with a majority of deaths related to disease relapse. The authors concluded that the inferior results observed as compared to that achieved with chronic myeloid leukemia (CML) and AML using the same conditioning regimen suggested an inferior graft versus disease effect in ALL.

In contrast, a Japanese study of 33 patients with ALL demonstrated relapse-free survival even in a subset of patients treated during disease relapse (5/14) [24]. The 1 year relapse free and overall survival was 30% and 39%, respectively. The authors suggested that despite a significant risk of relapse (51% at 3 years) an important graft versus disease effect was present. In a retrospective review by the EBMT, results of 97 patients with adult ALL who underwent reduced intensity conditioning transplantation were reviewed [25]. The 2-year leukemia-free survival in this high-risk population was 21%. Not surprisingly, relapse incidence was higher in patients with more advanced disease (greater than CR1). Of note, the presence of chronic GVHD was associated with improved survival consistent with the importance of a graft versus disease effect. These data suggest that while some patients may respond to alloreactive immunity, it is often insufficient in preventing relapse particularly in the setting of advanced disease.

Donor Lymphocyte Infusion

Treatment with donor lymphocytes infusion (DLI) post-transplant has been explored in an effort to reestablish a graft versus disease effect to eliminate minimal residual or relapsed disease [26]. In patients already manifesting complete donor chimerism, DLI represents the attempt to invigorate an alloreactive anti-tumor response by the introduction of lymphocytes that have not undergone tolerization in the patient in the presence of immunosuppressive therapy such as cyclosporine. The potency of DLI is highly variable and dependent on the disease setting and has shown the greatest promise in CML. Efficacy is likely due to the sensitivity to the alloreactive response as well as the kinetics of tumor growth and the ability to wait for the establishment of a graft versus disease effect that characteristically requires 1–3 months for full expression. Results for patients with ALL have been mixed. One of the first reports of the effective use of DLI was in a child with relapsed ALL who achieved a durable remission that has persisted for greater than 15 years [27]. However, in a review of the experience of the European Group for Blood and Marrow Transplantation, DLI was ineffective in generating durable remissions for a cohort of 22 patients with ALL [28]. Similarly, in a summary report of results from US centers, 44 patients with ALL were treated with either DLI alone or following chemotherapy-induced nadir [29]. Disappointingly, only two out of 15 patients receiving DLI alone achieved a CR and only three patients achieved long-term CR for the entire cohort. In a small cohort of seven patients with ALL undergoing DLI from unrelated donors two out of four evaluable patients achieved CR and disease-free survival was 30% at 1 year for the entire group.

These data raise the question as to why DLI is not more effective in ALL despite the evidence of a significant graft versus disease effect outlined above. One issue effecting both AML and ALL is the rapid growth kinetics of the disease that may not provide the necessary time to establish and immunologically based antitumor effect. In addition, there is evidence that ALL cells directly suppress the antitumor immune response through the induction of T cell anergy [30]. ALL cells may also serve as a more resistant target for donor alloreactivity because of their lack of effective antigen presentation due to the absence of costimulatory molecules and their intrinsic resistance to killing by natural killer (NK) cells [31, 32]. These findings point to the inherent weaknesses of immune-based targeting of ALL cells through alloreactivity. Concerns remain regarding the specificity and potency of this response and overcoming the intrinsic resistance offered by ALL cells. They raise the question as to whether ALL may be more effectively targeted by immunotherapy directed against leukemia specific targets in the context of efforts to alter the immunologic milieu to favor antitumor immune response.

Augmenting Alloreactive Immunity

One approach to reduce the risk of relapse following allogeneic transplantation is to pursue methods that heighten the alloreactive response that targets leukemia cells. In a murine model for B cell leukemia, investigators have demonstrated that the post-transplant infusion of recipient antigen-presenting cells increases allosensitization of donor lymphocytes with a resultant increase in GVHD and a concomitant clearance of BCL1+ cells [33]. In another murine model, investigators have examined a strategy to amplify the potency of DLI to eradicate leukemia cells using DLI from a partially HLA mismatched donor [34]. Animals underwent reduced intensity transplantation followed by inoculation with $1 \times 10(6)$ B cell leukemia cells (BCL1) and administration of mismatched DLI. Those animals who received DLI alone died of GVHD while those who received cyclophosphamide 14 days following DLI demonstrated no evidence of residual disease by PCR analysis while only experiencing self limited GVHD. These results suggest that the elimination of alloreactive cells following a period of activation may promote the graft versus disease effect. In a study using human cells, T cells derived from a haploidentical donor (parent) were cultured with the recipients ALL blasts and IL-2 [35]. The resultant cytotoxic lymphocyte (CTL) culture demonstrated a predominance of CD8+ T cells that demonstrated cytotoxicity against both ALL cells and allogeneic ConA-stimulated mononuclear cells suggesting the recognition of alloreactive targets. Infusion of these cells into a patient following haploidentical transplant resulted in clearance of circulating blasts without evidence of concurrent GVHD.

Another approach to augment the efficacy of donor lymphocytes is to amplify the alloreactive responses that more selectively target hematopoietic malignant cells. Minor histocompatiblity antigens have been identified that are uniquely expressed by hematopoietic cells and are targeted by donor lymphocytes. In a murine NOD/SCID model, animals infused with T cells generated against the HLA-A2-derived HA-1 peptide demonstrated delayed growth of leukemia cells [36]. In contrast, animals receiving CTLs directed against CMV did not show disease response. Of note, tumor growth was ultimately associated with the clearance of the HA-1 recognizing T cells.

Role of NK Cells

The role of innate immunity in targeting ALL cells remains under investigation. NK cells demonstrate cytotoxicity against infectious pathogens and malignant cells mediated by cytokine expression and antigen-dependent recognition not requiring activation of adaptive immunity. NK cell response is regulated by a series of cell surface receptors, which deliver inhibitory or stimulatory signals. The human killer Ig-like receptors (KIRs) are associated with HLA class I molecules and may deliver an inhibitory signal that prevents targeting of autologous tissue. Activation KIRs have also been identified, which may include non-HLA ligands. In addition, a series of other activation receptors are present such as NKG2D that mediate anti-tumor responses. Following haploidentical allogeneic transplantation, lack of KIR-mediated inhibitory signaling may result in the killing of leukemia cells by mismatched donor NK cells. This phenomenon has been best described in AML. In some studies, presence of KIR mismatch that facilitates NK cell activation is associated with improved outcomes in AML [37, 38]. In vitro studies demonstrate that alloreactive NK cells were capable of only lysing a minority of patient-derived ALL cells [39]. This may be due to a lack of stimulatory ligands present on ALL in contrast to AML. Despite these findings, a recent trial of suggested excellent outcomes in children with resistant ALL following haploidentical transplantation [40].

In preclinical models, investigators have examined approaches to enhance NK-cell-mediated killing of ALL cells. In a murine model, ALL cells were genetically engineered to express Murine B Defensin 2 (MBD2), a potent stimulator of innate immunity [41]. Administration of MBD2 expressing ALL cell line resulted in the production of IL-12 and IFNγ, activation of NK and CTL response, and tumor rejection. Animals were subsequently protected against challenge with the wild-type ALL cell line. Depletion of CD8 T cells or NK cells abrogated the response. These findings suggest that the intrinsic resistance of ALL cells to NK-mediated lysis may be overcome by the insertion of NK stimulatory signal.

Generation of Leukemia Specific Immunity

While allogeneic transplantation is effective for a subset of patients with ALL, the lack of specificity of the alloreactive response results in a significant risk of morbidity and mortality. In addition, a majority of patients with high risk and advanced disease relapse due to the lack of efficacy in eliminating the malignant clone. A major area of investigation is the identification of tumor-specific antigens that can be targeted selectively while minimizing the collateral damage on normal tissue. In addition, strategies to augment host immunity, reverse tumor-mediated immune suppression, and overcome tolerance are being pursued in an effort to develop effective immunotherapy for ALL.

Leukemia-Associated Targets for Antibody-Mediated Immunotherapy

Potential targets present in ALL cells include B lymphocyte-specific antigens such as CD19 and CD20, the latter of which is expressed in approximately 1/3 of B lineage precursor ALL. Correspondingly, Rituxamab has been shown to eliminate evidence of minimal residual disease in Ph+ after transplant [42]. In another study, 35 patients underwent treatment with Rituxamab in combination with cyclophosphamide and TBI in an effort to decrease risk of relapse as well as GVHD [43].While GVHD rates may have been impacted no clear effect on relapse was documented. One approach to enhance the efficacy of antibody-mediated therapy is the alteration of the Fc receptor to amplify antibody-dependent cytotoxicity. In one study, the mutated CD19 antibody known as XmAb5574 demonstrated markedly increased binding to the Fc receptor and a 100–1,000 fold increase in ADCC against a broad array of lymphoid leukemia and lymphoma lines [44]. In a murine study, the antibody was shown to significantly inhibit lymphoma growth in a mouse xenograft model.

Another potential immunologic target is CD25, a component of the IL-2 receptor, which is expressed on activated T cells and acute T cell leukemia. Daclizumab is an antibody with specificity to the α-subunit of the IL-2 receptor blocking its interaction with IL-2 [45]. Clinical trials with the murine antibody have demonstrated modest responses in a subset of patients but the humanized form of the antibody has demonstrated greater affinity toward the target. Conjugation of the daclizumab with the radioactive isotope ^{90}Y has resulted in clinical response in 10/18 evaluable patients. In a murine study, the combination of daclizumab and a histone deacetylase inhibitor demonstrated a markedly synergistic effect in the treatment of adult T cell leukemia [46].

The tyrosine kinase, FLT3, is expressed on leukemia cells in nearly all patients with B cell ALL and therefore may serve as a target for antibody therapy [47]. In a murine model, two anti-FLT3 antibodies (IMC-EB10 and IMC-NC7) were shown to prolong survival and reduce engraftment in animals challenged with ALL [48]. Responses were seen even when the antibody resulted in FLT3 activation and was abrogated by depletion of NK cells. Surviving cells after treatment remained sensitive to FLT3 antibody upon retransplantation in another animal.

T Cells Expressing Chimeric Antigen Receptors: Combined Humoral and Adoptive Immunotherapy

Another strategy is the development of adoptive immunotherapy that targets cell surface targets such as CD19 or CD20 while simultaneously utilizing the effector function of cellular immunity. Investigators have created chimeric antigen receptors (CARs) in which the heavy and light variable chains are joined into a single chain Fv and engrafted into the T cell receptor. In this manner, ligation of the CAR results in activation of the T cell receptor and initiation of signaling pathways that result in cytokine production and cell-mediated cytolysis. Using CARs specific for CD19, selective targeting of lymphoid malignancies has been demonstrated in animal models. To limit toxicity, T cells have been engineered to contain the suicide HY-TK gene allowing for the elimination of the infused cells using ganciclovir. In one study, primary human CD8+ cytotoxic T lymphocytes were genetically modified to express a CD19+-specific chimeric immunoreceptor. CD19+ expressing T cells were shown to proliferate, and secrete both TNF-α and interferon γ in response to stimulation by CD19+ but not CD19− tumors. In addition, genetically modified CD19+ T cells killed primary ALL tumors in a CTL assay [49].

Similarly, umbilical cord blood T cells genetically modified to express CD19 were shown to kill ALL blasts in vitro, and eliminate established tumor in a NOD/SCID mouse model [50]. In another study, human peripheral blood lymphocytes were transduced with a CD19-specific CAR called 19z1. Transduced T cells were expanded using a CD19 and CD80 expressing artificial antigen-presenting cell in conjunction with IL-15. SCID-Beige mice were inoculated with tumor and subsequently treated with 19z1+ T cells. T cell-treated mice had a significant survival advantage, demonstrating that genetically engineered human T cells can eradicate established tumors in vivo [51]. Use of T cells expressing CARs targeting CD19 eliminated cell lines that expressed the costimulatory molecule CD80 but were ineffective against an ALL cell line that did not provide co-stimulation. A series of second-generation CARs have been evaluated in vitro [52–58]. Addition of the CD28 transmembrane and signaling domain to the 19z1 CAR has been shown to enhance T cell proliferation, cytokine secretion, and survival in a murine model [52].

The sleeping beauty (SB) transposon system is an alternative, nonviral system used to genetically modify T cell populations [59]. In one study, human peripheral blood and umbilical cord blood T cells were transfected to co-express the CAR for CD19 and CD20. SB engineered T cells strongly co-expressed CD19 CAR and CD20, and effectively lysed two B ALL cell lines. Both peripheral blood and umbilical cord blood T cells engineered to express CD19 CAR and CD20 produced Th1

Table 22.1 Tumor associated antigens that may be immunologicaly targetted

Tumor associated antigen	Comment	References
MAGE	MAGE-A3 gene was shown to be expressed at the mRNA level in 20/53 ALL samples, and not in normal controls	[61]
Cancer-testis (CT) antigens	Testis specific antigen expression was demonstrated in 84.6% of bone marrow and peripheral blood samples obtained from patients with ALL	[62]
PRAME	A trend toward higher survival rates and lower WBC was seen in patients who over-expressed PRAME, possibly due to an immune response against this tumor antigen	[65, 69]
WT1	Native humoral immune responses to WT-1 have been detected in 45.5% of ALL patients suggesting that this is a tumor antigen that is recognized by the host immune repertoire	[66]
Her2/Neu	Her2/Neu specific CTLs were shown to kill ALL blasts, but not nonmalignant B cells, dendritic cells (DCs), bone marrow, or CD34+ progenitors from healthy donors indicating that Her2/Neu is selectively expressed by ALL blasts	[67]

but not Th2 cytokines. In addition, in a NOS/SCID mouse model, adoptive transfer of SB engineered T cells resulted in reduced tumor growth and prolonged survival.

Targeting Known Tumor-Associated Antigens

Known tumor-associated antigens found in other malignancies have also been identified in ALL blasts, including MAGE-A1 [60], MAGE-A3 [61], cancer-testis (CT) antigens [62], PRAME [63–65], WT-1 [66], and Her-2/neu [67, 68] (Table 22.1). In one study, MAGE-A3 gene was shown to be expressed at the mRNA level in 20/53 ALL samples, and not in normal controls [61]. Similarly, over-expression of PRAME was found in 42% of children with ALL [63]. A trend toward higher survival rates and lower WBC was seen in patients who over-expressed PRAME, possibly due to an immune response against this tumor antigen [65, 69]. However, in contrast to melanoma, PRAME-specific CTLs generated from normal subjects did not lyse ALL cells because of lower levels of antigen expression in these cells [70]. Native humoral immune responses to WT-1 have been detected in 45.5% of ALL patients suggesting that this is a tumor antigen that is recognized by the host immune repertoire [66]. The Her-2/neu antigen is also selectively expressed by ALL cells as evidenced by the observation that antigen-specific CTLs were shown to kill leukemic blasts from patients with ALL, but not nonmalignant B cells, dendritic cells (DCs), bone marrow, or CD34+ progenitors from healthy donors. Consistent with this finding, Her-2/neu specific CTLs generated using autologous DCs generated transfected with Her-2/neu mRNA effectively lyse ALL cells [67].

Enhancement of Antigen Presentation Using Dendritic Cells

Despite the presence of tumor-associated antigens potentially recognizable by the immune repertoire, the generation of an effective antitumor immune response remains elusive. The primary factors thought to be responsive include the lack of co-stimulation to support effective antigen presentation, tumor-mediated suppression of host immunity through the expression of inhibitory factors, and the increased presence of suppressor cells such as regulatory T cells. A major focus of investigation is to develop strategies to enhance antigen presentation and facilitate T cell responsiveness through the reversal of tumor-associated immune suppression.

One approach has been the use of dendritic cells (DCs) to enhance antigen presentation. DCs represent a complex network of cells that play a major role in maintaining the balance between immune activation and tolerance [71]. Mature myeloid DCs are uniquely capable of initiating primary immunity through their prominent expression of co-stimulatory and adhesion molecules. Vaccination of DCs loaded with leukemia-associated antigens has been shown to induce antitumor immune responses [72]. In one model, DCs were pulsed with HB-1, a B cell lineage specific antigen that is expressed on ALL cells and recognized by the T cell repertoire [73]. DCs were generated from normal volunteers, pulsed with a HB-1-B44 peptide and used to stimulate antigen-specific CTLs. Consistent with their tumor specificity, CTLs expressed IFNγ in response to exposure to HLA matched ALL cells. RNA encoding for leukemia associated genes has also been as a source of tumor antigens for DC-based vaccination. In one study, a highly efficient transfection system was developed to load RNA onto DCs generated from CD34+ cord blood [74]. HLA-A2+ DCs were pulsed with RNA derived from the HLA-A2+ Nalm-6 ALL cell line or autologous ALL cells and shown to stimulate ALL-specific cytotoxicity.

An alternative strategy involves the use of whole leukemia cells as a source of antigens. In one study, DCs were pulsed with lysate or apoptotic bodies generated from Jurkats cell line (T cell ALL) [75]. Exposure to lysate resulted in increased DC expression of costimulatory and maturation markers. Coculture of pulsed DCs and T cells induced T cell proliferation, IFNγ expression, CTL-mediated lysis of tumor target cells. Similarly, another study demonstrated that functionally active DCs may be generated from peripheral blood mononuclear cell (PBMCs) obtained from patients with ALL in remission [76]. The DCs were pulsed with apoptotic bodies derived from ALL cells and were highly effective in stimulating T cell responses.

Conversion of ALL Cells into Antigen Presenting Cells

Alternatively, leukemia cells can be directly transformed into more efficient antigen presenting cells. In a murine model, transduction of the Ph+ ALL cell line BM185 with CD80 resulted in its heightened immunogenicity and the capacity of animals to withstand tumor challenge with the altered cell line [77]. The protective effect was diminished by in vivo depletion of CD4 or CD8 T cells. However, this approach was ineffective in treating established disease. While transduction with IL-2 or GM-CSF was ineffective, cotransfection with CD80 and GM-CSF induced the most prominent CTL response directed against wild type BM185 and reduction of growth of subcutaneously implanted disease. Another approach is the transformation of ALL into antigen presenting cells with phenotypic features similar to DCs. In one study, strategies for generating dendritic cells from ALL blasts containing the 9;22 translocation were examined. They demonstrated that the combination of IL-1β, IL-3, IL-7, SCF, TNF-α, and CD40L most effectively differentiated t(9;22) lymphoblasts [78]. Upregulation of costimulatory molecule expression, CCR7 and CD54 was demonstrated. Differentiated blasts induced allogeneic T cell proliferation, and killing of leukemia cells in a CTL assay. Differentiated blasts were shown to be derived from the malignant clone by FISH analysis for t(9;22). Other groups have demonstrated that ALL blasts stimulated with CD40L strongly express MHC class I, co-stimulatory and adhesion molecules [30, 79, 80]. T cells stimulated by CD40L exposed blasts have been shown to lyse autologous tumor in CTL assays [79]. A phase I clinical trial was conducted in which patients with relapsed ALL were vaccinated with autolougous CD40L stimulated blasts. Vaccine was successfully generated in nine patients. Seven patients withdrew from study prior to vaccination, due to progressive disease (five patients) or to pursue other therapy (two patients). Two patients were vaccinated without evidence of toxicity, however, clinical responses were not seen [81]. This study highlights the difficulty of applying novel immunotherapeutic approaches in patients with rapidly growing disease.

Cytokine Therapy as Immune Adjuvants

Investigators have examined the role of cytokine therapy to reverse tumor mediate immune suppression and support the development of leukemia specific immunity. In a murine study, administration of rmIL-12 resulted in the eradication of established Ph+ ALL cells [82]. The schedule of treatment had a significant impact on efficacy. Depletion of CD4, CD8 or NK cells did not abrogate the response but combined removal of these cell types interfered with the activity of rmIL-12. Of note, administration of rmIL-12 did not result in immunologic memory such that animals remained susceptible to repeat challenge. However, combination of the rmIL-12 with vaccine consisting of leukemia cells modified to express CD40L/CD80/GM-CSF resulted in prolonged protection against secondary challenge with leukemia. Similarly, the role of toll-like receptor (TLR) signaling in promoting antitumor immunity has being examined [83]. In a preclinical study, B cell precursor ALL cell lines were exposed to TLR2, TLR7, and TLR9 agonists, which resulted in an increase in CD40 expression consistent with enhanced immunogenicity. Ligation of TLR2 on the ALL cell lines was most effective in altering T cell response in significantly increasing IFNγ production.

Summary

Chemotherapy-based strategies have been ineffective for many patients with ALL, particularly those with high-risk features or relapsed disease. In contrast, immunotherapeutic strategies hold potential promise as an approach to eliminate residual disease. The potency of immune based therapy in targeting ALL has been demonstrated in the allogeneic transplant setting. However, the lack of specificity of alloreactive T cells results in significant treatment associated toxicity and disease relapse remains a major concern. Investigators have examined approaches to enhance leukemia specific immunity. ALL associated antigens have been identified as targets for more selective forms of immunotherapy. Antibody therapy has been pursued and has been further augmented by the use of CARs to exploit anti-tumor cellular effector mechanisms. Efforts have also focused on stimulating anti-leukemia cellular immune responses by enhancing antigen presentation by the ALL cell or the introduction of ALL antigens onto professional antigen-presenting cells such as DCs. In addition, approaches to reverse tumor-associated immune suppression such as the use of cytokine are being examined. Defining the optimal timing of immunotherapy is of critical importance. Patients with relapsed/refractory disease demonstrate rapid disease progression, which may not allow sufficient time for an immunologic antitumor effect. As such, immunotherapeutic approaches will likely be most effective in patients with low tumor burden. Strategies that combine tumor-specific immunotherapy with chemotherapy or bone marrow transplantation warrant investigation in clinical trials.

References

1. Stein, A., & Forman, S. J. (2008). Allogeneic transplantation for ALL in adults. *Bone Marrow Transplantation, 41*, 439–446.
2. Davies, S. M., Ramsay, N. K., Klein, J. P., et al. (2000). Comparison of preparative regimens in transplants for children with acute lymphoblastic leukemia. *Journal of Clinical Oncology, 18*, 340–347.
3. Marks, D. I., Forman, S. J., Blume, K. G., et al. (2006). A comparison of cyclophosphamide and total body irradiation with etoposide and total body irradiation as conditioning regimens for patients undergoing sibling

allografting for acute lymphoblastic leukemia in first or second complete remission. *Biology of Blood and Marrow Transplantation, 12,* 438–453.

4. Blume, K. G., Forman, S. J., O'Donnell, M. R., et al. (1987). Total body irradiation and high-dose etoposide: A new preparatory regimen for bone marrow transplantation in patients with advanced hematologic malignancies. *Blood, 69,* 1015–1020.

5. Blume, K. G., Kopecky, K. J., Henslee-Downey, J. P., et al. (1993). A prospective randomized comparison of total body irradiation-etoposide versus busulfan-cyclophosphamide as preparatory regimens for bone marrow transplantation in patients with leukemia who were not in first remission: A Southwest Oncology Group study. *Blood, 81,* 2187–2193.

6. Moorman, A. V., Harrison, C. J., Buck, G. A., et al. (2007). Karyotype is an independent prognostic factor in adult acute lymphoblastic leukemia (ALL): Analysis of cytogenetic data from patients treated on the Medical Research Council (MRC) UKALLXII/Eastern Cooperative Oncology Group (ECOG) 2993 trial. *Blood, 109,* 3189–3197.

7. Hoelzer, D., Gokbuget, N., & Ottmann, O. G. (2002). Targeted therapies in the treatment of Philadelphia chromosome-positive acute lymphoblastic leukemia. *Seminars in Hematology, 39,* 32–37.

8. Jamieson, C. H., Amylon, M. D., Wong, R. M., & Blume, K. G. (2003). Allogeneic hematopoietic cell transplantation for patients with high-risk acute lymphoblastic leukemia in first or second complete remission using fractionated total-body irradiation and high-dose etoposide: A 15-year experience. *Experimental Hematology, 31,* 981–986.

9. Thomas, X., Boiron, J. M., Huguet, F., et al. (2004). Outcome of treatment in adults with acute lymphoblastic leukemia: Analysis of the LALA-94 trial. *Journal of Clinical Oncology, 22,* 4075–4086.

10. Bachanova, V., & Weisdorf, D. (2008). Unrelated donor allogeneic transplantation for adult acute lymphoblastic leukemia: A review. *Bone Marrow Transplantation, 41,* 455–464.

11. Weisdorf, D., Bishop, M., Dharan, B., et al. (2002). Autologous versus allogeneic unrelated donor transplantation for acute lymphoblastic leukemia: Comparative toxicity and outcomes. *Biology of Blood and Marrow Transplantation, 8,* 213–220.

12. Goldstone, A. H., Richards, S. M., Lazarus, H. M., et al. (2008). In adults with standard-risk acute lymphoblastic leukemia, the greatest benefit is achieved from a matched sibling allogeneic transplantation in first complete remission, and an autologous transplantation is less effective than conventional consolidation/maintenance chemotherapy in all patients: Final results of the International ALL Trial (MRC UKALL XII/ECOG E2993). *Blood, 111,* 1827–1833.

13. Horowitz, M. M., Gale, R. P., Sondel, P. M., et al. (1990). Graft-versus-leukemia reactions after bone marrow transplantation. *Blood, 75,* 555–562.

14. Appelbaum, F. R. (1997). Graft versus leukemia (GVL) in the therapy of acute lymphoblastic leukemia (ALL). *Leukemia, 11*(Suppl 4), S15–S17.

15. Doney, K., Fisher, L. D., Appelbaum, F. R., et al. (1991). Treatment of adult acute lymphoblastic leukemia with allogeneic bone marrow transplantation. Multivariate analysis of factors affecting acute graft-versus-host disease, relapse, and relapse-free survival. *Bone Marrow Transplantation, 7,* 453–459.

16. Passweg, J. R., Tiberghien, P., Cahn, J. Y., et al. (1998). Graft-versus-leukemia effects in T lineage and B lineage acute lymphoblastic leukemia. *Bone Marrow Transplantation, 21,* 153–158.

17. Marks, D. I., Bird, J. M., Cornish, J. M., et al. (1998). Unrelated donor bone marrow transplantation for children and adolescents with Philadelphia-positive acute lymphoblastic leukemia. *Journal of Clinical Oncology, 16,* 931–936.

18. Dombret, H., Gabert, J., Boiron, J. M., et al. (2002). Outcome of treatment in adults with Philadelphia chromosome-positive acute lymphoblastic leukemia – results of the prospective multicenter LALA-94 trial. *Blood, 100,* 2357–2366.

19. Dahlke, J., Kroger, N., Zabelina, T., et al. (2006). Comparable results in patients with acute lymphoblastic leukemia after related and unrelated stem cell transplantation. *Bone Marrow Transplantation, 37,* 155–163.

20. Fielding, A. K., & Goldstone, A. H. (2008). Allogeneic haematopoietic stem cell transplant in Philadelphia-positive acute lymphoblastic leukaemia. *Bone Marrow Transplantation, 41,* 447–453.

21. Arnold, R., Massenkeil, G., Bornhauser, M., et al. (2002). Nonmyeloablative stem cell transplantation in adults with high-risk ALL may be effective in early but not in advanced disease. *Leukemia, 16,* 2423–2428.

22. Martino, R., Giralt, S., Caballero, M. D., et al. (2003). Allogeneic hematopoietic stem cell transplantation with reduced-intensity conditioning in acute lymphoblastic leukemia: A feasibility study. *Haematologica, 88,* 555–560.

23. Gutierrez-Aguirre, C. H., Gomez-Almaguer, D., Cantu-Rodriguez, O. G., et al. (2007). Non-myeloablative stem cell transplantation in patients with relapsed acute lymphoblastic leukemia: Results of a multicenter study. *Bone Marrow Transplantation, 40,* 535–539.

24. Hamaki, T., Kami, M., Kanda, Y., et al. (2005). Reduced-intensity stem-cell transplantation for adult acute lymphoblastic leukemia: A retrospective study of 33 patients. *Bone Marrow Transplantation, 35,* 549–556.

25. Mohty, M., Labopin, M., Tabrizzi, R., et al. (2008). Reduced intensity conditioning allogeneic stem cell transplantation for adult patients with acute lymphoblastic leukemia: A retrospective study from the European Group for Blood and Marrow Transplantation. *Haematologica, 93*, 303–306.
26. Loren, A. W., & Porter, D. L. (2008). Donor leukocyte infusions for the treatment of relapsed acute leukemia after allogeneic stem cell transplantation. *Bone Marrow Transplantation, 41*, 483–493.
27. Slavin, S., Morecki, S., Weiss, L., & Or, R. (2002). Donor lymphocyte infusion: The use of alloreactive and tumor-reactive lymphocytes for immunotherapy of malignant and nonmalignant diseases in conjunction with allogeneic stem cell transplantation. *Journal of Hematotherapy & Stem Cell Research, 11*, 265–276.
28. Kolb, H. J., Schattenberg, A., Goldman, J. M., et al. (1995). Graft-versus-leukemia effect of donor lymphocyte transfusions in marrow grafted patients. *Blood, 86*, 2041–2050.
29. Collins, R. H., Jr., Goldstein, S., Giralt, S., et al. (2000). Donor leukocyte infusions in acute lymphocytic leukemia. *Bone Marrow Transplantation, 26*, 511–516.
30. Cardoso, A. A., Schultze, J. L., Boussiotis, V. A., et al. (1996). Pre-B acute lymphoblastic leukemia cells may induce T-cell anergy to alloantigen. *Blood, 88*, 41–48.
31. Galandrini, R., Albi, N., Zarcone, D., Grossi, C. E., & Velardi, A. (1992). Adhesion molecule-mediated signals regulate major histocompatibility complex-unrestricted and CD3/T cell receptor-triggered cytotoxicity. *European Journal of Immunology, 22*, 2047–2053.
32. Han, P., Story, C., McDonald, T., Mrozik, K., & Snell, L. (2002). Immune escape mechanisms of childhood ALL and a potential countering role for DC-like leukemia cells. *Cytotherapy, 4*, 165–175.
33. Hirshfeld, E., Weiss, L., Kasir, J., Zeira, M., Slavin, S., & Shapira, M. Y. (2006). Post transplant persistence of host cells augments the intensity of acute graft-versus-host disease and level of donor chimerism, an explanation for graft-versus-host disease and rapid displacement of host cells seen following non-myeloablative stem cell transplantation? *Bone Marrow Transplantation, 38*, 359–364.
34. Yang, I., Weiss, L., Abdul-Hai, A., Kasir, J., Reich, S., & Slavin, S. (2005). Induction of early post-transplant graft-versus-leukemia effects using intentionally mismatched donor lymphocytes and elimination of alloantigen-primed donor lymphocytes for prevention of graft-versus-host disease. *Cancer Research, 65*, 9735–9740.
35. Jurickova, I., Waller, E. K., Yeager, A. M., & Boyer, M. W. (2002). Generation of alloreactive anti-leukemic cytotoxic T lymphocytes with attenuated GVHD properties from haploidentical parents in childhood acute lymphoblastic leukemia. *Bone Marrow Transplantation, 30*, 687–697.
36. Hambach, L., Nijmeijer, B. A., Aghai, Z., et al. (2006). Human cytotoxic T lymphocytes specific for a single minor histocompatibility antigen HA-1 are effective against human lymphoblastic leukaemia in NOD/scid mice. *Leukemia, 20*, 371–374.
37. Aversa, F., Terenzi, A., Tabilio, A., et al. (2005). Full haplotype-mismatched hematopoietic stem-cell transplantation: A phase II study in patients with acute leukemia at high risk of relapse. *Journal of Clinical Oncology, 23*, 3447–3454.
38. Aversa, F. (2008). Haploidentical haematopoietic stem cell transplantation for acute leukaemia in adults: Experience in Europe and the United States. *Bone Marrow Transplantation, 41*, 473–481.
39. Pende, D., Spaggiari, G. M., Marcenaro, S., et al. (2005). Analysis of the receptor-ligand interactions in the natural killer-mediated lysis of freshly isolated myeloid or lymphoblastic leukemias: Evidence for the involvement of the Poliovirus receptor (CD155) and Nectin-2 (CD112). *Blood, 105*, 2066–2073.
40. Lang, P., & Handgretinger, R. (2008). Haploidentical SCT in children: An update and future perspectives. *Bone Marrow Transplantation, 42*(Suppl 2), S54–S59.
41. Ma, X. T., Xu, B., An, L. L., et al. (2006). Vaccine with beta-defensin 2-transduced leukemic cells activates innate and adaptive immunity to elicit potent antileukemia responses. *Cancer Research, 66*, 1169–1176.
42. Jandula, B. M., Nomdedeu, J., Marin, P., & Vivancos, P. (2001). Rituximab can be useful as treatment for minimal residual disease in bcr-abl-positive acute lymphoblastic leukemia. *Bone Marrow Transplantation, 27*, 225–227.
43. Kebriaei, P., Saliba, R. M., Ma, C., et al. (2006). Allogeneic hematopoietic stem cell transplantation after rituximab-containing myeloablative preparative regimen for acute lymphoblastic leukemia. *Bone Marrow Transplantation, 38*, 203–209.
44. Horton, H. M., Bernett, M. J., Pong, E., et al. (2008). Potent in vitro and in vivo activity of an Fc-engineered anti-CD19 monoclonal antibody against lymphoma and leukemia. *Cancer Research, 68*, 8049–8057.
45. Waldmann, T. A. (2007). Daclizumab (anti-Tac, Zenapax) in the treatment of leukemia/lymphoma. *Oncogene, 26*, 3699–3703.
46. Chen, J., Zhang, M., Ju, W., & Waldmann, T. A. (2009). Effective treatment of a murine model of adult T-cell leukemia using depsipeptide and its combination with unmodified daclizumab directed toward CD25. *Blood, 113*(6), 1287–1293.
47. Stam, R. W., Schneider, P., de Lorenzo, P., Valsecchi, M. G., den Boer, M. L., & Pieters, R. (2007). Prognostic significance of high-level FLT3 expression in MLL-rearranged infant acute lymphoblastic leukemia. *Blood, 110*, 2774–2775.

48. Piloto, O., Nguyen, B., Huso, D., et al. (2006). IMC-EB10, an anti-FLT3 monoclonal antibody, prolongs survival and reduces nonobese diabetic/severe combined immunodeficient engraftment of some acute lymphoblastic leukemia cell lines and primary leukemic samples. *Cancer Research, 66*, 4843–4851.

49. Cooper, L. J., Topp, M. S., Serrano, L. M., et al. (2003). T-cell clones can be rendered specific for CD19: Toward the selective augmentation of the graft-versus-B-lineage leukemia effect. *Blood, 101*, 1637–1644.

50. Serrano, L. M., Pfeiffer, T., Olivares, S., et al. (2006). Differentiation of naive cord-blood T cells into CD19-specific cytolytic effectors for posttransplantation adoptive immunotherapy. *Blood, 107*, 2643–2652.

51. Brentjens, R. J., Latouche, J. B., Santos, E., et al. (2003). Eradication of systemic B-cell tumors by genetically targeted human T lymphocytes co-stimulated by CD80 and interleukin-15. *Natural Medicines, 9*, 279–286.

52. Brentjens, R. J., Santos, E., Nikhamin, Y., et al. (2007). Genetically targeted T cells eradicate systemic acute lymphoblastic leukemia xenografts. *Clinical Cancer Research, 13*, 5426–5435.

53. Hombach, A., Wieczarkowiecz, A., Marquardt, T., et al. (2001). Tumor-specific T cell activation by recombinant immunoreceptors: CD3 zeta signaling and CD28 costimulation are simultaneously required for efficient IL-2 secretion and can be integrated into one combined CD28/CD3 zeta signaling receptor molecule. *Journal of Immunology, 167*, 6123–6131.

54. Maher, J., Brentjens, R. J., Gunset, G., Riviere, I., & Sadelain, M. (2002). Human T-lymphocyte cytotoxicity and proliferation directed by a single chimeric TCRzeta/CD28 receptor. *Nature Biotechnology, 20*, 70–75.

55. Imai, C., Mihara, K., Andreansky, M., et al. (2004). Chimeric receptors with 4-1BB signaling capacity provoke potent cytotoxicity against acute lymphoblastic leukemia. *Leukemia, 18*, 676–684.

56. Finney, H. M., Akbar, A. N., & Lawson, A. D. (2004). Activation of resting human primary T cells with chimeric receptors: Costimulation from CD28, inducible costimulator, CD134, and CD137 in series with signals from the TCR zeta chain. *Journal of Immunology, 172*, 104–113.

57. Pule, M. A., Straathof, K. C., Dotti, G., Heslop, H. E., Rooney, C. M., & Brenner, M. K. (2005). A chimeric T cell antigen receptor that augments cytokine release and supports clonal expansion of primary human T cells. *Molecular Therapy, 12*, 933–941.

58. Finney, H. M., Lawson, A. D., Bebbington, C. R., & Weir, A. N. (1998). Chimeric receptors providing both primary and costimulatory signaling in T cells from a single gene product. *Journal of Immunology, 161*, 2791–2797.

59. Huang, X., Guo, H., Kang, J., et al. (2008). Sleeping Beauty transposon-mediated engineering of human primary T cells for therapy of CD19+ lymphoid malignancies. *Molecular Therapy, 16*, 580–589.

60. Shichijo, S., Tsunosue, R., Masuoka, K., et al. (1995). Expression of the MAGE gene family in human lymphocytic leukemia. *Cancer Immunology, Immunotherapy, 41*, 90–103.

61. Martinez, A., Olarte, I., Mergold, M. A., et al. (2007). mRNA expression of MAGE-A3 gene in leukemia cells. *Leukemia Research, 31*, 33–37.

62. Mobasheri, M. B., Modarressi, M. H., Shabani, M., et al. (2006). Expression of the testis-specific gene, TSGA10, in Iranian patients with acute lymphoblastic leukemia (ALL). *Leukemia Research, 30*, 883–889.

63. Steinbach, D., Viehmann, S., Zintl, F., & Gruhn, B. (2002). PRAME gene expression in childhood acute lymphoblastic leukemia. *Cancer Genetics and Cytogenetics, 138*, 89–91.

64. Paydas, S., Tanriverdi, K., Yavuz, S., Disel, U., Baslamisli, F., & Burgut, R. (2005). PRAME mRNA levels in cases with acute leukemia: Clinical importance and future prospects. *American Journal of Hematology, 79*, 257–261.

65. Ikeda, H., Lethe, B., Lehmann, F., et al. (1997). Characterization of an antigen that is recognized on a melanoma showing partial HLA loss by CTL expressing an NK inhibitory receptor. *Immunity, 6*, 199–208.

66. Elisseeva, O. A., Oka, Y., Tsuboi, A., et al. (2002). Humoral immune responses against Wilms tumor gene WT1 product in patients with hematopoietic malignancies. *Blood, 99*, 3272–3279.

67. Muller, M. R., Grunebach, F., Kayser, K., et al. (2003). Expression of her-2/neu on acute lymphoblastic leukemias: Implications for the development of immunotherapeutic approaches. *Clinical Cancer Research, 9*, 3448–3453.

68. Buhring, H. J., Sures, I., Jallal, B., et al. (1995). The receptor tyrosine kinase p185HER2 is expressed on a subset of B-lymphoid blasts from patients with acute lymphoblastic leukemia and chronic myelogenous leukemia. *Blood, 86*, 1916–1923.

69. Kessler, J. H., Beekman, N. J., Bres-Vloemans, S. A., et al. (2001). Efficient identification of novel HLA-A(*)0201-presented cytotoxic T lymphocyte epitopes in the widely expressed tumor antigen PRAME by proteasome-mediated digestion analysis. *The Journal of Experimental Medicine, 193*, 73–88.

70. Griffioen, M., Kessler, J. H., Borghi, M., et al. (2006). Detection and functional analysis of CD8+ T cells specific for PRAME: A target for T-cell therapy. *Clinical Cancer Research, 12*, 3130–3136.

71. Avigan, D. (1999). Dendritic cells: Development, function and potential use for cancer immunotherapy. *Blood Reviews, 13*, 51–64.

72. Duncan, C., & Roddie, H. (2008). Dendritic cell vaccines in acute leukaemia. *Best Practice & Research. Clinical Haematology, 21*, 521–541.

73. de Rijke, B., Fredrix, H., Zoetbrood, A., et al. (2003). Generation of autologous cytotoxic and helper T-cell responses against the B-cell leukemia-associated antigen HB-1: Relevance for precursor B-ALL-specific immunotherapy. *Blood, 102*, 2885–2891.
74. Hsu, A. K., Kerr, B. M., Jones, K. L., Lock, R. B., Hart, D. N., & Rice, A. M. (2006). RNA loading of leukemic antigens into cord blood-derived dendritic cells for immunotherapy. *Biology of Blood and Marrow Transplantation, 12*, 855–867.
75. Schrauder, A., von Stackelberg, A., Schrappe, M., Cornish, J., & Peters, C. (2008). Allogeneic hematopoietic SCT in children with ALL: Current concepts of ongoing prospective SCT trials. *Bone Marrow Transplantation, 41*(Suppl 2), S71–S74.
76. Maggio, R., Peragine, N., Calabrese, E., et al. (2007). Generation of functional dendritic cells (DC) in adult acute lymphoblastic leukemia: Rationale for a DC-based vaccination program for patients in complete hematological remission. *Leukaemia & Lymphoma, 48*, 302–310.
77. Stripecke, R., Levine, A. M., Pullarkat, V., & Cardoso, A. A. (2002). Immunotherapy with acute leukemia cells modified into antigen-presenting cells: Ex vivo culture and gene transfer methods. *Leukemia, 16*, 1974–1983.
78. Lee, J., Sait, S. N., & Wetzler, M. (2004). Characterization of dendritic-like cells derived from t(9;22) acute lymphoblastic leukemia blasts. *International Immunology, 16*, 1377–1389.
79. Cardoso, A. A., Seamon, M. J., Afonso, H. M., et al. (1997). Ex vivo generation of human anti-pre-B leukemia-specific autologous cytolytic T cells. *Blood, 90*, 549–561.
80. Ghia, P., Transidico, P., Veiga, J. P., et al. (2001). Chemoattractants MDC and TARC are secreted by malignant B-cell precursors following CD40 ligation and support the migration of leukemia-specific T cells. *Blood, 98*, 533–540.
81. Haining, W. N., Cardoso, A. A., Keczkemethy, H. L., et al. (2005). Failure to define window of time for autologous tumor vaccination in patients with newly diagnosed or relapsed acute lymphoblastic leukemia. *Experimental Hematology, 33*, 286–294.
82. Gruber, T. A., Skelton, D. C., & Kohn, D. B. (2005). Recombinant murine interleukin-12 elicits potent antileukemic immune responses in a murine model of Philadelphia chromosome-positive acute lymphoblastic leukemia. *Cancer Gene Therapy, 12*, 818–824.
83. Corthals, S. L., Wynne, K., She, K., et al. (2006). Differential immune effects mediated by toll-like receptors stimulation in precursor B-cell acute lymphoblastic leukaemia. *British Journal Haematology, 132*, 452–458.

Chapter 23
Unique Subtypes in Acute Lymphoblastic Leukemia

Elisabeth Paietta

Until the advent of monoclonal antibodies, lineage affiliations were assigned solely based on morphologic and cytochemical features. Consequently, the thought that a leukemic blast could express phenotypic features from both the myeloid and lymphoid lineages was completely foreign. In 1982, Bettelheim and Paietta [1] demonstrated the expression of a myeloid-lineage-affiliated antigen on the surface of leukemic lymphoblasts. Shortly afterward, the same investigators distinguished between dual-lineage antigen expression by one single blast cell and the presence of distinct myeloid and lymphoid blasts within the same leukemia population [2]; the perception of "biphenotypic or hybrid" and "mixed" leukemias, respectively, had been born. These initial examples of unique subtypes in acute lymphoblastic leukemia (ALL) were generated 25 years ago using the first and then only myeloid monoclonal antibody available (VIM-D5/CD15), at a time when multicolor flow cytometry was a dream of the future, and our knowledge of antigen expression profiles was very limited. While the category of biphenotypic leukemia is still in use nowadays, its definition has changed completely [3, 4]. Several additional unique ALL antigen profiles have been described since then. Unfortunately, their definitions are often confounded by faulty or misinformed methodology or data interpretation. Among the most common flaws are the wrong selection of fluorochromes, poorly controlled permeabilization and fixation methods for intracytoplasmic antigen detection (e.g., myeloperoxidase), and an absent or unfortunate choice of blast gating strategies. The use of arbitrary cutoff points to define positive antigen expression is an unfortunate mistake that defies biologic relevance [5, 6]. Finally, it is still widespread practice among hematopathologists to assign blast cells to a certain lineage based on morphology and subsequently compare the antigen profile with the prior assessment. Rarely, this critical point is openly addressed as a drawback of a study [7]. Correctly, lineage-specific antigens, which are all intracellularly located, must be used to unequivocally assign lineage affiliations [3, 6, 8].

Increasingly, gene mutations or gene expression profiles are found to characterize subsets of patients with distinct prognosis. For most genetic lesions in ALL, particular surface marker profiles, which could serve as surrogates for specific genotype(s), have not yet been identified [9–11]. The recognition of a unique ALL subtype gains significance if it confers clinical relevance. Besides impact on response to standard therapy or overall survival, clinical relevance can also imply an association of pheno- or genotypic features with particular targeted therapy. Examples for the latter are the expression of the myeloid antigen (My Ag) CD33 by lymphoblasts, which predicts response to anti-CD33 antibody [12, 13], or the finding of FLT3 gene mutations in T-ALL blasts, which suggest the use of FLT3 kinase inhibitors [14].

E. Paietta (✉)
Montefiore Medical Center-North Division, 600 East 233rd Street, Bronx, NY 10466, USA
e-mail: epaietta@earthlink.net

A.S. Advani and H.M. Lazarus (eds.), *Adult Acute Lymphocytic Leukemia*, Contemporary Hematology,
DOI 10.1007/978-1-60761-707-5_23, © Springer Science+Business Media, LLC 2011

The rare T-ALL subset with activating FLT3 gene mutations [14] belongs to the few examples of gene mutations, which are predicted by the presence of a unique antigen expression pattern. Although it should be obvious that genotypes control the phenotypes of leukemic cells, it has been difficult and sometimes impossible to establish concordances between phenotypic and genotypic categories. Yagi et al. [15] demonstrated that FAB subtypes, which are predominantly based on morphology and cytochemical properties [16], and gene expression profiles measure fundamentally different characteristics of leukemic blast cells. In children, a gene expression profile specific for the E2A/PBX1 transcript was not specific for the Pre-B immunophenotype [17], although this genetic lesion is almost exclusively found in ALLs with that phenotype [3]. There are only a few examples of immune profiles that can reliably act as surrogate markers for genetic lesions in leukemia [18]. An excellent example is the association of CD25, the α-chain of the interleukin-2 receptor, with Philadelphia chromosome positivity in B-lineage ALL [19, 20]. Given the potential clinical efficacy of ABL tyrosine kinase inhibitors [21, 22], the detection of CD25 on lymphoblasts serves as an important therapeutic guide, even in the absence of cytogenetic or molecular proof for the Philadelphia chromosome or its genetic equivalent, the BCR/ABL transcript. While the antigen profile of FLT3-gene mutated T-lymphoblasts discussed before has prompted a postulate of a normal cellular equivalent in the thymus, the biologic link between CD25 expression and BCR/ABL positivity, to date, has remained unexplained.

Cytogenetic features with their relevant molecular equivalents are predictive of outcome in adult ALL [23–25]. However, vast genetic heterogeneity is starting to become apparent for individual genetic aberrations in ALL based on gene expression profiling, such as for BCR/ABL [26, 27] or NOTCH1-activating mutations [28]. On the other hand, although a core gene expression signature is associated with MLL gene rearrangements, cases segregate according to their lineage of origin, myeloblastic or lymphoblastic [29–31]. Since genomic or epigenetic classifiers predict and distinguish responders from failures under various treatment regimens, immunophenotypic correlates should be sought, making this gene expression–based classification of ALL more user-friendly. This chapter will restrict itself to discussing "unique immunophenotypes" that are either associated with a known genetic abnormality or otherwise carry prognostic information.

The first discussion will address My Ags in ALL in general, without emphasizing their association with prognostic genotypes. My Ag^{pos} ALL is the most commonly misdiagnosed disease and when considered isolated from other biologic parameters, it lacks clinical relevance.

Myeloid Antigen Expression in ALL

Several of the early reports on the finding of My Ags in ALL cannot be taken under consideration because immunophenotypic analysis of lineage affiliation was compared with a morphologic lineage assignment. In other words, leukemia populations were called lymphoid based on FAB criteria before antigen expression patterns were established. In fact, a positive correlation between morphology and immunophenotype is a rarity rather than the norm [3, 18, 32]. Cell lineage assignment must rely on the detection of lineage-specific rather than lineage-affiliated antigens, independent of morphologic criteria [3, 6, 8]. The 3 lineage-specific antigens are myeloperoxidase (MPO, myeloid lineage), intracytoplasmic CD3 (cCD3, T-cell lineage), and intracytoplasmic CD22 (cCD22, B-cell lineage) [3, 6, 8]. These intracytoplasmic antigens must be tested in combination with surface antigens that mark the individual leukemia population, such as CD34, CD117, CD10, etc. Based on the detection of lineage-specific antigens, true biphenotypic leukemias, defined as blast cells expressing MPO together with cCD3 or cCD22, or cCD3 together with cCD22, are extremely rare.

There are additional flaws with many investigations regarding My Ag expression in ALL. For instance, the testing of a limited number of myeloid antibodies (e.g., only CD33 and CD33, disregarding CD65, CD15) yields an underestimation of the incidence of My Ags. Most importantly, several studies rely merely on percent overlap of antigen expressions rather than demonstrating that My Ags are indeed expressed by the leukemic lymphoblasts. Gating on the blast cells and reporting antigen expression solely for those blasts is a prerequisite for valid data on unexpected antigen expression. If antibody binding is restricted to the blast gate, any level of antigen expression becomes significant. It is common for lymphoid leukemia populations to express My Ags on the majority of blasts, albeit often with low intensity. Any description of small My Ag[pos] ALL subpopulations requires that co-expression of lymphoid and myeloid antigens be unequivocally demonstrated to exclude contamination by small numbers of normal myeloid cells. Alternatively, it is feasible to consider the presence of a minor My Ag[pos] blast subpopulation, a finding that was originally termed "mixed leukemia" [2] as compared to "hybrid" leukemias [1] with co-expression of lymphoid and myeloid antigens. This nomenclature is outdated because irrelevant, unless lineage-specific, antigens can be demonstrated in distinct fractions of one leukemia population or within individual leukemic blasts; in either case, a true biphenotype should be diagnosed.

Finally, when investigators analyze the impact of My Ags in ALL without considering cytogenetic abnormalities, they ignore the established independent prognostic significance of karyotypes in adult ALL [23–25] by assigning prognostic significance to immunophenotypic parameters, which are part of an established genotype. The most common mistake seen is the implication that the combined expression of CD33 and CD13 is associated with poor outcome in ALL without realizing that the dual presence of these antigens is a characteristic feature of BCR/ABL positivity [18, 33], a major adverse prognostic factor in ALL [34, 35]. Thus, univariate analyses of immunophenotypic data nowadays are unacceptable.

As early as 1990, Ludwig and Thiel [36] postulated that the expression of 3 myeloid antigens, CD33, CD13, and CD65(s), were mandatory to distinguish ALL from poorly differentiated AML. Since then we have learned that undifferentiated AML frequently lacks CD65(s) [37]. This makes it essential to diagnose AML either by proving myeloid lineage affiliation through staining blasts with antibody to intracytoplasmic MPO or by disproving ALL through lack of reactivity for cCD22 (B-lineage) and cCD3 (T-lineage) antibodies [3, 18]. The same group of German investigators subsequently suggested that the expression of myeloid antigens in adult B-lineage ALL differs according to the level of B-lymphoblast differentiation [38], analogous to what was reported from pediatric ALL [39, 40]. Recently, the analysis of the largest adult ALL trial, E2993, to date replicated this observation [33]. In Pro-B ALL (CD10[neg]), lymphoblasts typically express CD65(s) and CD15(s), whereas in Early Pre-B ALL (CD10[pos]), lymphoblasts express CD33 and/or CD13. This correlation remained statistically significant even when BCR/ABL[pos] cases, which most frequently present as Early Pre-B ALL, were excluded from the analysis (Table 23.1). It is noteworthy that the incidence of CD15 expression is lower than that of CD15s, the sialylated CD15 variant. In other words, dependent upon whether CD15 or CD15s antibodies are used in ALL testing, disparate results can be obtained. Thus, there is a clear reverse association of the more mature My Ags, CD65(s) and CD15(s), with the more immature Pro-B/Pre-Pre-B ALL subtype, and of CD33 and/or CD13, the

Table 23.1 Myeloid antigen expression by B-lineage lymphoblasts in BCR/ABL[neg] patients on ECOG protocol, E2993 ($N=300$)

B-ALL maturation stage	N	Percentage of patients with My Ag expression on ≥30% of leukemic lymphoblasts				
		CD33	CD13	CD65(s)	CD15s	CD15
Pro-B/Pre-Pre-B	59	20	24	42	29	64
Early Pre-B	182	35	41	1	1	13
Pre-B; transitional Pre-B; Mature B	59	14	27	12	14	27

Pro/Pre-Pre B ALL, CD10[neg]; Early Pre-B ALL, CD10[pos]; Pre-B ALL, intracytoplasmic μ[pos]; Transitional Pre-B ALL, both intracytoplasmic and surface μ[pos]; Mature B-ALL, surface μ[pos] and surface immunoglobulin light chain monoclonal more immature My Ags, with CD10^{pos} Early Pre-B ALL. This suggests that the arbitrary scoring of myeloid antigens when expressed by lymphoblasts for the definition of biphenotypic acute leukemias, as suggested by the EGIL Scoring System [41], is ill-advised.

Overall, almost two-thirds of BCR/ABL^{neg} B-lineage ALL patients on E2993 expressed at least one myeloid antigen [33]. As in B-lineage ALL, the most commonly expressed My Ag in T-lineage ALL from E2993 was CD13, which in 52% of cases was present on the entire lymphoblast population, albeit sometimes with weak intensity. Vitale et al. [42] also demonstrated a prevalence of CD13 in adult T-ALL, though their incidence of CD13 was only 20%, probably due to differences in the interpretation of staining intensities. The Italian group found that positivity for CD13 decreased the likelihood of achieving complete remission (CR). Preliminary analysis from E2993 suggested that CD13 expression in T-lineage ALL was associated with inferior outcome [43], a result that is currently under review, using the final study data. Induction of CD13 expression as well as aminopeptidase-N activity on the surface of B-lymphoblasts has been observed following 72 h of culture [44]. Metabolic labeling studies have found that, at least in myeloid leukemia cells, the surface CD13 antigen is the posttranslationally differentially modified product of an intracellular form [45]. There is evidence suggesting that microenvironmental stimuli are responsible for the suppression of CD13 expression on the surface of normal and CD13^{neg} leukemic B-lymphoblasts, thus explaining its in vitro induction in the absence of marrow stroma [46]. That CD13 is the most common My Ag found in both B- and T-lineage ALL [33] is most likely explained by its transient appearance in the earliest stages of B- and T-cell differentiation [47].

While in pediatric ALL, My Ag expression when compared with My Ag^{neg} ALL lacks prognostic significance [40, 48, 49], results on the implication of My Ag expression in adult ALL are still controversial [50, 51]. One reason for this ongoing controversy in adults when compared with children may be the significantly higher incidence of BCR/ABL^{pos} disease in adults (1–4% in children versus up to 27% in adults). Any outcome analysis that refrains from excluding BCR/ABL^{pos} patients with their frequent expression of My Ags from the group of My Ag^{pos} ALL will invariably produce inferior results associated with the My Ag^{pos} ALL group. The recent final analysis of My Ag expression (MPO, CD33, CD13, CD65, CD15, CD11b, CD14) in 505 B-lineage ALL patients entered on the international E2993 trial failed to reveal any prognostic impact, provided that BCR/ABL^{pos} patients were excluded from the analysis cohort [33]. The analysis of T-lineage patients from that study is currently underway and will finally settle the question of a prognostic significance of My Ag expression also in this ALL subset.

It is reasonable to suggest that phenotypic features reflect the genetic makeup of leukemic cells [52, 53]. On the other hand, Serrano et al. [54] reported on the detection of MPO mRNA in ALL cases lacking MPO protein. Even more interesting, cDNA studies in pediatric ALL revealed the overexpression of several genes normally expressed only in the myeloid lineage in hematopoiesis, including the gene encoding the receptor for the granulocyte colony-stimulating factor [55]. These data sustain the intimate lineage relation between the development of myeloid and lymphoid cells, a notion supported by the existence of multipotential progenitors with lymphoid (both B and T), myeloid, and erythroid lineage potential in the CD34^{pos} CD1a^{neg} population in normal thymus [56].

My Ag^{pos} Genetic Subtypes

A logical follow-up to a discussion of My Ag^{pos} ALL in general are genetic subtypes, which are associated with My Ag expression, such as BCR/ABL^{pos} ALL, CD117^{pos} ALL with or without FLT3 gene mutations, NOTCH1-mutated My Ag^{pos} T-cell ALL, TEL/AML1^{pos} ALL, and MLL gene rearrangement in My Ag^{pos} Pro-B ALL.

Chapter 6
Acute Lymphoblastic Leukemia: Epidemiology

Matthew J. Hourigan and Anthony H. Goldstone

Demographic Patterns

Incidence

ALL accounts for approximately 1% of all adult cancers but nearly 25% of all childhood cancers. There is a slight male to female predominance of 1.3:1.0 (male to female ratio). In the USA, in 2008, there were approximately 5,400 new cases of ALL [1]. Among all ages, this represents 13% of all leukemias and 28% of all lymphocytic leukemias [1]. The overall age-adjusted incidence of ALL in the USA is 1.6 per 100,000 according to the most recent National Cancer Institute report based on cases between 2001 and 2005 [1]. This has gradually increased since 1976 when the incidence was 1.1 per 100,000. Age-adjusted rates of ALL do vary internationally with highest rates noted in Spain, Denmark, and Caucasians in Canada and New Zealand, with lowest rates in Asian and African populations [2]. Within the USA, the highest rates for both sexes are among Hispanics while those of black African descent are the lowest [1].

A majority of ALL cases occur in persons under the age of 15 years (Fig. 6.1) [3]. ALL is the most common malignancy in this age group (except in Africa and the Middle East). In the USA, the peak age group is between 1 and 4 years with an age-specific incidence of 7.7 per 100,000 between 2001 and 2005 [1]. For all children less than 5 years, this rate drops to 3.9 per 100,000. This represents 25.8% of childhood cancers and 78% of all childhood leukemias [1]. From 1975 to 2005, incidence rates of ALL in the US population have increased at a rate of about 0.9% per year [1]. Through until 1989, the rate was double this at 1.8% per year. However, it has been suggested that changes in diagnostic specificity with greater recognition of ALL from other leukemia subtypes may account, in part, for the apparent increase in incidence [4]. Since 1989, incidence rates for ALL and other leukemias have increased at only 0.3% per year [1].

Survival

Long-term survival rates for adult ALL cases have not significantly improved over the past two decades. Five-year survival is still only 30–40% for patients 20–60 years old, worsening to less than 15% for those older than 60 years and less than 5% for those older than 70 years [5–18].

M.J. Hourigan (✉)
Department of Haematology, University College Hospital, London, UK
e-mail: matthew.hourigan@uclh.nhs.uk

A.S. Advani and H.M. Lazarus (eds.), *Adult Acute Lymphocytic Leukemia*, Contemporary Hematology,
DOI 10.1007/978-1-60761-707-5_6, © Springer Science+Business Media, LLC 2011

By contrast, survival for childhood ALL has improved markedly over the past five decades. In the period of 1996–2004 in the USA, 5-year relative survival rates were 86.5%, which had improved from 56% in 1975–1977 and from 3% in 1962 [1, 19]. This represents the successful innovative approach with multidrug strategies.

Mortality

The age-adjusted death rate for all ALL cases in the USA was 0.5 per 100,000 people for the period 2001–2005 [1]. There has been a trend towards reduced mortality for all cases of ALL with a reduction in annual percentage change at 1.0% per annum. For all children less than 15 years, there has been a decline in mortality rates from 1975 to 2005 with a greater rate of decrease in the 1990s [1].

Sex Differences

As mentioned above, there is a slight male to female predominance of 1.3:1.0 male to female ratio. This predominance is noted across all age groups including childhood ALL [20]. The gender difference on US figures is more pronounced in white Caucasians than those of black African origin [1].

Race Differences

The incidence of ALL is higher in those of European descent than those of African descent. In adults in the USA, the incidence in whites is 1.7 per 100,000 compared to 0.9 per 100,000 for blacks. The difference is even more marked in children with a peak excess rate of over 150% between 1 and 4 years with comparative rates of 8.4 vs 3.3 per 100,000 for whites and blacks, respectively. As noted prior, within the USA, the racial subgroup with highest incidence is that of Hispanic males at a rate of 2.4 per 100,000 [1].

Age Differences

There is a clear peak of incidence of ALL between 2 and 4 years old followed by falling rates during later childhood, adolescence, and early childhood [21]. There is a bimodal pattern with a smaller secondary peak gradually trending up beyond 60 years old (Fig. 6.1) [1]. Interestingly, the sharp peak in early childhood was first noted in the UK and USA in the 1930s, then subsequently in Japan, China, and among children of African descent in the USA [22]. The peak appears to be absent in many parts of the developing world. This change in incidence with industrialization and affluence may provide an answer to the leukemogenic etiological agents that give rise to ALL.

Parental and Birth Characteristics

Epidemiological studies have revealed a variety of parental patterns and birth characteristics of ALL cases. Firstborn babies and high birth-weight babies have a higher risk of ALL [23]. Maternal age over 35 years, maternal cigarette smoking, and history of prior fetal loss have also

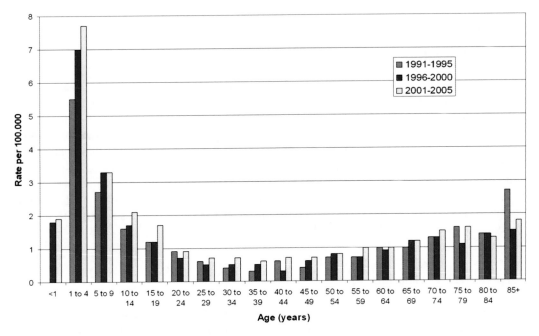

Fig. 6.1 Age-specific incidence rates for acute lymphoblastic leukemia by observation period. Data based on Surveillance, Epidemiology, and End Results (SEER) Program Cancer Statistics Review (Data from [1])

been shown to impart subsequent increased risk of ALL on offspring [24, 25]. Breast feeding has been suggested to be protective against ALL but has not been shown in more recent studies [25].

Socioeconomic Status

The predominance of ALL among white European and Westernized populations has led to the suggestion that ALL may be associated with higher socioeconomic status (SES). Greenberg and colleague [26] reviewed six studies conducted prior to 1983 where five of the six revealed a positive association between SES and childhood ALL. More recently, Poole and colleagues [27] reviewed 47 studies concluding that connections of SES measures to childhood leukemia are likely to vary with place and time and that different socioeconomic measures (such as income and education) and individual-level and community-level measures may represent different risk factors. They advised researchers to report these measures separately rather than in summary indices of social class.

Etiology

The cause of ALL in adults remains largely unknown. In children, genetic predisposition syndromes and ionizing radiation are known risk factors. Many risk factors have been suggested but hitherto are under investigation including chemical exposure to benzenes, pesticides, automobile exhausts, cigarette smoking, and magnetic fields.

Biological Factors

Genetic Syndromes

Inherited, predisposing genetic syndromes are associated with less than 5% of ALL cases. Germ-line abnormalities associated with ALL include Down syndrome (trisomy 21), ataxia-telangiectasia, Fanconi's anemia, Nijmegen breakage syndrome, Klinefelter's syndrome, Bloom syndrome, and neurofibromatosis [28]. Patients with Down syndrome have a 10–30 times greater risk of leukemia where acute megakaryocytic leukemia predominates in those less than 3 years old, while ALL occurs in older age groups with B cell precursor ALL being the most common subtype [29]. Patients with ataxia-telangiectasia have a 70 times greater risk of developing leukemia, particularly T cell ALL. The causative gene, termed *ATM* (ataxia-telangiectasia mutated), is involved in DNA repair, regulation of proliferation, and apoptosis; alterations in this gene have been associated with susceptibility to sporadic cases of T cell ALL children [30].

Acquired Genetic Abnormalities

Cytogenetic abnormalities are the most important independent prognostic factor for predicting outcome in adult ALL. These abnormalities have been detected in 62–85% of cases [31, 32], but with improved collection, transportation, and preservation techniques, identification of clonal abnormalities can be achieved in greater than 90% of cases.

The major cytogenetic abnormalities are clonal translocations. The most common of these in adults is t(9;22), or the Philadelphia chromosome, resulting in the *BCR-ABL* fusion gene, occurring in 11–29% of adult ALL [31, 32]. This results in an activated kinase that confers a proliferative advantage.

In children, the most common clonal translocation is t(12;21), which generates the *TEL-AML1* fusion gene (found in about 20–25% of B-lineage childhood ALLs) [33–37]. Other clonal translocations include t(4;11) giving rise to the *MLL-AF4* fusion gene, t(1;19) giving rise to *E2A-PBX1* fusion gene, t(8;14), and t(10;14).

Other structural abnormalities include abnormalities in 9p, 6q, and 12p. Somatic abnormalities resulting in numerical abnormalities include hypodiploidy (<46 chromosomes), hyperdiploidy (47–50), high hyperdiploidy (51–67), and near tri/tetraploidy. Aneuploidy, in any of the above forms, is much more common in children and is noted in 92% of childhood ALL cases [38, 39], but in only 20–35% of adult cases [31, 32].

Infectious Etiology

Observations of a peak age of development of childhood ALL of 2–5 years, an association of industrialization and modern or affluent societies with increased prevalence of the disease, and the occasional clustering of childhood leukemia cases (especially in new towns) have lead to three variations on the infection-based hypotheses by British investigators: Kinlen's population-mixing hypothesis [40, 41], Smith's perinatal-infection hypothesis [42, 43], and Greaves' delayed-infection hypothesis [44, 45]. No specific virus has definitely been linked with human childhood leukemia, and there is no evidence of genomic inclusions within leukemic cells.

Kinlen's hypothesis [40, 41] predicts that clusters of childhood cases of ALL result from exposure of susceptible (nonimmune) individuals to common but fairly nonpathological infections after unusual population mixing with carriers. The agent would be a currently unrecognized but mild infectious agent, and the outcome of leukemia would be a rare event. Kinlen and colleagues [40] that HOX11/TLX1-T-ALL is closely associated with the early cortical thymocyte developmental stage in all age groups: CD1^{pos}, CD4/CD8 double^{pos}, surface CD3$^{low\ or\ neg}$ [63, 76]. My Ag expression in HOX11^{pos} T-ALL is poorly investigated. Ferrando et al. [63] reported that none of the pediatric HOX11^{pos} cases ($n=8$) expressed either the CD33 or CD13 My Ag. Analysis of a subset of E2993 adult ALL patients confirmed that HOX11/TLX1-overexpression cases forms a low-risk subgroup [10]. Remarkably, however, these 11 cases demonstrated extensive antigenic heterogeneity, including lack of CD1 (two cases), strong surface CD3 expression (four cases), three single CD8^{pos}, and seven double CD4/CD8^{pos} cases, and infrequent though varied expression of My Ags. This observation suggests that the prognostic significance of HOX11/TLX1 overexpression is independent of the stage of T-lymphoblast maturation arrest.

TEL/AML1^{pos} ALL

The TEL/AML1 fusion gene, created by the cryptic (12;21)(p13;q22) translocation, encodes a chimeric transcription factor, which interferes with the pattern of HOX-gene expression during normal hematopoiesis [79, 80]. The TEL/AML1 hybrid is the most common genetic aberration in pediatric ALL (>20%) but only accounts for <1–3% of adult ALL [58, 80–82]. Children with TEL/AML1 have an excellent outcome, especially with high-intensity treatment [83], while in adults prognostic data are not available, due to the low incidence of this genetic lesion. In children, it has been demonstrated that the TEL/AML1 fusion occurs exclusively in CD10^{pos} B-lineage ALL. Early on, Borowitz et al. [84] suggested a TEL/AML1-associated phenotype negative for CD9 and CD20 and likely positive for CD13. Subsequently, De Zen et al. [85] improved the predictive value of this phenotype by demonstrating a higher intensity of CD10 and HLA-DR, and lower expression levels of CD20, CD135, CD45, and CD34 in TEL/AML1^{pos} cases. Microarray analysis found high mRNA levels for CD10, consistent with high CD10 protein expression [17]. The significantly higher staining intensity for HLA-DR and a frequent occurrence of CD13 and CD33 have been confirmed, together with a stronger expression of CD40 and lower expression of CD86 [86]. These unique patterns in the expression of components of antigen presentation may suggest that TEL/AML1^{pos} blasts have enhanced ability to stimulate the immune system. Immunophenotypic information in TEL/AML1^{pos} adults is scarce. In the nine TEL/AML1^{pos} cases found among ECOG E2993 patients (1.4%), Paietta et al. [82] found support for a CD10^{pos} Early-Pre-B phenotype, lacking CD20 and predominantly CD34, and with frequent expression of CD33+CD13. However, in comparison to Early Pre-B ALL with normal cytogenetics and molecularly negative for BCR/ABL, MLL/AF4, or E2A/PBX1, there was no difference in CD45 intensity, and CD40 intensity was higher than the median value in normal karyotype controls in only half of the patients. Although based on small numbers of patients, the most predictive immune profile for TEL/AML1^{pos} adult B-lineage ALL to date is CD10^{pos}, CD20^{neg}, CD34^{neg}, cIgM^{neg}, frequently CD33+CD13^{pos}.

MLL/AF4^{pos} ALL

MLL/AF4^{pos} ALL is the typical subtype of infant ALL and the most prevalent of the diverse MLL fusion proteins in adult ALL [31, 87, 88]. Although usually associated with poor response to chemotherapy [23, 24, 49, 89], intensification of postremission therapy may improve outcome in adult patients [38]. MLL/AF4^{pos} ALL is associated with CD10^{neg} Pro/Pre-Pre-B ALL [18, 23, 38, 49, 89, 90]. Uniquely among all ALL phenotypes, MLL/AF4^{pos} lymphoblasts show a propensity to express the My Ags CD65 and CD15, while lacking CD33 and CD13 [49, 82, 89, 90]. In the large adult ALL trial, E2993, 15% of patients were found to express MLL/AF4 transcripts [82]. Two-thirds of these patients fit the CD10^{neg} Pro/Pre-Pre-B phenotype and all of them co-expressed either both CD65+CD15 (87%) or CD15 alone (13%). Although five patients were CD10^{pos} B-lineage ALLs, four of them still co-expressed CD65 and CD15, contrary to what is usually seen at this maturation stage in B-lineage ALL [33, 38–40]. Though based on small numbers of patients, these observations suggest that My Ag expression in B-lineage ALL is determined by the underlying genetic defect rather than B-lymphoid developmental stage.

Genotypes with Unique Antigenic Features Other Than My Ags

CALM/AF10^{pos} T-ALL and Γδ-T-Cell Receptor Expression

Fusion transcripts that involve the MLL gene at 11q23 and the AF10 gene on the short arm of chromosome 10 lead to the MLL/AF10 fusion transcript, which is commonly associated with AML [31, 88]. This event must be carefully distinguished from another genetic aberration that also involves the long arm of chromosome 11, though at a band other than q23 (location of the MLL gene). In the rare t(10;11)(p13–14;q14–21), the resulting fusion transcript is the CALM/AF10 hybrid gene, which has been found in hematologic malignancies of various kinds [91, 92].

T-cell receptor genes undergo ordered rearrangements in normal thymic precursors with the TCRδ locus being the first to rearrange [93, 94]. Precursors, which undergo β-selection (TCRαβ precursors) correlate with the CD1^{pos}, surface CD3^{neg}, CD4/CD8 double^{pos}, cytoplasmic TCRβ protein^{pos} cortical thymocyte stage. Thymocytes, which have not yet undergone TCR gene rearrangements are CD1^{neg} and surface CD3/CD4/CD8 triple^{neg} [59]. However, TCRγδ-precursors do not have a known characteristic marker profile [95]. Asnafi et al. [92] suggested that CALM/AF10 transcripts occur in approximately 10% of pediatric and adult T-ALL and are restricted to TCRγδ-T-ALLs, either the mature form with surface TCRγδ protein expression or precursors still lacking surface TCR-chain expression. CALM/AF10^{pos} TCRγδ-precursors differed from both CALM/AF10^{pos} mature TCRγδ-T-ALLs and from all other T-ALLs by their CD5^{pos}/CD2^{neg} immunophenotype.

Marks et al. [77] found that the 5/79 adult T-ALL patients who tested positive for surface TCRγδ expression in the E2993/UKALLXII intergroup study demonstrated a very heterogenous phenotype except for CD10 positivity in every single case. This heterogeneity in terms of T-cell antigen expression agrees with the data reported by Langerak et al. in 30 cases of TCRγδ T-ALL [96]. Among >600 patients which were both centrally immunophenotyped and cytogenetically evaluated by ECOG [77], only three T-ALL cases with t(10;11)(p13–14;q14–21) were identified, all of which lacked CD2 and surface TCRγδ expression, consistent with the alleged TCRγδ-precursor antigen profile suggested by Asnafi and coworkers [92, 95].

E2A/PBX1^{pos} B-Lineage ALL

The translocation (1;19)(q23;p13) is found in 3–5% of ALLs and results in the expression of an E2A/PBX1 hybrid transcription factor with oncogenic potential [97]. Although closely associated with the Pre-B Immunophenotype [98], expression of cytoplasmic IgM, the phenotypic hallmark of the Pre-B subtype, is not consistently found in E2A/PBX1^{pos} ALL [99]. In support of this flow cytometric data, the strong specific gene expression profile for the E2A/PBX1 lesion does not correlate with the Pre-B immunophenotype [17]. Along the same line, the lack of CD34 expression, which is commonly seen in Pre-B ALL, is not invariably found in E2A/PBX1^{pos} ALL [100]. Without fail, however, lymphoblasts with the E2A/PBX1 fusion lack the My Ags, CD33 and CD13, but express the B-lymphoid affiliated surface antigens CD19, CD10, CD9, and CD22 [99–101].

TCRβ-HOXA Rearranged T-ALL

A unique genotype, which occurs in about 5% of pediatric and adult T-ALL, involves the HOXA locus on the short arm of chromosome 7 (7p15) and the TCRβ gene at 7q34 [102, 103]. Among HOXA cluster genes, HOXA10b appears to be particularly upregulated under the control of the TCRβ gene locus [103]. The typical immune profile of lymphoblasts containing TCRβ-HOXA rearrangements consists of CD2 negativity and single CD4 expression without CD8; TCR surface proteins are most commonly absent, consistent with arrest at an immature stage of thymic development [93].

Unique ALL Subtypes without Invariably Apparent Genetic Correlates

CD56^{pos} ALL

ALL with expression of the natural killer (NK) cell marker CD56, a member of the immunoglobulin family of adhesion molecules, is rare. In 2001, ECOG issued a preliminary report on CD56^{pos} adult ALL with an incidence of 3% among 194 cases from ALL trial, E3993 [104]. In that report, 4/6 CD56^{pos} cases belonged to the T-cell lineage. Of the two CD56^{pos} B-lineage ALLs, one had a normal karyotype, the other was positive for the Philadelphia chromosome.

Now, among a total of 619 patients immunophenotyped for CD56 on E2993, 28 cases expressed CD56 on 75–99% of lymphoblasts, the largest series of CD56^{pos} ALL described ever [77, 82]. Of these, 15 cases were T-ALLs and 13 were B-ALLs. As described previously, CD56^{pos} T-ALLs were phenotypically very heterogenous, sharing only intracytoplasmic CD3 and surface CD7 expression, with lack of CD5 (1/15), CD2 (7/15), surface CD3 (8/15), CD4/CD8 double^{neg} (8/15), CD4/CD8 double^{pos} (2/15), CD4^{neg}CD8^{pos} (5/15), CD1^{pos} (4/15). Three of the T-ALL cases expressed CD19, five were positive for CD10, and one for CD24. My Ags expression was just as varied and included CD33, CD13, CD65, or CD15. Three cases were positive for CD117, eight for CD34. CD57, another NK-cell marker, was not found on any of the cases. The finding of intracytoplasmic CD3 in all lymphoblasts from these patients clearly confirmed their association with the T-cell lineage. This is in stark contrast to cCD3^{neg}CD5^{neg}CD56^{pos} phenotype typical for NK-cell lymphomas with T-cell features [105].

Although CD56 is encoded by a gene located at 11q23 [106], there is no apparent association between CD56 expression in ALL and cytogenetic aberrations affecting 11q23. MD Anderson reported that CD56 expression in adult ALL predicted the occurrence of CNS disease in a series of 200 patients [107]. Although these investigators did not provide any details on immunophenotypic or cytogenetic features of their patients, they stated that no correlation existed between CD56 expression and Pre-B, B- or T-immune profile, or karyotype. Though anectodal, other reports regarding CD56^{pos} T-ALL (cCD3^{pos}) confirm a heterogenous pattern of antigen expression from various lineages [108]. These observations support the notion of the existence of common precursor cells for T, B, and NK-cells [109–111].

On the other hand, in B-lineage ALL, CD56 expression appears to be associated with BCR/ABL positivity [82]. Of the 13 CD56^{pos} B-lineage cases on E2993, nine were positive for BCR/ABL transcripts and a 10th BCR/ABL[neg] patient expressed CD25 on the majority of blasts, a surrogate marker for BCR/ABL positivity in ALL [19, 20]. The three remaining patients had 20 normal diploid metaphases, were negative for BCR/ABL, and lacked CD25 expression. Without fluorescence-in-situ hybridization (FISH) studies, an occult genetic event affecting the ABL gene cannot be excluded. All of these CD56[pos] B-lymphoblasts demonstrated Early-Pre-B or Pre-B (intracytoplasmic μ[pos]) levels of B-cell differentiation, lacked T-cell antigens and expressed CD13 alone or together with CD33 in every single case [82]. Based on these unifying pheno- and genotypic features, CD56[pos] B-ALL should be considered as a distinct disease entity.

In chronic myeloid leukemia (CML), CD56 expression is commonly detected on myeloid elements in the bone marrow or peripheral blood and could affect the cell homing mechanisms in this disease [112]. Eight of the nine CD56[pos] B-lineage ALL cases in E2993 expressed the e1a2 (p190) BCR/ABL transcript form, while in CML blast crisis, the b2a2 or b3a2 (p210) transcript form is dominant [113], arguing against the concept that CD56[pos] B-lineage ALL may represent lymphoid blast crisis of CML.

CD2[pos] B-Lineage ALL

The incidence of CD2[pos]CD19[pos] ALL approximates 4% in children [114] and has only recently been established in adults (3% of ALL on E2993) [82]. Although earlier reports failed to establish a firm affiliation of CD2[pos]CD19[pos] ALL with the B-cell lineage, overall immunophenotypic and genotypic features pointed in that direction [114, 115]. CD2[pos]CD19[pos] ALL in E2993 could be clearly assigned to the B-cell lineage based on expression of intracytoplasmic CD22 and absence of cytoplasmic CD3. This, CD2[pos]CD19[pos] ALL must not be considered an example for biphenotypic ALL. CD2 expression spanned all levels of B-cell maturation, and My Ag expression followed the established pattern associated with B-cell differentiation in ALL [33, 38]. In pediatric B-ALL, CD2 expression was associated with favorable outcome potentially due to good prognostic presenting features, such as low white blood cell counts and high platelet counts; cytogenetic and molecular analyses were only limited in that study [114]. A possible clinical impact of CD2 expression in adult B-lineage ALL must await the completed analysis of E2993 data [82].

Comments for the Future

This chapter does not claim to be all inclusive. Its purpose is to emphasize that ALL subsets with unique immunophenotypes are commonly associated with distinct genetic lesions and vice versa. In some instances, the proven prognostic significance of such genotypic aberrations clearly enhances the clinical relevance of surrogate marker profiles. Alternatively, the common genetic denominator for some recurrent unique phenotypes, e.g., in CD2[pos] B-lineage ALL, has not yet been discovered. Then again, there are a multitude of novel molecular risk markers, such as ERG and BAALC gene expression levels in T-ALL [11] or constitutive activation of ERK1/2, a mitogen-responsive kinase participating in cell-cycle progression and differentiation, in B- or T-ALL [116], for which surrogate markers or marker profiles remain undefined.

The characterization of ALL subtypes has only two goals, to improve prognostic knowledge or define subsets with therapeutic relevance. With increasingly better insights into oncogenic pathways derived from gene expression or epigenetic studies, the classification of the acute leukemias, including ALL, has become a moving target.

References

1. Bettelheim, P., Paietta, E., Majdic, O., et al. (1982). Expression of a myeloid marker on TdT-positive acute lymphocytic leukemic cells: Evidence by double-fluorescence staining. *Blood, 60,* 1392–1396.
2. Paietta, E., Bettelheim, P., Schwarzmeier, J. D., et al. (1983). Distinct lymphoblastic and myeloblastic populations in TdT positive acute myeloblastic leukemia: Evidence by double-fluorescence staining. *Leukemia Research, 7,* 301–307.
3. Paietta, E. (2003). Immunobiology of acute leukemia. In P. Wiernik, J. Dutcher, J. Goldman, & E. Kyle (Eds.), *Neoplastic diseases of the blood* (4th ed., pp. 194–231). Cambridge: Cambridge University Press.
4. Craig, F. E., & Foon, K. A. (2008). Flow cytometric immunophenotyping for hematologic neoplasms. *Blood, 111,* 3941–3967.
5. Paietta, E., Andersen, J., & Wiernik, P. H. (1996). A new approach to analyzing the utility of immunophenotyping for predicting clinical outcome in acute leukemia. *Leukemia, 10,* 1–4.
6. Campana, D., & Behm, F. G. (2000). Immunophenotyping of leukemia. *Journal of Immunological Methods, 243,* 59–75.
7. Boucheix, C., David, B., Sebban, C., et al. (1994). Immunophenotype of adult acute lymphoblastic leukemia, clinical parameters, and outcome: An analysis of a prospective trial including 562 tested patients (LALA87). *Blood, 84,* 1603–1612.
8. Kaleem, Z., Crawford, E., Pathan, H., et al. (2003). Flow cytometric analysis of acute leukemias. *Archives of Pathology & Laboratory Medicine, 127,* 42–48.
9. Chiaretti, S., Li, X., Gentleman, R., et al. (2004). Gene expression profile of adult T-cell acute lymphocytic leukemia identifies distinct subsets of patients with different response to therapy and survival. *Blood, 103,* 2771–2778.
10. Ferrando, A. A., Neuberg, D. S., Dodge, R. K., et al. (2004). Prognostic importance of HOX11 oncogene expression in adults with T-cell acute lymphoblastic leukemia. *Lancet, 363,* 535–536.
11. Baldus, C. D., Martus, P., Burmeister, T., et al. (2007). Low ERG and BAALC expression identifies a new subgroup of adult acute T-lymphoblastic leukemia with a highly favorable outcome. *Journal of Clinical Oncology, 25,* 3739–3745.
12. Golay, J., Di Gaetano, N., Amico, D., et al. (2005). Gemtuzumab ozogamicin (Mylotarg) has therapeutic activity against CD33+ acute lymphoblastic leukemias in vitro and in vivo. *British Journal Haematology, 128,* 310–317.
13. Cheung, K., Wong, L., & Yeung, Y. (2008). Treatment of CD33 positive refractory acute lymphoblastic leukemia with Mylotarg. *Leukemia & Lymphoma, 49,* 596–597.
14. Paietta, E., Ferrando, A. A., Neuberg, D., et al. (2004). Activating FLT3 mutations in CD117/KIT positive T-cell acute lymphoblastic leukemia. *Blood, 104,* 558–560.
15. Yagi, T., Morimoto, A., Eguchi, M., et al. (2003). Identification of a gene expression signature associated with pediatric AML prognosis. *Blood, 102,* 1849–1856.
16. Bennett, J. M., Catovsky, D., Daniel, M. T., & Flandrin, G. (1976). Proposals for the classification of the acute leukemias. *British Journal Haematology, 33,* 451–458.
17. Yeoh, E.-J., Ross, M. E., Shurtleff, S. A., et al. (2002). Classification, subtype discovery, and prediction of outcome in pediatric acute lymphoblastic leukemia by gene expression profiling. *Cancer Cell, 1,* 133–143.
18. Paietta, E. (2006). In manual of molecular and clinical laboratory Immunology. In B. Detrick, R. G. Hamilton, & J. D. Folds (Eds.), *Phenotypic correlates of genetic abnormalities in acute and chronic leukemia* (7th ed., pp. 201–214). Washington: ASM Press.
19. Paietta, E., Racevskis, J., Neuberg, D., et al. (1997). Expression of CD25 (interleukin-2 receptor α chain) in adult acute lymphoblastic leukemia predicts for the presence of BCR/ABL fusion transcripts: Results of a preliminary laboratory analysis of ECOG/MRC Intergroup Study E2993. *Leukemia, 11,* 1887–1890.
20. Paietta, E., Li, X., Richards, S., et al. (2008). Outcome in Philadelphia chromosome positive (Ph+) adult ALL patients (Pts) may be more determined by CD25 expression than by Ph status per se. *Blood, 112,* 533.
21. Kurzrock, R., Kantarjian, H. M., Druker, B. J., & Talpaz, M. (2003). Philadelphia chromosome-positive leukemias: From basic mechanisms to molecular therapeutics. *Annals of Internal Medicine, 138,* 819–830.
22. de Labarthe, A., Rousselot, P., Huguet-Rigal, F., et al. (2007). Imatinib combined with induction or consolidation chemotherapy in patients with de novo Philadelphia chromosome-positive acute lymphoblastic leukemia: Results of the GRAAPH-2003 study. *Blood, 109,* 1408–1413.
23. Cimino, G., Elia, L., Mancini, M., et al. (2003). Clinico-biologic features and treatment outcome of adult pro-B-ALL patients enrolled in the GIMEMA 0496 study: Absence of the ALL1/AF4 and of the BCR/ABL fusion genes correlates with a significantly better clinical outcome. *Blood, 102,* 2014–2020.
24. Moorman, A. V., Harrison, C. J., Buck, G. A. N., et al. (2007). Karyotype is an independent prognostic factor in adult acute lymphoblastic leukemia (ALL): Analysis of cytogenetic data from patients treated on the Medical

Research Council (MRD) UKALLXII/Eastern Cooperative Oncology Group (ECOG) 2993 trial. *Blood, 109,* 3189–3197.

25. Pullarkat, V., Slovak, M. L., Kopecky, K. J., et al. (2008). Impact of cytogenetics on the outcome of adult acute lymphoblastic leukemia: Results of Southwest Oncology Group 9400 study. *Blood, 111,* 2563–2572.

26. Primo, D., Tabernero, M. D., Perez, J. J., et al. (2005). Genetic heterogeneity of BCR/ABL + adult B-cell precursor acute lymphoblastic leukemia: Impact on the clinical, biological and immunophenotypical disease characteristics. *Leukemia, 19,* 713–720.

27. Juric, D., Lacayo, N. J., Ramsey, M. C., et al. (2007). Differential gene expression patterns and interaction networks in BCR-ABL-positive and -negative adult acute lymphoblastic leukemias. *Journal of Clinical Oncology, 25,* 1341–1349.

28. Dose, M., & Gounari, F. (2008). Fifty ways to NOTCH T-ALL. *Blood, 112,* 457–458.

29. Armstrong, S. A., Kung, A. L., Mabon, M. E., et al. (2003). Inhibition of FLT3 in MLL: Validation of a therapeutic target identified by gene expression based classification. *Cancer Cell, 3,* 173–183.

30. Ross, M. E., Mahfouz, R., Onciu, M., et al. (2004). Gene expression profiling of pediatric acute myelogenous leukemia. *Blood, 104,* 3679–3687.

31. Kohlmann, A., Schoch, C., Dugas, M., et al. (2005). New insights into MLL gene rearranged acute leukemias using gene expression profiling: Shared pathways, lineage commitment, and partner genes. *Leukemia, 19,* 953–964.

32. Riley, R. S., Massey, D., Jackson-Cook, C., et al. (2002). Immunophenotypic analysis of acute lymphocytic leukemia. *Hematology/Oncology Clinics of North America, 16*(2), 245–299.

33. Paietta, E., Li, X., Richards, S., et al. (2008). Implications for the use of monoclonal antibodies in future adult ALL trials: Analysis of antigen expression in 505 B-lineage (B-lin) ALL patients (pts) on the MRC UKALLXII/ECOG2993 intergroup trial. *Blood, 112,* 666.

34. Hoelzer, D., & Goekbuget, N. (2003). Diagnosis and treatment of adult acute lymphoblastic leukemia. In P. Wiernik, J. Dutcher, J. Goldman, & E. Kyle (Eds.), *Neoplastic diseases of the blood* (4th ed., pp. 273–305). Cambridge: Cambridge University Press.

35. Goldstone, A. H., Chopra, R., Buck, G., et al. (2003). The outcome of 267 Philadelphia positive adults in the international UKALL12/ECOG E2993 study. Final analysis and the role of allogeneic transplant in those under 50 years. *Blood, 102,* 80a.

36. Ludwig, W.-D., & Thiel, E. (1990). Routine immunophenotyping of acute leukemias. *Blut, 60,* 48–50.

37. Paietta, E., Neuberg, D., Bennett, J. M., et al. (2003). Low expression of the myeloid differentiation antigen CD65s, a feature of poorly differentiated AML in older adults: Study of 711 patients enrolled in ECOG trials. *Leukemia, 17,* 1544–1550.

38. Ludwig, W.-D., Rieder, H., Bartram, C. R., et al. (1998). Immunophenotypic and genotypic features, clinical characteristics, and treatment outcome of adult Pro-B acute lymphoblastic leukemia: Results of the German multicenter trials GMALL 03/87 and 04/89. *Blood, 92,* 1898–1909.

39. Borowitz, M. J., Carroll, A. J., Shuster, J. J., et al. (1993). Use of clinical and laboratory features to define prognostic subgroups in B-precursor acute lymphoblastic leukemia: experience of the Pediatric Oncology Group. In W.-D. Ludwig & E. Thiel (Eds.), *Recent results in cancer research. Recent advances in cell biology of acute leukemia* (pp. 257–265). Berlin: Springer.

40. Putti, M. C., Rondelli, R., Cocito, M. G., et al. (1998). Expression of myeloid markers lacks prognostic impact in children treated for acute lymphoblastic leukemia: Italian experience in AIEOP-ALL 88-91 studies. *Blood, 92,* 795–801.

41. Bene, M. C., Castoldi, G., Knapp, W., et al. (1995). Proposals for the immunological classification of acute leukemias. *Leukemia, 9,* 1783–1786.

42. Vitale, A., Guarini, A., Ariola, C., et al. (2006). Adult T-cell acute lymphoblastic leukemia: Biologic profile at presentation and correlation with response to induction treatment in patients enrolled in the GIMEMA LAL 0496 protocol. *Blood, 107,* 473–479.

43. Paietta, E., Kim, H., Rowe, J. M., et al. (2001). Prognostic significance of immunophenotyping and cytogenetics in adult acute lymphoblastic leukemia (ALL): Interim analysis of ECOG/MRC phase III intergroup trial E2993. *Blood, 98*(11), 841a.

44. Makrynikola, V., Favaloro, E. J., Browning, T., et al. (1995). Functional and phenotypic upregulation of CD13/aminopeptidase-N on precursor-B acute lymphoblastic leukemia after in vitro stimulation. *Experimental Hematology, 23,* 1173–1179.

45. Ashmun, R. A., Holmes, K. V., Shapiro, L. H., et al. (1995). CD13 (aminopeptidase N) cluster workshop report. In S. F. Schlossman, L. Boumsell, W. Gilks, et al. (Eds.), *Leucocyte typing V. White cell differentiation antigens* (pp. 771–775). New York: Oxford University Press.

46. Saito, M., Kumagai, M., Okazaki, T., et al. (1995). Stromal cell-mediated transcriptional regulation of the CD13/aminopeptidase N gene in leukemic cells. *Leukemia, 9,* 1508–1516.

47. Riemann, D., Kehlen, A., & Langner, J. (1999). CD13-not just a marker in leukemia typing. *Immunology Today, 20*, 83–88.
48. Schrappe, M., Reiter, A., Ludwig, W.-D., et al. (2000). Improved outcome in childhood acute lymphoblastic leukemia despite reduced use of anthracyclines and cranial radiotherapy: Results of trial ALL-BFM 90. *Blood, 95*, 3310–3322.
49. Pui, C.-H., & Evans, W. E. (2003). Acute lymphoblastic leukemia. *The New England Journal of Medicine, 339*, 605–615.
50. Boldt, D. H., Kopecky, K. J., Head, D., et al. (1994). Expression of myeloid antigens by blast cells in acute lymphoblastic leukemia of adults. The Southwest Oncology Group experience. *Leukemia, 8*, 2118–2126.
51. Larson, R. A., Dodge, R. K., Burns, C. P., et al. (1995). A five-drug remission induction regimen with intensive consolidation for adults with acute lymphoblastic leukemia: Cancer and Leukemia Group B study 8811. *Blood, 85*, 2025–2037.
52. Hrušak, O., & Porwit-MacDonald, A. (2002). Antigen expression patterns reflecting genotype of acute leukemias. *Leukemia, 16*, 1233–1258.
53. Kern, W., Kohlmann, A., Wuchter, C., et al. (2003). Correlation of protein expression and gene expression in acute leukemia. *Cytometry. Part B: Clinical Cytometry, 55B*, 29–36.
54. Serrano, J., Román, J., Jiménez, A., et al. (1999). Genetic, phenotypic and clinical features of acute lymphoblastic leukemias expressing myeloperoxidase mRNA detected by RT-PCR. *Leukemia, 13*, 175–180.
55. Niini, T., Vettenranta, K., Hollmén, J., et al. (2002). Expression of myeloid-specific genes in childhood acute lymphoblastic leukemia – a cDNA array study. *Leukemia, 16*, 2213–2221.
56. Weerkamp, F., Baert, M. R. M., Brugman, M. H., et al. (2006). Human thymus contains multipotent progenitors with T/B lymphoid, myeloid, and erythroid lineage potential. *Blood, 107*, 3131–3137.
57. Tabernero, M. D., Bortoluci, A. M., Alaejos, I., et al. (2001). Adult precursor B-ALL with BCR/ABL gene rearrangements displays a unique immunophenotype based on the pattern of CD10, CD34, CD13 and CD38 expression. *Leukemia, 15*, 406–414.
58. Mancini, M., Scappaticci, D., Cimino, G., et al. (2005). A comprehensive genetic classification of adult acute lymphoblastic leukemia (ALL): Analysis of the GIMEMA 0486 protocol. *Blood, 105*, 3434–3441.
59. Broudy, V. C. (1997). Stem cell factor and hematopoiesis. *Blood, 90*, 1345–1364.
60. Sperling, C., Schwartz, S., Buchner, T., et al. (1997). Expression of the stem cell factor receptor c-KIT (CD117) in acute leukemias. *Haematologica, 82*, 617–621.
61. Gilliland, D. G., & Griffin, J. D. (2002). The roles of FLT3 in hematopoiesis and leukemia. *Blood, 100*, 1532–1542.
62. Bertho, J.-M., Chapel, A., Loilleux, S., et al. (2000). CD135 (Flk2/Flt3) expression by human thymocytes delineates a possible role of FLT3-ligand in T-cell precursor proliferation and differentiation. *Scandinavian Journal of Immunology, 52*, 53–61.
63. Ferrando, A. A., Neuberg, D. S., Staunton, J., et al. (2002). Gene expression signatures define novel oncogenic pathways in T cell acute lymphoblastic leukemia. *Cancer Cell, 1*, 75–87.
64. Van Vlierberghe, P., Meijerink, J. P. P., Stam, R. W., et al. (2005). Activating FLT3 mutations in CD4+/CD8− pediatric T-cell acute lymphoblastic leukemias. *Blood, 106*, 4414–4415.
65. Nishii, K., Kita, K., Miwa, H., et al. (1992). c-kit gene expression in CD7-positive acute lymphoblastic leukemia: Close correlation with expression of myeloid-associated antigen CD13. *Leukemia, 6*, 662–668.
66. Perry, S. S., Wang, H., Pierce, L. J., et al. (2004). L-selectin defines a bone marrow analog to the thymic early T-lineage progenitor. *Blood, 103*, 2990–2996.
67. Leong, K. G., & Karsan, A. (2006). Recent insights into the role of Notch signaling in tumorigenesis. *Blood, 107*, 2223–2233.
68. Weng, A. P., Ferrando, A. A., Lee, W., et al. (2004). Activating mutations of NOTCH1 in human T cell acute lymphoblastic leukemia. *Science, 306*, 269–271.
69. Breit, S., Stanulla, M., Flohr, T., et al. (2006). Activating NOTCH1 mutations predict favorable early treatment response and long-term outcome in childhood precursor T-cell lymphoblastic leukemia. *Blood, 108*, 1151–1157.
70. Malyukova, A., Dohda, T., von der Lehr, N., et al. (2007). The tumor suppressor gene hCDC4 is frequently mutated in human T-cell acute lymphoblastic leukemia with functional consequences for Notch signaling. *Cancer Research, 67*, 5611–5616.
71. Mansour, M. R., Sulis, M. L., Duke, V., et al. (2010). Prognostic implications of NOTCH1 and FBXW7 mutations in adult patients with T-cell acute lymphoblastic leukemia treated on the MRC UKALLXII/ECOG E2993 protocol. *Journal of Clinical Oncology, 27*, 4352–4356.
72. Pullen, J., Shuster, J. J., Link, M., et al. (1999). Significance of commonly used prognostic factors differs for children with T cell acute lymphocytic leukemia (ALL), as compared to those with B-precursor ALL: A Pediatric Oncology Group (POG) study. *Leukemia, 13*, 1696–1707.

73. Niehues, T., Kapun, P., Harms, D. O., et al. (1999). A classification based on T cell selection-related phenotypes identifies a subgroup of childhood T-ALL with favorable outcome in the COALL studies. *Leukemia, 13,* 614–617.

74. Kees, U. R., Heerema, N. A., Kumar, R., et al. (2003). Expression of HOX11 in childhood T-lineage acute lymphoblastic leukemia can occur in the absence of cytogenetic aberration at 10q24: A study from the Children's Cancer Group (CCG). *Leukemia, 17,* 887–893.

75. Cavé, H., Suciu, S., Preudhomme, C., et al. (2004). Clinical significance of HOX11L2 expression linked to t(5;14)(q35;q32), of HOX11 expression, and of SIL-TAL fusion in childhood T-cell malignancies: Results from EORTC studies 58881 and 58951. *Blood, 103,* 442–450.

76. Bergeron, J., Clappier, E., Radford, I., et al. (2007). Prognostic and oncogenic relevance of TLX1/HOX11 expression level in T-ALLs. *Blood, 110,* 2324–2330.

77. Marks, D., Richards, S., Paietta, E., et al. (in preparation).

78. Wouters, B. J., Jordà, M. A., Keeshan, K., et al. (2007). Distinct gene expression profiles of acute myeloid/T-lymphoid leukemia with silenced CEBPA and mutations of NOTCH1. *Blood, 110,* 3706–3714.

79. Look, A. T. (1997). Oncogenic transcription factors in the human acute leukemias. *Science, 278,* 1059–1064.

80. Pui, C.-H., Relling, M. V., & Downing, J. R. (2004). Mechanisms of disease. Acute lymphoblastic leukemia. *The New England Journal of Medicine, 350,* 1535–1548.

81. Aguiar, R. C. T., Sohal, J., van Rhee, F., et al. (1996). TEL-AML1 fusion in acute lymphoblastic leukemia in adults. *British Journal Haematology, 95,* 673–677.

82. Paietta, E., Racevskis, J., Ketterling, R., et al. Immunophenotypic features of molecular subsets of B-lineage adult acute lymphoblastic leukemia: Analysis of phase III adult ALL intergroup trial E2993/UKALLXII (in preparation).

83. Rubnitz, J. E., Pui, C.-H., & Downing, J. R. (1999). The role of TEL fusion genes in pediatric leukemias. *Leukemia, 13,* 6–13.

84. Borowitz, M. J., Rubnitz, J., Nash, M., et al. (1998). Surface antigen phenotype can predict TEL-AML1 rearrangement in childhood B-precursor ALL: A Pediatric Oncology Group study. *Leukemia, 12,* 1764–1770.

85. De Zen, L., Orfeo, A., Cazzaniga, G., et al. (2000). Quantitative multiparametric immunophenotyping in acute lymphoblastic leukemia: Correlation with specific genotype. I. ETV6/AML1 ALLs identification. *Leukemia, 14,* 1225–1231.

86. Alessandri, A. J., Reid, G. S., Bader, S. A., et al. (2002). ETV6 (TEL)-AML1 pre-B acute lymphoblastic leukemia cells are associated with a distinct antigen-presenting phenotype. *British Journal Haematology, 116,* 266–272.

87. Ayton, P. M., & Cleary, M. L. (2001). Molecular mechanisms of leukemogenesis mediated by MLL fusion proteins. *Oncogene, 20,* 5695–5707.

88. Harper, D. P., & Aplan, P. D. (2008). Chromosomal rearrangements leading to MLL gene fusions: Clinical and biological aspects. *Cancer Research, 68,* 10024–10027.

89. Gleissner, B., Goekbuget, N., Rieder, H., et al. (2005). CD10⁻ pre-B acute lymphoblastic leukemia (ALL) is a distinct high-risk subgroup of adult ALL associated with a high frequency of MLL aberrations: Results of the German Multicenter Trials for Adult ALL (GMALL). *Blood, 106,* 4054–4056.

90. Janssen, J. W. G., Ludwig, W.-D., Borkhardt, A., et al. (1994). Pre-Pre-B acute lymphoblastic leukemia: High frequency of alternatively spliced ALL1-AF4 transcripts and absence of minimal residual disease during complete remission. *Blood, 84,* 3835–3842.

91. Bohlander, S. K., Muschinsky, V., Schrader, K., et al. (2000). Molecular analysis of the CALM/AF10 fusion: Identical rearrangements in adult acute myeloid leukemia, acute lymphoblastic leukemia and malignant lymphoma patients. *Leukemia, 14,* 93–99.

92. Asnafi, V., Radford-Weiss, I., Dastugue, N., et al. (2003). CALM-AF10 is a common fusion transcripts in T-ALL and is specific to the TCRγδ lineage. *Blood, 102,* 1000–1006.

93. Blom, B., Verschuren, M. C., Heemskerk, M. H., et al. (1999). TCR gene rearrangements and expression of the pre-T cell receptor complex during human T-cell differentiation. *Blood, 93,* 3033–3043.

94. Spits, H., Blom, B., Jaleco, A. C., et al. (1998). Early stages in the development of human T, natural killer and thymic dendritic cells. *Immunological Reviews, 165,* 75–86.

95. Asnafi, V., Beldjord, K., Boulanger, E., et al. (2003). Analysis of TCR, pTα, and RAG-1 in T-acute lymphoblastic leukemias improves understanding of early human T-lymphoid lineage commitment. *Blood, 101,* 2693–2703.

96. Langerak, A. W., Wolvers-Tettero, I. L. M., van den Beemd, M. W. M., et al. (1999). Immunophenotypic and immunogenotypic characteristics of TCRγδ⁺ T cell acute lymphoblastic leukemia. *Leukemia, 13,* 206–214.

97. Aspland, S. E., Bendall, H. H., & Murre, C. (2001). The role of E2A-PBX1 in leukemogenesis. *Oncogene, 20,* 5708–5717.

98. Hunger, S. P. (1996). Chromosomal translocations involving the E2A gene in acute lymphoblastic leukemia: Clinical features and molecular pathogenesis. *Blood, 87,* 1211–1224.

99. Troussard, X., Rimokh, R., Valensi, F., et al. (1995). Heterogeneity of t(1;19)(q23;p13) acute leukemias. *British Journal Haematology, 89*, 516–526.
100. Piccaluga, P. P., Malagola, M., Rondoni, M., et al. (2006). Poor outcome of adult acute lymphoblastic leukemia patients carrying the (1;19)(q23;p13) translocation. *Leukemia & Lymphoma, 47*, 469–472.
101. Foa, R., Vitale, A., Mancini, M., et al. (2003). E2A-PBX1 fusion in adult acute lymphoblastic leukemia: Biological and clinical features. *British Journal Haematology, 120*, 484–487.
102. Soulier, J., Clappier, E., Cayuela, J. M., et al. (2005). HOXA genes are included in genetic and biologic networks defining human acute T-cell leukemia (T-ALL). *Blood, 106*, 274–286.
103. Cauwelier, B., Cave, H., Gervais, C., et al. (2007). Clinical, cytogenetic and molecular characteristics of 14 T-ALL patients carrying the TCRβ-HOXA rearrangement: A study of the Groupe Francophone de Cytogenetique Hematologique. *Leukemia, 21*, 121–128.
104. Paietta, E., Neuberg, D., Richards, S., et al. (2001). Rare adult acute lymphocytic leukemia with CD56 expression in the ECOG experience shows unexpected phenotypic and genotypic heterogeneity. *American Journal of Hematology, 66*, 189–196.
105. Jaffe, E. S., Lee Harris, Z. N., Stein, H., & Vardiman, J. W. (Eds.). (2001). *World Health Organization classification of tumours. Tumours of haematopoietic and lymphoid tissues.* Lyon: IARC Press.
106. Gower, H. J., Barton, C. H., Elsom, V. L., et al. (1988). Alternative splicing generates a secreted form of N-CAM in muscle and brain. *Cell, 55*, 955–964.
107. Ravandi, F., Cortes, J., Estrov, Z., et al. (2002). CD56 expression predicts occurrence of CNS disease in acute lymphoblastic leukemia. *Leukemia Research, 26*, 643–649.
108. Ino, T., Tsuzuki, M., Okamoto, M., et al. (1999). Acute leukemia with the phenotype of a natural killer/T cell bipotential precursor. *Annals of Hematology, 78*, 43–47.
109. Spits, H., Lanier, L. L., & Phillips, J. H. (1995). Development of human T and natural killer cells. *Blood, 85*, 3654–3670.
110. Miller, J. S., McCullar, V., Punzel, M., et al. (1999). Single adult human CD34+/Lin-/CD38- progenitors give rise to natural killer cells, B-lineage cells, dendritic cells, and myeloid cells. *Blood, 93*, 96–106.
111. Reynaud, D., Lefort, N., Manie, E., et al. (2003). In vitro identification of human pro-B cells that give rise to macrophages, natural killer cells, and T cells. *Blood, 101*, 4313–4321.
112. Lanza, F., Bi, S., Castoldi, G., & Goldman, J. M. (1993). Abnormal expression of N-CAM (CD56) adhesion molecule on myeloid and progenitor cells from chronic myeloid leukemia. *Leukemia, 7*, 1570–1575.
113. Wong, S., & Witte, O. N. (2001). Modeling Philadelphia chromosome positive leukemias. *Oncogene, 20*, 5644–5659.
114. Uckun, F. M., Gaynon, P., Sather, H., et al. (1997). Clinical features and treatment outcome of children with biphenotypic CD2+CD19+ acute lymphoblastic leukemia: A Children's Cancer Group study. *Blood, 89*, 2488–2493.
115. Lenormand, B., Vannier, J. P., Bene, M. C., et al. (1993). CD2+ CD19+ acute lymphoblastic leukemia in 16 children and adults: Clinical and biological features. *British Journal Haematology, 83*, 580–588.
116. Gregorj, C., Ricciardi, M. R., Petrucci, M. T., et al. (2007). ERK1/2 phosphorylation is an independent predictor of complete remission in newly diagnosed adult acute lymphoblastic leukemia. *Blood, 109*, 5473–5476.

Index